About the Authors

BARBARA LUKE, Sc.D., M.P.H., R.N., R.D., is Professor of Obstetrics, Gynecology, and Reproductive Biology at Michigan State University. She has published numerous studies on multiple pregnancy and is the recipient of the 2005 Agnes Higgins Award from the March of Dimes for distinguished lifetime achievement in maternal-fetal nutrition. Dr. Luke also is the author of *Every Pregnant Woman's Guide to Preventing Premature Birth,* coauthor with Tamara Eberlein of *Program Your Baby's Health,* and coauthor with Roger B. Newman, M.D., of *Multifetal Pregnancy: A Handbook for Care of the Pregnant Patient.* Dr. Luke has held leadership positions in the Society for Pediatric and Perinatal Research and the Academy of Nutrition and Dietetics, including chairing the Women's Health and Reproductive Nutrition Dietetic Practice Group.

TAMARA EBERLEIN, an award-winning health journalist and editor, has published hundreds of articles on health, parenting, and psychology in national magazines. She is the author of *Sleep: How to Teach Your Child to Sleep Like a Baby* and *Whining: Tactics for Taming Demanding Behavior.* She is also the mother of twins.

ROGER B. NEWMAN, M.D., is Professor of Obstetrics and Gynecology and Maas Endowed Chair for Reproductive Sciences at the Medical University of South Carolina (MUSC). A nationally recognized expert in high-risk obstetrics and the care of women pregnant with multiples, Dr. Newman has directed the MUSC Prenatal Wellness Center Multiple Pregnancy Program (Twin Clinic) since its inception in 1987. He has published nearly 150 scientific articles and 20 book chapters, primarily on the care of multiples, as well as the medical mystery novels *Occam's Razor* and *Two Drifters.* Dr. Newman has held leadership positions in the American Congress of Obstetrics and Gynecology and is a past president of the Society for Maternal-Fetal Medicine.

When You're Expecting Twins, Triplets, or Quads: Fourth Edition

WILLIAM MORROW

An Imprint of HarperCollins*Publishers*

When You're Expecting Twins, Triplets, or Quads

PROVEN GUIDELINES FOR A
HEALTHY MULTIPLE PREGNANCY

Fourth Edition

Dr. Barbara Luke, Tamara Eberlein,
and Dr. Roger B. Newman

WHEN YOU'RE EXPECTING TWINS, TRIPLETS, OR QUADS (FOURTH EDITION). Copyright © 2017 by Dr. Barbara Luke, Tamara Eberlein, and Dr. Roger B. Newman. All rights reserved. Printed in the United States of America. No part of this book may be used or reproduced in any manner whatsoever without written permission except in the case of brief quotations embodied in critical articles and reviews. For information, address HarperCollins Publishers, 195 Broadway, New York, NY 10007.

HarperCollins books may be purchased for educational, business, or sales promotional use. For information, please email the Special Markets Department at SPsales@harpercollins.com.

A paperback edition of this book was published in 2011 by William Morrow, an imprint of HarperCollins Publishers.

First edition printed in 1999.

FOURTH EDITION

Designed by Jennifer Ann Daddio

Library of Congress Cataloging-in-Publication Data is available upon request.

ISBN 978-0-06-237948-1

17 18 19 20 21 RRD 10 9 8 7 6 5 4 3 2 1

To the children in our family—
my son, Peter Martin Wissel,
my sister's son, daughter, and grandchildren,
Nathaniel Lane Pearson, Alisa Christine Pearson,
Willa Bee Hudson, and Sebastian Lane Pearson,
and my brother's daughters,
Megan Rand Luke and Julia Ann Luke

—BARBARA LUKE

For my twins,
James and Samantha Garvey,
and my singleton, Jack

—TAMARA EBERLEIN

For my loving and beautiful wife, Diane,
and the wonderful children we have had together,
Bryan Forest, Taylor Holmes, and Sarah Haley

—ROGER NEWMAN

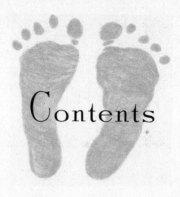

Contents

Acknowledgments

BARBARA LUKE, Sc.D., M.P.H., R.N., R.D.

I would like to thank the following individuals for their help in the development of this book.

First and foremost, special thanks to Timothy R.B. Johnson, M.D., for his support over many years. When Dr. Johnson was the Director of Maternal-Fetal Medicine in the Department of Gynecology and Obstetrics at Johns Hopkins Hospital, he supported my doctoral studies by hiring me as a Research Associate, serving as a member of my dissertation committee, and obtaining funding and resources to facilitate my research on twins. As the chairman of the Department of Obstetrics and Gynecology at the University of Michigan, he supported the creation of the Multiples Clinic and the University Consortium on Multiple Births, and provided funding and resources to ensure my success.

Sincerest thanks also to the following people at the University of Michigan Health Systems, in Ann Arbor, Michigan: Suzanne Wanty, M.S.N., R.N., Family Nurse Practitioner, for her dedication, expertise, and creativity in helping to establish the Multiples Clinic at the University of Michigan. Clark Nugent, M.D., for his careful reading of and thoughtful comments on the entire manuscript, and for his support in making the Multiples Clinic a success. Elaine Anderson, P.T., M.P.H., Physical Therapist and Research Associate at the University of Michigan, the developmental specialist who evaluated all of our twins and triplets in our follow-up study, and who developed many of the exercises recommended in this book. Mary Ann Zettelmeier, M.S.N., M.S., R.N., Clinical Nurse Specialist in Perinatal Nursing, for her review of and suggestions on the labor and delivery section of this book. Eileen J. Wright, M.S.N., R.N., Clinical Nurse Specialist in Neonatal Nursing, and Steven M. Donn, M.D., Professor of Pediatrics, Division of Neonatal-Perinatal Medicine, for their help on the section about the nursery and the neonatal intensive care unit. The obstetricians and midwives who have referred patients to the Multiples Clinic. And all the families who invited us into their lives by participating in the Multiples Clinic and follow-up.

At the University Consortium on Multiple Births: Frank R. Witter, M.D., at the Department of Gynecology and Obstetrics at Johns Hopkins University in Baltimore, Maryland; Roger B. Newman, M.D., at the Department of Obstetrics and Gynecology at the Medical University of South Carolina in Charleston; and Mary Jo O'Sullivan, M.D., at the Department of Obstetrics and Gynecology, Jackson Memorial Hospital, University of Miami, Florida, for their commitment to improving the outcomes of multiple-gestation pregnancies. Many of the recommendations in this book are based upon our collaborative research.

At the Rush–Presbyterian–St. Luke's Medical Center in Chicago, Illinois: Hal Bigger, M.D., for his review of and advice regarding the neonatal and newborn sections of this book, and for his help in obtaining newborn footprints; and the nursing staff in the neonatal intensive care unit for their assistance with the footprints.

At Valley Perinatal Services in Scottsdale, Arizona: John Elliott, M.D., for his review of the section on the obstetrical care of women pregnant with triplets and quadruplets.

My coauthors and I also gratefully acknowledge the invaluable contributions of the many parents of multiples who freely shared their experiences and expertise in the course of lengthy interviews. Our thanks in particular go to Meredith Alcott, Helen Armer, Michelle Brow, Marcy Bugajski, Karen Danke, Lydia Greenwood, Erin Justice, Kelly Kassab, Katy Lederer, Judy Levy, Allison MacDonald, Arlene and Kevin McAndrew, Kelly McDaniel, Lisa McDonough, Amy Maly, Ruth Markowitz, Stacy Moore, Benita Moreno, Heather Nicholas, Joni Quinn, Hannah-Beth Rhodes, Dr. Megan Smirti Ryerson, Anne Seifert, Ginny Seyler, Miriam Silverstein, Dr. Hannah Bosdell Steele, Joanie Stevens, Sarah Turner, Elin Wackernagel-Slotten, and Tessa Walters. We also appreciate the many readers who wrote to us, either by letter or via their reviews on www.amazon.com, to share their experiences.

Special thanks go to Tanya Leonello and Ginny Canady for their beautiful illustrations.

Introduction

BARBARA LUKE, Sc.D., M.P.H., R.N., R.D.

What Is the University Consortium on Multiple Births?

Back in 1988, I began graduate studies toward my doctorate degree at Johns Hopkins University School of Hygiene and Public Health in Baltimore, Maryland. Years before, I had conducted a pilot study examining the relationship between maternal weight gain and twin birthweight—evaluating the effect of weight gained by specific weeks' gestation on twin birthweight.[1] For my dissertation, I reviewed the medical records of all twin births at Johns Hopkins Hospital during a ten-year period (between 1979 and 1989) and found a strong relationship between twin birthweights and (1) how much a woman weighed before she became pregnant and (2) how much weight she gained by 24 weeks' gestation, and overall.[2,3] I also examined many other factors that influence this relationship: whether or not the woman smoked during her pregnancy; whether she became anemic; her height; her race and ethnic background; whether she had been pregnant before, and the outcomes of those prior pregnancies.

1. Luke B. Twin births: Influence of maternal weight on intrauterine growth and prematurity. Federation Proceedings 1987; 46:1015.
2. Luke B, Minogue J, Abbey H, Keith L, Witter FR, Feng TI, et al. The association between maternal weight gain and the birthweight of twins. Journal of Maternal-Fetal Medicine 1992; 1:267–76.
3. Luke B, Minogue J, Witter FR, Keith LG, Johnson TRB. The ideal twin pregnancy: Patterns of weight gain, discordancy, and length of gestation. American Journal of Obstetrics & Gynecology 1993; 169(3):588–97.

After earning my doctorate in 1991, I continued to do research on improving outcomes in twin pregnancies. I also expanded my interest to include triplets and quadruplets.

When I joined the Department of Obstetrics and Gynecology at the University of Michigan at Ann Arbor in 1995, I continued to work with obstetricians at Johns Hopkins University, as well as those at the University of Miami and the Medical University of South Carolina. Although the number of multiple pregnancies has increased greatly over the past several decades, no single center has enough data to conduct research alone—so we pooled our data. This alliance is known as the University Consortium on Multiple Births.

In recent years, other centers have joined us, including the University of Texas Medical Branch at Galveston, the University of Pennsylvania, the University of Kansas, and Columbia University. Every year we present our research on multiple pregnancies at the Society for Maternal-Fetal Medicine, the scientific society of high-risk obstetricians.

For six years, I ran a clinic for women pregnant with multiples at the University of Michigan. The goal: To improve outcomes for women pregnant with multiples by providing special prenatal care, patient education, risk screening, and intensive nutrition therapy. This is the clinic we refer to as the Multiples Clinic throughout the book, and many of the mothers quoted have participated in this program. I am now a professor of obstetrics, gynecology, and reproductive biology at Michigan State University in East Lansing, where I continue to conduct research on improving outcomes in multiple pregnancy, as well as evaluating the health of men, women, and their children after infertility treatments.

The advice in this book is designed to allow readers to reap the same rewards—including easier pregnancies and healthier babies—as Multiples Clinics' patients do.

One reader of a previous edition of this book asked how medical advice comes to be—how recommendations are formulated, updated, and disseminated to the public. This is an excellent question and very relevant to the advice in this book. Our philosophy in writing *When You're Expecting Twins, Triplets, or Quads* was to utilize *evidence-based medicine*—the very best and most up-to-date evidence from the most reliable sources—as the basis for our recommendations. This evidence comes from published studies and reviews that have undergone rigorous peer review, including the Cochrane Database of Systematic Reviews, position papers and professional guidelines from expert committees, and the most recent guidelines from respected national health organizations. To this list we add our own published research studies, many of which have been incorporated into the official recommendations from these other sources.

Professional health organizations—including the American College of Obstetricians and Gynecologists, the Society for Maternal-Fetal Medicine, the American Dietetic Association, the American Diabetes Association, the American Heart Association, and the World Health Organization, to name a few—issue position papers summarizing the latest study findings in specific areas and also offer guidelines for health care practitioners and the public. Periodic publications update these guidelines, providing more in-depth analyses and more details on clinical practice. For example, *Guidelines for Perinatal Care* (7th edition, 2012) is published jointly by the American Academy of Pediatrics Committee on the Fetus and Newborn and the American College of Obstetricians and Gynecologists Committee on Obstetric Practice. These guidelines include the most current scientific information, professional opinions, and clinical practices.

In addition, the National Academy of Sciences' Institute of Medicine (IOM) convenes inter-disciplinary committees of experts to review the scientific literature and formulate recommendations on contemporary health issues. In 1970, the IOM issued the report *Maternal Nutrition and the Course of Pregnancy*. Its 1990 report, *Nutrition During Pregnancy: Weight Gain and Nutrient Supplements,* was updated with the 2009 report, *Weight Gain During Pregnancy: Reexamining the Guidelines.* In this report the IOM, for the first time, included weight-gain guidelines for expectant mothers of twins based on women's pre-pregnancy weight—recommendations based on research from our University Consortium on Multiple Births. Our work with the Consortium is one reason why I received the March of Dimes' Agnes Higgins Award in 2005, given in recognition of distinguished lifetime achievements in research, education, and clinical service in the field of maternal-fetal nutrition.

Information from all of these sources has been incorporated into every edition of *When You're Expecting Twins, Triplets, or Quads*—including this most recent one. Throughout the book you will see footnotes citing selected references to particularly pertinent research. While the footnoted material represents just a small portion of the evidence-based data used in writing this book, these citations will be helpful for readers who want more in-depth information on some recent scientific findings. The footnoted references also are included among the hundreds of studies listed in the extended bibliography, covering dozens of relevant topic areas, which appears at the end of this book.

ROGER B. NEWMAN, M.D.

What Is the Twin Clinic at the Medical University of South Carolina?

After completing my fellowship in Maternal-Fetal Medicine at the University of California, San Francisco, in 1986, I returned to Charleston, South Carolina, and joined the ob/gyn faculty at the Medical University of South Carolina (MUSC). One of my first orders of business was to establish a specialized, multidisciplinary antepartum clinic for women carrying twins, triplets, or more. The MUSC Prenatal Wellness Center Multiple Pregnancy Program (often called simply the Twin Clinic) opened in 1987, and since then we have cared for thousands of expectant mothers and their multiples—including almost 2,000 pairs of twins, more than 200 sets of triplets, four sets of quadruplets, and one set of quintuplets.

Over the years I have been blessed to work with some fantastic residents and maternal-fetal medicine fellows. Among these are Jen Little, M.D.; E. Ramsey Unal, M.D.; Hannah Steele, M.D.; Carlton Schwab, M.D.; and Jennifer L. Burgess, M.D.—all of whom not only worked in the Twin Clinic but also became parents of twins themselves!

Our Twin Clinic model also includes certified nurse midwives as part of the care team because we do not want to give up high-touch care in order to achieve high-tech care. Over the years, I have had the pleasure of working with three fabulous midwives who are as much responsible for the success of our program as any other element.[4, 5] Special thanks go to Janna Ellings, C.N.M.; Mary Myers, C.N.M.; and Amelia Rowland, C.N.M.

Besides being a valuable clinical resource for our own patients, the Twin Clinic also has allowed us to answer a number of important research questions that affect the care of all women pregnant with multiples. Various publications over the past 25 years have documented improvements in obstetrical and newborn outcomes associated with the model of care that we offer in our Twin Clinic. In addition, it was in developing our program that we were drawn to the work of Dr. Barbara Luke on the relationships between optimal maternal nutrition in multifetal gestations and improved outcomes for mothers and babies. This led to our participation in Dr. Luke's University Consortium on Multiple Births and the critical clinical research advancements that this group has been able to achieve.

I have been honored to speak at numerous local, regional, and national meetings on the topic of best practices for women carrying twins, triplets, or more. We were asked by the Society for Maternal-Fetal Medicine to author an expert opinion paper for the journal *Obstetrics & Gynecology* on optimal nutrition for women with multiples.[6] The MUSC Twin Clinic was also selected to be a participating site for the National Twin Growth Study

---

4. Ellings JM, Newman RB, Hulsey TC, et al. Reductions in very low birth weight deliveries and perinatal mortality in a specialized multi-disciplinary twin clinic. Obstetrics & Gynecology 1993; 81:387–91.

5. Newman RB, Ellings JM. Antepartum management of the multiple gestation: The case for specialized care. Seminars in Perinatology 1995; 19:387–403.

6. Goodnight W, Newman R; for the Society for Maternal-Fetal Medicine. Optimal nutrition for improved twin pregnancy outcome. Obstetrics & Gynecology 2009; 114:1121–34.

sponsored by the National Institutes of Health's National Institute for Child Health and Human Development.[7] My staff and I are very proud of the fact that the MUSC Twin Clinic has been used as a model for the establishment of several other specialized obstetrical practices for the care of multiples—all geared toward optimizing health for moms and their multiples.

7. Burgess JL, Unal ER, Nietert PJ, Newman RB. Risk of late preterm stillbirth and neonatal morbidity for monochorionic and dichorionic twins. American Journal of Obstetrics & Gynecology 2014; 210:578–86.

Chapter One

Your Unique Pregnancy

TAMARA: As I lay flat on the examining table, the radiology technician turned the ultrasound screen toward me. I was about to catch my first glimpse of the baby that had been growing inside me for 18 weeks. But after a moment, she pushed the screen to one side to block my view, then stepped into the hall to summon a doctor. Together, they manipulated the dials of the ultrasound machine, whispering and pointing. Anxiously, I asked, "Is everything okay?"

The doctor turned the screen toward me again and, with a huge grin, said, "Here's what we've got. This is a leg, and an arm, and this is the head. And now, over here, we see a foot, and a back, and *another* head—twins! And they look just fine."

If you, too, have joined the ranks of expectant mothers of multiples—twins, triplets, even quadruplets or more—congratulations! You're now in a special group whose membership is swelling more and more each year. In the past four decades, the number of twins born yearly in the United States has more than doubled—from 59,122 infants in 1972 to 135,336 infants in 2014. Over that same period of time, the frequency of twin births has risen from approximately 1 percent of all births to just over 3 percent. Additionally, the birthrate of higher-order multiples (meaning three or more babies born together) has increased more than fivefold—from 907 infants in 1972 to 4,526 infants in 2014.

You've probably got a thousand questions about your pregnancy but have been frustrated by a lack of answers—because, unfortunately, reliable sources of information have not kept up with the explosion in the number of multiple births. "As soon as I found out that I was going to have twins, I read everything I could find on the subject. Yet most pregnancy books have only a page or two about multiples, and the books devoted to twins focus mostly on taking care of the babies after they're born," says Judy Levy, mother of twin girls and an older daughter.

Or perhaps you succeeded in finding some material on multiple pregnancies but were put off by its gloom-and-doom tone. "Everything I read about having twins seemed so frightening, as if the writers were saying, 'You will definitely have all sorts of problems—and your babies will too.' I couldn't bear to read that scary stuff," says Stacy Moore, mother of twin boys. "What I really needed was some sensible advice on the specific steps I could take to lower the risk of complications and give my babies the best possible start in life. And I found it—at a special clinic for expectant mothers of multiples, where I learned that many problems associated with multiple births are preventable. I did everything they told me to do, and my whole pregnancy went very smoothly. My twins were born big and healthy at full term, weighing 6 lb., 11 oz., and 6 lb., 1 oz."

DR. LUKE: As a Professor of Obstetrics and Gynecology at the University of Michigan Medical School in Ann Arbor, and a researcher and nutritionist, I founded the clinic that Stacy Moore attended, and directed it for six years. This is the Multiples Clinic we refer to throughout the book, and many of the mothers quoted participated in this program.

For family reasons, I've since moved around the country and am now a professor in the Department of Obstetrics, Gynecology, and Reproductive Biology at Michigan State University in East Lansing, where I continue to work with experts from universities across the country, as the University Consortium on Multiple Births. We have pooled data on multiple pregnancies from several universities (including Johns Hopkins University, Medical University of South Carolina, University of Michigan, University of Miami, and others) to publish studies ranging from maternal weight-gain guidelines to fetal growth standards to the optimal timing of delivery. The results of these studies have been used in the Multiples Clinic and many other prenatal programs throughout the United States, and even in establishing national prenatal care guidelines for multiples. In 2009, the National Academy of Sciences' Institute of Medicine issued the first-ever official weight-gain guidelines for women pregnant with multiples—based on our research with the University Consortium on Multiple Births.

Our goal has always been to improve pregnancy outcomes—in other words, to help women have the healthiest pregnancies and the healthiest babies—whether by providing in-person patient care at the Multiples Clinic at the University of Michigan in Ann Arbor, improving the guidelines for prenatal care of multiples by publishing in the professional literature for physicians, or offering information directly to families expecting multiples through Web-based consultations (www.drbarbaraluke.com) and the previous editions of this book.

At the Multiples Clinic we provided special prenatal care, including patient education, risk factor screening and risk reduction, and intensive nutrition therapy—and it worked. Our clinical success proved it. Compared to the average mother of multiples, women who followed our guidelines experienced significantly fewer complications before the birth of their children. For instance:

- Our expectant mothers developed fewer infections.
- They had less trouble with high blood pressure and preeclampsia.
- They had a lower incidence of preterm premature rupture of the membranes.
- Our patients were hospitalized for preterm labor less frequently, and spent fewer days in the hospital if they were admitted.

For infants born to our moms, the results were even more exciting:

- Triplets born to mothers in our program weighed 35 percent more at birth, on average, than triplets typically do. That's very significant, given that the average birthweight for triplets is just half that of a singleton—3 lb., 10 oz. versus 7 lb., 4 oz.
- Our twins were born about 20 percent heavier than the average twins delivered at the same gestational age.
- Two out of three of our twins weighed more than 5½ pounds at birth (the average birthweight for twins), and one out of four weighed more than 6 pounds. These birthweight figures demonstrate that you can break the rule that says twins are always born small.
- Sixty percent of our mothers of twins delivered at 37 weeks or later, compared to only about 40 percent of twin moms nationwide.
- Our babies were healthier at birth, regardless of when they were born, because they had grown well right from the start of the pregnancy.
- Infants born to patients in our program went home sooner than the average multiple-birth baby, spending only half as much time in the hospital. (Their hospital bills were only half the average, too!)

What's more, the benefits are long term. Follow-up studies of children born to mothers in our program reveal that, at age three, our children had significant advantages:

- Children from our program were less likely than nonprogram children to have delays in mental development.
- Delays in motor development were also less common.
- Our youngsters grew better.
- Hospitalizations were less frequent among program children.

To describe our research from the University Consortium on Multiple Births and the Multiples Clinic at the University of Michigan in complete detail, I've teamed up with Tamara Eberlein, a professional writer and mother of twins. Our first edition of *When You're Expecting Twins, Triplets, or Quads*, published in 1999, garnered accolades from readers and health care professionals alike and an Outstanding Book of the Year Award from the American Society of Journalists and Authors.

In this revised fourth edition, we are joined by Roger B. Newman, M.D., Director of the Prenatal Wellness Center Multiple Pregnancy Program, also known as the Twin Clinic, at the Medical University of South Carolina (MUSC) in Charleston. The Twin Clinic, which Dr. Newman established in 1987, has provided specialized, multidisciplinary care for about 2,000 twin pregnancies and 200 triplet pregnancies, as well as four sets of quadruplets and one set of quintuplets. Dr. Newman is a maternal-fetal medicine specialist who has had the honor of serving as president and executive board member of the Society for Maternal-Fetal Medicine, a national organization of obstetricians with additional training in the area of high-risk, complicated pregnancies. We are delighted to offer readers the benefit of Dr. Newman's medical expertise.

DR. NEWMAN: The Twin Clinic at MUSC has collaborated for years with Dr. Luke and the University Consortium on Multiple Births and has contributed to much of the research cited above. As with Dr. Luke's Multiples Clinic at the University of Michigan, the success of the Twin Clinic has been well documented. The Twin Clinic model includes consistent, close pregnancy surveillance by a dedicated maternal-fetal medicine specialist, a certified nurse-midwife, a nutritionist, and an ultrasonographer. Benefits to our patients include:

- Reductions in early preterm births (births prior to 32 weeks' gestation).
- Reductions in very low birthweight deliveries (less than 3 lb., 3 oz.).

- Reductions in the rates of preterm premature rupture of the membranes.
- Improved fetal growth and birthweight through an emphasis on optimal maternal nutrition.
- Dramatic reductions in the rates of stillbirth and neonatal mortality for both identical and fraternal twins.

Having recommended *When You're Expecting Twins, Triplets, or Quads* to my patients on a routine basis for more than a decade, I am excited to be coauthoring this new fourth edition. Here we include updates on the latest scientific studies and advances in obstetrical care for multiples, provide new information on the special challenges of identical twins, expand our recommendations on late-pregnancy surveillance of multiples, offer evidence-based advice on the optimal timing of delivery, and provide updated information on the care of newborn multiples. We also provide a new appendix, geared toward physicians, that discusses in detail some of the current research involving the major issues in the obstetrical management of multiple gestations.

The guidelines in this book are not based on opinion, speculation, or individual anecdotes but, rather, on years of research involving thousands of twin, triplet, and quadruplet pregnancies.

Following the advice in this book can help you and your babies reap the same rewards as our own patients do.

The Information You Need

"I'd had a typical, routine pregnancy with my first child a year and a half earlier," says Judy Levy. "So when I learned I was carrying twins, I figured it would be just like a regular pregnancy, only more so. But it turned out to be more challenging than just 'more so.'"

Why shouldn't a woman who's expecting twins, triplets, or quads just follow the same standard advice given to a woman pregnant with one baby (a singleton)? Because when you're carrying multiples, your pregnancy requirements go beyond what is standard.

You have specific medical requirements that must be considered in choosing health care providers. You have special nutritional needs. You have distinct concerns about physical exertion and workday demands. You face a higher risk of medical complications, and your babies face a greater chance of prematurity and other health problems. Psychologically, your pregnancy presents extraordinary joys as well as extraordinary challenges. Circumstances surrounding your labor, delivery, and recovery may be more complex. And your babies' experiences after birth may be markedly different from those of most singletons.

This note of caution must be sounded not only when triplets or quadruplets are on the way, but also in the case of twins. "With all the triplets and quads being born now, our society has become blasé about twins," says Amy Maly, mother of identical twin girls. "We've been programmed to think that it's no big deal to be expecting 'just two.' But as someone who's been there, I can attest to the fact that a twin pregnancy can be tricky. It pays to be careful."

TAMARA: I want to tell you my story to motivate you to do everything in your power to help ensure that your pregnancy goes well. And you *do* have a lot of power! You'll be making many decisions daily that can affect your unborn babies. Armed with the appropriate information, you can make the best possible choices.

When I learned I was expecting twins, I read everything I could find on the subject—which, unfortunately, at the time, wasn't much. Most books and articles were devoted to post-pregnancy concerns: what to name your twins, how to feed them, whether to dress them in matching outfits. I was disappointed to find little in-depth information on the pregnancy itself. The material that did cover gestation seemed to say that a can-do mind-set was the key to having healthy multiples. Readers were urged to "make a double effort to stay in shape," to regard with skepticism the "inflated reports" of complications in multiple pregnancies, and to be wary of obstetricians who might impose "unnecessary restrictions" on activities.

Thus persuaded that a happy outcome was practically assured, I felt pleased by my own doctor's upbeat, unbossy, laissez-faire attitude. There were no special nutritional recommendations or weight-gain guidelines, even after I lost 16 pounds in my second trimester during a two-week bout of food poisoning. There was no suggestion that I cut back at the office, despite my long workdays. And there were no instructions on how to recognize the subtle warning signs of preterm labor.

So I was completely unprepared when, two full months before my due date, my water broke and my twins were born. My 3-pound son and 2-pound daughter had to spend a month in the neonatal intensive care unit. Thank goodness, in the end they were fine—but that was a very difficult month for us all.

I firmly believe that, if I'd had access to the information that Dr. Luke's patients receive, my pregnancy would have lasted longer and my babies would have been born bigger and healthier. So when Dr. Luke invited me to coauthor this book, I jumped at the chance. I wanted to write the book I wish I'd been able to read when I was pregnant—a book that can help other mothers-to-be of multiples give their babies a healthier start than my own twins had.

DR. LUKE: Over the past four decades I've counseled thousands of pregnant women and helped generations of children begin their lives healthy and strong. Our goal with this book is to give you the benefit of these years of experience, with sensible guidelines geared specifically toward expectant mothers of multiples.

Here you'll learn about the common risks and how to avoid them. You'll understand the need to educate not only yourself but also your partner, your boss, your friends, maybe even your doctor. You'll get the information and support needed to guide you through this extra-special experience of being pregnant with multiples.

You'll also read about some of the mothers from our clinical programs in Ann Arbor, Michigan, and Charleston, South Carolina, as well as other mothers of multiples from around the country, including readers of earlier editions of *When You're Expecting Twins, Triplets, or Quads* who wrote to us about their experiences. You'll hear from women who sailed through their multiple pregnancies with a minimum of discomfort or inconvenience, and women who had to alter their lifestyle significantly for the sake of their babies. Women who began their pregnancy with a good understanding of nutrition, and women who reformed poor dietary habits to help their unborn babies thrive. Women who conceived multiples the first time they tried to get pregnant, and women who underwent years of infertility treatments before finally conceiving. Their experiences can help you as well.

I also invite you to visit my website, www.drbarbaraluke.com, for personalized nutrition counseling based on our research and clinical program.

Conception: A Miracle Multiplied

"I had always been fascinated with the science of conception. It seemed like an utter miracle. Once I learned that I was carrying twins, I imagined over and over the amazing moment when two lives began inside of me. Just thinking about it filled me with awe and a fierce determination to protect these babies who were coming into being," says Lydia Greenwood, mother of boy/girl twins.

You can put to good purpose your wonder at the miracle of a multiple conception. The more clearly you understand the biological changes occurring inside you, the easier it will be to dedicate the next months to nurturing your unborn babies. Start by reviewing the basics of how babies are conceived.

Every month during a woman's childbearing years (from menarche to menopause), her ovaries release a mature egg. This process is called ovulation. The egg travels down the fallopian tubes, where fertilization (also known as conception) occurs if the egg unites with the father's sperm. During fertilization, the genetic material, or chromosomes, from both mother and father combine. Then the fertilized egg begins to divide. Within a week after fertilization, this dividing egg, which is now called a zygote, embeds itself in the lining of the uterus.

The dividing egg, bathed in nutrient-rich fluid, begins to separate into outer and inner layers. The outer layer grows to form the major portion of the placenta, the vascular organ that will continue to provide nutrients as the unborn baby grows and develops. The inner layer becomes the embryo, which develops into the baby itself. By the second week of life, the embryo is firmly implanted in the endometrium (lining of the uterus) and is surrounded by tissues rich in carbohydrates.

The conception and development of multiples is similar to that of a singleton baby, but with a few essential differences. Of primary importance is twin type—in other words, whether the multiples are identical or fraternal.

THE BIG QUESTION: IDENTICAL OR FRATERNAL?

Identical twins begin the same way as a singleton, with one egg and one sperm. But the resulting zygote divides an extra time, producing two separate but identical zygotes. If one zygote then divides yet again, identical triplets will form. An additional division will result in identical quadruplets (though these are exceedingly rare). Identical twins, triplets, or quads are also called monozygotic (MZ), indicating that they developed from a single zygote.

The timing of this additional division determines the structure of the fetal membranes—the *amnion* or inner membrane, which will hold the amniotic fluid and developing embryo, and the *chorion* or outer membrane, which establishes the connection with the internal lining of the uterus. A part of the chorion proliferates to form the placenta, which is the vascular exchange organ that allows maternal blood to provide nourishment for a fetus. Here's what happens:

- If the split occurs within three days of conception, while the original zygote is still traveling down the fallopian tube, these identical twins will have two separate placentas, two chorions, and two amnions. The two placentas may be well separated, or they may form side by side and appear to be fused. This is a diamniotic, dichorionic (or di/di, for short) twin pregnancy.

- If the extra division of the zygote occurs between three and seven days after conception, the twins will have separate amnions but will share one chorion. The two fetuses will share a single placenta. This is termed a diamniotic, monochorionic (di/mo) twin pregnancy.
- If the split occurs after the eighth day following conception, the identical twins will share the same placenta, chorion, and amnion. This is described as a monoamniotic, monochorionic (mo/mo) twin pregnancy.
- For identical triplets, the structure of the fetal membranes varies. Sometimes all three have separate amnions, chorions, and placentas, referred to as triamniotic and trichorionic. In other cases, two babies share membranes, while the third has separate membranes. This is called a triamniotic, dichorionic triplet pregnancy. Very rarely, all three share the same placenta, chorion, and amnion. This is called a monoamniotic, monochorionic triplet pregnancy.

Approximately one-third of all twin pairs are identical. Because identical twins share 100 percent of their genes, they are always of the same sex and have the same basic physical features, such as hair color and eye color. Some pairs are mirror-image—one is right-handed, the other left-handed; their hair whorls are reversed; they may have matching birthmarks on opposite sides of their bodies. Though identical twins can vary significantly in size at birth if one baby received a greater share of nourishment in utero (while growing inside the uterus), adult height usually differs by less than 2 inches. Identical twins typically have very similar IQs and often share many personality characteristics. (Interestingly, identical twins have similar but not entirely identical fingerprints because fingerprints are affected by the uterine environment prior to birth.)

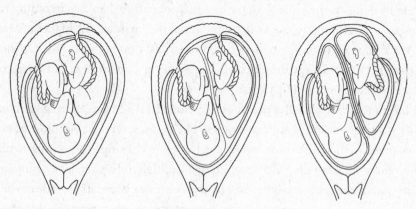

Left: *Monoamniotic, monochorionic (mo/mo) twin pregnancy.* Center: *Diamniotic, monochorionic (di/mo) twin pregnancy.* Right: *Diamniotic, dichorionic (di/di) twin pregnancy.*

Fraternal twins result when the mother produces two eggs instead of one in the normal monthly cycle, and each egg is fertilized by separate sperm. Fraternal triplets form from three eggs and three separate sperm; fraternal quads form from four eggs and four sperm. These fertilized eggs travel independently through the fallopian tubes, and each embeds in the lining of the uterus. Fraternal twins always have separate placentas, chorions, and amnions, although if they embed close to each other, their placentas may appear to be fused. All fraternal twins are dizygotic (DZ), meaning that they developed from two separate zygotes. In addition, each dizygotic twin has its own placenta, chorion, and amnion—so they are all diamniotic, dichorionic (di/di).

About two-thirds of all twins are fraternal. Half of these pairs are boy/girl, one-fourth are girl/girl, and one-fourth are boy/boy. Sharing, on average, 50 percent of their genes, fraternal twins are no more alike genetically than are nontwin siblings. That's why fraternal twins should not be expected to have the same appearance, personality, intelligence level, or rate of growth and development.

Unfortunately, there are no official national data on twin type among higher-order multiples. One survey of families with triplets, however, suggests that only about 6 percent of triplet sets are identical. Most are composed either of three fraternal siblings (who are thus triamniotic, trichorionic) or of an identical pair plus one fraternal sibling.

Who's Having Multiples?

Prior to the advent of infertility treatments several decades ago, the natural incidence of twins was 1 in 89 births. Yet by the year 2014 (the most recent year for which statistics are available), the birthrate of twins in the United States had skyrocketed to 1 in 29, according to the National Center for Health Statistics. At the same time, the birthrate for higher-order multiples surged upward from its 1972 rate of 1 in 3,593 to its 2014 rate of 1 in 881. Of these, triplet births account for 1 in 942, quadruplet births account for 1 in 16,212, and births of quintuplets or more account for 1 in 84,853.

What has caused this explosive rise in multiple births? And who is giving birth to all these twins, triplets, and quadruplets? To answer these questions, several factors must be considered.

Some women are naturally prone to producing more than one egg during ovulation and are therefore more likely to give birth to fraternal multiples. This tendency runs in families, and you can inherit the trait through either your mother's or your father's side of the family.

Your male partner and his family history have no influence on your chances of conceiving fraternal multiples. That makes sense, given that it is the woman's ovulation pattern alone that sets the stage for this type of twinning. In other words, it doesn't matter one bit how many pairs of fraternal twins are perched on your husband's family tree. (Most people are unaware of this fact, as you'll realize long before you are asked for the hundredth time, "Which side of the family do twins run on, yours or your husband's?")

Race and ethnicity are other factors that influence who has multiples—or at least who has fraternal multiples. With one exception (discussed later), monozygotic twinning is completely random, and monozygotic twin rates worldwide are remarkably constant at about 3 to 4 per 1,000 live births. However, the dizygotic twinning rate can vary a great deal based on ethnicity.

For instance, in the United States in 2014, the rate for twin births (per 1,000 live births) is highest for non-Hispanic blacks at 40.0, followed by non-Hispanic whites at 36.7, and Hispanics at 24.1.[1] The rate for triplets and higher-order multiples (per 100,000 live births) is highest among non-Hispanic whites at 140.9, followed by non-Hispanic blacks at 89.7, and Hispanics at 64.3.

A factor estimated to be responsible for about one-fourth of the recent rise in the rate of multiple births is that women today tend to have children later in life than did previous generations. Between the years 1980 and 2014, among women age 30 and older, the proportion of all births more than doubled (from 19.8 percent to 42.8 percent), while the proportion of women giving birth for the first time increased more than threefold (from 8.6 percent to 30.2 percent).

That is significant because biologically an older woman is more prone to conceiving multiples. For instance, a woman who is 35 to 40 years old is three times more likely to give birth to fraternal twins than a woman between the ages of 20 and 25. This effect may be compounded when a woman waits until her thirties to marry, because twins are more often conceived in the first months after marriage—perhaps owing to more frequent sex!

The use of oral contraceptives plays a part, too. A woman's chances of having twins double if she conceives in the first month after discontinuing birth control pills.

The primary cause of the current rise in multiple births, however, has been the use of modern infertility treatments, also known as assisted reproductive technologies (ART). These treatments include in vitro fertilization or IVF (when a woman's eggs are fertilized by sperm in the laboratory) and non-IVF procedures such as ovulation induction. An estimated 12 percent of American women of childbearing age have some type of fertility problem, and the treatments used to overcome these conditions vastly increase the odds of a multiple pregnancy.[2]

---

1. Hamilton BE, Martin JA, Osterman MJK, Curtin SC, Mathews TJ. Births: Final data for 2014. National Vital Statistics Report, vol. 64, no. 12, December 23, 2015.
2. Chandra A, Copen CE, Stephen EH. Infertility service use in the United States: Data from the National Survey of Family Growth, 1982–2010. National Health Statistics Report, no. 73, January 22, 2014.

For instance, about 20 percent of women who conceive while taking an ovulation-stimulating drug such as Pergonal have multiples, as do about 10 percent of those who get pregnant using Clomid or a similar medication.

In 2014 there were 139,862 infants born from multiple-gestation pregnancies in the United States. In the past four decades, the number of twins born yearly in the United States more than doubled—from 59,122 infants in 1972 to 135,336 infants in 2014. During that same period, the birthrate of higher-order multiples increased more than fivefold—from 907 infants to 4,526 infants. Approximately three-fourths of this rise is attributable to ART. In 2012, 26 percent of all live births from ART were multiples, a decrease from the 2004 rate of 33 percent. On a national basis, it is estimated that 20 percent of all multiple births, including 19 percent of twins and 33 percent of triplet and other higher-order multiples, are the result of ART.[3]

The majority of multiples conceived through ART are fraternal, because they form from separate eggs that have been fertilized by separate sperm. However, certain factors with infertility treatments can increase the likelihood that the embryo will split, making a woman treated for infertility more likely than the average woman to give birth to identical twins.[4] Fortunately, a number of recent studies have demonstrated that twins conceived through ART are no more likely to have problems than twins who were conceived spontaneously.

DR. LUKE: The proportion of multiples conceived through ART compared to those conceived spontaneously varies greatly around the country, as shown by the statistics from the University Consortium on Multiple Births. In the University of Miami program, only about 6 percent of twins were the result of infertility treatments, and 94 percent were spontaneous. At Johns Hopkins University and the Medical University of South Carolina, about 12 to 15 percent of twin pregnancies were from ART, and the other 85 to 88 percent were spontaneous. In comparison, at the University of Michigan, about 37 percent of twin pregnancies were due to ART, and only about 63 percent were spontaneous.

3. Sunderam S, Kissin DM, Crawford S, Anderson JE, Folger SG, Jamieson DJ, et al. Assisted reproductive technology surveillance—United States, 2010. Morbidity and Mortality Weekly Report, vol. 62, no. 9, December 6, 2013; 1–28.
4. Luke B, Brown MB, Wantman E, Stern JE. Factors associated with monozygosity in assisted reproductive technology pregnancies and the risk of recurrence using linked cycles. Fertility and Sterility 2014; 101:683–9.

Getting the News: How and When Multiples Are Diagnosed

One of the earliest clues that a woman is carrying more than a single baby is that she's experiencing excessive nausea and vomiting. Though it may seem like small consolation at the time, morning sickness can be a good sign. As the placenta or placentas begin to grow, they provide the hormones needed to maintain the pregnancy. Only about one-third of mothers with singleton babies experience nausea, compared to one-half or more of mothers-to-be of multiples. This is believed to be related to the larger placental mass and the higher production of the placental hormone called human chorionic gonadotropin (HCG). Other first-trimester signs of a possible multiple pregnancy include extreme fatigue, greatly increased appetite, and higher-than-expected weight gain. "I could tell early on that this pregnancy was different from my two previous pregnancies. The morning sickness was much worse, and I felt woozy and lethargic. When we went for an ultrasound, my husband looked at the big screen where the ultrasound image was being projected and said to the doctor, 'Am I counting *three*?' Sure enough, we had spontaneously conceived triplets," says Allison MacDonald.

Another hint that multiples may be present is when a woman's uterus is larger than expected for a particular stage of pregnancy. With twins, this is often evident by the 14th week of pregnancy. With triplets or quadruplets, the larger-than-average uterus is frequently noted even earlier. Stacy Moore says, "My obstetrician said my belly was bigger than one would normally see at 17 weeks. Thinking that we might have miscalculated my due date, she scheduled an ultrasound. That's when we saw two heads."

DR. LUKE: How much larger is the uterus of a woman carrying multiples? For the sake of comparison, imagine that four women are lined up in a row, and you are looking at them in profile. Each is 24 weeks pregnant.

1. For the expectant mother of a singleton, her growing uterus has lifted up from her pelvis and has created a mound that rises about as high as her navel. In other words, her pregnancy has only recently begun to show. Her uterus is the size of a ball about 20 inches around (imagine a football with its pointy ends cut off).
2. The twin mom is larger—the size you'd expect to see at 32 weeks if she were carrying just one baby. Her uterus, the size of a basketball, is about 30 inches around.
3. The triplet mother looks like she's 36 weeks into a singleton pregnancy. Her uterus is the size of a smallish beach ball, about 33 inches around.

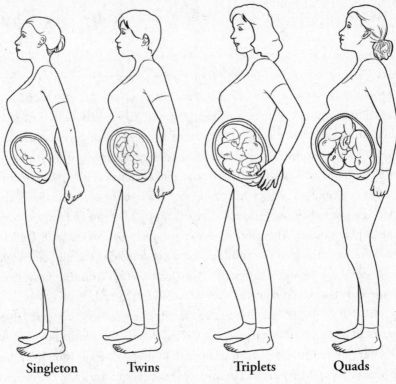

Singleton   **Twins**   **Triplets**   **Quads**

Sideways view at 24 weeks' gestation

4. And the woman expecting quadruplets is as large as a singleton mom would be at 40 weeks. As big as an average beach ball, her uterus is about 36 inches around—in other words, full-term size.

Another indication of multiple pregnancy that can be detected as early as 10 to 12 weeks into the pregnancy is the sound of two hearts beating. Using a sensitive device called a Doppler that amplifies sound, an obstetrician can hear a baby's heartbeat. The fetal heart rates are easily distinguished from the mother's because they are much more rapid. Twins are suspected when the doctor hears two distinct rapid heartbeats. Often, though, this clue is overlooked until some later test reveals the truth. Amy Maly says, "It was fortunate I was lying down during that first ultrasound when the radiologist asked me, 'Did your obstetrician hear two heartbeats? Because I see two babies.'"

Multiples also may be suspected when a woman feels more fetal movement than she did with a previous pregnancy. This alone is not conclusive evidence of a multiple pregnancy, however. A woman already familiar with the feeling of a baby moving inside her is generally more sensitive to fetal movement. She may notice those first kicks earlier in a second pregnancy—perhaps by the 14th week rather than the average of 18 to 22 weeks—even if she is carrying only one baby. Or the baby may simply be more active than his or her older sibling was.

Some women receive their first hint that multiples may be present when they get the results of their alpha-fetoprotein (AFP) test. This test, generally performed 15 to 20 weeks into the pregnancy, measures the level of a protein produced by the growing fetus that is present in the amniotic fluid and, in smaller amounts, in the mother's blood. A high AFP suggests several possibilities: that the pregnancy is more advanced than had been believed, that the baby has a serious medical problem such as spina bifida (a defect of the spinal column) or an abdominal wall defect, or that there's more than one normal fetus growing. To determine the specific reason for the high AFP reading, the doctor will order additional diagnostic tests.

No matter what hints may or may not have come before, these days the majority of multiple pregnancies are definitively diagnosed through ultrasound, a technology that uses sound waves to project a picture of a fetus onto a monitor screen. Ultrasound can detect the baby's heartbeat, estimate gestational age, track fetal growth, reveal gender, identify certain birth defects, and confirm the presence of multiples. In a national study performed to compare routine ultrasound screening versus the selective use of ultrasound, one of the most significant differences between the two groups was the nearly universal detection of multiples in the routine scanning group.[5] Without the routine use of ultrasound, a substantial number of twins are not diagnosed until the third trimester—and some are not identified until the first twin is delivered and it becomes clear that there is still a second baby waiting to be born!

Because ultrasound can be done at any point in a pregnancy, many mothers learn early on that they are carrying multiples. This is especially likely to occur if a woman's pregnancy is being closely monitored for some reason—for instance, because she is older or has had infertility treatments—and is sent for her first ultrasound within a month or two of conception. "We had done intrauterine insemination, and then some of the early blood test levels were unexpectedly high, so my wife had an ultrasound at six weeks. That's when we got the news that triplets were on the way," says Kevin McAndrew. "My wife was thrilled, but I was worried. I knew that a twin pregnancy was high risk, and I figured that a triplet pregnancy would be even riskier, perhaps exponentially so."

---

5. Crane JP, LeFevre ML, Winborn RC, et al. A randomized trial of prenatal ultrasonographic screening: Impact on the detection, management, and outcome of anomalous fetuses. American Journal of Obstetrics & Gynecology 1994; 171:392–9.

DR. NEWMAN: In a multiple pregnancy, it is no longer considered sufficient simply to determine how many babies are present. In order to provide you with optimal prenatal care, your doctor also must determine the babies' twin type, chorionicity, and amnionicity—because the risks and the medical management differ, depending on these factors. For instance, certain monozygotic twins require special surveillance because they are at increased risk for various pregnancy complications. Timely detection of such a complication provides the best chance for these monozygotic twins to be born healthy.

In many cases, ultrasound provides a clear answer to the question of twin type early in pregnancy. For example, if the ultrasound image reveals that both babies share only one chorion, the twins are identical; when the image reveals boy/girl twins, clearly the babies are fraternal.

Sometimes, though, ultrasound does not provide clear-cut proof of twin type. For instance, same-sex twins with two separate placentas and separate amniotic and chorionic sacs may be fraternal—or they may be identical if the zygote split in the first three days after fertilization.

Also, it can be difficult on ultrasound to tell the difference between a single placenta (indicating identical twins) and two fused placentas (most likely indicative of fraternal twins). In such a case, a physician should check for the *lambda* or *twin peak* sign. In a monochorionic twin pregnancy (which always indicates identical twins), the two amniotic membranes separating the twins come together and are flat against the surface of the single placenta, forming a T-shaped intersection. However, in a fused dichorionic twin pregnancy (which probably indicates fraternal twins but could be di/di identical twins), the two amniotic and two chorionic membranes separating the twins come together near the point of fusion of the two placentas—and as the membranes come together, a small amount of placental tissue will curve upward to meet the approaching membranes, creating a lambda or mountain peak–shaped point of intersection. You can see this in the ultrasound image on page 17.

If ultrasound examination is not enough to determine twin type, you may want to consider additional prenatal testing such as chorionic villus sampling and amniocentesis (described in Chapter 2). Otherwise, questions may remain. "My health care providers did not hazard a guess as to my unborn babies' twin type. But because the boys were each in separate sacs, I was told that they most likely were fraternal. Yet one day when the twins were close to a month old, my partner and I mixed them up for hours because they looked so similar. That's when we did a mail-order DNA test and found out that they're identical after all," says Erin Justice.

If you, too, are left with questions about twin type after your babies are born, you can order

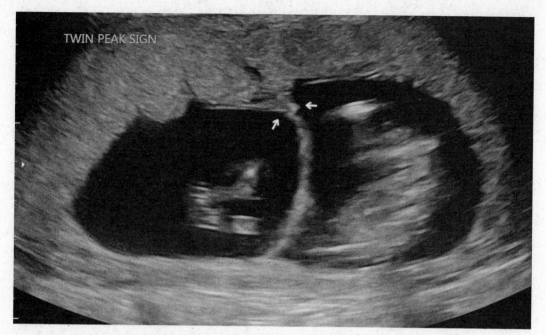

TWIN PEAK SIGN

In a diamniotic, dichorionic pregnancy the thick dividing membrane forms a lambda or twin-peak sign (see arrows) as it approaches the fused placental surfaces.

a DNA test kit from Affiliated Genetics at www.affiliatedgenetics.com. You use swabs to collect samples of cells from the inside of each child's cheek, then mail these to a lab for analysis. The DNA of fraternal multiples will show many differences, whereas the DNA of identicals will match completely. The cost is $150 plus $10 handling for twins; add $75 for each additional multiple.

How Your Unborn Babies Grow

"I had a ritual I did weekly throughout my pregnancy," says Lydia Greenwood, mother of boy/girl twins. "Every Sunday, I sat down with a wonderful book entitled *A Child Is Born* by Lennart Nilsson. It shows the most amazing photographs of babies at various stages of prenatal development, from the earliest embryonic days onward, and explains when each part of the body develops. I loved to envision my own twins inside me and track all the changes they would be going through in the coming week."

You may experience a similar satisfaction in tracking your babies' development as they grow week by week. This understanding can help you to feel closer emotionally to your unborn babies. And it can help make the restrictions that go along with a multiple pregnancy—the guidelines on what and when to eat, the limits on physical activity and work hours, for instance—seem far less onerous and easier to follow.

It is important to understand that, because the exact date of conception usually is not known (except in the case of infertility treatments), a pregnancy is dated from the first day of a woman's last menstrual period—which typically occurs two weeks *before* the actual moment of conception. In other words, when your doctor says you're 12 weeks pregnant, your babies have in fact been growing inside you for about 10 weeks.

EARLY PREGNANCY: THE EMBRYONIC PERIOD

DR. NEWMAN: The first two weeks after fertilization are considered an *all-or-none period of development.* The cells of the early zygote are duplicating themselves, but have not yet begun to form specific organs or fetal parts. Environmental contaminants, infections, radiation, medications, or drugs to which the mother is exposed will either cause the loss of the embryo (the *all* part of the all-or-none phrase) or will have no effect at all (the *none* part).

The third through the eighth week of fetal life is a critical time in human development, because it is when the body's essential internal and external structures form. This is referred to as the embryonic period. Anything that disrupts normal development at this stage could lead to structural malformations (birth defects) or even pregnancy loss. That's why any woman who is trying to conceive or believes she may have just become pregnant should take extra care to avoid exposure to potentially harmful influences, such as viruses, radiation, medications, and alcohol.

Miscarriage is also most common during the embryonic stage of development, usually due to a genetic abnormality or physiologic problem such as poorly controlled diabetes. Sometimes the loss of the embryo occurs so early that the woman does not even realize she was pregnant; she may simply believe her menstrual period was a few days late that month.

In a normal, healthy pregnancy, however, the embryo or embryos continue to develop in predictable ways. Here's what is happening to your unborn multiples as they grow week by week. (Remember that these weeks are calculated from the date of your last menstrual period, about two weeks before actual conception.)

Week 1: Your monthly menstruation begins. Pregnancy is calculated from day one of your period (referred to as the LMP, or last menstrual period).

Week 2: After your menstrual period ends, the endometrium, or lining of the uterus, begins to build up again in preparation for a possible pregnancy. Ovulation, or the release of a mature egg from the ovary, usually occurs at the end of this second week. The released egg is drawn in by the fallopian tube, which has small tentacle-like appendages to guide the egg into the tube. Conception occurs if the father's sperm fertilizes the mature egg as it travels through the fallopian tube to the uterus.

Week 3: The week-old fertilized egg (now called a zygote) or eggs embed in your endometrium, which has reached its greatest thickness and maximum richness in blood supply and nutrients. This is also the first week of fetal life.

Week 4: The placenta or placentas have grown deeper into the endometrium. As the mother's blood supply bathes the outside of the placentas and the unborn babies' circulation flows within the placentas, nutrients are passed to the babies and their waste products are carried away. By this time, the developing placentas have begun producing HCG (the hormone detected by home and office-based pregnancy tests) in rapidly increasing amounts. The primary role of HCG at this point is to support the production of progesterone by the ovaries, which is essential for preventing miscarriage until about 7 weeks' gestation, when placental production takes over.

Week 5: The organs and tissues of the growing embryos are evolving, particularly the spinal cord and nervous system and the heart and circulatory system. The heart is the first organ to form. Once their blood supply has been established, the embryos are no longer dependent on the meager store of nutrients from the eggs, and growth can begin in earnest. By the end of this week, each baby's umbilical cord—the vital link to the placenta—has formed.

Week 6: By now, the early stages of heart formation are complete and each baby's heart has begun to beat! Soon the embryos will start to produce their own blood. Meanwhile, the limbs are forming. By the 26th day after conception, your babies have the beginnings of arms. By day 28, budding legs are visible.

Weeks 7 and 8: Rapid cellular growth during this time causes a significant event to occur—a folding of the developing embryos, which now assume a more tubular C-shaped curvature. The eyes develop and become pigmented. Fingers and outer ears start to take shape, and soon after the early beginnings of toes become apparent.

Weeks 9 and 10: The fingers, toes, and outer ears become more developed. By the close of the 10th week—the end of the embryonic period—all major organs have been formed. A space called the amniotic cavity, which had formed between the embryo and the inner lining

Growth of Your Embryos

Days after Conception	Length of Embryo (inches)	Main External Characteristics
22	0.06–.08	Embryos are still straight.
26	0.12–.14	Embryos have become C-shaped. Arms appear as small swellings. Eyes begin to develop.
28	0.16–.20	Hands begin to form. Legs appear as small swellings. The lens of the eye starts to develop.
33	0.32–.40	Fingers are forming; wrists and elbows become apparent. Feet begin to develop. Eyes and nostrils are clearly defined.
35	0.48–.56	Ears begin to form. Eyes become pigmented.
40	0.84–.88	Fingers are formed. Eyelids are clearly visible. Toes begin to be defined.
45	1.00–1.08	The external ear becomes apparent. Toes are short and stubby. Fingers become elongated.
48	1.12–1.20	Fingers and toes are clearly defined. The head, trunk, and limbs have a distinctly human appearance.

Table 1.1

of the placenta, has gradually filled with fluid to become the amniotic sac, or bag of waters. The developing embryos float in their sacs as they grow, cushioned from shocks from the outside environment and kept at an even temperature.

If you could peer inside yourself and see your babies' faces, you would notice clearly recognizable eyes, eyelids, noses, mouths, and ears. You would also see that each baby has a well-developed head, neck, arms, and legs, with clearly defined fingers and toes. In other words, each of your babies now has an unquestionably human appearance.

Weeks 11 and 12: From the 8th to the 12th week, the length of each baby has increased fourfold, to reach about 4 inches, and the weight has increased tenfold, to about 1.5 ounces. The buds for the primary, or baby, teeth are present, and the nail beds are beginning to form. Each baby's fingers and toes, as well as external genitalia, are becoming distinct. The baby's eyelids are formed but closed. As early as the 12th week your babies may even start sucking their thumbs. All the organ systems have fully formed, with one important exception—the fetal brain continues to grow and develop throughout gestation and at birth is only about one-fourth of its adult weight. Although the human brain is most impressionable through late adolescence,[6] it continues to develop over a person's lifetime.

> **DR. LUKE:** Throughout the embryonic period—in fact, throughout all of growth and development before birth—the upper portions of the body mature earlier than the lower portions. In other words, your babies' heads, hearts, arms, and hands develop more quickly than their legs, feet, and urinary and reproductive systems. After birth, this rule still applies. Babies can raise their heads long before they can sit up; they are able to push up on their hands and arms long before they learn to stand.

LATER PREGNANCY: THE FETAL PERIOD

The fetal period includes the last month of the first trimester, plus the entire second and third trimesters. Although it is also a period of rapid growth, the fetal period is different from the embryonic period in that, other than the fetal brain and nervous system, no new structures are being formed; development is mainly in size. For this reason, the unborn babies are less susceptible to harm caused by external factors such as X-rays, drugs, and viruses—though, of course, they still can be adversely affected.

Many factors influence your babies' growth and their ultimate size and health at birth. Genetics plays a large part, as does the mother's weight prior to conception and her pattern of weight gain during pregnancy.

Here's how your multiples grow and develop, month to month, during the fetal period:

Weeks 13 to 16: Your babies are becoming even more human in appearance as the eyes move from the sides of the head to the front of the face and the outer ears develop further. The brain has been developing rapidly, so that the head accounts for about half of each baby's sitting length, or crown–rump length. Arms and legs grow to reach their relative length in proportion to the rest of the body, although the development of the lower limbs still lags behind that of the upper body. Your babies move around actively within the uterus, stretching their arms and kicking their legs, but these movements are usually too faint for you to feel. By the end of this month, the kidneys are functioning and excreting urine into the amniotic fluid, and the babies'

---

6. Raznahan A, Greenstein D, Lee NR, Clasen LS, Giedd JN. Prenatal growth in humans and postnatal brain maturation into late adolescence. Proceedings of the National Academy of Sciences. USA, 2012; 109:11366–71.

external genitals are clearly developed. Growth is very rapid, with each baby gaining about 3.5 ounces and achieving a total weight of about 4.25 ounces. Body length increases threefold to reach about 6.5 inches by the end of the 16th week.

Weeks 17 to 20: The babies more than double their weight this month, reaching about 10 ounces, and grow in length to about 9 inches by the 20th week. Lower-body development is beginning to catch up to the upper body; by now, each baby's head is only about one-third of his or her crown–rump length. The babies' skin is covered with a fine, downy growth of hair and a white, slippery, protective material called vernix. The eyebrows, eyelashes, and scalp hair begin to form, and the nails become visible on their fingers and toes. By the end of this month the muscles have become well developed, and the babies are quite active. Most exciting, the babies' kicks are strong enough for you to feel them!

Weeks 21 to 24: Each baby's weight gain during this month is substantial, doubling again to about 20 ounces (1.25 pounds), while length reaches about 12 inches. The babies' skin appears red, wrinkled, and almost translucent because of the absence of fat beneath the skin. By the end of the month, distinctive footprints and fingerprints have formed. The respiratory and nervous systems are developing quickly, yet are still too immature to function adequately outside the womb.

Weeks 25 to 28: The babies' rapid growth continues this month, with a doubling in weight to about 42 to 46 ounces (about 2.5 to 3 pounds each) and their length averaging about 14 inches by the 28th week. Their skin becomes less red and wrinkled as more fat is laid down. Their fingernails and toenails are fully formed. The babies' eyelids are open and the eyelashes are present. By the end of the month, the scalp hair is well developed. All the parts of the respiratory system have developed by now (although babies born at this point often cannot breathe on their own due to the lack of pulmonary surfactant, a chemical that keeps the air cells of the lungs from collapsing).

Weeks 29 to 32: During this month the babies each gain an additional 16 to 20 ounces, reaching a weight of about 4 pounds each, and have a length of about 16 inches by the end of the 32nd week. The babies' skin is smooth and pink—even babies of dark-skinned races, since the color changes develop after exposure to sunlight. The babies' bones are developed but are soft and flexible, since the storage of calcium and iron doesn't occur until the final weeks before birth.

Weeks 33 to 36: By this time each of your babies weighs about 5 pounds and is about 18 inches in length. They will continue to gain nearly half a pound a week. The babies have a plumper, rounded appearance. The fine, downy growth of hair has all but disappeared, and the nails have grown to reach the end of the fingers and toes. Sometime during this period, the air cells in the lungs get the signal to begin an accelerated production of pulmonary surfactant in anticipation of delivery.

Weeks 37 to 40: During the last few weeks before birth there is a slowing down of growth. The babies may be less active because they have less space to move around. At birth, full-term babies typically weigh between 6½ and 8½ pounds or even more, and are usually about 20 to 22 inches in length. Their skin is smooth, pale pink, and thickly covered with vernix. The fingernails are firm and may extend beyond the fingertips. All babies' eyes have a slate-blue color at birth but will change to their true color within the first six months of life.

From the moment of conception to the moment of birth, each baby has increased in size about 200 billion times to become a complex, unique individual.

Average Fetal Growth

Weeks	Head Circumference		Abdominal Circumference		Femur Length	
	(Inches	Millimeters)	(Inches	Millimeters)	(Inches	Millimeters)
12	3	78	2.5	64	0.4	9.5
16	5	126	4.5	115	0.8	22
20	7	178	6.25	158	1.3	34
22	8	198	7	175	1.5	38
24	9	223	8	200	1.75	45
26	10	248	8.75	223	1.9	49
28	11	272	9.75	246	2.1	53
30	11.5	285	10	256	2.2	56
32	12	303	11	283	2.4	62
34	12.5	312	12	302	2.5	64
36	13	327	12.75	322	2.7	69
38	13.5	331	13.25	336	2.8	70
40	14	347	14.25	366	3	75

Table 1.2

The growth of multiples basically parallels that of a singleton, but with several important differences. One of these differences works to your babies' advantage—multiples generally develop slightly faster than singletons do. For example, the average triplet is more mature at 30 weeks than is the typical 30-week singleton. Multiples' lungs, in particular, tend to be ready sooner to deal with the challenges of the world outside the womb.

But in another important way, multiples are at a developmental disadvantage. Whereas an unborn singleton's weight climbs until 40 weeks' gestation before slowing down, in multiples this slowing-down of the growth rate occurs much earlier—typically after 34 weeks for twins, 30 weeks for triplets, and 26 to 27 weeks for quadruplets. As a result, multiples tend to be born at a lighter weight compared to a singleton born at the same gestational age. This compounds the problems caused by the fact that multiples are also more likely to be born prematurely.

Certain multiples are at particular risk for low birthweight:

- Identical twins—monozygotic siblings tend to be lighter than their fraternal counterparts.
- Girls—the hormone testosterone generally gives boys a boost in terms of weight.
- Infants born to short and/or lightweight mothers—such children have a genetic propensity toward smaller size.
- Higher-order multiples—the more babies sharing space in the uterus, the smaller each is likely to be. The average birthweight for twins, for example, is 5 lb., 3 oz. For triplets, the typical birthweight is 3 lb., 10 oz. Quadruplets are born weighing an average of just 2 lb., 14 oz., and quintuplets average 2 lb., 9 oz.

Fortunately, there is a lot you can do to minimize the effects of these risk factors. Those specific steps are the focus of this book and are described in detail in subsequent chapters.

DR. LUKE: You'll notice that, in many instances, our guidelines differ depending on how many babies you're expecting. That's because the demands of a triplet pregnancy are not the same as those of a twin pregnancy; the demands of a quadruplet pregnancy are not the same as those of a triplet pregnancy.

I've found that many women are much better able to follow our daily guidelines on diet, rest, and physical activity once we translate the data on fetal growth into terms they can easily understand. For instance, a woman may be tempted to skip breakfast or work overtime. But when she has a graphic illustration of the difference in size between babies born prematurely and those born closer to full term, she is more motivated to not cut corners in her care and the care of her babies.

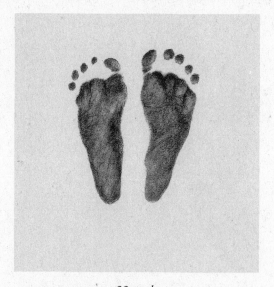

22 weeks

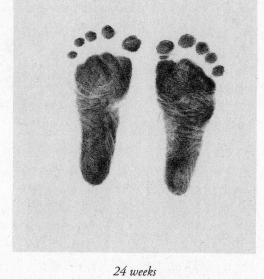

24 weeks

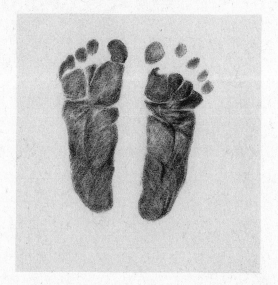

26 weeks

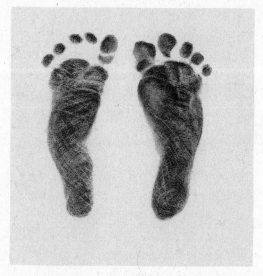

28 weeks

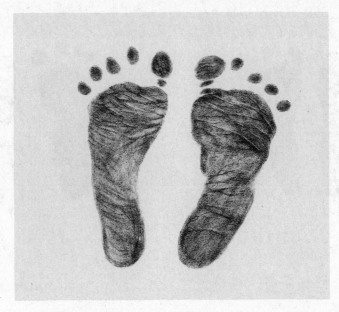

30 weeks

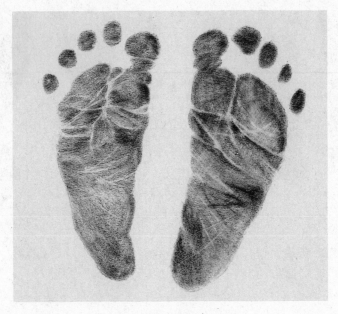

34 weeks

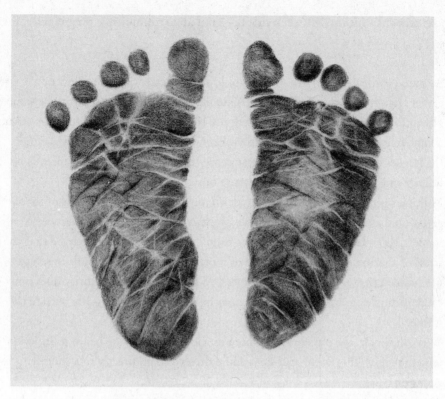

40 weeks

One of the most helpful tools we've developed is a chart that compares actual footprints of babies born at various gestational ages, from 22 weeks all the way to 40 weeks. As Amy Maly said to me, "The footprints of the preemies were so tiny. They were scary—but inspiring, too. Every time I thought, 'Ugh, I can't eat right now,' or, 'I'm supposed to stay in bed, but maybe it wouldn't hurt to do a little housecleaning,' I'd look at those footprints and feel renewed determination to do whatever was best for my babies." We've reproduced these footprints here, in the hope that you will find inspiration in them, too.

Countdown to Due Date

In a singleton pregnancy, birth typically occurs about 280 days after the first day of the woman's last menstrual period. This is equal to 40 weeks, 10 lunar months, or approximately

9 calendar months. But this 40-week rule does not apply to multiple pregnancies, for several reasons:

- As stated earlier, the growth rate for multiples typically begins to slow down earlier than it does for singletons—particularly when they are sharing the same placenta. The more babies, the sooner growth slows. Although the reasons are not completely clear, there is evidence that when babies are growing poorly, either the fetuses or the mother or both may sense that the uterine environment is not a healthy one and signal for the premature onset of labor.
- Multiples generally are more mature developmentally than singletons of the same gestational age, and they are therefore prepared for birth two to three weeks sooner. Though the physiology of this is not well understood, it may be that the stress of sharing the womb with one or more siblings triggers a built-in safety mechanism that accelerates development. While this added maturity does not cause multiples to be born sooner, it does help prepare them for life outside the womb.
- With multiples, the placentas age more quickly and therefore begin to function less efficiently. This factor may contribute directly or indirectly to a shorter gestation.
- The uterus can stretch only so far, and an overdistended uterus spontaneously contracts more often. The combined weight of several babies, several placentas, and a whole lot of amniotic fluid eventually signals to the body that it's time for labor to start, no matter how much longer the calendar says the pregnancy should continue. By the time she reaches 32 weeks, the uterus of a woman carrying twins is already as large as that of a singleton mom at the full 40 weeks. For the mother of triplets, the uterus is stretched to full-term size by 28 weeks. And with quadruplets on board, a woman's uterus reaches full-term size as early as 24 weeks.

Anne Seifert, mother of quadruplets, knows from personal experience how these factors can combine to limit the length of a multiple pregnancy. "My obstetrician originally said we would aim for me to carry the quads to 34 weeks," says Anne. "But by week 24, my uterus was already stretched beyond the size a singleton's mother would be at full term. We both realized there was no way I'd be able to make it to 34 weeks. It was all I could do to get to 31."

If a due date based on 40 weeks' gestation is not realistic for mothers-to-be of multiples, when should you expect to deliver? Here are the averages:

- Twins, on average, are born at 35.4 weeks' gestation.
- Triplets, on average, arrive at 31.8 weeks.
- Quadruplets, on average, are born at 29.7 weeks.

Keep in mind, though, that these figures are averages. Your pregnancy may be longer—or labor may begin sooner than average. Consider these statistics:

- Ten percent of singletons are born before 37 weeks; fewer than 2 percent are born before 32 weeks.
- Sixty percent of twins arrive prior to 37 weeks; 12 percent arrive prior to 32 weeks.
- Ninety-two percent of triplets are delivered before 37 weeks; more than 36 percent are delivered before 32 weeks.
- Ninety-five percent of quadruplets are born before 37 weeks; 79 percent are born before 32 weeks.

Your own obstetrical history plays a part, too.[7] If you've already given birth at least once, you're at an advantage during your multiple pregnancy. Research indicates the following:

- Your risk of delivering twins prior to 35 weeks' gestation is only half that of a woman for whom a twin pregnancy is her first.
- Your risk of delivering triplets prior to 30 weeks' gestation is only one-fourth that of a woman for whom a triplet pregnancy is her first.[8] Also, if your previous singleton pregnancy lasted at least 37 weeks, your triplets are likely to grow faster and be born heavier than triplets born to a first-time mother.

Another factor to consider is your age.[9] Surprisingly, although younger women tend to do better during singleton pregnancies, older moms-to-be of multiples may have an advantage over younger ones. For instance:

7. Luke B, Brown MB, Wantman E, Baker VL, Grow DR, Stern JE. Second try: Who returns for additional assisted reproductive technology treatment and the effect of a prior assisted reproductive technology birth. Fertility and Sterility 2013; 100:1580–4.
8. Luke B, Nugent C, van de Ven C, Martin D, O'Sullivan MJ, Eardley S, et al. The association between maternal factors and perinatal outcomes in triplet pregnancies. American Journal of Obstetrics & Gynecology 2002; 187:752–7.
9. Luke B, Brown MB. Contemporary risks of maternal morbidity and adverse outcomes with increasing maternal age and plurality. Fertility and Sterility 2007; 88:283–93.

- Women age 30 or older are significantly more likely to carry their twins for at least 35 weeks than are younger women.
- Triplets born to mothers age 40 and over tend to be among the healthiest. This may be due in part to higher socioeconomic status and earlier prenatal care.

So think of your due date as a goal, not a given. Focus on maximizing your odds of getting as close as possible to full term by carefully following your doctor's instructions as well as the guidelines in this book.

If that seems like a difficult challenge at times, try to think positively and proactively. It's understandable if you feel concerned when you learn about potential problems in multiple pregnancies, but remind yourself that knowledge equals power. The more you know about your unique pregnancy, the more you can do to ensure an optimal outcome.

As one twin mom says, "I bought this book shortly after my multiples were diagnosed because I didn't want advice on whether to give the babies rhyming names or let them sleep in the same crib—I wanted guidance on how to get through my high-risk pregnancy with as few complications as possible, so that I would be able to go home with two healthy babies. I wanted to be educated about any potential problems and, more important, about the concrete and do-able things that would maximize my chances of avoiding these problem areas."

If you do experience setbacks, don't let them erode your confidence or discourage you from making proactive efforts to optimize your pregnancy outcome. "I had a worrisome pregnancy. I experienced some bleeding, my cervix was weak, and I was having contractions from 18 weeks onward. Preterm labor was a serious threat, and I had to stay on bed rest for more than four months," says Heather Nicholas, mother of boy/girl twins. "But I ended up carrying those babies to 38 and a half weeks. At birth, Madeleine weighed 7 lb., 3 oz., and Benjamin weighed 6 lb., 15 oz.—so both were heavier than the average singleton at that gestational age."

You may experience various complications, as Heather did—or you may sail through your pregnancy with a minimum of trouble. Either way, remember that your actions can have a strongly positive influence on your babies' health and well-being.

Chapter Two

The Best Medical Care for Expectant Mothers of Multiples

When Ginny Seyler and her husband, David, first tried to start a family, Ginny conceived easily—but, sadly, that pregnancy ended in miscarriage. Then followed nearly four years of infertility. Finally, with the use of Clomid, Ginny conceived again—but severe bleeding at seven weeks threatened to end this pregnancy as well. The fertility specialist who was treating Ginny immediately scheduled an ultrasound.

"I expected to be told that I was miscarrying again. Instead, on the screen we saw a healthy baby growing. Then we saw another healthy baby, and we were thrilled! But when the doctor saw a *third* baby, our excitement turned to shock. I have a master's degree in maternal-child health, so I knew more than the average person about the challenges a triplet pregnancy presents," Ginny explains. "I realized that, this very day, I would have to begin a quest for the best obstetrician I could find."

Assembling Your Health Care Team

Ginny was right on target. A multiple pregnancy carries a greater potential for problems than does a singleton pregnancy. The most important step you can take to minimize risk is to select a doctor with enough experience managing multiple gestations to anticipate these potential problems, detect them early, and treat them in the most effective way possible. General practitioners, family doctors, midwives, and even many general obstetricians may not have the extra training, years of experience, or volume of twins or triplets in his or her practice necessary to provide the most advanced and appropriate care for an expectant mother of multiples.

That's why you should seriously consider receiving your obstetrical care from a maternal-fetal medicine specialist—an obstetrician who has received extensive specialized training and put it to use in the management of high-risk pregnancies.

> **DR. LUKE:** If you're expecting triplets or quadruplets, you're probably already convinced of the need for specialized care. But if you're carrying twins, you may think a specialist is unnecessary.
>
> I urge you to think again. Because twin pregnancies are fairly common, not all doctors recognize the unique needs of women who are carrying two babies. The truth is that *all* multiple pregnancies involve increased risk, as reported in many studies from researchers across the country and around the world, including our research group, the University Consortium on Multiple Births. Anyone who tells you otherwise is misinformed.
>
> This is not to say that you necessarily will have difficulties during this pregnancy. You may experience no complications whatsoever. Still, it's smart to be prepared. Think of a medical specialist as an insurance policy—you hope you never need to make a claim, but if tough times do arise you'll be happy to have that policy in place. One reader reports, "I'm so glad that I followed the advice to put myself into the care of a group of maternal-fetal medicine specialists. Because of their proactive approach, when I began to show signs of preterm labor, my twins arrived at 31 weeks instead of 26 weeks, as they were threatening to do."
>
> As Judy Levy said to me during one of her prenatal visits to the University of Michigan Multiples Clinic, "I appreciate that my obstetrician never treats me like I'm sick or implies that I will definitely have problems just because I'm expecting twins. Yet it's a relief to know that, because he specializes in high-risk pregnancies, he's well qualified to deal with any complications that might develop. I would feel much more anxious if I didn't have him on my team."

IF YOU ALREADY HAVE A DOCTOR—BUT HE OR SHE IS NOT A SPECIALIST

Often a woman does not learn that she is carrying multiples until well into the second trimester. By that time, she has already been someone's patient for several months. The big question then is whether to switch to a high-risk specialist or stick with her current doctor.

In some cases, the doctor makes the decision for you. "We very much liked the regular obstetrician who had delivered our older son. But when the ultrasound revealed that my wife was carrying triplets this time, the obstetrician told us right away that we should transfer to a high-risk practice. We had no sense of being disloyal by switching, especially since we were following her guidance," says Kevin McAndrew, father of fraternal triplets and an older son.

What if your regular doctor does *not* suggest transferring? You may feel embarrassed at the thought of saying to a physician, "I'm going elsewhere for my prenatal care." But don't let that stop you from doing what is best for you and your babies—especially if you have not been 100 percent thrilled with your care so far.

"I'd been warned against switching obstetricians in the middle of a pregnancy because it was important that a doctor have time to really get to know the patient. That's why I stuck with my original doctor even after I learned I was expecting twins, though he did not specialize in multiple gestation," says Meredith Alcott, mother of identical twin girls. "In hindsight, though, I do wish I had changed to a specialist. I received the standard care you'd expect during a single-ton pregnancy—but what I needed went beyond standard. For instance, my obstetrician gave only perfunctory answers to my questions about diet and other special needs of a twin preg-nancy. And he never saw me more than once a month, even after I developed complications."

Recognize, too, that even if your regular obstetrician can offer quality care for a multiple pregnancy, other health care providers in his or her practice may not be as capable. "My own doctor was terrific. But the disadvantage in not going to a specialist was that the rest of the of-fice staff wasn't as up-to-speed on multiple pregnancy as they might have been," explains Benita Moreno, mother of fraternal twin boys. "The nurses, for instance, were supposed to advise me on what to eat, help me learn to recognize contractions, teach me about warning signs to watch for, and so on. But they weren't helpful at all. They even made critical remarks about how heavy I was getting, though both my doctor and my nutritionist had urged me to gain weight quickly!"

Switching doctors under circumstances similar to Meredith's or Benita's should not cause you more than a few moments of discomfort. But it is admittedly much more difficult to leave your current physician if you already have a close, trusting relationship with him or her—and particularly if that doctor has cared for you during a previous pregnancy.

DR. NEWMAN: As soon as it is known that you're carrying more than one baby, there are several points that you and your doctor should promptly discuss. Among those are the need to identify the type of multiple gestation (whether it is dichorionic versus monochorionic), the risks that may be encountered with that type of pregnancy, and your specific nutritional requirements. That conversation, combined with your own knowledge of your past health and obstetrical history, as well as the information in this book, should help you judge whether or not your current doctor is prepared to deal with any of the various complications that your multiple pregnancy may present.

Important questions to ask your doctor include the following:

- How many expectant mothers of multiples have you cared for in the last year? How many over the course of your career?
- Do you have any special nutritional recommendations for women pregnant with multiples?
- Does the hospital with which you are affiliated provide care for babies born earlier than 34 weeks' gestation?
- Do you routinely consult with a maternal-fetal medicine specialist prior to the development of any pregnancy problems?
- If a pregnancy does become complicated, whom do you consult at that point?
- Do you differentiate between monochorionic and dichorionic twins?
- Do you manage monochorionic and dichorionic twins any differently?

A primary goal of this conversation is to help you gauge whether your doctor and those who share his or her practice are experienced enough in caring for women expecting twins, triplets, or quads; recognize the need for an elevated level of care; and are prepared to facilitate a transition of your care to a maternal-fetal medicine specialist if complications arise. Many general obstetricians do have years of experience caring for multiples, large practices that allow them to keep their skills sharp, and an interest in caring for these special pregnancies. If this is your situation, then you are fortunate and ahead of the game.

However, if you do *not* feel that your current doctor has enough experience in these areas, you would do well to transfer to a maternal-fetal medicine specialist or a regional center that offers a specialized program for multiple gestations.

DR. LUKE: We all see many health professionals over the years—general practitioners for sore throats and earaches, dentists for chipped teeth and regular cleanings, perhaps an orthopedist or physical therapist for back problems. But for most women, our obstetrician holds a special place in our hearts. He was the one who confirmed our pregnancies, saw us through bouts of nausea and vomiting, and told us we looked radiant when we were eight months pregnant and felt huge. He was there with words of encouragement when labor was painful and we wanted to give up. And it was our obstetrician who, with patience and skill, brought our precious children into the world.

It's natural you would feel reluctant to defect from the doctor you trust by turning your care over to an unknown doctor, even though you know it's advisable to see a specialist. In this case, there is another option: the team approach. Ask your primary care provider to arrange a consultation with a local or regional maternal-fetal medicine specialist. It should be possible to work out an effective collaborative care arrangement between your current physician and the multiples specialist. The team approach also provides you with an opportunity to meet with the high-risk pregnancy specialist, evaluate his or her style, and determine if there are any gaps in the care that you have been receiving so far.

It is common for general obstetricians, family practitioners, or midwives to work together with maternal-fetal medicine specialists when their patients are carrying multiples. If your pregnancy is going well, the maternal-fetal medicine specialist may advise you to continue seeing your original health care provider during the early months, then transfer your care to the specialist later in pregnancy. It is best to receive this consultation by your 18th week. Most complications develop after 20 to 24 weeks, so you would want to be established in your specialist's care by then. And, of course, the specialist should be in charge of all the additional monitoring that occurs during the last months preceding the delivery of your babies.

The team tactic worked well for Judy Levy. "I used our family doctor during my first pregnancy and was very pleased with my obstetric care, so I had planned to use her again the second time I got pregnant. I had already scheduled my first prenatal checkup with her when, a few weeks before the appointment, an ultrasound showed twins. After much consideration, I decided to take advantage of the extra measure of care a specialist could provide, yet I still wanted my family doctor to be involved," Judy explains. "And she did stay involved. For instance, at 28 weeks, I scheduled a consultation with her to discuss the pros and cons of attempting a vaginal birth after a cesarean. And I continued to see her for all non-pregnancy-related problems, like a bad case of bronchitis. My family doctor was very supportive of this cooperative approach. She even came to my delivery to cheer me on! And now that the twins have been born, she's their family physician, too."

How to Find a Maternal-Fetal Medicine Specialist

Fortunately, maternal-fetal medicine specialists are now available in most midsize and larger communities in the United States. However, there are areas where access could still be a problem. Here are a number of ways to go about finding a qualified maternal-fetal medicine provider:

- Ask for a referral from your family doctor or regular obstetrician/gynecologist.
- If you achieved your multiple pregnancy through infertility treatments, your reproductive endocrinology/infertility specialist can be a valuable resource. He or she will know which providers or groups in your area have the most experience and success in providing obstetrical care for patients expecting multiples.
- Most medium-to-large hospitals with busy obstetrical services have an affiliated maternal-fetal medicine provider or group practice on staff. These providers should have a great deal of experience dealing with complicated twin pregnancies and pregnancies involving higher-order multiples. Call the obstetrics department of hospitals in your area and ask for the names of maternal-fetal medicine specialists affiliated with the facility.
- Contact the Society for Maternal-Fetal Medicine: 409 12th Street, SW, Washington, DC 20024. Telephone 202-863-2476; website www.smfm.org (click on "Find an MFM").
- Appendix D of this book includes a list of well-respected prenatal programs for multiples in the United States, as well as fetal therapy providers. This list is not meant to be all-inclusive—certainly there are many other health care providers and groups who have had accumulated a great deal of experience in managing multiple pregnancies—but it does give you a place to start your search.
- Ask for referrals from other mothers of multiples in your area. Many communities have local chapters of Multiples of America (also known as the National Organization of Mothers of Twins Clubs), so check their website at www .multiplesofamerica.org.
- To confirm the credentials of any doctor you're considering, call the American Board of Medical Specialties' toll-free hotline at 866-ASK-ABMS, or check their website at www.abms.org. You can find out if a particular doctor is a board-certified specialist, the year he or she became certified, and when recertification is due.

When you call to make your first prenatal appointment, be sure to specify that yours is a multiple pregnancy. You want to be seen promptly, so don't accept any lengthy delays. "When I phoned the high-risk obstetrician who had been recommended to me, the receptionist said that the doctor had no time available for another six weeks. I said, 'Oh please, this is *quadruplets*!' She gave me an appointment for the following week," says Anne Seifert.

If there are several qualified specialists in your area, try to check out each one personally before making your selection. Even a five-minute visit or phone call can help you assess which doctor's style suits you best. Does he or she seem like the type of physician who establishes a personal relationship with each patient—or the type who's too busy to give you the extra time you may need?

"I picked my obstetrician because he was the director of women's health at a top hospital. But I learned that credentials aren't everything," says one mother of twins. "You need someone who makes you feel comfortable, someone who listens to you. Yet my doctor had his hand on the doorknob at every appointment. I felt too rushed to ask all my questions, and too flustered by his obvious impatience to remember his hurried answers."

You may have to look and look again before you find the doctor who's right for you. "The first obstetrician I saw diagnosed my triplet pregnancy based on the ultrasound, but he had no experience with triplets. He even told me that it didn't matter whether or not I gained any weight before week 20, which I knew couldn't be right. Next I consulted a maternal-fetal medicine specialist, but he had such a negative outlook that my husband called him Dr. Gloom-and-Doom," says Allison MacDonald. "Then I wrote to Dr. Luke, and she referred me to a wonderful maternal-fetal specialist who saw me that very same day and with whom I felt completely comfortable. Though her office was an hour from my home, it was worth making the trek."

DR. NEWMAN: Keeping that standard in mind will help you find a physician who can provide both the high-tech care and the high-touch attention that you and your babies deserve.

Hospital Options

TAMARA: I didn't give much thought, during my twin pregnancy, to the hospital where I'd be delivering. My obstetrician had told me the name and location of the hospital with which he was affiliated, and, of course, I made certain I knew how to get there without getting lost. I even timed the drive from my home to the hospital—19 minutes—many months before my due date, in anticipation of the exciting journey that would occur once I went into labor. But it didn't cross my mind to ask whether the hospital had any special facilities or capabilities when it came to caring for babies born early.

So when my water broke unexpectedly only 31 weeks into my pregnancy, and my doctor ordered me to rush to the hospital at 2 A.M., I didn't have the slightest idea of what to expect. As I gave birth to my tiny twins just two hours later, the staff of the small community hospital responded capably and kindly—yet clearly the facility was not equipped to take care of my premature newborns. As soon as my son and daughter were stable enough to be moved, ambulances whisked them to a major medical center 30 miles away.

Left behind at the little community hospital, I did not get to see or touch or hold my precious babies until I was discharged two days later. Those were long, lonely, anxiety-filled days.

It is difficult under any circumstances to learn that your newborns have medical problems. But you'll be even more upset if you are separated from them. To ensure that this doesn't happen, you need some basic information about hospitals.

Hospital obstetrical services and newborn nurseries are divided into four categories, according to the level of care they can provide. Here's how it breaks down:[1, 2]

- *Level I:* Most hospitals in the country are classified at this level. These facilities can manage routine, uncomplicated labors and deliveries and care for healthy full-term newborns. They can also handle mild complications an infant may develop, such as jaundice. In addition, they are able to provide neonatal resuscitation at delivery, care for infants born at 35 weeks or later who remain stable, and stabilize infants born at less than 35 weeks until those infants can be transferred to a higher level of care.
- *Level II:* These hospitals have the staff and equipment to take care of many complications that newborns may experience if born prematurely, including mild to moderate respiratory distress syndrome and the need for gavage feeding (feeding through a tube inserted through the nose and into the stomach). They also provide care for infants convalescing after intensive care (in what is sometimes called step-down care). In addition, they can stabilize infants born prior to 32 weeks' gestation and those born weighing less than about 3.3 pounds (1,500 grams) until the babies can be transferred to a neonatal intensive care unit.

    Level II hospitals frequently do care for infants who weigh 3.3 pounds to 5.6 pounds (1,500 grams to 2,500 grams) and who are born as early as 32 to 34 weeks' gestation. However, it's important to note that approximately 10 percent to 15 percent of twins are delivered prior to 32 weeks' gestation, and as many as one-third are delivered prior to 34 weeks.

---

1. Committee on Fetus and Newborn. Levels of neonatal care. Pediatrics 2012; 130:587–97.
2. American Academy of Pediatrics; American College of Obstetricians and Gynecologists. Guidelines for perinatal care. 7th edition. Elk Grove, IL, 2012; 21–59.

You should also realize that there is great variability among Level II hospitals. Some have on-staff maternal-fetal medicine specialists and neonatologists (pediatricians who specialize in the care of newborns), while others do not. Some have an established neonatal intensive care unit with the capability to ventilate babies for more than a brief period of time, but others do not. If your obstetrical care provider is affiliated with a Level II hospital, it would be wise to inquire about the facility's capabilities, including the number of neonatal intensive care patients the unit typically handles at any given time—because the more experienced the staff is at caring for sick newborns, the better at it they are likely to be.

- *Level III:* Typically found in large cities and/or affiliated with universities, these facilities are equipped to care for very sick or very small babies. Along with a regular nursery for well newborns and a special-care nursery for infants with mild to moderate medical problems, these hospitals include a full neonatal intensive care unit, or NICU (sometimes pronounced *nick-you*). Staff includes full-time neonatologists as well as pediatric neurologists, surgeons, and developmental experts. These NICUs can care for premature or full-term infants who require complex care, including life-support techniques such as long-term mechanical ventilation. These facilities can also care for infants requiring inhaled nitric oxide therapy and high-frequency ventilation, and the chronically technology-dependent infant. In addition, Level III NICUs can care for infants requiring extracorporeal membrane oxygenation (ECMO), essentially a state-of-the-art infant heart-lung machine.

- *Level IV:* Located within major medical centers, these NICUs have all the capabilities of the Level III NICUs, with the additional resources and experience to provide care for the most complex and critically ill newborns, including those needing surgery. Level IV NICUs (also known as regional NICUs) have on-site staffs that include a full range of pediatric medical subspecialists, such as pediatric surgeons, pediatric cardiothoracic surgeons, and pediatric anesthesiologists.

In light of the fact that newborn multiples are at risk for needing special medical care, the best way to guarantee that you and your babies remain in the same hospital after delivery is to give birth at a Level III or Level IV facility. This is not as difficult to ensure as it may sound, because most maternal-fetal medicine specialists are affiliated with such hospitals. If you've already found a physician qualified to manage your multiple pregnancy, chances are that he or she has admitting privileges at the type of hospital you need.

If you haven't yet found a doctor, call your area hospitals and ask what level nursery they have. Once you identify the closest Level III or Level IV facility, ask for a referral to a maternal-fetal medicine specialist on their staff. "I chose my hospital *before* I chose my obstetrician," says Karen Danke. "I knew this facility had a great reputation, especially for its NICU. I wanted to make sure that if my twins needed extra care after birth, they would already be in the hospital best qualified to help them." Your babies may never need such care—many multiples do not—but it's important that it be available, just in case.

Not only your babies but you, too, can benefit from this. That's because hospitals with Level III or Level IV nurseries also generally have the most advanced facilities for treating problems that women might develop during the course of a high-risk pregnancy or after delivery.

Once you have chosen an obstetrician and a hospital, it's a good idea to take a tour. Usually run by the nursing staff in obstetrics, a hospital tour gives you an opportunity to ask questions, see the actual labor and delivery rooms, and perhaps visit the NICU. Familiarizing yourself with the facilities under relaxed, calm conditions will help you feel less anxious should you need to be admitted during your pregnancy, as well as allow you to approach labor and delivery with more confidence.

Nurses: The Heart and Soul of Health Care

An integral part of every aspect of medicine, from prevention to acute care, is the nursing staff. During the course of your pregnancy, you'll meet many nurses. Some work in your doctor's office or clinic. Others care for you during labor and delivery, and during your recovery from childbirth. The nursing staff is also a vital component of your babies' hospital health care team. Many of these professionals, such as nurse practitioners, clinical specialists, and midwives, have received additional specialized training and are qualified to perform a variety of duties that were previously done only by doctors.

Take advantage of the knowledge and skills of the nurses you encounter. They can educate you and your partner on what to expect during this important time in your life, teach you how to watch for danger signs, and translate confusing data into practical and usable information. Equally important, nurses provide the warm, caring, emotional support that is so comforting during a potentially complicated pregnancy.

A Vital Team Member: Your Dietitian

When you're expecting a team of babies, you need a *team* of health care providers. That team is led, of course, by your obstetrician. But a key member of your team is a registered dietitian.

Prenatal nutrition—what you eat when you're pregnant—has long been recognized as a critical factor in your health and the health of your unborn babies. For more than 40 years, the American College of Obstetricians and Gynecologists (a professional organization for medical doctors who specialize in women's reproductive health care) has said that nutrition assessment and dietary counseling is a vital part of prenatal care. Since most medical doctors have little training in nutrition, your best bet is to ask your physician for a referral to someone who specializes in this field.

A registered dietitian (RD) is the type of health care professional best equipped to evaluate your diet. She or he can make sure you're getting the right varieties of foods, in the right quantities, to promote optimal growth and development of your unborn babies. Your dietitian can also offer advice for the postpartum period to help ensure success in breast-feeding and to help you regain your figure after delivery.

"Having access to the nutrition counseling offered by the Multiples Clinic was a real advantage," says Helen Armer, mother of triplets. "My babies were all a good size when they were born—one weighed almost 6 pounds, and the others were close to 5 pounds. I don't think that would have happened without Dr. Luke's nutrition program."

Not just any nutritionist will do, however. Many lack the additional training and experience needed to counsel mothers-to-be of multiples. "I made an appointment with a dietitian, but as it turned out, she was used to taking care of heart patients. She didn't know much about obstetrical patients, and she knew even less about the nutritional demands of unborn triplets," Ginny Seyler laments.

DR. LUKE: It is unfortunately true that it's often tough to find a dietitian who has much experience with multiples. Look for someone who specializes in obstetrics; she will be most familiar with the nutritional demands of pregnancy and can properly adjust upward the requirements for certain nutrients, depending on how many babies you're carrying.

As Judy Levy says, "For me, having the benefit of a nutritionist who was knowledgeable about multiple pregnancy was a real plus. She gave me the kind of specific menu-planning advice and concrete details one doesn't typically get from an obstetrician. And she was seeing me more often too—once a week, compared to only once a month for the obstetrician."

To find a qualified professional in your area, check the website of the Academy of Nutrition and Dietetics (formerly called the American Dietetic Association) at www .eatright.org/programs/rdnfinder/. In the "Search by Expertise" box, click on "Maternal Nutrition." You can also get personalized nutrition advice directly from me through my website, www.drbarbaraluke.com.

In today's mobile society, women often live far away from the mothers and sisters who might be able to help them learn to breast-feed. And in many cases, these mothers and sisters themselves may not have had the experience of nursing their children, and therefore are not the best breast-feeding advocates and teachers for expectant and new mothers, particularly those facing the challenges of nursing multiples.

That's why one of the best ways to prepare for successful breast-feeding is to meet with a lactation consultant while you are still pregnant. If you then have difficulties once you do begin breast-feeding, you will have already established a relationship with this important health professional and can call upon her again for assistance.

An International Board Certified Lactation Consultant (IBCLC) specializes in helping mothers to breast-feed successfully. IBCLCs are certified by the International Board of Lactation Consultant Examiners (www.iblce.org), under the direction of the U.S. National Commission for Certifying Agencies. IBCLCs work in a wide variety of health care settings, including hospitals, pediatricians' offices, public health clinics, and private practice. IBCLCs provide:

- Prenatal counseling about factors that may affect breast-feeding, such as fatigue and stress.
- Information on practices that promote successful breast-feeding, such as appropriate diet, adequate hydration, and support from the babies' father.
- Specific instructions on preventing and managing common concerns, such as problems with latching on, inadequate milk supply, and nipple or breast pain, as well as techniques for calming fussy babies.
- Advice on milk expression and storage.
- Tips for breast-feeding after returning to work.
- Strategies for challenging situations, such as breast-feeding multiples or infants who are premature or have special medical needs.

To find a lactation consultant in your area, go to the International Lactation Consultant Association website at www.ilca.org and click on "Find a Lactation Consultant," or phone 888-ILCA-IS-U (888-452-2478) or 919-861-5577.

DR. NEWMAN: Many hospitals are now undertaking the challenge of becoming certified as Baby-Friendly health care facilities. In order to receive this certification, hospital facilities must remove all barriers to the rapid initiation of breast-feeding and have lactation consultants on staff to assist new mothers. Given the unquestioned health benefits of breast-feeding, I suggest that you investigate whether the hospital where you plan to deliver is certified as Baby-Friendly—and if it is not, ask why not. (For more information on Baby-Friendly facilities, see Chapter 11.)

PHYSICAL THERAPIST

This is another health professional you may want to add to your team. A physical therapist provides services that help restore physical function, improve mobility, relieve pain, and prevent or limit physical disabilities. Typically, a master's degree from an accredited physical therapy program is the minimum level of education for a practicing physical therapist.

Treatment often includes special exercises designed to increase flexibility, range of motion, strength, balance, coordination, and endurance, improving how an individual functions at work and at home. Physical therapists also may use hot packs, cold compresses, deep-tissue massage, and/or ultrasound therapy to relieve pain, reduce swelling, and improve circulation and flexibility.

Because a multiple pregnancy places additional strain on a woman's body, physical therapy may be particularly helpful in relieving discomfort. To find a physical therapist in your area, go to the website of the American Physical Therapy Association at www.apta.org and click on "Find a PT," or phone 800-999-APTA (800-999-2782) or 703-684-2782.

The Doctor-Patient Partnership

You and your obstetrician are partners for this very unique period in your life. That partnership involves rights and responsibilities for both of you, as outlined in the American College of Obstetricians and Gynecologists' book on prenatal care *Planning Your Pregnancy and Birth*.

You have a right to:

- Quality care without discrimination.
- Privacy.
- Know the professional status of your health care providers and their fees.
- Advice about your diagnosis, treatment, options, and the expected outcome.
- Active involvement in decisions about your care.

- Refuse treatment.
- Agree or refuse to participate in any research that affects your care.

You have a responsibility to:

- Provide accurate and complete health information.
- Let your doctor know whether you understand the medical procedures and what you are expected to do.

PREPARING FOR YOUR FIRST PRENATAL VISIT

The more your obstetrician knows about you and your pregnancy, the better prepared he or she will be to detect and treat any potential health problems. Yet it's not always easy to remember every detail when you're sitting in a doctor's office.

The Prenatal Care Questionnaire that follows can help. Spend some time filling in the answers before your first prenatal visit. This overall picture of your medical history and current health can help your obstetrician plan the prenatal care that's right for you and your unborn babies.

Also call any other physicians you have seen—your family doctor, gynecologist, previous obstetrician, fertility specialist (if applicable)—and request that your medical records be forwarded to your new obstetrician as soon as possible. Be sure to provide your obstetrician with complete information regarding any prior pregnancies, whether or not they resulted in a birth. This is particularly important if any of your pregnancies ended three or more weeks before your due date, or if any of your children weighed less than 5½ pounds at birth. Studies show that there is a strong tendency to repeat the birthweight and gestational age at birth of previous pregnancies. If you had a prior singleton pregnancy in which you delivered a premature or low-birthweight baby, your risk of doing so again is magnified even further now that you're pregnant with multiples.

You'll also want to talk to your female relatives about their childbearing experiences, because genetics may play an important role in the course and outcome of your pregnancy. For example, there is evidence that the risk of prematurity may be carried through the maternal side of the family tree. Ask your mother, sisters, and maternal aunts if their pregnancies ended earlier than expected, and make note of their babies' birthweights. Find out if anyone experienced complications such as a blood clot during pregnancy or heavy bleeding during delivery. Also be sure to inform your doctor of any history of genetic diseases in your family or your husband's family. Forewarned with this knowledge, your obstetrician may order additional tests and take extra precautions to reduce the risks associated with such a family history.

Finally, promise yourself to be completely honest with your obstetrician about any sensitive issues such as sexually transmitted diseases or alcohol and drug use. Remember, it can be very dangerous to your unborn babies if you fail to disclose that you have herpes, for example, or that you are tempted to drink even though you're pregnant.

Prenatal Care Questionnaire:
Information You Should Provide to Your Doctor

Family Health History

Your ethnic background _____

Your partner's ethnic background _____

Inherited genetic disorders _____

Any previous children born with a birth defect _____

Medical and Surgical History

Current medications taken _____

Current dietary/herbal supplements taken _____

Past medications taken _____

Allergies and allergic reactions _____

Current medical conditions _____

Past medical conditions _____

History of fertility treatments _____

Prior surgeries _____

Exposure to infectious diseases _____

Menstrual History

Age at your first menstrual period _____

Date of your last menstrual period _____

History of use of birth control pills _____

Other methods of contraception used _____

Lifestyle Habits

Type and place of employment _____

Alcohol use _____

Cigarette/e-cigarette/other tobacco use _____

Recreational drug use _____

Exposure to toxic substances _____

Past Pregnancies

Miscarriages or induced abortions _____

Length of gestation of any previous pregnancies _____

Complications before delivery _____

Length of labor _____

Method of delivery (vaginal or cesarean) _____

Complications after delivery _____

Newborn's birthweight _____

Newborn's medical condition _____

PRENATAL CHECKUP PRIMER

What's the major difference in prenatal care for an expectant mother of multiples? You will have more frequent checkups with your obstetrician than a woman pregnant with a single baby. Though the schedule of prenatal appointments varies according to the doctor and the patient's needs, here is a typical checkup routine:

Frequency of Prenatal Checkups

Weeks of Pregnancy	Mother of Singleton	Mother of Multiples
0–24 weeks	Monthly	Monthly*
24–28 weeks	Monthly	Every other week
28–32 weeks	Every other week	Every other week
32–36 weeks	Every other week	Weekly
36 weeks–delivery	Weekly	Weekly

*Exception: A woman pregnant with monochorionic twins should be seen every other week between weeks 16 and 26 to check for twin-twin transfusion syndrome (TTTS), as discussed in Chapter 7.

Table 2.1

It is vital that you not skip any of your appointments with the obstetrician. Babies born to mothers who do not receive adequate prenatal care tend to do much worse than those whose mothers were closely followed by medical professionals. "I realized that the best way to give my triplets a good chance of being born healthy was to keep all my prenatal appointments and follow every single instruction from my obstetrician and from the Multiples Clinic," explains Helen Armer, who carried her triplets to an impressive 36 weeks.

Because the laboratory tests and medical history you provide at your first prenatal checkup will establish your personal database for this entire pregnancy, it is typically a long visit. Allow plenty of time.

Subsequent visits are much shorter. These usually involve the following:

- Measuring the growth of the uterus.
- Estimating the babies' sizes, positions, and relative growth.

- Listening to the babies' heart rates.
- Monitoring your blood pressure.
- Recording your weight and calculating your weight gain.
- Testing your urine.
- Performing additional tests and evaluations, depending on how many weeks pregnant you are.
- Reviewing any symptoms you may be experiencing.
- Answering your questions.

This last point is an essential aspect of quality prenatal care, so prepare for it in advance. "I arrived at each appointment with a list of questions and a notepad for recording the doctor's answers," says Judy Levy. "I think this made the doctor take my concerns more seriously. He spent a lot of time with me, and even photocopied articles from medical journals for me, because he knew I wasn't going to stop asking questions until I had the information I wanted." (Use the Prenatal Care Fact Sheet that follows as a guide to questions you should ask and to have a record of your doctor's answers.)

If you have trouble asserting yourself, bring your partner along for moral support. "My doctor always seemed to be in a hurry, so I was intimidated about taking up his time with a lot of questions," says Meredith Alcott. "Luckily, my husband is more outspoken than I am. He came with me to every appointment and told the obstetrician, 'We have a list of questions here, and we're not leaving until they're all answered.'"

What if you have a question that seems too important to save for your next checkup? Don't hesitate to call your doctor with any pressing concerns. Knowledge is power—and as the mother-to-be, you are your babies' best advocate.

Prenatal Care Fact Sheet: Information Your Doctor Should Provide to You

Office Procedures

The type of care given in the office or clinic _____

Necessary laboratory tests _____

Schedule of routine examinations _____

Basic Pregnancy Information

Your due date _____

Nonemergency symptoms to report at your next checkup _____

Emergency Action Plan

Symptoms to report to the doctor immediately _____

How to recognize contractions _____

What to do if you feel contractions _____

What to do if bleeding occurs _____

What to do if fluid trickles from your vagina _____

What to do if fluid gushes from your vagina _____

Labor Plan

Plans for hospital admission _____

Circumstances under which vaginal delivery will be attempted _____

Circumstances under which cesarean delivery will be performed _____

Analgesic and anesthetic options for labor _____

Additional Information/Instructions

Recommended educational literature _____

Referral to childbirth preparation class _____

Referral to infant care class _____

Referral to local support group for parents of multiples _____

Referral to tours of labor and delivery ward, newborn nursery, NICU _____

Prenatal Tests for Moms-to-Be of Multiples

Women carrying multiples generally undergo more types of prenatal tests, and with greater frequency, than do mothers of singletons. Knowing what to expect and thinking of the tests as an opportunity to be reassured that all is well can make the process easier. Here's what you should know about prenatal tests:

PELVIC EXAMINATIONS

During the first prenatal visit, the obstetrician performs a digital pelvic examination by placing two gloved fingers inside your vagina to feel your cervix and other internal organs. This allows the doctor to estimate how many weeks pregnant you are and to check for any cervical, uterine, or ovarian problems. She or he may also perform a Pap smear by using a small brush or swab to scrape a few cells from your cervix. These are examined under a microscope to detect any abnormal cervical changes. Along with the Pap smear, cervical-vaginal cultures are usually taken to screen for gonorrhea and chlamydia. If a discharge is present, a cotton swab is used to collect a sample, which is then examined under a microscope for infections such as yeast, trichomonas, and nonspecific vaginosis.

The pelvic examination is generally not repeated until after the 24th week of pregnancy. However, if you are experiencing symptoms of preterm labor, such as uterine contractions, pelvic pressure, or vaginal discharge, your obstetrician may perform a pelvic exam to check for changes in the cervix. Although a transvaginal ultrasound is very effective in determining cervical length, a manual pelvic exam can give additional information regarding other indicators of preterm labor, such as cervical dilatation, position and softness, and the descent of the baby closest to the cervix.

URINE TESTS

At each prenatal visit, your urine is tested for the presence of ketones (by-products of fat breakdown), which indicate that your diet does not include sufficient carbohydrates and/or calories. Urine is also tested for protein, which may be a sign of kidney disease or preeclampsia (a serious pregnancy complication related to blood pressure). If you experience pain or other urinary symptoms, urine is analyzed for bacteria; if an infection is found, it is treated with antibiotics.

Blood Tests

To check for iron-deficiency anemia, or low iron in the blood, your doctor draws a blood sample to evaluate the levels of hemoglobin (the oxygen-carrying, iron-containing component of red blood cells) and hematocrit (the percentage of red blood cells in the blood). Because the drain on your iron stores is greater when you're carrying more than one baby—and because adequate iron is so important to your babies' growth as well as your own health—you're checked more frequently for anemia than is a singleton mom. If you are anemic, you can increase your iron stores by eating iron-rich foods (see Chapters 4 and 5).

Your blood is also evaluated for blood type and any antibodies you may have developed against red blood cell proteins. It's particularly important that your blood be checked for a protein called the Rh factor. If your blood is Rh negative (as is the case for 10 to 15 percent of the population) and your partner is Rh positive, this can potentially cause problems for your unborn babies. To prevent you from making antibodies against your babies, you need injections of a drug called RhoGAM at about 28 weeks' gestation and immediately after delivery if any of your babies prove to be Rh positive. RhoGAM should also be administered to Rh-negative women after any episode of vaginal bleeding and following certain procedures such as amniocentesis or chorionic villus sampling.

RhoGAM contains antibodies directed against Rh-positive red blood cells (from one or more of the babies) that might have entered your bloodstream. The antibodies neutralize the Rh-positive cells and prevent your immune system from identifying them as foreign. Over the past half century, RhoGAM has proven highly effective, reducing Rh-factor incompatibility from being the number-one cause of stillbirth in the United States in the 1960s to being a rare cause today.

Your blood is also tested for rubella, hepatitis B, syphilis, and HIV antibodies, because these infections can be passed on to your unborn babies and cause serious harm. These blood tests may also be repeated later in pregnancy, if necessary.

In addition, your blood pressure is taken at each checkup. Women who have high blood pressure (hypertension) are more likely to deliver preterm and to have babies whose growth has been restricted. Preexisting hypertension also increases a woman's risk for developing preeclampsia, a pregnancy complication in which there is protein in the urine, rapid weight gain, rapid rise in blood pressure, and swelling from fluid retention. In severe cases, preeclampsia can lead to serious risks for the mother (see Chapter 7).

GLUCOSE TOLERANCE TEST[3]

Between the 24th and 28th weeks of your pregnancy, you are tested for gestational diabetes. First you are given a special high-carbohydrate beverage to drink; one hour later, blood is drawn and its sugar content measured. If your blood glucose (blood sugar) level is high during this screening test, you are scheduled for an oral glucose tolerance test (OGTT). This test is administered over a period of three hours. First you fast overnight, then blood is drawn and analyzed to measure your fasting blood sugar level. Next you drink the special high-carbohydrate beverage, and then have your blood drawn again after one, two, and three hours. If the results show two or more high levels of blood glucose, you may be given a special diet, started on an oral hypoglycemic agent, and/or placed on insulin until the end of your pregnancy.

The incidence of gestational diabetes is about 4 percent for singleton pregnancies, 7 percent for twin pregnancies, 9 percent for triplet pregnancies, and 11 percent for quadruplet pregnancies. The increased incidence among women pregnant with multiples is due in large part to the actions of hormones produced by the placenta (primarily human placental lactogen) on carbohydrate metabolism during the second half of pregnancy. These actions are greater in a twin, triplet, or quad pregnancy because of the larger size or greater number of placentas present. For this reason, many physicians and nutritionists recommend screening expectant mothers of multiples for gestational diabetes early in pregnancy, when prenatal care first begins, and then repeating the tests again later if the initial test was normal.

ALPHA-FETOPROTEIN TEST

Alpha-fetoprotein (AFP) is a type of protein produced only by an unborn baby or its yolk sac. The test for AFP, which is performed between 15 and 20 weeks' gestation, involves analyzing the level of this protein in the mother's blood.

High levels of AFP may indicate that a woman is carrying more than one baby—or that the twins she had been told to expect are in fact triplets or quads! Elevated AFP can also mean that the pregnancy is further along than previously estimated. Or it may indicate that an unborn baby has a fetal anomaly, specifically a neural tube defect (such as open spina bifida) or an abdominal wall defect (such as gastroschisis or omphalocele).

---

3. Standards of Medical Care in Diabetes—2014. Diabetes Care, vol. 37, suppl. 1, January 2014; S1–S67.

QUAD SCREENING TEST

The AFP test can be offered by itself as a screening test for fetal anomalies as previously described. However, it is often offered in combination with other hormonal measures as a screening test for chromosomal problems such as Down syndrome. This combination blood test, which is also performed between the 15th and 20th weeks of pregnancy, is usually referred to as the quad test—not because it has anything to do with quadruplets but, rather, because it measures four separate substances:

- AFP.
- Unconjugated estriol (UE), a hormone produced by the placenta and the fetal liver working in conjunction.
- Human chorionic gonadotropin (HCG), a hormone produced by the placenta.
- Inhibin-A, another hormone produced by the placenta.

There are expected amounts of each of these substances in a woman's bloodstream that vary slightly for each week of gestation. In the case of a twin or triplet gestation, these amounts are proportionately higher, which is to be expected.

Blood test results that reveal amounts of these substances that vary from the expected levels may indicate a problem. For instance, when a baby has Down syndrome, the levels of HCG and inhibin-A are higher than normal, and the levels of AFP and unconjugated estriol are lower than normal. In a singleton pregnancy, the quad screen detects approximately 75 percent of Down syndrome cases when the mother is under age 35 and more than 80 percent of Down syndrome cases when the mother is over 35 (however, there also is a 5 percent false positive rate).

In twin pregnancies, the ability of the quad test to accurately detect Down syndrome and other genetic abnormalities is reduced by about 15 percent. That's because the unaffected twin may mask the abnormalities of the affected twin, given that the test results reflect the combination of proteins and hormones from both babies and both placentas.

In triplet pregnancies, this masking effect is even more pronounced, so the test results are even less accurate. For this reason, the quad test is not recommended for women expecting triplets.

DR. NEWMAN: It is important to remember that both the AFP test alone and the quad test are only screening tests, not diagnostic procedures. Think of these like a cholesterol test. Your cholesterol level is a screening tool that helps predict the risk of heart disease—but an elevated cholesterol level does *not* necessarily mean that you do have heart disease.

In the same way, abnormal AFP or quad test results should not lead you to panic or assume the worst. Instead, such results indicate the need for further follow-up diagnostic testing, such as ultrasound, amniocentesis, or chorionic villus sampling (described on pages 55–59). In addition, it is often helpful to obtain a consultation with a genetic counselor to help you understand the results of your screening test.

First-Trimester Nuchal Translucency (NT) Screening

Assuming that you begin your prenatal care early enough, the first trimester nuchal translucency (NT) test is probably the best routine screening test for Down syndrome when you are having twins. The nuchal translucency test also helps screen for certain congenital heart defects. This test is offered between 11 and 13 weeks' gestation.

The first trimester NT screen involves two steps. First, a blood sample is collected to measure HCG and pregnancy-associated plasma protein-A (PAPP-A), similar to the quad screen described earlier. Then a special ultrasound examination is performed to measure a fluid-filled space called the nuchal translucency at the back of each baby's neck. A thickened space with a lot of fluid has been associated with both chromosomal abnormalities and fetal heart defects. The NT measurement is a technically difficult measurement to do correctly, and small differences in the measurement can significantly change your risk estimate, making your results far less accurate. That's why it is important for your sonographer and the physician reading the scan to be certified to perform the NT measurement.

Because the NT measurement applies specifically to each individual twin, this part of the screening test is more accurate than the quad screen for twin pregnancies, with approximately a 75 to 85 percent detection rate for Down syndrome and a 5 percent false positive rate. Again, this test does not diagnose problems—it only tells you if your risk is greater than average. If this test is positive, further counseling is advised to discuss the available diagnostic testing options.

Whether you get the first-trimester NT screen or a second-trimester quad screen, or neither, is totally your choice. Some expectant parents prefer to know about potential health concerns ahead of time so that they can consider whether to continue the pregnancy. Others want the option of notifying friends and family prior to the delivery, undergoing increased fetal surveillance during the pregnancy, and/or arranging to deliver at a hospital with NICU capabilities. However, some expectant parents are not interested in such testing, feeling that the test results would not influence their ultimate decision and course of action.

ULTRASOUND EXAMINATIONS

Ultrasound allows doctors to safely look inside the uterus. Many parents find that these glimpses into the world inside the womb enhance the emotional bond they feel to their unborn babies. This effect can be even more pronounced with the relatively recent development of three-dimensional ultrasound imaging. "My husband and I looked forward to our monthly ultrasounds. When we saw over time how both boys were keeping right up with the average growth rate for *singletons*, we felt really encouraged. That did a lot to make up for the aches and inconveniences of pregnancy," says twin mom Stacy Moore.

Ultrasound technology uses sound waves to create a picture of your unborn babies, the fluid surrounding them, the membranes separating them (if present), and the placenta or placentas. It is performed either by inserting a lubricated probe into the vagina or by moving a lubricated transducer back and forth across the woman's abdomen. The probe or transducer records the echoes of sound waves bouncing off the babies and projects the resulting images onto a video screen.

By measuring the various images, your doctor can more accurately determine your due date, gauge each baby's growth and development, and identify potential problems. Ultrasound

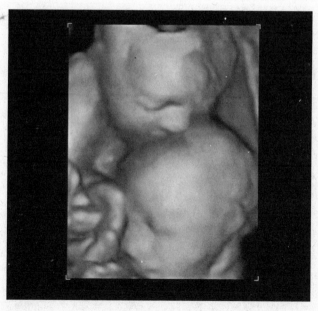

This three-dimensional ultrasound of a twin pregnancy shows the babies in amazing detail. Such ultrasound images are believed to promote parental bonding prenatally.

is also used as a guide for amniocentesis and chorionic villus sampling (described on page 59), greatly reducing the risk of these procedures.

For a woman pregnant with a singleton, ultrasound examinations are typically performed only once or twice—around the 18th week of pregnancy and perhaps again at 32 to 36 weeks. As the mother-to-be of multiples, however, you can expect to have more frequent ultrasounds. If your pregnancy was the result of infertility treatments, you may have your first ultrasound examination within the first six weeks of your pregnancy. An early ultrasound also may be ordered to gauge a woman's due date. Or it may be done if a woman experiences vaginal bleeding, to confirm the viability of the pregnancy.

At around 18 weeks, your doctor performs what is called a structural ultrasound or anatomic survey. This involves a very thorough evaluation of the internal and external organs of each baby as well as the structure of the placenta or placentas. At this point, the children's gender can usually be detected.

If your babies' twin type has not already been determined, it can be assessed at the 18-week ultrasound—and the results are likely to affect the scheduling of future ultrasounds, as well as the frequency of prenatal visits. For instance:

- Diamniotic, dichorionic twins (two separate or fused placentas, a double-thickness separating membrane, and same-sex or opposite-sex twins) usually receive an ultrasound examination about every four weeks following the anatomic survey. This allows the doctor to monitor the growth of each baby, check the volume of amniotic fluid, and assess the location and functioning of the placenta or placentas.

- Diamniotic, monochorionic twins (one placenta, a thin diamniotic separating membrane, and same-sex twins) are at risk for an uncommon complication called twin-twin transfusion syndrome (TTTS), in which abnormal vascular connections allow blood to move from one twin to the other. TTTS is most serious when it has its onset in the middle trimester (16 to 26 weeks). Most doctors perform ultrasound examinations of monochorionic twins every two weeks following the anatomic survey until about 24 to 26 weeks' gestation. The major reason for this is that the most effective treatment for TTTS, which is laser ablation of the abnormal vascular connections, is offered only up to 24 to 26 weeks' gestation in most treatment centers. After 26 weeks, it is reasonable to space out the frequency of ultrasound exams to every three weeks in monochorionic pregnancies.

- Monoamniotic, monochorionic twins generally receive the same schedule of ultrasound examination as diamniotic, monochorionic twins because they are also at risk for TTTS. In some cases, however, women with this type of pregnancy are admitted to the hospital for daily fetal testing in the late second trimester.

An important additional use of ultrasound is to estimate the length of a woman's cervix. It is usually performed for the first time during the anatomic survey at about 18 weeks, and is probably the most predictive when done between 22 and 24 weeks' gestation. (Prior to 16 weeks' gestation, the cervical length measurement is not very reliable and should not be done.) Because the cervix shortens and softens as labor approaches, this measurement helps to predict which women are likely to deliver prematurely. For example, research has shown that a cervical length of less than 20 millimeters at 23 weeks occurred in only 8 percent of twin pregnancies, but accounted for 40 percent of cases in which twins were born before 33 weeks.[4] Having this information about cervical length will help your doctor assess your risk for preterm labor and, if necessary, take appropriate steps to help prevent your babies from being born early.

Fetal Fibronectin Test

Fetal fibronectin is a protein produced during pregnancy that functions as biological glue, attaching the fetal sac to the uterine lining. During the first half of pregnancy (up to about 22 weeks' gestation), it is normal for fetal fibronectin to be found in vaginal secretions. In most cases, after 22 weeks, this protein is no longer present until a few weeks before labor. When fetal fibronectin is detected after 22 weeks, it indicates a possible increased risk of preterm delivery.

If your doctor recommends the fetal fibronectin test, he or she uses a cotton swab to collect a sample of your vaginal secretions, which is sent to a lab for analysis. Some office-based tests may not be available for 24 hours, but most hospitals can perform the test within one to two hours. Your doctor will usually collect the test sample before performing a digital pelvic examination, because the lubricating jelly will invalidate the test results. If the pelvic examination is completely reassuring, the collected sample can be discarded.

Most doctors use the fibronectin test in women who are experiencing symptoms of preterm labor. If the results are negative, you can feel reassured that the risk of preterm delivery in the next one to two weeks is very low. If the results are positive, you and your doctor have the opportunity to take preventive measures to help delay labor or to prepare for a possible early delivery.

---

4. Souka AP, Heath V, Flint S, et al. Cervical length at 23 weeks in twins in predicting spontaneous preterm delivery. Obstetrics & Gynecology 1999; 94:450–4.

Amniocentesis

This procedure has been used for more than 50 years to detect genetic abnormalities. It is routinely recommended for women 35 and older, when the risks of age-related pregnancy problems increase significantly. Amniocentesis is also commonly recommended when there is a family history of a neural tube defect or an inherited disorder (such as sickle-cell disease, cystic fibrosis, or Tay-Sachs disease).

In addition, amniocentesis may be done when an ultrasound or other test suggests an increased risk for some type of fetal aneuploidy, meaning a condition in which there are missing or extra chromosomes. The most common aneuploidy is trisomy, in which there is an extra chromosome, including trisomy 21 (Down syndrome), trisomy 13 (Patau syndrome), and trisomy 18 (Edwards syndrome). Monosomy is a condition in which there is a missing chromosome—for instance, with Turner syndrome, a female has a missing or damaged X chromosome.

Amniocentesis typically is performed during the second trimester, after about 15 weeks. It also may be performed toward the end of a pregnancy in the event of premature labor, to determine if the babies' lungs are mature enough to function. Late amniocentesis can also reveal various medical problems that may make it advisable to deliver the babies early because they would do better outside the womb.

Here's how the test works: As the fetuses grow, cells from their skin and lungs are discarded into the amniotic fluid. During amniocentesis, fluid containing these discarded cells is retrieved. The procedure is guided by ultrasound. After cleaning your skin with antiseptic, the obstetrician inserts a long, very thin needle through your abdomen and into your uterus, and then withdraws some of the amniotic fluid from each baby's amniotic sac. The cells are grown in a culture over 10 to 14 days, and then the chromosomal number of dividing cells is analyzed by a cytopathologist. A more rapid technique called FISH (fluorescence in situ hybridization) has been developed to look at a few specific chromosomes in about 48 hours. The babies' gender is also determined, should the parents want to know.

Most women experience nothing more than slight cramping from amniocentesis. However, in a small number of cases, the procedure can trigger an infection, bleeding, or premature labor. Amniocentesis also does carry a slight risk of pregnancy loss, usually as a result of rupture of the membranes. In singleton pregnancies, the loss rate following amniocentesis is about 1 in 400 to 500 procedures. The risk in a twin pregnancy is not as well established, but is estimated to be somewhere between 1 in 100 to 200 procedures. This risk should be considered in deciding whether or not to have the test.

Chorionic Villus Sampling

Chorionic villi are tiny projections from the chorion, a membrane that eventually gives rise to the placenta. Because villi contain the same genetic material as the baby, a sampling can be tested for a wide variety of congenital conditions. This test is called chorionic villus sampling (CVS).

The procedure is similar to amniocentesis. Guided by ultrasound, the obstetrician inserts a long, thin needle into the uterus, either through the abdomen or through the vagina and cervix, to collect a sampling of villi from each fetus. As with amniocentesis, in a twin pregnancy, an important technical issue is to make sure that both fetuses are being independently sampled, as opposed to one of the fetuses being sampled twice. Most women undergoing CVS experience only slight spotting or none at all. However, as with amniocentesis, there is a small risk (approximately 1 percent) that the procedure will trigger pregnancy loss.

An advantage of CVS over amniocentesis is that it can be done earlier in the pregnancy, between 10 and 13 weeks of gestation. Test results are ready within two weeks. If the results are abnormal, parents have the option of considering whether to end the pregnancy during the first trimester, when it would be safest. This earlier diagnosis also allows parents greater privacy, since family and friends may not yet even be aware of the pregnancy.

Nonstress Test

Many women carrying a singleton never undergo a nonstress test. But as a mother-to-be of multiples, you are more likely to have this test, which is done during the third trimester. However, if the estimated weight of one or more of your unborn babies is below the 10th percentile, the nonstress test may be performed earlier and/or more frequently.

In addition, the frequency and timing of the test depend on your babies' twin type and number. Here's a typical schedule:

- Diamniotic, dichorionic twins (two separate or two fused placentas, a double-thickness separating membrane, or opposite-sex twins): weekly beginning at 34 weeks.
- Diamniotic, monochorionic twins (one placenta, a single-thickness separating membrane, and same-sex twins): weekly beginning at 30 to 32 weeks.
- Monoamniotic, monochorionic twins (one placenta, no separating membrane): two or three times weekly beginning as early as the 24th to 26th week. Once

viability is achieved, a doctor may choose to hospitalize a patient who is pregnant with monoamniotic twins in order to perform more frequent nonstress testing—as often as three times per day. If it is determined, based on abnormal fetal heart rate tracings, that the babies would have a better chance of surviving outside the womb at this point, they can be delivered by cesarean.

- With triplets or quadruplets, the nonstress test is usually done after 30 to 32 weeks, depending on fetal growth and other clinical factors.

The purpose of the nonstress test is to evaluate your unborn babies' heartbeats and movements, as well as the frequency of uterine contractions, using external fetal monitors. If the heart rate of one or more babies does not react to movement or other stimuli, or if a baby does not move at all, or if other abnormalities are noted, fetal distress may be present.

BIOPHYSICAL PROFILE

This profile includes an assessment of your unborn babies' heart rates, breathing patterns, body movements, muscle tone, and amount of surrounding amniotic fluid. The heart rates are measured using the nonstress test, and ultrasound is used to determine the other components of the biophysical profile: fetal movement, fetal breathing, normal fetal body tone, and amniotic fluid volume. Each of these measures is given a score and totaled. A score of 8 to 10 is normal. A biophysical profile score of 8 after the ultrasound is equivalent to a reassuring nonstress test, so the nonstress test is frequently omitted. If any baby scores lower than 8, your doctor will probably repeat the test or recommend some other form of fetal assessment. The complete evaluation takes about half an hour.

DOPPLER FLOW STUDIES

Doppler is a form of ultrasound that uses sound wave movement and the velocity of that movement. In a multiple pregnancy, Doppler flow studies are used to evaluate the quality of blood flow through the umbilical cords of your unborn babies.

An umbilical cord contains one vein and two arteries. The umbilical vein carries oxygenated blood and nutrients from the placenta to the fetus. Once the oxygen and nutrients have been used, the umbilical arteries transfer the deoxygenated blood and waste from the fetus back to the placenta. There should always be a forward flow through the umbilical arteries to the placenta—more during a fetal heartbeat (systolic flow) than in between fetal heartbeats (diastolic flow). This can be evaluated as a ratio of systolic to diastolic flow (S/D ratio). If the placenta becomes damaged or dysfunctional, the amount of diastolic flow decreases, resulting in a progressive rise in the S/D ratio. Even more serious is an absence or a reversal of diastolic flow, which occurs when placental injury is severe.

Doppler flow studies are recommended toward the end of pregnancy if growth has slowed for one or more of the babies. If the test reveals problems with fetal blood flow, more intensive fetal surveillance may be recommended, or a decision may be made to deliver the babies.

A Test to Avoid: The X-Ray

X-rays are not a part of the normal battery of prenatal tests. The ionizing radiation used in X-rays can harm your unborn babies. Postpone elective X-rays (such as those routinely taken during a dental checkup) until after delivery. If you do need the procedure—because you've broken a bone, for instance—be sure to tell the doctor that you're pregnant. The doctor should then take extra precautions to protect your babies, such as placing a lead shield over your abdomen.

Childbirth Preparation Classes

Childbirth classes are designed to help first-time parents get ready, physically and mentally, for the rigors of labor and delivery. Common methods, such as Lamaze, Bradley, and Grantly Dick-Read, center on the premise that much of the pain felt during childbirth stems from fear and tension. Although the specific techniques vary, the courses share the goal of relieving discomfort through knowledge, relaxation techniques, and emotional support. Other programs, such as Hypnobabies, offer instruction in medical hypnosis techniques to make labor more comfortable.

Childbirth education instructors can also help you evaluate your labor options and prepare a birth plan (for instance, positions you'd like to try and people you'd like to be present). Provided you discuss these preferences with your obstetrician well ahead of time, chances are that he or she will try to accommodate them if possible.

Even if you've given birth before, consider taking a refresher course. The classroom environment offers an opportunity to practice the breathing and relaxation exercises and to receive updated information on any hospital policies that might have changed since your last delivery.

For the most rewarding experience, shop around for a class designed for expectant parents of multiples. "My instructor had never dealt with a twin pregnancy before. She had little knowledge of how my labor and delivery might be different from a singleton mother's. But still, it was worthwhile. The breathing techniques didn't help me much, but the focusing and relaxing strategies were useful," Stacy Moore says. Be sure your course includes information and advice on cesarean delivery, since about half of all twins and nearly all triplets and quadruplets are delivered this way.

For more information, contact the following organizations:

- Bradley Method (American Academy of Husband-Coached Childbirth): P.O. Box 5524, Sherman Oaks, CA 91413-5224. Telephone 800-4-A-BIRTH (800-422-4784); website www.bradleybirth.com.
- Hypnobabies: Telephone 714-894-BABY (714-894-2229); email info@hypnobabies .com; website www.hypnobabies.com.
- International Childbirth Education Association: 2501 Aerial Center Parkway, Suite 103, Morrisville, NC 27560. Telephone 800-624-4934; website www .icea.org.
- Lamaze International (American Society for Psychoprophylaxis in Obstetrics): 2025 M Street NW, Suite 800, Washington, DC 20036-3309. Telephone 800-368-4404; website www.lamaze.org.

Keep in mind that it's wise to schedule the class for your second trimester in case you end up delivering early, as many mothers of multiples do. If you need to go on bedrest—another fairly common occurrence in multiple pregnancies—consider hiring an instructor to come to your home for private lessons. Not only will you feel more prepared for childbirth, but the tedium of bedrest will be alleviated by the companionship and sense of purpose such instruction can provide.

Chapter Three

Your Weight-Gain Goals

Feeling like your life is not completely under your control right now? No wonder. Starting from the day you get the big news that not just one but two or more babies are on the way, your pregnancy is prone to surprises. Your delivery date is harder to predict. It's possible you'll have to stop working sooner than you'd anticipated. You may need to go on bedrest unexpectedly. If you're normally a careful planner or a take-charge type, it's disconcerting to feel suddenly that you are no longer directing the action.

But there's one aspect of this surprise-filled pregnancy over which you do have *total control:* your diet. That's terrific, because what you eat and how much weight you gain are among the most important factors affecting your own health and that of your unborn babies.

This isn't mere speculation. Decades of research, involving thousands of twin and triplet pregnancies, support this statement: The quality and quantity of the food you eat in the coming months will determine, to a significant extent, the size and health of your babies at birth—and beyond. Consider this:

- Babies who are well nourished before they are born weigh significantly more and are healthier at birth than less well-nourished babies born at the same gestational age. Among mothers carrying twins, those who meet pregnancy weight-gain recommendations deliver babies that are heavier. Their twins also are less likely to have low birthweights (of less than 5½ pounds), to be growth-restricted (below the 10th percentile for gestational age, meaning that 90 percent of babies of that age weigh more), or to require specialized newborn intensive care after delivery.[1, 2, 3, 4]

- Good intrauterine growth may reduce the likelihood of premature birth. Evidence suggests that some survival mechanism detects when babies are not growing well before birth and may trigger labor. For instance, twins whose rate of growth during pregnancy is among the lowest 10 percent are 10 times more likely to be born before 33 weeks.[5] Triplets whose rate of growth during pregnancy is among the lowest 25 percent are likely to be born five weeks earlier than average, whereas triplets whose growth is among the highest 25 percent are likely to be delivered nearly three weeks later than average.[6]

- Even if they are born prematurely (before 37 weeks' gestation), babies who have been well nourished in the womb have fewer illnesses and recover from them more quickly than do infants whose mothers had inadequate diets.

- Because the prenatal period involves the most rapid growth of the entire life span, optimal nutrition now provides your babies with the best blueprint for a healthy childhood. And that, in turn, gives them a running start on being healthy adults. In fact, research in the field of metabolic programming (also known as the Barker hypothesis or fetal determinants of adult disease) has revealed that many adult illnesses that have long been blamed on genetic influences or an unhealthy lifestyle, such as heart disease and diabetes, are attributable in part to the uterine environment and nutrition *before birth*. Developing babies who don't receive adequate nutrition during pregnancy modify their development in an attempt to cope. Some of these adaptations include changes in vascular modeling, leading to an increased risk of

1. Fox NS, Rebarber A, Roman S, et al. Weight gain in twin pregnancies and adverse outcomes examining the 2009 Institute of Medicine guidelines. Obstetrics & Gynecology 2010; 116:100–6.
2. Gonzalez-Quintero VH, Kathiresan ASQ, Tudela FJ, et al. The association of gestational weight gain per Institute of Medicine guidelines and prepregnancy body mass index on outcomes of twin pregnancies. American Journal of Perinatology 2012; 29:435–40.
3. Fox NS, Stern E, Saltzman DH, et al. The association between maternal weight gain and spontaneous preterm birth in twin pregnancies. Journal of Maternal-Fetal & Neonatal Medicine 2014; 27:1652–5.
4. Pettit KE, Lacoursiere DY, Schrimmer DB, et al. The association of inadequate mid-pregnancy weight gain and preterm birth in twin pregnancies. Journal of Perinatology 2015; 35:85–9.
5. Hediger ML, Luke B, Gonzalez-Quintero VH, et al. Fetal growth rates and the very preterm delivery of twins. American Journal of Obstetrics & Gynecology 2005; 193:1498–1507.
6. Luke B, Nugent C, van de Ven C, et al. The association between maternal factors and perinatal outcomes in triplet pregnancies. American Journal of Obstetrics & Gynecology 2002; 187:752–7.

hypertension, heart disease, and stroke in adulthood; the formation of fewer nephrons in the kidneys, which increases the long-term risk of kidney failure; fewer islet cells in the pancreas, which increases the risk of diabetes; and hormonal changes affecting metabolism that favor the storage of energy rather than the mobilization of energy, which increases the risk of obesity when the nutrient supply is plentiful.

Each of your unborn babies has the same genetic potential as any other unborn baby—the likelihood to weigh 6, 7, even 8 pounds or more at birth. For multiples, certain factors can limit the realization of that goal: the length of your pregnancy, your height, outcomes of prior pregnancies, and your level of physical activity. Adequate diet and weight gain help to minimize the negative influences of these factors, so that each of your babies can come as close as possible to reaching his or her genetic potential for a healthy birthweight.

So try not to think of the special nutritional needs of multiple pregnancy as a burden. Instead, see them as a means of empowerment. When you decide to make every bite count, your babies reap the benefits. "The nutrition program at the Multiples Clinic gave me an element of control over my pregnancy and increased my confidence in my ability to carry my twins to term," says Stacy Moore, mother of fraternal twin boys. "I firmly believe that my careful attention to diet and weight gain was the major reason why my twins had such healthy birthweights—Steven was 6 lb., 11 oz., and Brandon was 6 lb., 1 oz."

DR. LUKE: I tell moms-to-be that pregnancy has a lot in common with gardening. You can't just throw seeds into soil, forget to feed or water them, and still expect blue-ribbon roses. You have to nurture and nourish your future showstoppers. So it's only logical that nutrition would play an important role in pregnancy.

Multiples are not automatically born small. There are lots of 6- and 7-pound twins out there to prove it. The moms who deliver the largest and healthiest multiples are in general the ones who are diligent about meeting their prenatal dietary goals, gaining an appropriate amount of weight based on a healthy diet.

Every time I walked into the newborn nursery or NICU, the nurses would say that they could immediately tell which infants were born to mothers from our clinic and which were not—because our babies were usually bigger and more mature. Our statistics proved it: Our triplets weighed 35 percent more at birth, on average, than triplets typically do. And our twins were generally born 20 percent heavier than the average twins delivered at the same gestational age.

Your multiples can benefit from our nutrition program, too. It's simple:

- Follow the weight-gain and dietary guidelines in this chapter and in Chapters 4 and 5.
- Use the highly nutritious recipes at the back of the book.
- Visit my website, www.drbarbaraluke.com, for personalized nutrition counseling.
- For even more in-depth information on nutrition during pregnancy, as well as throughout your babies' childhood, consult another of our books, *Program Your Baby's Health: The Pregnancy Diet for Your Child's Lifelong Well-being*. This book also provides an in-depth look at the fascinating field of metabolic programming, mentioned above.

What's Your Weight-Gain Target?

TAMARA: When an ultrasound unexpectedly revealed that I was carrying twins, my obstetrician gave me a big bear hug and his heartiest congratulations. What he didn't give me was any particular advice related to my new status as an expectant mother of multiples. Finally I asked him if I needed to change my diet or increase the weight-gain goal he'd given me at the beginning of my pregnancy. He replied, "Oh, just keep on eating what you've been eating. And maybe you should plan to gain an extra 5 pounds, just to be safe. Let's aim for a total of about 30 pounds instead of 25." I followed that advice to the letter, putting on precisely 30 pounds.

But it wasn't enough. Staring at my 3 lb., 6 oz. son and my 2 lb., 5 oz. daughter as they lay in their isolettes in the NICU, I realized it wasn't *nearly* enough.

DR. NEWMAN: Lack of schooling on nutrition is frequently cited as one of the greatest deficiencies in the education of medical students and residents-in-training, especially in obstetrics and gynecology. Very few continuing-education conferences in obstetrics are dedicated to addressing this limited nutritional knowledge base. Even doctors who have years of experience with multiple pregnancies are not always aware of the extent of the increased nutritional needs of women like you.

This educational deficit has been slow to change. For instance, despite having provided nutritional recommendations for pregnant and lactating women for decades, the Institute of Medicine did not issue its first body mass index–specific weight-gain recommendations for expectant mothers of twins until 2009.[7]

The unfortunate result is that many expectant mothers of multiples receive little or no nutritional advice from their physicians. Those who are given a diet to follow may discover that it's the same diet prescribed for all the pregnant patients in a doctor's practice—most of whom are, of course, expecting singletons. One reader writes, "My obstetrician told me next to nothing about diet, other than to say, 'Theoretically, you get to eat more food.'"

"The other physicians in my obstetrician's practice were not as knowledgeable about multiple pregnancy as she was," says Benita Moreno, mother of fraternal twin boys. "One time when my own doctor was out of town, I had to see one of her associates. Because I'm plump to begin with and had gained another 5 pounds that month, this doctor belittled me for eating too much! When I told my dietitian what had happened, she was appalled and said, 'No one should *ever* tell a pregnant mother of multiples not to gain weight.'"

Such misinformation stems from the fact that most research on weight gain during pregnancy has focused on singletons—because in the past, multiple births were rare. But now the data on twins, triplets, and quadruplets are beginning to add up. And, not surprisingly, prenatal weight gain seems to be even more important when a woman is pregnant with multiples. In a singleton pregnancy, a woman can gain anywhere from 20 to 60 pounds and still have a 7-pound baby born at full term. But with multiples, a much narrower range of weight gain (and a shorter length of gestation in which to achieve it) is associated with a good outcome.

Stated simply:

- You probably need to *gain more* than you imagined—and certainly more than your friends expecting singletons have been counseled to gain.
- You also need to put on those pounds *more quickly* than a singleton mom does.
- The more babies you're carrying, the more you need to gain—and the *less time* you have to gain it, because the shorter your pregnancy probably will be. Remember, you're very unlikely to go a full 40 weeks.

---

7. Institute of Medicine. Weight gain during pregnancy: Reexamining the guidelines. Food and Nutrition Board, National Academy of Sciences. Washington, DC; 2009.

Weight-Gain Guidelines for Moms-to-Be of Multiples

If You're Expecting . . .	Your Total Weight-Gain Goal Is . . .
Twins	40–56 lb. (for a normal-weight woman)
Triplets	58–75 lb.
Quadruplets	70–80 lb.

Table 3.1

DR. NEWMAN: Many expectant mothers of multiples, upon first hearing these pregnancy weight-gain targets, fear that they will wind up retaining lots of extra weight after their babies are born. We promise you, this will not be the case! It has been our experience—both at the Multiples Clinic at the University of Michigan and at the Twin Clinic at the Medical University of South Carolina—that as long as you do not exceed our recommended weight-gain range, you will be back to within a few pounds of your prepregnancy weight within a few months of delivery—or even sooner if you are breast-feeding.

Hannah Steele, mother of identical twin girls, confirms that: "Even though I'm a physician and was in the third year of my residency in obstetrics when I got pregnant with my twins, I was shocked when Dr. Newman told me how much weight I was supposed to gain. It seemed like a *very* big number! But I followed his instructions—and to my amazement, by the time of my 6-week postpartum checkup, I actually weighed a little *less* than I had before I got pregnant. That, along with my twins' healthy birthweights, is why I am now a firm believer in these weight-gain guidelines."

DR. LUKE: The number of babies you're carrying is the most important factor in determining your weight-gain goals, but it's not the only factor. Your prepregnancy weight is a vital consideration, too.

The thinner you were before you conceived, the more you need to gain now. That's because if you are underweight, the first pounds you put on will go primarily to correcting your own weight deficit, rather than to promoting the growth of your babies. You should therefore aim to gain the amount it would take to bring you within the normal weight range for your height and body build, *plus* the amount recommended for the number of babies you're expecting. My coauthor, Tamara, for example, would have been well advised to aim for a weight gain of 50 to 66 pounds, given that she began her twin pregnancy about 10 pounds underweight.

What if you were overweight when you conceived? Sometimes women with curves look at pregnancy as an opportunity to slim down. Overweight patients have said to me, "I know I'll lose weight automatically when the babies are born. So if I can just maintain my current weight during the pregnancy, in nine months I'll be 25 pounds thinner." This faulty reasoning is "penny-wise and pound-foolish." The mom's body may be in better shape after delivery, but what shape will the babies' bodies be in? To keep your babies growing well, you need to gain a reasonable amount of weight from eating the right foods. An overweight woman who is carrying twins can get by with gaining somewhat less than a normal-weight woman. However, if you're expecting triplets or quadruplets, you should stick with our recommendations, even if you were overweight when you conceived.

In setting weight-gain goals, expectant mothers of multiples need to consider several additional factors:

- Is this your *first pregnancy*? For women who have not given birth before, the uterus has not yet been stretched. Higher weight gain will help to ensure better growth for your babies. Try to gain an additional 5 to 7 pounds as quickly as possible.
- Was your pregnancy the result of *infertility treatments*? If so, you should aim to gain an additional 4 to 6 pounds during the first half of your pregnancy. Though the exact reason is not known, evidence suggests that this extra weight can reduce the risk of miscarriage in pregnancies resulting from assisted reproductive technologies.
- Are you a *smoker*, or did you recently quit smoking? Smokers have lower levels of many essential nutrients. Smokers in general are also thinner. If you're still smoking, you've never had a better reason to stop. If you quit when you became pregnant, good for you! But remember that your body needs time to replenish those nutrients that cigarettes siphoned off. Be particularly careful to eat a balanced diet, and plan on gaining an additional 5 to 7 pounds.

Your Weight-Gain Pattern: Why It Matters So Much

Pregnant women are often told that there's no need to gain a lot of weight early on, because the baby is so small that it doesn't yet require much in terms of calories. This could not be further from the truth, particularly for multiple gestations—this has been supported by clinical research. There are a number of reasons why it is vital for mothers-to-be of multiples to put on a significant number of pounds in the first one-half to two-thirds of their pregnancy:

- Your weight gain prior to 28 weeks has the greatest influence on the babies' rate of growth. Research on twin pregnancies has shown that the amount you gain *before* 28 weeks' gestation significantly influences your babies' growth rates both before and *after* 28 weeks—and all the way up to their delivery date.[8, 9, 10, 11] With triplets and quadruplets, the weight you gain before 24 weeks has the greatest effect on your babies' rate of growth, while weight gained after 24 weeks has less effect on growth rate.[12] (For instance, triplets whose moms gain at least 36 pounds by week 24 generally are born nearly half a pound heavier than triplets whose moms did not hit this early weight-gain goal.) Therefore, your pattern of weight gain may actually be more important than your total weight gain.
- Certain hormonal changes of pregnancy are expressly intended to facilitate maternal weight gain long before the babies themselves gain any significant amount of weight. (That's why pregnant women feel so ravenous, often even before they realize they have conceived!) The purpose is to increase your body stores of fat and other nutrients during the first half of pregnancy, thereby providing a nutritional reserve for the second half of pregnancy, when diet alone can't keep pace with the nutritional demands. In other words, a significant portion of the weight you gain early on is needed to sustain your babies' growth later.

---

8. Luke B, Minogue J, Abbey H, Keith L, Witter FR, Feng TI, et al. The association between maternal weight gain and the birthweight of twins. Journal of Maternal-Fetal Medicine 1992; 1(5):267–76.
9. Luke B, Minogue J, Witter FR, Keith LG, Johnson TRB. The ideal twin pregnancy: Patterns of weight gain, discordancy, and length of gestation. American Journal of Obstetrics & Gynecology 1993; 169(3):588–97.
10. Luke B, Gillespie B, Min S-J, Avni M, Witter FR, O'Sullivan MJ. Critical periods of maternal weight gain: Effect on twin birthweight. American Journal of Obstetrics & Gynecology 1997; 177(5):1055–62.
11. Luke B, Min S-J, Gillespie B, Avni M, Witter FR, Newman RB, et al. The importance of early weight gain on the intrauterine growth and birthweight of twins. American Journal of Obstetrics & Gynecology 1998; 179(5):1155–61.
12. Luke B, Bryan E, Sweetland C, Keith L. Prenatal weight gain and the birthweight of triplets. Acta Geneticae Medicae Gemellologiae 1995; 44(2):93–101.

- It becomes harder to gain weight as your pregnancy progresses. The bigger your babies grow, the less room there is for your stomach to expand. As anyone who has given birth to a full-term singleton can attest, by the time a woman reaches 40 weeks, there's scarcely any room left for food. With multiples, that 40-week size arrives much sooner—at around 32 weeks for twins, 28 weeks for triplets, and 24 weeks for quads.
- You won't have a full nine months in which to gain, since multiples are almost always delivered before 40 weeks. The more babies you're carrying, the less time you'll have to put on the needed pounds.
- Research has shown that emphasizing the importance of early weight gain and following this pattern of weight gain with multiples results in not only higher birthweights and longer gestations, but also less extra weight retained postpartum. By gaining most of your pregnancy weight prior to 28 weeks, then slowing down the rate of gain from 28 weeks to delivery, much of the added weight is mobilized—so that there is less to lose in the months after delivery.[13]

To ensure that your weight-gain pattern is optimal, you'll want to set *three weight-gain goals*. The cutoffs are a little different from the traditional trimesters of pregnancy, but based on years of research, they have been found to be more physiologically important in terms of fetal nutrition and growth:

- The first target is the amount you need to gain by the 20th week of pregnancy.
- The second target is the amount you need to gain by the 28th week.
- The third is the amount you need to gain between week 28 and your delivery date (ideally, about 37 to 38 weeks for most twins, 34 to 36 weeks for triplets, and 32 to 34 weeks for quads).

Here are the recommended targets, along with the optimal length of gestation for the number of babies expected. (Singleton pregnancy is included for the sake of comparison.) It is important to note that these recommendations are for normal-weight women. Recommendations that adjust for differences in prepregnancy body size are presented later in this chapter.

---

13. Luke B, Hediger ML, Min L, Nugent C, Newman R, Hankins G, et al. The effect of weight gain by 20 weeks gestation on twin birthweight and postpartum weight. American Journal of Obstetrics & Gynecology 2006; 195 (Supplement):S85.

Optimal Weight-Gain Patterns During Pregnancy

Type of Pregnancy	Weight Gain by 20 Weeks	Weight Gain by 28 Weeks	Total Weight Gain	Optimal Length of Gestation
Singleton	12 lb.	20 lb.	25–35 lb.	39–40 weeks
Twins	25 lb.	38 lb.	40–56 lb.	37–38 weeks
Triplets	35 lb.	54 lb.	58–75 lb.	34–36 weeks
Quadruplets	45 lb.	65 lb.	70–80 lb.	32–34 weeks

Table 3.2

If you were underweight when you became pregnant, or if you lost weight during the first trimester owing to morning sickness or other illness, you should make up that deficit early in your pregnancy. "I got a bad stomach virus shortly after conceiving my twins, and I lost 7 pounds. Since I'm slender to begin with, Dr. Luke was very concerned. She told me I needed to gain 40 pounds by my 24th week of pregnancy," says Judy Levy, mother of fraternal twin girls.

Note: *Even if you were overweight* before becoming pregnant, if you're expecting triplets or quads, the recommended weight gain by 20 weeks remains the same—35 pounds for triplets, and 45 pounds for quadruplets.

Do these guidelines sound excessive? Truly, they are not. "I managed to gain 24 pounds by week 20, even though I had terrible morning sickness. My efforts to pack in the protein and calories really paid off, because my twins had astounding birthweights. My daughter was 7 lb., 11 oz., and my son was a whopping 9 lb., 4 oz.," says Kelly McDaniel, mother of boy/girl twins and three older children. "At the hospital where I delivered, doctors and nurses and even janitors kept coming by to see the 'huge twins.' Best of all, the babies had no health problems whatsoever—and they both came home from the hospital with me three days after their birth."

WHERE DOES THE WEIGHT GAIN GO?

Many women think that the weight gained during pregnancy just goes to their baby or babies: "If I gain 7 pounds, then I'll have a 7-pound baby." But Mother Nature didn't plan it that way.

In actuality, the weight gained in pregnancy reflects not only the weight of the baby or babies but also all the supporting tissues that ensure a healthy pregnancy, plus adequate nutritional stores to successfully breast-feed.

Following is a breakdown of the components of pregnancy weight, based on the number of babies you are expecting. This list may surprise you! And you'll probably be delighted to realize that, even though you are being encouraged to gain more weight than you may have expected, you will have very little pregnancy weight left to lose after your babies are born.

What Accounts for Weight Gained During Pregnancy

	Singleton	Twins	Triplets	Quads
Baby (or babies)	**8 lb.**	**10–16 lb.**	**12–18 lb.**	**12–20 lb.**
Placenta(s)	2–3 lb.	4–6 lb.	6–8 lb.	10–12 lb.
Amniotic fluid	2–3 lb.	4–6 lb.	6–8 lb.	10–12 lb.
Breast tissue	2–3 lb.	3–5 lb.	3–5 lb.	3–5 lb.
Uterine tissue	2–5 lb.	3–8 lb.	3–8 lb.	3–8 lb.
Additional blood	4 lb.	8 lb.	8–10 lb.	8–10 lb.
Stored fat for breast-feeding	5–9 lb.	6–10 lb.	10–12 lb.	10–12 lb.
TOTAL	**25–35 lb.**	**38–59 lb.**	**48–69 lb.**	**56–79 lb.**
Weight-gain recommendations for normal-weight women	25–35 lb.	40–56 lb.	58–75 lb.	70–80 lb.

Table 3.3

UNDERSTANDING BMI: THE BODY MASS INDEX

A healthy weight is more than just a number on the bathroom scale. It's a balance between your body's proportions of muscle and fat. The amount of body fat associated with good overall health ranges from 20 to 25 percent.

Body mass index, or BMI, is a calculation based on your weight and height. Although it is not an accurate reflection of body fat, and does not account for racial and ethnic differences in body build or relative amounts of muscularity, the BMI does give a useful estimate of your degree of underweight/normal weight/overweight.

To determine your BMI, see the online calculator at http://www.nhlbi.nih.gov/health/educational/lose_wt/BMI/bmicalc.htm or use the following table. To calculate your prepregnancy BMI, locate your height in the far left column of Table 3.4, then move across that row to find your weight. At the top of your weight column is your body mass index.

Here are the BMI categories:

- Less than 18.5 is underweight.
- 18.5 to 24.9 is normal weight.
- 25.0 to 29.9 is overweight.
- 30.0 or more is obese. Among obese individuals, additional categories include:
  o Class I, BMI of 30.0 to 34.9.
  o Class II, BMI of 35.0 to 39.9.
  o Class III, BMI of 40.0 or greater.

In terms of BMI, being underweight before conception holds greater risk for subsequent poor fetal growth and prematurity than being at a normal weight. That's why in the guidelines that follow, the suggested cutoff for defining underweight is a BMI of less than 20.0 instead of less than 18.5. This may seem like a small difference—but the higher weight-gain guidelines recommended for underweight women are also beneficial for women on the border between being underweight and normal weight, particularly when pregnant with multiples.

For example, consider a woman who is 5 feet, 4 inches tall. At 108 pounds, her BMI is 18.5; at 116 pounds, her BMI is 20.0. If her prepregnancy weight falls into this in-between range of 108 to 116 pounds, she would do best to follow the weight-gain guidelines for underweight women rather than those for normal-weight women.

Determining Your Body Mass Index (BMI)

Body Mass Index

Height (inches)	17	18	19	20	21	22	23	24	25
				Body Weight (pounds)					
58	82	87	91	96	100	105	110	115	119
59	85	90	94	99	104	109	114	119	124
60	87	93	97	102	107	112	118	123	128
61	90	96	100	106	111	116	122	127	132
62	93	99	104	109	115	120	126	131	136
63	96	102	107	113	118	124	130	135	141
64	99	105	110	116	122	128	134	140	145
65	103	109	114	120	126	132	138	144	150
66	106	112	118	124	130	136	142	148	155
67	109	115	121	127	134	140	146	153	159
68	112	119	125	131	138	144	151	158	164
69	116	122	128	135	142	149	155	162	169
70	119	126	132	139	146	153	160	167	174
71	122	130	136	143	150	157	165	172	179
72	126	133	140	147	154	162	169	177	184
73	129	137	144	151	159	166	174	182	189
74	133	141	148	155	163	171	179	186	194
		Underweight			Normal Weight				

Determining Your Body Mass Index (BMI)

Body Mass Index

Height (inches)	26	27	28	29	30	31	32	33	34	35
					Body Weight (pounds)					
58	124	129	134	138	143	149	154	159	163	168
59	128	133	138	143	148	154	159	164	169	174
60	133	138	143	148	153	159	165	170	175	180
61	137	143	148	153	158	165	170	175	181	186
62	142	147	153	158	164	170	176	181	187	192
63	146	152	158	163	169	176	181	187	193	198
64	151	157	163	169	174	181	187	193	199	205
65	156	162	168	174	180	187	193	199	205	211
66	161	167	173	179	186	193	199	205	212	218
67	166	172	178	185	191	199	205	212	218	224
68	171	177	184	190	197	205	211	218	225	231
69	176	182	189	196	203	211	218	224	231	238
70	181	188	195	202	209	217	224	231	238	245
71	186	193	200	208	215	223	230	238	245	252
72	191	199	206	213	221	230	237	244	252	259
73	197	204	212	219	227	236	244	251	259	266
74	202	210	218	225	233	243	250	258	266	274
	Overweight				Obese/Class I					

Determining Your Body Mass Index (BMI)

Body Mass Index

36	37	38	39	40	41	42	43	44	45
				Body Weight (pounds)					
172	177	181	186	191	196	201	205	210	215
178	183	188	193	198	203	208	212	217	222
184	189	194	199	204	209	215	220	225	230
190	195	201	206	211	217	222	227	232	238
196	202	207	213	218	224	229	235	240	246
203	208	214	220	225	231	237	242	248	254
209	215	221	227	232	238	244	250	256	262
216	222	228	234	240	246	252	258	264	270
223	229	235	241	247	253	260	266	272	278
230	236	242	249	255	261	268	274	280	287
236	243	249	256	262	269	276	282	289	295
243	250	257	263	270	277	284	291	297	304
250	257	264	271	278	285	292	299	306	313
257	265	272	279	286	293	301	308	315	322
265	272	279	287	294	302	309	316	324	331
272	280	288	295	302	310	318	325	333	340
280	287	295	303	311	319	326	334	342	350
	Obese/Class II			Obese/Class III					

Table 3.4

DR. NEWMAN: I know that some obstetricians advise very obese pregnant women to limit their weight gain to 20 pounds or less, regardless of the number of babies they are carrying. This advice is misguided and has no scientific basis. Until research is available on pregnant women in the Class II or Class III obesity category, the best strategy for such women is to follow the weight-gain guidelines for obese women, as outlined in this chapter. Instead of imposing unproven and potentially harmful weight-gain restrictions, the focus should be on maintaining optimal blood glucose levels in the mother, and on ensuring steady and adequate growth for the babies.

DR. LUKE: Many readers have expressed an interest in knowing how our weight-gain recommendations were formulated. Here is a brief description of the science behind the numbers.

The challenge of determining the optimal pattern and amount of weight gain in multiple pregnancies that would result in the best birthweights has been a focus of my professional life for more than four decades. Back in 1974, after earning my master's degree in nutrition, I started a prenatal nutrition clinic at Columbia-Presbyterian Medical Center in New York City. Most of the women I counseled were pregnant with singletons. Birthweights were good for babies born to women who'd had adequate weight gain, particularly those who had not been underweight before getting pregnant. For women expecting twins, though, both their prepregnancy weight and the amount and pattern of weight gain during pregnancy seemed to have a much greater influence—not only on birthweight but also on the length of gestation. It was clear—and logical—that the usual amount and pattern of weight gain for a singleton pregnancy would not be enough for a twin pregnancy.

In 1987, I published the results of a pilot study I had done, which indicated that attaining a certain weight (as a combination of prepregnancy weight plus pregnancy weight gain) by a certain point in gestation was associated with better twin birthweights.[14] Results of this pilot were included in the 1990 report from the Institute of Medicine on weight gain in pregnancy, as part of their recommendations for twin pregnancies.[15] This pilot was also the basis for my doctoral dissertation, which used data on twin births that occurred over the course of a decade at Johns Hopkins Hospital in Baltimore, Maryland. Basically, the findings from my dissertation showed that

---

14. Luke B. Twin births: Influence of maternal weight on intrauterine growth and prematurity. Federation Proceedings 1987; 46:1015.
15. Institute of Medicine. Nutrition during pregnancy. National Academy of Sciences. Washington, DC: National Academy Press; 1990.

gaining 24 pounds by 24 weeks' gestation was associated with significantly better twin birthweights and longer gestations.[16, 17]

Because no single medical center had enough multiple pregnancies to publish meaningful research, I formed the University Consortium on Multiple Births soon after finishing my doctorate in 1991. The research I had completed at Johns Hopkins University provided the foundation for this consortium, and clinicians and researchers at three other universities—the Medical University of South Carolina, the University of Michigan, and the University of Miami—joined in. We added more clinical data every year to our original twin database and periodically tested our findings with larger sample sizes. Today our database includes comprehensive data on nearly 4,000 multiple pregnancies.

In my original research, I evaluated weight gain before and after 24 weeks' gestation, based on 205 twin pregnancies. Although obstetrics has traditionally classified pregnancy into trimesters (three equal time periods of about 13 weeks each), when we statistically modeled maternal weight gain and fetal growth, we concluded that the more significant time period classifications were actually from conception to 20 weeks (the first half of pregnancy), 20 to 28 weeks, and 28 to 38 weeks (38 weeks is considered full term for twins). In 1997, we published our initial findings using these divisions to assess data on 646 twin pregnancies. We showed that weight gain before 20 weeks' gestation had a significant effect on twin birthweight—with the greatest effect among infants of underweight women and the least effect among infants of overweight women.[18]

In 1998 we published a subsequent and larger study based on 1,564 twin pregnancies, using the same gestational periods.[19] This study showed that maternal weight gain during the early period (conception to 20 weeks) benefited the babies' growth during the middle period (20 to 28 weeks) and the late period (28 to 38 weeks). Weight gain during the middle period had a similar effect, immediately influencing fetal growth and continuing to do so throughout the late period as well. Weight gain in the late

16. Luke B, Minogue J, Abbey H, Keith L, Witter FR, Feng TI, et al. The association between maternal weight gain and the birthweight of twins. Journal of Maternal-Fetal Medicine 1992; 1(5):267–76.

17. Luke B, Minogue J, Witter FR, Keith LG, Johnson TRB. The ideal twin pregnancy: Patterns of weight gain, discordancy, and length of gestation. American Journal of Obstetrics & Gynecology 1993; 169(3):588–97.

18. Luke B, Gillespie B, Min S-J, Avni M, Witter FR, O'Sullivan MJ. Critical periods of maternal weight gain: Effect on twin birthweight. American Journal of Obstetrics & Gynecology 1997; 177(5):1055–62.

19. Luke B, Min S-J, Gillespie B, Avni M, Witter FR, Newman RB, et al. The importance of early weight gain on the intrauterine growth and birthweight of twins. American Journal of Obstetrics & Gynecology 1998; 179(5):1155–61.

period had the smallest effect on birthweight, although it was still significant. Like money in the bank earning interest, adequate early- and mid-pregnancy weight gain benefited fetal growth throughout pregnancy.

We then took these findings one step further. In 2003, based on 2,324 twin pregnancies (4,648 infants), we published guidelines for maternal weight gain—based on maternal prepregnancy body mass index (BMI)—that were associated with optimal fetal growth and birthweights in twins.[20] We studied the rates of maternal weight gain in uncomplicated twin pregnancies with birthweights between the singleton 50th percentile and the twin 90th percentile born at 36 weeks or greater (2,850 to 2,950 grams, or 6 lb., 5 oz. to 6 lb., 8 oz.). For comparison, the average twin birthweight in the United States is only 5 lb., 2 oz. Using the same three gestational periods, we calculated the rates of weight gain and the cumulative weight gain that resulted in optimal birthweights for twins born to women who were underweight, normal weight, overweight, and obese. These are the weight-gain guidelines you see in Table 3.5.

20. Luke B, Hediger ML, Nugent C, Newman RB, Mauldin JG, Witter FR, et al. Body mass index-specific weight gains associated with optimal birth weights in twin pregnancies. Journal of Reproductive Medicine 2003; 48:217–24.

Week-by-Week Weight-Gain Recommendations for Women Pregnant with Twins, Based on BMI

Weeks' Gestation	10	12	14	16	18	**20**	22	24	26	**28**	30	32	34	36	**38**
BMI below 20.0															
Advised Gain (lb.)	1.25–1.75 lb./week					1.5–2.0 lb./week				1.25–1.5 lb./week					
Advised Range (lb.)															
Upper	18	21	25	29	32	**35**	39	43	47	**51**	54	57	60	63	**66**
Lower	13	15	18	21	23	**25**	28	31	34	**37**	40	42	45	47	**50**
BMI 20.0–24.9															
Advised Gain (lb.)	1.0–1.5 lb./week					1.25–2.0 lb./week				1.0 lb./week					
Advised Range (lb.)															
Upper	15	18	21	24	27	**30**	34	38	42	**46**	48	50	52	54	**56**
Lower	10	12	14	16	18	**20**	23	25	27	**30**	32	34	36	38	**40**
BMI 25.0–29.9															
Advised Gain (lb.)	1.0–1.25 lb./week					1.0–1.5 lb./week				1.0 lb./week					
Advised Range (lb.)															
Upper	13	15	18	20	23	**25**	28	31	34	**37**	39	41	43	45	**47**
Lower	10	12	14	16	18	**20**	22	24	26	**28**	30	32	34	36	**38**
BMI 30.0 or higher															
Advised Gain (lb.)	0.75–1.0 lb./week					1.0 lb./week				0.75 lb./week					
Advised Range (lb.)															
Upper	10	12	14	16	18	**20**	22	24	26	**28**	30	31	33	34	**36**
Lower	8	9	11	12	14	**15**	17	19	21	**23**	25	26	28	29	**31**

Table 3.5

We also calculated similar guidelines for women pregnant with triplets and quadruplets, although these were based on a much smaller number of pregnancies.[21, 22, 23] These guidelines are shown in Table 3.6 and in Table 3.7.

Week-by-Week Weight-Gain Recommendations for Women Pregnant with Triplets

Weeks' Gestation	10	12	14	16	18	20	22	24	26	28	30	32	34
Advised Gain (lb.)	1.5–2.0 lb./week					2.0–2.5 lb./week							
Advised Range (lb.)													
Upper	20	24	28	32	36	40	45	50	55	60	65	70	75
Lower	15	18	21	24	27	30	34	38	42	46	50	54	58

Table 3.6

Week-by-Week Weight-Gain Recommendations for Women Pregnant with Quadruplets

Weeks' Gestation	10	12	14	16	18	20	22	24	26	28	30	32
Advised Gain (lb.)	2.0–2.5 lb./week					2.5 lb./week						
Advised Range (lb.)												
Upper	25	30	35	40	45	50	55	60	65	70	75	80
Lower	20	24	28	32	36	40	45	50	55	60	65	70

Table 3.7

21. Luke B, Bryan E, Sweetland C, Keith L. Prenatal weight gain and the birthweight of triplets. Acta Geneticae Medicae Gemellologiae 1995; 44(2):93–101.
22. Luke B, Nugent C, van de Ven C, Martin D, O'Sullivan MJ, Eardley S, et al. The association between maternal factors and perinatal outcomes in triplet pregnancies. American Journal of Obstetrics & Gynecology 2002; 187:752–7.
23. Luke B, O'Sullivan MJ, Martin D, Nugent C, Witter FW, Newman RB. Outcomes in quadruplet pregnancies: Role of maternal nutrition. American Journal of Obstetrics & Gynecology 2001; 185:S105.

In 2009, the Institute of Medicine's Committee on the Reexamination of IOM Pregnancy Weight Guidelines[24] asked us to reanalyze our twin data using the traditional trimesters and an optimal birthweight of at least 2,500 grams (5 lb., 8 oz.) at 37 to 42 weeks' gestation. In addition, they asked us to use the newer BMI definitions of less than 18.5 as underweight, 18.5 to 24.9 as normal weight, 25.0 to 29.9 as overweight, and 30.0 or above as obese. Based on these criteria, we calculated the weight-gain guidelines for expectant mothers of twins shown in Table 3.8. (There was not enough data available to calculate guidelines for underweight women based on a BMI cutoff of less than 18.5.)

IOM Weight-Gain Guidelines for Women Pregnant with Twins

	To 13 weeks	To 26 weeks	To 37–42 weeks
Normal Weight	8 lb.	29 lb.	46 lb.
Overweight	5 lb.	25 lb.	42 lb.
Obese	4 lb.	19 lb.	35 lb.

Table 3.8

The IOM Committee then asked us to calculate ranges of weight gain and cumulative gain by trimesters, based on the 25th through 75th percentiles. Shown in Table 3.9, these are the newest weight-gain guidelines for expectant mothers of twins from the Institute of Medicine—and they are based on our research.

IOM Weight-Gain Ranges for Women Pregnant with Twins

	To 13 weeks	To 26 weeks	To 37–42 weeks
Normal Weight	3–12 lb.	22–36 lb.	37–54 lb.
Overweight	1–9 lb.	17–31 lb.	31–50 lb.
Obese	2–8 lb.	11–25 lb.	25–42 lb.

Table 3.9

24. Institute of Medicine. Weight gain during pregnancy: Reexamining the guidelines. Washington, DC: National Academy Press; 2009.

DR. LUKE: Some readers have asked why our weight-gain recommendations are different from the recommendations of the Institute of Medicine. First, understand that both sets of recommendations were derived from the same population of women with uncomplicated twin pregnancies. That said, our recommendations are based on: (1) defining underweight as a BMI of less than 20.0; (2) defining optimal birthweight and gestation as 2,850 to 2,950 grams or higher (6 lb., 5 oz. to 6 lb., 8 oz.), which is between the singleton 50th percentile and the twin 90th percentile at 36 weeks or greater; and (3) gestational periods of 0 to 20 weeks, 20 to 28 weeks, and 28 to 38 weeks.

In contrast, the recommendations from the Institute of Medicine are based on: (1) defining underweight as a BMI less than 18.5; (2) defining optimal birthweight as 2,500 grams or higher (5 lb., 8 oz.) at 37 to 42 weeks (full term for singletons); and (3) traditional trimesters of 0 to 12 weeks, 13 to 26 weeks, and 27 to 42 weeks.

As you can see, this has been a long journey—spanning four decades—to determine the optimal pattern and amount of weight gain that would result in the best birthweights for multiples. Based on our years of research, we have concluded that *adequate maternal weight gain is associated with significantly better fetal growth, longer length of gestation, and higher birthweights, as well as better childhood development.*

We have also conducted research on the causes and effects of slowed fetal growth and reduced birthweights in twins and triplets. In twins, we evaluated data on twins whose growth placed them among the lowest 10th percentile, as measured by ultrasound at 28 weeks' gestation.[25] Factors associated with reduced growth included:

- Smoking during pregnancy—ninefold increased risk.
- Fetal reduction or fetal loss—fivefold risk.
- Maternal height of less than 62 inches—threefold risk.
- Low maternal weight gain during the first half of pregnancy (less than 0.65 pound per week before 20 weeks' gestation)—threefold risk.

This reduced fetal growth by 28 weeks' gestation was associated with significantly reduced birth length and birthweight, which persisted through three years of age.

---

25. Luke B, Brown MB, Hediger ML, Nugent C, Misiunas RB, Anderson E. Fetal phenotypes and neonatal and early childhood outcomes in twins. American Journal of Obstetrics & Gynecology 2004; 191:1270–6.

In triplets, we evaluated factors associated with fetal growth, birthweight, and length of gestation.[26] We found that triplets born to women who had a prior pregnancy with a good outcome (birthweight over 5 lb., 8 oz. and length of gestation greater than 37 weeks) had longer gestations (by about 8 days), better rates of fetal growth, and higher birthweights. Inadequate maternal weight gain (less than 36 pounds by 24 weeks' gestation) was associated with significantly lower rates of fetal growth and lower birthweights. Triplets whose growth was among the lowest 25 percent were born about five weeks earlier, on average, compared to triplets with better growth.

The link between slowed fetal growth and prematurity in singleton pregnancies has been shown by many researchers. In 2005, based on 1,612 twin pregnancies, we evaluated the risks for preterm delivery by the rates of fetal growth.[27] This study confirmed in multiples what had been previously shown in singletons—that babies growing slowly are at much greater risk of being born prematurely.

Every child has the growth potential to be big and healthy at birth—and that outcome has a lasting positive effect throughout childhood and even into adulthood. Interestingly, at 18 to 20 weeks' gestation, nearly all unborn babies measure about the same size. The growth curves we developed for twins and triplets demonstrated that the overall pattern of fetal growth for well-grown multiples does not differ from that of singletons until late in pregnancy, when the growth rate for multiples begins to slow down. In our study of more than 3,600 twins,[28] those growing at the twin 90th percentile had birthweights equal to the singleton 50th percentile by 38 weeks, which is full-term for twins. These data are represented in Table 3.10.

26. Luke B, Nugent C, van de Ven C, Martin D, O'Sullivan MJ, Eardley S, et al. The association between maternal factors and perinatal outcomes in triplet pregnancies. American Journal of Obstetrics & Gynecology 2002; 187:752–7.
27. Hediger ML, Luke B, Gonzalez-Quintero VH, Witter FR, Mauldin J, Newman RB. Fetal growth rates and very preterm birth of twins. American Journal of Obstetrics & Gynecology 2005; 193:1498–507.
28. Min S-J, Luke B, Gillespie B, Newman RB, Mauldin JG, Witter, FR, Salman FA, et al. Birthweight references for twins. American Journal of Obstetrics & Gynecology 2000; 182 (5):1250–7.

Growth Curves of Singletons and Twins
10th, 50th, and 90th Percentiles

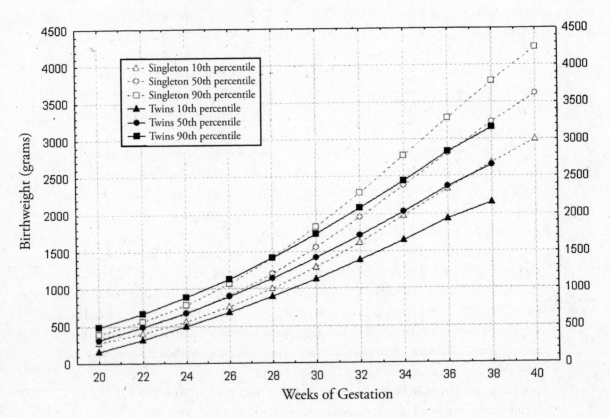

Legend:
- ⟁ Singleton 10th percentile
- ◇ Singleton 50th percentile
- □ Singleton 90th percentile
- ▲ Twins 10th percentile
- ● Twins 50th percentile
- ■ Twins 90th percentile

Y-axis: Birthweight (grams)
X-axis: Weeks of Gestation

Table 3.10

In our study of 564 triplets,[29] those growing at the triplet 90th percentile had birthweights equal to the singleton 50th percentile by 34 weeks, which is term for triplets. These data are shown in Table 3.11. The actual birthweight references for twins and triplets are shown in Appendices B and C.

---

29. Min S-J, Luke B, Min L, Misiunas R, Nugent C, van de Ven C, et al. Birthweight references for triplets. American Journal of Obstetrics & Gynecology 2004; 191:809–18.

Growth Curves of Singletons and Triplets
10th, 50th, and 90th Percentiles

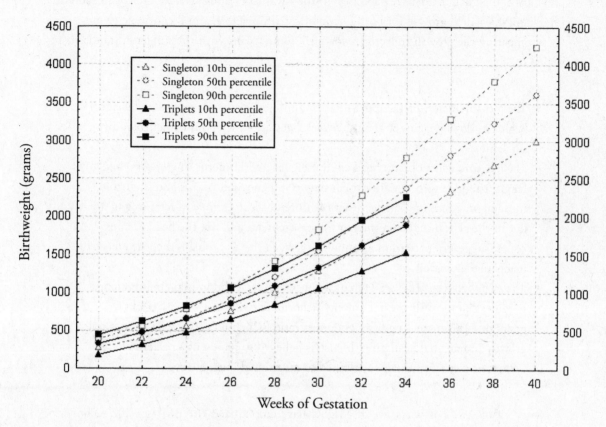

Table 3.11

Bottom line: This extensive research, conducted over many years with data from *thousands* of multiple pregnancies, confirms the following:

- The amount and pattern of maternal weight gain has a substantial effect on the rate of fetal growth and ultimate birthweight.
- The rate of fetal growth is, in turn, significantly associated with length of gestation.
- Babies who are born well-grown and at a good gestational age are healthier at birth and throughout childhood.

The recently concluded Fetal Growth Study from the National Institute of Child Health and Human Development revealed similar fetal growth patterns as those described previously. The goal of this NIH-sponsored study was to establish a standard for intrauterine ultrasound-measured growth for both uncomplicated singletons and dichorionic twins.

Comparing the growth trajectories for dichorionic twins with the singleton standards revealed the following:

- The measurement of fetal abdominal circumference and estimated fetal weight begins to slow in twins at about 33 weeks' gestation, which is earlier than for singletons.
- The measurements of fetal head circumference and humerus (upper arm) and femur (thigh) length remain similar between dichorionic twins and singletons throughout gestation. The fact that the differences in estimated fetal weight are due to the abdominal circumference measurement, and not the head or long bones, suggests a pattern of asymmetric growth that is probably a consequence of inadequate nutrition.
- The ratio between fetal head circumference and fetal abdominal circumference becomes significantly greater among dichorionic twins at about 31 weeks' gestation. This increasing head/abdomen ratio (which reflects slower abdominal growth and normal head growth) also is believed to represent a pattern of asymmetric growth usually attributed to nutritional inadequacy.

DR. NEWMAN: For years, we at MUSC have emphasized the BMI-specific recommendations on weight gain developed by Dr. Luke. Recently we decided to compare outcomes of women who achieved their weight-gain targets against those who did not. We looked back at twin pregnancies over 10 years, representing experience with almost 600 sets of twins followed in our Twin Clinic. Here's what we found:

- Women who achieved their BMI-specific recommended pregnancy weight gain (about half of our twin mothers) delivered *two weeks* later than did those who failed to meet the weight-gain guidelines.
- 48 percent of the women who failed to achieve their recommended weight gain delivered prior to 32 weeks' gestation, while only 21 percent who gained the recommended amount of weight delivered that early. Conversely, 29 percent of the women who met their weight-gain goals

delivered after 37 weeks of pregnancy, while only 13 percent of those who failed to gain adequate weight delivered after 37 weeks.

- Among babies whose moms achieved their weight-gain targets, birthweights averaged 2,223 grams (4 lb., 14 oz.). This was more than a pound larger per twin compared to the average birthweight of 1,779 grams (3 lb., 14 oz.) for twins whose mothers gained inadequate weight. In addition, the likelihood of being small for gestational age was substantially reduced among babies whose mothers gained enough weight.

Not surprisingly, babies born later and larger were much healthier than twins born earlier and smaller. For instance:

- Significant newborn complications (such as respiratory distress syndrome, severe intraventricular hemorrhage, necrotizing enterocolitis, sepsis, or death) were *twice as common* among twins whose mothers did not achieve recommended weight-gain targets.
- Newborn twins whose mothers did not reach their weight-gain milestones also were twice as likely to be admitted to the NICU (44.3 percent versus 22.6 percent), and they had an average newborn length of stay in the hospital that was more than twice as long (22.9 days versus 10.5 days).

To make sure that the benefits of achieving maternal weight-gain goals applied to women of different sizes, we also looked at our patients based on their prepregnancy BMI. This was especially important in two BMI categories—underweight and obese. Here's why: Even though underweight women are probably at greatest risk if they fail to gain enough weight during pregnancy, the Institute of Medicine has not yet issued gestational weight-gain recommendations for underweight women. As for obese women, there is controversy because many health care providers are under the mistaken impression that maternal weight gain is not all that important for women whose prepregnancy BMI places them in the obese category.

However, among our patients at MUSC, we found the following:

- In *all* BMI categories, achieving maternal weight-gain goals resulted in higher birthweights and fewer deliveries prior to 35 weeks.

- Among underweight women, those who met weight-gain goals were *three times less likely* to deliver before 32 weeks' gestation.
- Among obese women, those who achieved weight-gain targets had significant reductions in the risk of preterm delivery prior to 32 weeks, as well as significant reductions in the likelihood of major newborn health complications.

The lesson in all this is that by achieving your BMI-specific pregnancy weight-gain goals, you can vastly improve your chances of having healthy multiples. Paying attention to your nutrition is a self-empowering and tremendously important way to safeguard your own health as well as your babies' futures.

A Better Way Than the Bathroom Scale to Plot Your Progress

The bathroom scale is not necessarily the best way to plot your weight-gain progress, because it does not really indicate how your babies are growing. A better method is to use anthropometric measures to evaluate your nutritional status during pregnancy. A simple way for you to periodically monitor these changes is to use a tape measure to track your upper-arm circumference midway between elbow and shoulder.

Remember that pregnancy hormones cause you to put on pounds long before your babies gain any significant amount of weight. The fat your body stores during the first half of pregnancy serves as a nutritional reserve for the second half, when it's difficult to take in enough calories to meet your babies' metabolic demands for growth.

Most women find this a fascinating phenomenon to track, because weight gain (as measured by the bathroom scale) and your babies' growth (as measured by ultrasound) rapidly increase after about 28 weeks of pregnancy, while body fat (as measured at the upper arm) remains the same or even decreases. Twin mom Judy Levy says, "It was interesting to see that my upper-arm measurement stayed at 10 inches from 28 weeks all the way to when I delivered at 37½ weeks, even though I gained 20 pounds during that time."

An additional measurement done at each prenatal visit is an assessment of your fundal height, or an estimate of the size of your uterus. While lying on your back, the doctor or nurse measures the distance from the top of your belly to your pubic bone. This provides an indirect measure of your babies' growth. For a singleton pregnancy, this figure (measured in centimeters) is typically about the same as the length of the pregnancy in weeks. For example, 26 weeks into her pregnancy, the average expectant mother of a singleton has a fundal height of 26 centimeters.

When you're pregnant with multiples, of course, your uterus grows much faster. Table 3.12 shows how the fundal height measurement changes based on plurality (the number of babies) and the weeks of gestation. Notice how a multiple pregnancy compares to a singleton pregnancy. For instance, by 24 weeks the fundal height is at 33-week size with twins, at 36-week size with triplets, and at 39- to 40-week size with quads. By 28 weeks, the fundal height is at 37-week size with twins, at 40-week size with triplets, and at what would be 44-week size with quads.

Changes in Fundal Height by Plurality and Weeks' Gestation

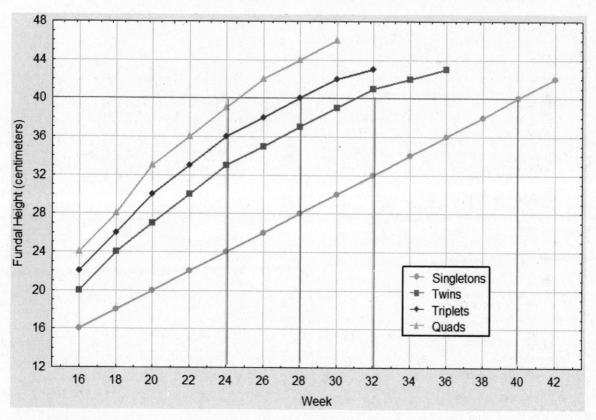

Table 3.12

A convenient way to keep track of your own fundal height and other measurements, as well as your weight-gain progress and the results of various tests, is to use the following chart, Table 3.13.

Plotting Your Progress

DATE

WEEK	10	12	14	16	18	20	21	22
Fundal height								
Cervical exam								
Blood pressure								
Upper-arm circumference								
Weight								
Net gain								
Hemoglobin								
Hematocrit								
Glucose (one-hour)								
Rho-Gam								
Urine culture								

ULTRASOUND DATE

WEEK	10	12	14	16	18	20	21	22
50th percentile (grams)	35	58	93	146	223	331	399	478
50th percentile (ounces)	1.2	2	3.3	5.1	7.9	11.7	14	17
Baby A								
Baby B								
Baby C								
Baby D								

Plotting Your Progress

DATE

WEEK	23	24	25	26	27	28	29	30
Fundal height								
Cervical exam								
Blood pressure								
Upper-arm circumference								
Weight								
Net gain								
Hemoglobin								
Hematocrit								
Glucose (one-hour)								
Rho-Gam								
Urine culture								

ULTRASOUND DATE

WEEK	23	24	25	26	27	28	29	30
50th percentile (grams)	568	670	785	913	1,055	1,210	1,379	1,559
50th percentile (lb./oz.)	1 lb., 4 oz.	1 lb., 8 oz.	1 lb., 12 oz.	2 lb., 0 oz.	2 lb., 5 oz.	2 lb., 11 oz.	3 lb., 0 oz.	3 lb., 7 oz.
Baby A								
Baby B								
Baby C								
Baby D								

Plotting Your Progress

DATE

WEEK	31	32	33	34	35	36	37	38
Fundal height								
Cervical exam								
Blood pressure								
Upper-arm circumference								
Weight								
Net gain								
Hemoglobin								
Hematocrit								
Glucose (one-hour)								
Rho-Gam								
Urine culture								

ULTRASOUND DATE

WEEK	31	32	33	34	35	36	37	38
50th percentile (grams)	1,751	1,953	2,162	2,377	2,595	2,813	3,028	3,236
50th percentile (lb./oz.)	3 lb., 14 oz.	4 lb., 5 oz.	4 lb., 12 oz.	5 lb., 4 oz.	5 lb., 11 oz.	6 lb., 3 oz.	6 lb., 11 oz.	7 lb., 2 oz.
Baby A								
Baby B								
Baby C								
Baby D								

Table 3.13

DR. LUKE: It is a common fear that the weight gain and diet we recommend will just make women fat, and that the weight won't be lost after delivery. Yet time and time again, it has been shown that this is not what happens. If you gain weight by consuming appropriate foods (primarily protein-rich choices, fiber-rich carbohydrates, and healthy fats) and gain in the right pattern (with most of your weight gain occurring in the first 28 weeks of pregnancy, then plateauing until delivery), you will build strong placentas through which to nourish your babies. With this foundation, as the babies' growth takes off in the second half of pregnancy, you will actually mobilize a considerable amount of your fat stores. If you breast-feed, this mobilization continues after delivery, particularly from fat stored on your hips and thighs, slimming you down—and giving your babies the absolute best start in life.

DR. NEWMAN: I wholeheartedly agree. At the Medical University of South Carolina, we looked at maternal weight retention at the time of their first postpartum checkup for women who had delivered twins. By six weeks postpartum, women who gained the recommended amount of weight during their twin pregnancy, regardless of BMI, were carrying an average of *just 5 extra pounds* over their prepregnancy weight, while those who gained less than the recommended amount were carrying an average of 2.5 extra pounds. In other words, there was scarcely any difference in the amount of weight retained.

However, the women who achieved their pregnancy weight-gain goals had significant benefits. On average, their pregnancies lasted two weeks longer, they delivered babies who were more than a pound heavier, and their babies experienced fewer newborn complications after birth. That is quite a bargain, considering the paltry few extra pounds of postpartum weight.

The only women who had a problem with an excessive amount of retained weight by six weeks postpartum were those who exceeded the recommended weight-gain goals during their pregnancy. But even they were carrying only an extra 10 to 15 pounds over their prepregnancy weight. And these women, too, eventually lost the extra weight—it just took a little longer.

It is important to realize that the weight-gain recommendations in this book are based on a pregnancy diet with balanced proportions of proteins, carbohydrates, and fats, as well as lots of fluids (mostly water). Wholesome, healthy foods will fill you up, make you feel energized, and keep your babies growing stronger every day. On the other hand, a diet based on French fries and chocolate cake may enable you to gain 50 or 65 pounds—or much more—but you'll feel sluggish and run-down, and your babies won't grow very well. And you'll still be left with 20, 30, or 40 extra pounds to lose, months after you deliver. So go ahead and enjoy your cheeseburger, but go light on the fries. Treat yourself to an occasional candy bar, but only after you've finished your grilled salmon and salad.

Following the food plan in Chapters 4 and 5 is the best way to promote optimal growth for your unborn babies, while ensuring that you'll be able to regain your figure after delivery. This holds true even if you have struggled with your weight in the past. "I have never been a skinny person. I did manage to lose 55 pounds the year before I conceived, but it required paying attention to every single calorie," says Erin Justice, mother of identical twin boys. "When I got pregnant, it was a relief to learn that my babies would benefit if I gained 40 or 50 pounds rather than trying to starve myself. So I focused on eating nutritious foods and didn't worry about getting fat. I figured that, once the biological symphony of growing my babies was done, I could 'clean up the auditorium,' so to speak, and work on losing the weight. The result was that my pregnancy lasted 39 weeks and my boys were born big and healthy—Felix weighed 7 lb., 4 oz., and Emerson weighed 6 lb., 12 oz. And guess what? Of the 40 pounds I gained during my pregnancy, 35 pounds were gone before the babies were two weeks old."

If you are still worried about being too heavy after this pregnancy, set your mind at ease by reading Chapter 12, "A Better Body after Babies." It describes specific diet, exercise, and lifestyle strategies that can help new mothers of multiples lose their pregnancy weight after delivery. Follow these guidelines after your babies are born—and you will soon look and feel better than ever.

Chapter Four

Need-to-Know Nutrition

Now that you know how much weight to gain and when to gain it in order to maximize your babies' growth, the next step is to learn when and what to eat. Yet it can be very difficult to find practical advice that can transform dietary guidelines from a confusing array of grams and milligrams into a workable, day-to-day eating plan. As one mother of triplets says, "I loved my obstetrician, but I admit he didn't give me much in the way of specific suggestions on how often or how much to eat, or even on which foods would be most beneficial."

> **DR. LUKE:** In designing the optimal diet for women pregnant with multiples, I began with a diet about which we know a great deal—the *diabetic diet*. It was originally designed for individuals with diabetes as the primary therapy before the discovery of insulin in 1922—and it is still the foundation of diabetes therapy today. Maintaining a normal blood glucose level through an appropriate diet is at the core of the national recommendations from the American Diabetes Association,[1, 2, 3] the American Heart

---

1. Wheeler ML, Dunbar SA, Jaacks LM, et al. Macronutrients, food groups, and eating patterns in the management of diabetes. Diabetes Care 2012; 35:434–5.
2. Evert AB, Boucher JL, Cypress M, et al. Nutrition therapy recommendations for the management of adults with diabetes. Diabetes Care 2013; 36:3821–42.
3. Evert AB, Boucher JL. New diabetes nutrition therapy recommendations: what you need to know. Diabetes Spectrum 2014; 27:121–30.

Association,[4, 5] and the Academy of Nutrition and Dietetics.[6, 7] You may be surprised to learn that the diabetic diet is the basis for a number of very popular, very healthy eating plans, including the Weight Watchers Diet, the South Beach Diet, and the Zone Diet.

During pregnancy, many women develop a temporary form of diabetes known as gestational diabetes. For this reason, it has long been standard practice to give a *glucose tolerance test* in the second trimester or early in the third trimester of pregnancy to screen women for gestational diabetes—and to prescribe a diabetic diet if the test result is positive. The primary purpose of a diabetic diet is to achieve and maintain blood glucose levels within a normal range. This is important because elevated blood glucose levels, even in the absence of gestational diabetes, are associated with an increased risk for complications, including unhealthy fetal growth, preterm birth, and *chorioamnionitis* (infection of the placental membranes) in singletons[8] as well as twins.[9]

Given that a stable blood glucose level is associated with fewer pregnancy complications, why wait until the third trimester and a failed glucose tolerance test to start following a blood sugar–stabilizing diabetic diet? My strategy is to put all women expecting multiples on a diabetic diet from the very first prenatal visit—and to maintain that regimen throughout pregnancy. As you will read in Chapter 12, this is also the basis for our postpartum diet—because it is also the very best way to get back in shape after you've delivered.

4. Gidding SS, Lichtenstein AH, Faith MS, et al. Implementing American Heart Association pediatric and adult nutrition guidelines. Circulation 2009; 119:1161–75.
5. Lichtenstein AH, Appel LJ, Brands M, et al. Diet and lifestyle recommendations revision 2006. A scientific statement from the American Heart Association Nutrition Committee. Circulation 2006; 114:82–96.
6. Academy of Nutrition and Dietetic. Position paper. Nutrition and lifestyle for a healthy pregnancy outcome. Journal of the Academy of Nutrition and Dietetics 2014; 114:1099–1103.
7. Academy of Nutrition and Dietetics. Practice paper. Nutrition and lifestyle for a healthy pregnancy outcome. July 2014; 1–13.
8. Scholl TO, Sowers MF, Chen X, Lenders C. Maternal glucose concentration influences fetal growth, gestation, and pregnancy complications. American Journal of Epidemiology 2001; 154:514–20.
9. Luke B, Brown MB, Misiunas RB, Mauldin JG, Newman RB, Nugent C, et al. Elevated maternal glucose concentrations and placental infection in twin pregnancies. Journal of Reproductive Medicine 2005; 50:241–5.

The Basics of the Diet

The prescription for a diabetic diet includes getting 20 to 25 percent of your daily calories from protein, 30 percent from fats, and 45 to 50 percent from carbohydrates. Here is a simple way to apply the diabetic principles for stable blood sugar levels to a pregnancy diet for multiples:

- Eat often—at least three meals plus two to three snacks per day.
- Eat at least every three to four hours if you are expecting twins; eat at least every two to three hours if you are expecting triplets or quads, or if you were underweight before your twin pregnancy.
- Eat lean proteins, especially those rich in iron (such as lean red meats), as well as fish, poultry, dairy, and nuts.
- Eat healthy fats, such as mono- and polyunsaturated fats (found in olive oil, canola oil, nuts, seeds) and omega-3 fatty acids (found especially in fish). Limit saturated fats and high-fat dairy. Avoid all sources of trans fats (such as hydrogenated vegetable shortening and some margarines).
- Eat carbohydrate-rich foods that are unrefined or minimally processed whenever possible. Focus on fresh fruits and vegetables, legumes, and whole grains, which are nutritious and high in fiber; avoid refined carbohydrates (cookies, pastries, white bread) and starchy foods.
- Eat protein and carbohydrates together in every snack and every meal.
- Eat a bedtime snack that includes dairy.

Planning your prenatal diet doesn't need to be complicated if you follow the simple rule to eat three meals plus two or three snacks a day. Most women find a workable schedule to be breakfast, midmorning snack, lunch, midafternoon snack, dinner, and a bedtime snack. Understand that a snack does *not* mean carrots and celery sticks. It means something substantial, a mini-meal—for instance, a small bowl of cereal and milk, half a tuna fish sandwich, yogurt and fresh fruit, a small portion of macaroni and cheese, or a small whole-grain muffin with a glass of milk.

If this sounds like you should be eating almost all the time, you're right! Remember that the central issue is blood glucose control, which means maintaining a stable blood sugar level. Your unborn babies' nervous systems need a constant supply of glucose in order to develop properly. When you skip meals or go too long without eating, your blood sugar level drops and your babies are deprived of the glucose they need. Fasting is particularly dangerous during pregnancy because it leads to extremely low blood sugar, or hypoglycemia, which can trigger preterm labor and even preterm birth. Eating sweet foods can have a similar effect because sweets cause your blood sugar to initially spike, then plunge. Such instability in blood sugar levels is especially problematic for a woman expecting multiples.

DR. NEWMAN: Glucose is the primary fetal fuel. The placenta has many important functions, but none is more essential than maintaining an uninterrupted supply of glucose flowing from the maternal side to the fetal side.

A hormone called *human placental lactogen* (HPL) is produced by the placenta in quantities that are greater than those of any other hormone produced by human beings at any point in their lives. The bigger the placenta gets as your pregnancy progresses, and the more placentas there are nourishing your multiples, the more HPL is produced. All of this HPL is dumped into your circulation—none goes into the fetal circulation.

The action of HPL is one important way that your unborn babies control your metabolism to create an optimal environment for their growth and development. A primary function of HPL is to mobilize glucose from your liver and muscle, and to then block your insulin receptors so that any circulating glucose stays available for the developing babies for a longer period of time.

At the same time, HPL stimulates lipolysis (the breakdown of fat into fatty acids), thereby providing you with an alternative energy source while leaving the glucose available for the babies. However, if you go too long without eating, the utilization of fatty acids as an energy source will create ketone by-products—and the resulting metabolic state called ketosis is a problem for several reasons. First, it indicates that your intake of carbohydrates (the glucose source) may be inadequate to meet your babies' needs. Second, maternal ketosis may be associated with an increased risk for fetal malformations and other possible adverse effects on the babies' development.

Fortunately, eating so often won't be as much of a challenge as you may think, because being pregnant with multiples makes you feel much hungrier than usual. "Before I even realized I was pregnant, and long before I knew it was twins, I couldn't understand why I was suddenly so famished all the time. For instance, I was stopping to pick up a sandwich or burger every afternoon, though I'd never done that before. I guess my body knew that my babies needed the extra food, even if my brain hadn't yet gotten the message," says Stacy Moore.

Don't wait for hunger to signal that it's time to fuel up, though. To take in enough calories to support a multiple pregnancy, you need to *eat at least every three to four hours if you are expecting twins; eat at least every two to three hours if you are expecting triplets or quads or if you were underweight before your twin pregnancy.*

"I knew I couldn't rely on hunger pangs to tell me when to sit down to a meal or snack. When you're supposed to eat every two hours, you never get much chance to feel truly hungry. Instead, I just watched the clock," says Helen Armer, mother of triplets. "I was very disciplined about doing exactly what the Multiples Clinic staff had told me to do, so I never ever missed a meal or snack." Helen's dedication paid off: At birth, her largest baby weighed 5 lb., 13 oz., and even the smallest weighed a respectable 4 lb., 11 oz. Compared to the national average for triplets of just 3 lb., 10 oz., the Armer trio were downright hefty.

Eating frequently also keeps you feeling your best. Stacy Moore explains, "I knew that if I felt woozy, it meant my blood sugar had dropped because I had gone too long without food. I learned to keep a snack with me at all times, in case I became light-headed."

Conscientiously following this eating schedule will help to ensure that your babies are well grown at birth, even if they arrive early. As one reader reports, "I was very careful about my diet and weight-gain goals, and my identical twin girls were born healthy at 36 weeks. My pediatrician exclaimed excitedly during their first exam, 'They're so strong. They're behaving like full-term newborns!'"

DR. LUKE: The metabolic and hormonal changes that occur with pregnancy are all geared toward creating and maintaining the environment most favorable for fetal growth and development. These changes include an increased requirement for all nutrients—but the need for *certain* nutrients is far greater than for others.

That's why the National Academy of Sciences' Food and Nutrition Board publishes recommended dietary allowances (RDAs) for pregnant women, setting a standard for how much of each specific nutrient an expectant mother should take in each day. These RDAs, however, are geared toward women pregnant with singletons. No guidelines have yet been established for women pregnant with twins, triplets, or quadruplets. So how can you know how much of each nutrient you need to nourish your unborn babies?

In our clinic, we advised moms-to-be of twins to increase their intake of each nutrient by 50 to 100 percent over the RDAs for a singleton pregnancy. Women carrying triplets and quads need to increase their nutrient intake even more. Table 4.1, "Estimated Nutrient Requirements and Recommended Servings per Day for Expectant Mothers of Multiples," lists my own educated estimates of the nutritional requirements for women pregnant with multiples. A guideline for twin pregnancies of eating 1,000 calories over nonpregnant requirements has been used successfully in a number of specialized multiples programs, including the Montreal Diet Dispensary,[10] our Multiples Clinic at the University of Michigan,[11] and Dr. Newman's Twin Clinic at the Medical University of South Carolina. Until more extensive research can provide us with better answers, these figures are your best bet.

Here's an important note: You most likely will not be able to eat this much food throughout your entire pregnancy—but *eating this well before 28 weeks is the primary goal*. After 28 weeks with twins, and after 20 weeks with triplets or quads, just try to come as close to these goals as you can by eating smaller meals throughout the day.

10. Dubois S, Dougherty C, Duquette M-P, Hanley JA, Moutquin J-M. Twin pregnancy: The impact of the Higgins Nutrition Intervention Program on maternal and neonatal outcomes. American Journal of Clinical Nutrition 1991; 53:1397–1403.
11. Luke B, Brown MB, Misiunas R, Anderson E, Nugent C, van de Ven C, et al. Specialized prenatal care and maternal and infant outcomes in twin pregnancy. American Journal of Obstetrics & Gynecology 2003; 189:934–8.

Estimated Nutrient Requirements and Recommended Servings per Day for Expectant Mothers of Multiples

			Pregnancy			
		Nonpregnant	Singleton Pregnancy	Twin Pregnancy	Triplet Pregnancy	Quad Pregnancy
Calories per day		2,200	2,500	3,500	4,000	4,500
Protein (grams)	20–25% of calories	110–138	125–156	175–219	200–250	225–281
Carbohydrate (grams)	45–50% of calories	248–275	281–313	394–438	450–500	506–563
Fat (grams)	30% of calories	73	83	117	133	150

Food groups	Serving size					
Dairy (nonfat or low fat)	8 oz. milk or yogurt, or 1 oz. cheese	6	8	10	12	14
Lean meat, poultry, fish, eggs	1 oz., or 1 medium egg	8	9	12	14	16
Vegetables	½ cup cooked or 1 cup fresh	4	4	6	7	8
Fruits	1 medium fruit or ½ cup sliced	4	4	6	7	8
Grains & starchy vegetables*	1 slice bread, or ½ cup	8	9	12	14	14
Fats, oils, and nuts	1 tablespoon oil or butter, or 12 nuts	8	8	14	14	16

*Starchy vegetables include corn, potatoes, chickpeas, beans, and peas

Table 4.1

DR. LUKE: In the top half of Table 4.1, you'll notice that the proportion of calories you should get from protein, fat, and carbohydrates remains the same, no matter how many babies you're carrying. But the required total calorie counts increase with each additional baby.

Rather than thinking of the daily diet in terms of these percentages, however, most women find it easier to think of servings from the basic food groups. That's why I've translated the requirements to create the menu guidelines included in the bottom half of Table 4.1, listing the appropriate number of servings per day from each food group. These guidelines also reflect a pregnant woman's need to increase her intake of calcium, iron, and other tissue-building nutrients, depending on the number of babies she's expecting.

When you are using Table 4.1, be sure to check the serving sizes. For instance, look at the recommendation for an expectant mother of twins to eat 12 servings of protein daily. Since a serving of protein equals 1 ounce, the recommended daily intake is 12 *ounces* of protein—not 12 big steaks!

What if you know from past experience that, prior to your pregnancy, you needed to eat significantly less than 2,200 calories per day in order to maintain a normal weight? A small percentage of women, particularly those over age 35, do have slower metabolisms. If that is your situation, rather than aiming for 3,500 calories per day during your twin pregnancy, you can aim for your normal prepregnancy calorie count *plus* an additional 1,000 to 1,300 calories. For instance, if you normally consume 1,700 calories a day, you should take in 2,700 to 3,000 calories per day when pregnant with twins.

But remember, this guideline applies to you *only* if:

- You are consistently reaching the weight-gain goals outlined in Chapter 3.
- Ultrasound exams show that your babies are growing well and achieving the expected growth targets for their gestational age.
- Your prepregnancy BMI was normal or overweight, *not underweight*.
- You closely adhere to a nutrient-rich diet with the proper proportion of protein, carbohydrates, and fats, as described in this chapter.
- You are pregnant with twins. (Regardless of their prepregnancy calorie needs, expectant mothers of triplets and quads should strive to meet the calorie goals listed in Table 4.1.)

Katy Lederer, mother of boy/girl twins, shares her experience: "I've always needed to eat a lot less than the average women in order to maintain a normal weight. Before I conceived, I had a BMI of 25 and I ate about 1,400 calories per day. If I ate more than that, I gained weight. When I got pregnant with the twins at age 40, it was a struggle to take in more than 2,400 calories per day because even with just that amount of food, I constantly felt full. Plus I was on bedrest, so I wasn't using up many calories on physical activity," says Katy. "Even so, I made certain that I was reaching each weight-gain target, and ultrasounds showed that my twins were growing quite well. By the time I delivered at 37 weeks, I had gained 55 pounds. And my babies were big—at birth, Zoe weighed 7 lb., 8 oz., and Isaac weighed 7 lb., 11 oz."

WHAT'S SO IMPORTANT ABOUT THESE NUTRIENTS?

It's wise to keep a detailed record of what you eat for a week and to review it with your dietitian. Says Anne Seifert, mother of quadruplets: "Dr. Luke had me keep a log of every bite I ate. Then she analyzed it to make sure I was getting enough of everything I needed, particularly protein and fat."

Fat? That's right. The purpose of including some moderate-fat, calorically dense foods is to make sure that the protein in your diet is used for building tissue—your own, your babies', and that of the placentas. Fat is the most concentrated source of calories, so it helps you meet your caloric requirements during the first half of pregnancy, when the vital placentas are forming. And later on, when it becomes difficult to eat as much because the babies are taking up so much space inside you, calorically dense foods help reduce the volume of food you need to eat to keep up with demands.

To motivate yourself to achieve the right balance of protein, carbohydrates, and fats, it helps to understand how each contributes to the well-being of your unborn babies.

Proteins are the body's basic building blocks.

Proteins are made up of amino acids, structural units that are essential for building and repairing tissue as well as forming blood, bones, and the brain. Amino acids are also vital components of enzymes, hormones, and antibodies (part of the immune system). Once you're pregnant, you need extra protein to build the placentas, to allow for increases in breast and uterine tissue and blood volume, and, of course, to promote your babies' growth. Some of the amino acids in protein cannot be made by the body. These are called the essential amino acids, and they must be obtained through your diet. For this reason, the *quality* of the protein you eat during pregnancy is as important as the *quantity*. Protein foods that contain all essential amino acids—called complete proteins—include meat, seafood, poultry, eggs, milk, and cheese.

It is wise to include some form of protein with every meal and every snack. Not only does this promote optimal development for your babies, it also stabilizes your blood sugar so you can feel your best.

Fats promote proper nerve development and help prevent pregnancy complications.

Fat provides a carrier for the fat-soluble vitamins A and D. It also plays a critical role in nerve development and tissue growth. In fact, fat is an integral part of nearly every cell in your babies' bodies.

As with protein, some of the structural components of fat—called the essential fatty acids—cannot be manufactured by the body and must be supplied from food. Omega-3 fatty acids are especially important. Good sources include all seafood and fish, egg yolks, and oils such as flaxseed, canola, and olive. During pregnancy, omega-3 fatty acids provide many benefits to mothers and babies:

- They significantly lessen a mother's risk of developing preeclampsia, a serious complication of pregnancy characterized by a rapid rise in blood pressure (see Chapter 7 for details).
- Omega-3s help to reduce the risk of preterm delivery, perhaps by inhibiting the synthesis of certain prostaglandins, substances that initiate labor.
- They promote the development of your unborn babies' nervous systems and vision.
- Omega-3s may help reduce the risk of maternal depression during pregnancy as well as postpartum depression in the weeks after delivery.
- Evidence suggests that babies born to mothers who got adequate amounts of omega-3s have a reduced risk of developing high blood pressure as well as diabetes in the future.

Carbohydrates provide energy.

Every living creature needs an energy source. Carbohydrates provide the primary energy source for humans, including unborn babies—and they provide the *only* energy source that can be used for fetuses' developing nervous systems. Carbohydrates come in two forms: simple and complex. Simple carbohydrates are found in fruits, honey, milk, and refined sugar. Complex carbohydrates include potatoes, corn, wheat, and rice.

Adequate intake of carbohydrates also helps prevent several common problems of pregnancy. The first is constipation. Fiber, a nondigestible form of carbohydrate, absorbs water as it passes through the digestive system and aids in proper bowel function. There also is some evidence that fiber reduces the risk of developing preeclampsia. High-fiber foods include breads and cereals made from bran or whole grain, and raw fruits and vegetables. The Institute of Medicine has issued guides for good nutrition called dietary reference intakes (DRIs), which take into account age, gender, and other factors. The DRI for dietary fiber is 14 grams per

1,000 calories.[12] For the average adult, that translates to a daily fiber recommendation of 38 grams for a man and 25 grams for a nonpregnant woman. For a woman pregnant with multiples, the DRI translates to about 50 to 60 grams of fiber per day. Unfortunately, few people reach these goals—in fact, the average American only gets about 15 grams of fiber per day.

Another common pregnancy problem that carbohydrates help to prevent is hypoglycemia, or a sudden drop in blood sugar. This afflicts expectant mothers of multiples even more often than it does other pregnant women. Symptoms include shakiness, dizziness, sweating, fatigue, irritability, and mood swings. At night, hypoglycemia can trigger fitful sleeping, night sweats, and disturbing dreams. Carbohydrates combat hypoglycemia by helping to maintain a regular blood sugar level, especially when eaten in combination with protein foods—for instance, crackers with peanut butter or cheese, or cereal with milk, or melon with prosciutto.

The Food Groups Demystified

"It seemed like a nuisance at first to keep track of the food groups. I'd lose count by mid-afternoon—was I up to four servings of grains and five of dairy, or was it five grains and four dairy?" admits Lydia Greenwood, mother of boy/girl twins. "But after my dietitian filled me in on how each type of food was helping my babies, I was careful to tally up my day's intake and make sure the scores came out right."

One reader shares an excellent suggestion for keeping track and staying motivated: "I made flash cards for each serving of food per food group and for each serving of water, and laid them out at the start of each day. My goal by the end of the day was to have all the cards moved over into the 'eaten' pile. It was a lot of food and water, and it wasn't always easy to get it all—but it worked. I gained what I needed to, and my twins were born big and healthy. What's more, I lost all my pregnancy weight by six months postpartum, which is quicker than I lost the weight after my prior two singleton births."

Here is the information that can help you have a similarly positive experience:

WHAT DAIRY DOES FOR YOU AND YOUR BABIES

Dairy products are your diet's richest source of calcium, a mineral needed to build your babies' bones and teeth. Dairy foods also contain other important vitamins and minerals, and are a

---

12. Institute of Medicine, Food and Nutrition Board. Dietary reference intakes: Energy, carbohydrates, fiber, fat, fatty acids, cholesterol, protein, and amino acids. Washington, DC: National Academies Press; 2002.

good source of complete proteins. Some dairy foods, such as yogurt with active cultures, contain *probiotics* (beneficial digestive bacteria) that help maintain a healthy balance of flora in the intestinal tract and may also stimulate the immune system. Except for their lack of iron, dairy products are considered by many nutritionists to be the perfect food.

It's not hard to get enough dairy if you get creative. "My dietitian told me to drink at least a quart of milk every day," says twin mom Judy Levy. "All that milk went down more easily once I started warming it up and stirring in some chocolate, vanilla, or honey. I actually looked forward to drinking a big thermos of flavored milk during my morning commute to work." For an added boost, try a calcium-fortified brand of milk such as Lactaid, which has 500 milligrams of calcium per glass.

Is ice cream an acceptable option for some of your daily dairy servings? Sure! "I would never have thought it was wise to have milkshakes every night if Dr. Luke hadn't told me to. But those really helped me put on the weight I needed, while providing a calcium boost, too," reports Heather Nicholas, mother of boy/girl twins.

Yogurt is another good choice. For probiotic benefits, be sure to choose yogurt that contains live and active cultures (check the label). Try Greek yogurt, such as the brand Fage. Unlike typical yogurt, it is triple-strained to remove the watery whey. As a result, Greek yogurt is thick and creamy like sour cream and sweet like fromage blanc.

Dairy foods also make excellent bedtime snacks. Because they are digested slowly, they can prevent hunger-induced awakenings in the middle of the night. Good options include a grilled-cheese sandwich, cereal with milk, or a small bowl of ice cream. Place a small carton of milk in a cooler next to your bed in case you do wake up hungry. The amino acids in the milk will help you fall asleep again quickly.

Facts About Fruits and Vegetables

Produce has lots of fiber, which aids digestion and helps prevent irregularity. Fruits and vegetables also have a high water content, which keeps you hydrated. And they are excellent sources of water-soluble vitamins, such as folic acid and the B vitamins as well as vitamin C.

When it comes to produce, color is generally the key to nutrient density—the deeper the color, the more nourishing the food. For example, romaine and red-leaf lettuce have more nutrients than iceberg; carrots and broccoli have more than cauliflower. So fill your shopping cart with the darkest, brightest fruits and vegetables you can find. Create a colorful salad every day, using a variety of dark green lettuces, purple cabbage, tomatoes, red and green peppers, and other veggies.

Just be careful not to overdo produce at the expense of protein. Says Judy Levy, "I love fruits and vegetables, but overdosing on them made me uncomfortably full. If I ate too big a salad, I couldn't find much room for meat."

GOING WITH THE GRAIN

Whole-grain cereal, bread, pasta, rice, and other products are rich in the B vitamins that are essential to good health. And because they often are fortified, they help to ensure that you get the nutrients you need. For instance, fortified grain products are good sources of folic acid, which helps prevent neural tube defects such as spina bifida and may reduce the risk of miscarriage.

Remember that whole grains also are rich in fiber, which helps to stabilize blood sugar levels and prevent constipation. Check package labels to see if you're getting enough fiber: A good source should provide at least 2 to 3 grams per serving; an excellent source will provide 5 grams or more. For easy identification while shopping, look for the Whole Grain stamp (a stylized sheaf of grain on a golden-yellow background with a bold black border) issued by the Whole Grains Council (www.wholegrainscouncil.org). It signifies that a product contains 8 grams or more of whole grain per serving.

Grain products have the added advantage of being portable, versatile, and inexpensive. Nutritious and convenient options include microwaveable rice and grain dishes from Seeds of Change (www.seedsofchangefoods.com), such as Tigris—A Mixture of Seven Whole Grains, or Uyuni Quinoa and Whole Grain Brown Rice. For a snack, try two slices of Wasa crispbread with two tablespoons of peanut butter, which provide 5 grams of fiber plus 9 grams of protein for about 250 calories.

FATS AND OILS: HEROES, NOT VILLAINS, DURING PREGNANCY

When you don't take in enough calories from carbohydrates, your body must get its energy from fat—either from the foods you eat or from your body fat. This is a problem because by-products of the breakdown of fat, called ketones, can be toxic to your unborn babies. So even though you're probably used to thinking of fat as bad, during a multiple pregnancy you need to readjust your viewpoint.

Don't be surprised, though, if other people fail to understand this. Meredith Alcott, mother of identical twin girls, recalls, "Even after we realized I was carrying twins, my obstetrician told me to stick to a low-fat diet. But my dietitian had other ideas. She said, 'Forget low-fat for now! Go get yourself some ice cream.'"

Not just any type of fat will do, however. The best fats to emphasize are flaxseed, canola, and olive oils, which are rich in omega-3 fatty acids. You should avoid trans fats (also known as trans fatty acids). These are manufactured when liquid oils are made into solid fats through a process called partial hydrogenation. Check the ingredients list on processed foods—trans fats are usually listed as partially hydrogenated oils. This type of fat increases low-density lipoprotein (LDL, or the bad cholesterol) and reduces high-density lipoprotein (HDL, or the good cholesterol), thereby increasing your risk for coronary heart disease, stroke, and diabetes. What's more, the intake of trans fat during pregnancy has been linked to an increased risk of fetal loss.[13]

THE EXCELLENCE OF EGGS

Eggs are a powerhouse of nutrition, packed with a wide variety of vitamins, minerals, and other essential nutrients. Egg protein is of the highest biologic value, because it provides all the essential amino acids in sufficient amounts. In fact, egg protein is the gold standard against which all other proteins are judged. About 40 percent of the egg's protein is in the yolk. Eggs also provide substantial amounts of vitamins A, D, E, and the B vitamins (including folate); the minerals copper, zinc, magnesium, iron, calcium, and phosphorus; and the nutrients choline, lutein, and zeaxanthin, which are essential for eye health.

For maximum nutrition, try eggs that are enriched with omega-3 fatty acids, marketed under brand names such as Eggland's Best and Wilcox Farms. These eggs come from chickens whose all-vegetarian feed contains healthy grains, canola oil, and an all-natural supplement of rice bran, alfalfa, sea kelp, and vitamin E. Compared to regular eggs, these enriched eggs contain two to six times as much omega-3 and vitamin E.

One caution: Do not eat raw or undercooked eggs. These can be a source of bacterial food poisoning.

THE MANY BENEFITS OF MEATS, POULTRY, AND SEAFOOD

A number of the essential nutrients needed in larger quantities during a multiple pregnancy are supplied by red meats, pork, poultry, and fish. These foods are excellent sources of the complete protein that's vital to your babies' growth. They are also rich in vitamin B_{12} as well as iron, which protects against anemia and its complications. That's why you should aim to eat these lean protein foods often—at least twice a day—if you are pregnant with twins, and even more often if you are pregnant with triplets or quads. (If you are a vegetarian, see Chapter 5 for more information about following a vegetarian diet during a multiple pregnancy.)

---

13. Morrison JA, Glueck CJ, Wang P. Dietary trans fatty acid intake is associated with increased fetal loss. Fertility and Sterility 2008; 90:385–90.

Some women aren't accustomed to eating this much protein, particularly red meat—so if it seems challenging at first, try increasing your protein intake gradually. "I was used to mainly meatless meals, so it was tough to find high-protein foods that both my stomach and my taste buds could tolerate," says Judy Levy. "But through trial and error, I discovered some good strategies. For instance, pasta-and-protein combinations made meat much more enjoyable. My favorites were lasagna with ground beef, spaghetti with meatballs, and eggs with ham on an English muffin."

Poultry is an excellent source of protein and other nutrients. The breast meat has the lowest fat content, but even dark meat is relatively low in fat—and in any event, a substantial portion of the fat in chicken and turkey is the heart-healthy unsaturated kind. Poultry also is high in the B vitamins (especially B_6, B_{12}, pantothenic acid, and niacin), iron, phosphorus, magnesium, and zinc. "I had been a vegetarian for years before I got pregnant, so chicken seemed like the best 'entry-level' meat to reintroduce into my diet. I integrated it slowly—for instance, I wouldn't eat a whole roasted chicken, but it was easy to add some ground chicken to my vegetable stir-fry," says Megan Ryerson, mother of boy/girl twins.

Seafood is especially important for your pregnancy diet. It provides high-quality protein, essential vitamins and minerals, and polyunsaturated fats. Fish also is rich in the omega-3 fatty acids—particularly docosahexaenoic acid (DHA) and eicosapentaenoic acid (EPA)—needed for your babies' neurological development. The fish you eat now promotes your children's visual acuity, cognitive abilities, and verbal and motor development. Later, if you breast-feed, the DHA you consume will pass through your breast milk to your babies and continue to benefit their development. Eating fish also benefits you directly, because the demands of pregnancy (particularly a multiple pregnancy) can drain a mother's own levels of omega-3.[14, 15] Although the body can convert a substance called alpha-linolenic acid (found in flaxseeds, walnuts, and canola oil) to DHA, the conversion is not efficient, and the converted form is far less beneficial to brain development than the preformed DHA found in fatty fish.

Certain types of seafood are more highly recommended than others. One concern has to do with environmental contaminants, such as mercury and polychlorinated biphenyls (PCBs). A mother's consumption of seafood contaminated with these substances may pose health risks to her babies before birth and during breast-feeding. The Institute of Medicine report called

---

14. Foreman-van Drongelen MMHP, Zeijdner EE, Houwelingen ACV, et al. Essential fatty acid status measured in umbilical vessel walls of infants born after a multiple pregnancy. Early Human Development 1996; 46:205–15.

15. Zeijdner EE, Houwelingen ACV, Kester ADM, et al. Essential fatty acid status in plasma phospholipids of mother and neonate after multiple pregnancy. Prostaglandins, Leukotrienes, and Essential Fatty Acids 1997; 56:395–401.

Seafood Choices: Balancing Benefits and Risk[16] is based on the recommendations of an expert panel. These guidelines suggest that women who are or may become pregnant or who are breast-feeding:

- May benefit from consuming seafood, especially those with relatively higher concentrations of EPA and DHA.
- Can safely consume 12 ounces of seafood per week.
- Can consume up to 6 ounces of canned light tuna per week.
- Should avoid large predatory fish such as shark, swordfish, tilefish, or king mackerel.

The Food and Drug Administration (FDA) and Environmental Protection Agency (EPA) recommendations, which are in line with those of the Institute of Medicine, suggest that the best choices are low-mercury species like anchovies, Atlantic mackerel, canned light tuna, catfish, cod, freshwater rainbow trout, monkfish, pollack, sardines, shrimp, and wild Alaskan salmon.

An FDA report on the net effect of eating fish on brain development and heart health is based on an evaluation of research studies to date.[17] According to this report, at every level of consumption the benefits far outweighed the risks, indicating better child development—including higher IQs, better visual acuity, and better memory—among children whose mothers ate more fish and seafood before their birth.

How can you translate these various recommendations to a usable plan for your pregnancy diet? Aim to eat seafood several times per week, choosing from the recommended sources and avoiding large predatory fish (as described above). For more help in making the best seafood choices, go to the Seafood Selector on the Environmental Defense Fund website (www.edf.org).

A final important point: Make sure that all meats, poultry, and seafood are sufficiently cooked. Raw dishes (such as sushi) and undercooked products (such as rare hamburgers and underdone chicken or turkey) are a potential source of parasites or bacterial food poisoning.

---

16. Institute of Medicine. Seafood choices: Balancing benefits and risks. Washington, DC: National Academies Press; 2006.
17. Food and Drug Administration Center for Food Safety and Nutrition. Draft risk and benefit assessment of quantitative risk and benefit assessment of consumption of commercial fish, focusing on fetal neurodevelopmental effects (measured by verbal development in children) and on coronary heart disease and stroke in the general population; www.cfsan.fda.gov/~dms/mehgrb.html.

Putting Your Food Plan into Action

DR. LUKE: I've often heard moms-to-be of multiples say, "I understand how much weight I should gain and how often I should eat. But exactly *what* should I be eating? How can I plan my daily menus? What recipes will help my babies get the nutrients they need? It all seems so complicated."

To answer those questions as simply and completely as possible, this book provides lots of information about nutrition. For instance, in this chapter and in Chapters 5, 11, and 12, the easy-to-follow advice on food choices includes:

- Top 25 Food All-Stars that make nutritious eating easy.
- 75 original recipes, each designed for maximum nutrition as well as great taste.
- 120 specific menu suggestions for meals and snacks, organized trimester-by-trimester and targeted to maximize your babies' development during each stage of pregnancy—plus a section for the postpartum period (sometimes called the fourth trimester) designed to provide the nutrients you need to successfully breast-feed multiples *and* to regain your figure (as explained in Chapters 11 and 12).
- Strategies for making smart food choices in all kinds of situations—at home, at the office, and on the road.
- Updated recommendations, based on the latest studies, for the specific vitamins and minerals that are most beneficial during a multiple pregnancy.
- Information on the use of dietary supplements during pregnancy.
- Tips on how to stay motivated to eat right.

Superstar Foods

The simplest way to get many of the nutrients you and your unborn babies need, starting today, is to eat more of the Top 25 Food All-Stars. Foods earn a spot on this list based on four criteria: high nutrient content, flavor, versatility as an ingredient in recipes, and low glycemic index. The glycemic index is a ranking system on a scale of 0 to 100 that indicates the degree to which a carbohydrate-containing food raises the blood glucose level compared to an equal amount of pure sugar. A score of 55 or less is considered low (good), a GI of 56 to 69 is medium, and a GI of 70 or greater is high (bad).

Table 4.2 lists the Top 25 winners, along with the benefits of each.

Top 25 Food All-Stars

Food Group	Food	Nutritional Benefits
Dairy	Yogurt	Easily digested, high-quality protein; low-glycemic-index carbohydrate; calcium; phosphorus; zinc; riboflavin; vitamins B_{12} and D; immunologic qualities; probiotic health-promoting lactic acid bacteria (Lactobacillus, Bifidobacterium).
	Milk	High-quality protein; low-glycemic-index carbohydrate; calcium; iodine; magnesium; phosphorus; potassium; vitamins A, B_{12}, and D; riboflavin; niacin; conjugated linolenic acid (CLA).
	Cheese	High-quality protein; calcium; phosphorus; magnesium; zinc; vitamin A.
Protein	Coldwater fish	High-quality protein; biotin; calcium; niacin; omega-3 essential fatty acids (DHA and EPA); riboflavin; vitamins A and B_{12}.
	Shellfish	High-quality protein; low-fat; calcium; copper; iodine; manganese; vitamin D.
	Eggs	High-quality protein; choline; lutein; zeaxanthin; folate; biotin; iron; chromium; selenium; phosphorus; vitamins A, B_6, and D; zinc.
	Lean beef	High-quality protein; conjugated linolenic acid (CLA); iron; chromium; selenium; zinc; thiamin; pantothenic acid; vitamin B_{12}.
	Lean pork	High-quality protein; iron; chromium; thiamin; pantothenic acid; vitamin B_{12}.
	Lean poultry	High-quality protein; iron; chromium; selenium; zinc; thiamin; pantothenic acid; pyridoxine; vitamin B_{12}.
	Tofu	Protein; low-fat; fiber; vitamin A; thiamin; folic acid; calcium; zinc; phytonutrients.
Legumes	Beans, peas, lentils, chickpeas	Protein; low-fat; fiber; low-glycemic-index carbohydrate; folic acid; thiamin; pyridoxine; calcium; copper; iron; zinc; potassium.
Nuts	Peanuts, cashews, walnuts, pecans, almonds	Protein; fiber; copper; magnesium; manganese; zinc; pyridoxine; biotin; monounsaturated fatty acids.
Vegetables	Asparagus	Fiber; vitamins A, C, and E; riboflavin; folic acid; thiamin; copper; magnesium; potassium.

Food Group	Food	Nutritional Benefits
	Broccoli	Fiber; vitamins A, C, and K; riboflavin; folic acid; calcium; chromium; magnesium; manganese.
	Cabbage	Fiber; vitamins A, C, and K; riboflavin; folic acid; sulforaphane.
	Pumpkin	Fiber; vitamins A and C; chromium.
	Spinach	Calcium; chromium; iron; magnesium; manganese; potassium; vitamins A, C, and K; riboflavin; folic acid.
	Sweet potatoes, yams	Fiber; vitamin A; low-glycemic-index carbohydrate; chromium.
Fruits	Apples	Fiber; chromium; low-glycemic-index carbohydrate; flavanols; proanthocyanidin.
	Avocados	Fiber; B vitamins; vitamins A and E; copper; magnesium; potassium; pyridoxine.
	Cherries	Low-glycemic-index carbohydrate; vitamins A and C; anthocyanins.
	Citrus (oranges, grapefruit)	Fiber; low-glycemic-index carbohydrate; vitamins A and C; folic acid; potassium; flavanols.
	Tomatoes	Vitamins A and C; carotenoids (especially lycopene and lutein).
Grains	Oatmeal	Protein; fiber; low-glycemic-index carbohydrate; iron; magnesium.
	Wheat germ	Protein; fiber; low-fat; vitamin E; thiamin; folic acid; magnesium; phosphorus; zinc.

Table 4.2

RECIPES YOU (AND YOUR BABIES) WILL LOVE

Take a look at the Best Recipes for Moms-to-Be of Multiples in Appendix A. Each of these recipes includes at least one if not two, three, four, or even more of the Top 25 Food All-Stars. For easy reference, check the All-Star Rating at the bottom of each recipe to see how many All-Stars it offers.

Some of the common Food All-Stars—eggs, milk, vegetables, meat—are ingredients readily found in many recipes. Other All-Stars—pumpkin, legumes, nuts, tofu—appear less frequently in typical cookbooks. That's why so many of the original recipes included in this book contain these often-overlooked nutritional powerhouses.

You'll also want to take note of each recipe's Blue-Ribbon Rating. This indicates the number of nutrients the recipe provides, per serving, at a level of 20 percent or more of the recommended dietary allowance for pregnancy. Some recipes earn as many as 15 ribbons!

Menus for Moms-to-Be of Multiples

The following Master List of Menu Suggestions includes 120 nutritious and flavorful menu items. Let this list be an inspiration as you plan your weekly menus and prepare your shopping lists. Note: An asterisk indicates that the item is included among the 75 original recipes given in Appendix A at the back of the book. For other suggested menu items, consult your favorite cookbook.

Master List of Menu Suggestions

BEEF AND LAMB ENTRÉES
*Asian-Style Meatballs
Beef and Barley Soup
*Beef and Bean Chili
Beef Brisket
*Beef Stew
*Beef Stroganoff
Beef Tacos
Beef Teriyaki
Cheeseburgers
Corned Beef and Cabbage
Hamburgers
*Lamb and Lentil Stew
*Lamb Salad
London Broil
*Mini Meat Loaves
Pepper Steak
Pot Roast
Spaghetti and Meatballs

*Spicy Beef
*Steak and Arugula Salad
*Vietnamese Steak Salad

PORK ENTRÉES
Baked Ham
*French Toast with Ham and
   Cheese
Grilled Ham and Cheese Sandwich
Grilled Pork Chops
*Ham and Pumpkin Quiche
*Lentil and Ham Salad with Walnuts
*Maple Pork and Spinach Salad
Marinated Pork Tenderloin
*Pasta with Peas and Ham
*Pork and Cashew Bok Choy
Pork Roast
*Pork with Apple Stuffing
Quiche Lorraine

*Spicy Pork with Peanut Sauce
Sweet and Sour Pork

POULTRY ENTRÉES
*Cashew Chicken
*Chicken and Dumplings
*Chicken and Sweet Potatoes
*Chicken and Wild Rice Casserole
*Chicken-Barley Soup
*Chicken-Citrus Salad
Chicken Pot Pie
*Chinese Chicken Salad
*Cobb Salad
*Golden Chicken Salad
*Greek Lemon Chicken
Grilled Chicken
*Honey Chicken Salad with Cherries
*Pasta with Chicken and Peanut Sauce
*Seasoned Baked Chicken
*Waldorf Chicken Salad

SEAFOOD ENTRÉES
*Caesar Salad with Shrimp
*Citrus Salmon
Gefilte Fish
Grilled Salmon
*Linguine with Clams and Dried Tomatoes
Manhattan Clam Chowder
New England Clam Chowder
*Salad Niçoise
*Salmon and Asparagus Salad
*Salmon Burgers
*Shrimp and Scallop Grill
Shrimp Egg Foo Yung
*Spicy Shrimp Salad

Tuna Casserole
*Tuna Salad with White Beans
Whitefish Salad

DAIRY AND VEGETARIAN ENTRÉES
*Arugula and Pear Salad
*Asparagus Quiche
*Autumn Pancakes
*Avocado Salad with Orange and Grapefruit
Baked Manicotti
*Beet Salad with Goat Cheese
*Caprese Salad
Cheese Lasagna
Deviled Eggs with Toast
Egg Burritos
French Toast with Applesauce
*Ginger Stir-Fry
*Greek Salad
*Greek Spinach and Cheese Pie
Grilled Cheese and Tomato Sandwich
*Lentil Soup
*Mediterranean Sauté
*Oatmeal-Almond Pancakes
Oatmeal with Dried Cherries
*Pasta with Green Sauce
*Pumpkin Waffles
*Ratatouille
*Salsa Frittata
Scrambled Eggs and Raisin Toast
*Spinach and Pumpkin Casserole
*Tomato Apricot Salad
*Vegetarian Lasagna
*Vegetarian Stroganoff
Whole-wheat Pancakes
*Wild Rice Omelet

SIDE DISHES AND SNACKS

Apple Slices and Peanut Butter

Apple, Walnut, and Cheese Salad

Baked Apples with Cheddar Cheese

Blueberry Muffins

*Chickpea Salad

Cottage Cheese and Fruit

Fruit Salad with Cheese and Crackers

*Harvest Muffins

Oatmeal-Walnut Cookies with Yogurt

*Powerhouse Granola

*Pumpkin Custard

*Pumpkin-Fruit Muffins

*Pumpkin Loaf

*Sunrise Bread Pudding

*Tabbouleh

Vanilla Yogurt with Walnuts and Wheat Germ

*Weekend Hash Browns

Whole-wheat Toast with Peanut Butter

*Yogurt Guacamole

SMOOTHIES

*Basic Fruit Smoothie

*Basic Vegetable Smoothie

*Ginger Smoothie

Take menu planning a step further by selecting dishes that best suit your stage of pregnancy. The menus that follow are specifically designed to satisfy the nutritional needs of your unborn babies (as well as your own body), depending on whether you're in your first, second, or third trimester.

FIRST TRIMESTER: FOCUS ON FOLIC ACID AND OTHER B VITAMINS

The first trimester, also called the embryonic period, includes the time from conception to the 12th week of pregnancy. During these weeks, 70 percent of the nutrients you supply to your unborn babies are devoted to their brain growth and neurological development. An adequate intake of folic acid now helps to prevent neural tube defects such as spina bifida, and also may protect against congenital heart disease. All vital organs are also forming at this time, and folic acid promotes their proper growth. Good sources of folic acid (also called folate or vitamin B_9) include fortified rice, pasta, breads, cereals, grains, poultry, lentils and beans, green leafy vegetables, avocados, tomatoes and tomato juice, oranges, and papayas.

With some creativity, you can easily up your intake of folic acid–rich foods. Tessa Walters, mother of fraternal twin boys, reports, "I wasn't big on fruits and veggies before I got pregnant, but I found some simple ways to increase my intake of folic acid. For instance, I doubled the beans in my chili recipe, added avocado to my tacos, and started topping my salads with diced peppers and chickpeas."

Research suggests that vitamin B_{12} also may help prevent neural tube defects.[18] In fact, many of the B vitamins are important during the first trimester because they are involved in the formation and growth of all tissues. B vitamins are known as water-soluble vitamins because they are not stored in the body for very long. That means you must eat a steady supply to promote your babies' optimal growth.

Following are the B vitamins you need, and the foods that provide them:

- Thiamin (B_1): beans, enriched whole grains, fish, nuts, peas, pork, soy.
- Riboflavin (B_2): dairy foods, green leafy vegetables, legumes, meat, nuts.
- Niacin (B_3): dairy foods, eggs, fortified cereals, meat, poultry, shellfish.
- Pantothenic acid (B_5): mushrooms, peanuts, salmon, whole grains.
- Pyridoxine (B_6): bananas, eggs, fish, legumes, meat, nuts, poultry, yams.
- Biotin (B_7): barley, corn, egg yolks, fortified cereals, milk, peanuts, soybeans, walnuts.
- Folate (B_9): fortified cereals and breads, pasta, poultry, lentils and beans, green leafy vegetables, oranges.
- Cobalamin (B_{12}): fish, fortified cereals and breads, grains, meat, nuts, poultry.

Remember, too, that the placentas are developing rapidly during this time. As the vital middleman between mother and baby, the placenta delivers nutrients from your bloodstream and carries away the waste products. Any factors that interfere with placental growth now will adversely affect your babies' growth later in the pregnancy. To help the placentas develop properly, be sure to get plenty of protein and foods rich in iron.

Use the following menus to help plan your daily diet for the first trimester. This way, you'll get the nutrients your unborn babies need most right now, at their most critical period of development. (An asterisk indicates that the recipe is included in Appendix A at the back of this book.)

18. Molloy AM, Kirke PN, Troendle JF, et al. Maternal vitamin B_{12} status and risk of neural tube defects in a population with high neural tube defect prevalence and no folic acid fortification. Pediatrics 2009; 123:917–23.

Menu Suggestions for the First Trimester

BREAKFAST

*Asparagus Quiche

Grilled Cheese and Tomato Sandwich

*Powerhouse Granola

*Pumpkin-Fruit Muffins

Whole-wheat Pancakes

LUNCH OR DINNER

*Arugula and Pear Salad

*Avocado Salad with Orange and Grapefruit

Baked Ham

*Cashew Chicken

*Chicken-Barley Soup

*Chicken-Citrus Salad

*Ginger Stir-Fry

*Golden Chicken Salad

*Greek Salad

Grilled Chicken

*Lamb and Lentil Stew

*Lentil and Ham Salad with Walnuts

*Linguine with Clams and Dried Tomatoes

Marinated Pork Tenderloin

*Pasta with Chicken and Peanut Sauce

*Pork and Cashew Bok Choy

*Pork with Apple Stuffing

*Spicy Beef

*Spicy Pork with Peanut Sauce

*Tomato Apricot Salad

SNACKS

Baked Apples with Cheddar Cheese

*Basic Fruit Smoothie

*Basic Vegetable Smoothie

*Ginger Smoothie

Pear, Walnut, and Cheese Salad

*Sunrise Bread Pudding

SECOND TRIMESTER: FOCUS ON IRON AND FIBER

The second trimester includes the fourth, fifth, and sixth months of pregnancy. Your babies have now graduated from embryo to fetus status. The main difference between the embryonic and fetal periods is that now, in the fetal period, no new structures are being formed (other than brain development, which continues throughout pregnancy, into childhood and even into adulthood). Your babies' growth now is mainly in size. Yet proper nutrition—supplied through your diet—is still a powerfully positive force in their development.

An adequate intake of iron is very important during this middle trimester. Because you are carrying multiples, your blood volume has increased by 100 percent or more over your prepregnancy levels. Red blood cells, which carry oxygen throughout the body, have increased by 50 to 60 percent. If the availability of iron is inadequate to support this increase in the number of red blood cells, iron-deficiency anemia develops. Symptoms include fatigue, light-headedness, dull headache, pallor, and shortness of breath. Untreated, anemia can adversely affect the growth of your babies, increase the risk for preterm birth, and also increase your own risk for complications both during and after the birth. The best way to avoid anemia is to eat foods rich in heme iron—lean red meats, pork, fish, poultry, and eggs—and to get additional iron from enriched or fortified grains and breads, nuts, beans and lentils, spinach, dried fruits, and wheat germ.

Fiber is also important now. During the second trimester, your gastrointestinal system slows down to absorb more nutrients from the foods you eat. This can lead to constipation. Fiber-rich foods help to keep you regular. Best bets include fruits such as oranges, apples, raisins, figs, prunes, and pears, and vegetables such as beans, broccoli, tomatoes, and potatoes.

Though the fatigue of early pregnancy has probably passed, there may be times when you need a quick pick-me-up. If you find yourself dragging, select a snack in the 200- to 250-calorie range that provides an immediate energy boost to sustain you until your next big meal. Two healthy, convenient, and delicious snack choices are LäraBars (www.larabar.com) and Kind Bars (www.kindsnacks.com). They provide fiber, protein, and low-glycemic-index carbohydrates. Here are other suggestions that also fit the bill:

- Spread a small banana with peanut butter.
- Top yogurt with a spoonful of crunchy granola.
- Make a trail mix of nuts, raisins, and flaked coconut.
- Eat low-fat cottage cheese with fresh grapes and high-fiber crackers.
- Melt low-fat cheese on fresh apple or pear slices.

Find more snack suggestions, as well as midpregnancy mealtime menu ideas, in the following list. (Items marked with an asterisk are included in the recipe section at the back of this book.)

Menu Suggestions for the Second Trimester

BREAKFAST
Egg Burritos
*Harvest Muffins
*Pumpkin Loaf
Scrambled Eggs and Raisin Toast
*Wild Rice Omelet

LUNCH OR DINNER
*Asian-Style Meatballs
*Beef and Bean Chili
Beef Brisket

*Beef Stew
Beef Tacos
Beef Teriyaki
*Caprese Salad
*Chicken and Sweet Potatoes
*Chinese Chicken Salad
*Cobb Salad
Corned Beef and Cabbage
*Greek Lemon Chicken
*Greek Spinach and Cheese Pie
*Honey Chicken Salad with Cherries

*Lamb Salad

*Lentil Soup

*Mediterranean Sauté

*Pasta with Green Sauce

*Seasoned Baked Chicken

*Shrimp and Scallop Grill

*Steak and Arugula Salad

*Vegetarian Stroganoff

*Waldorf Chicken Salad

SNACKS

Apple, Walnut, and Cheese Salad

*Basic Fruit Smoothie

*Basic Vegetable Smoothie

*Chickpea Salad

*Ratatouille

*Tabbouleh

*Yogurt Guacamole

THIRD TRIMESTER: FOCUS ON CALCIUM AND OMEGA-3 FATTY ACIDS

The third trimester includes the seventh, eighth, and ninth months of pregnancy. During this time, your babies' bones and teeth require a steady supply of calcium. Although this mineral has been important right from the beginning of your pregnancy, it is even more critical now. If your diet does not contain adequate amounts, calcium is mobilized from your own bones in order to meet the needs of your babies. If this occurs, your ultimate risk for osteoporosis increases significantly. The older you are, the more problematic this becomes, since you have fewer years to rebuild bone density before the onset of menopause weakens your bones further. Calcium is also an important element in the prevention of preeclampsia. Dairy foods such as milk, cheese, and yogurt are excellent sources of calcium. Boost your calcium intake further by eating sardines and salmon with bones, eggs, tofu, spinach, beans, and peanuts. Also try these tips:

- Substitute nonfat evaporated milk or calcium-fortified milk for regular milk in recipes, doubling the calcium content.
- Mix plain yogurt with dried onion soup mix to create a tasty, calcium-rich dip for vegetables.
- Try fruit-flavored yogurt on top of pancakes.
- Bake quiche for breakfast or lunch.
- Have pudding or custard for a midmorning snack.
- Choose calcium-fortified orange juice rather than regular juice.
- Go for creamy, milk-based soups rather than broth-based varieties.

DR. NEWMAN: In order for your body to absorb the calcium you eat, you need sufficient vitamin D. The sun's energy turns a substance present in the skin into vitamin D—

but because many people today spend little time outdoors without sunscreen, vitamin D deficiency is common.

That's why your obstetrician should give you a blood test to check your levels of *25-hydroxy vitamin D*. An optimal level is from 40 to 60 ng/ml. If your blood level is lower than this, your doctor can recommend an appropriate dosage of vitamin D supplementation to correct the deficiency. This will allow you to adequately absorb and use the calcium in your diet. (For more on vitamin D, see Chapter 5.)

The third trimester is also when you have a greater need for the omega-3 fatty acids. Here's why:

- Omega-3s are critical to your babies' vision and neurological systems, which are developing most rapidly during this period.
- Through a biochemical mechanism, omega-3 fatty acids block the formation of factors that can lead to premature labor.
- They may also protect your own brainpower. During pregnancy, the mother's blood level of omega-3 fatty acids drops by almost two-thirds, as compared to her prepregnancy level—probably as a result of the growing babies' drain of this vital nutrient. Studies show that the expectant mother's brain shrinks by about 3 percent during the last trimester. This may explain the memory loss that has long been associated with pregnancy, and may be linked to postpartum depression as well.

Coldwater fish and other seafood are the best sources for the essential fatty acids: 5 grams in a 7-ounce serving of Pacific salmon, 4.2 grams in Atlantic herring, 4.1 grams in canned anchovies, 3.4 grams in canned salmon, and 3 grams in canned tuna. Aim for at least two servings per week of fish.

You'll also benefit from using olive or canola oil when cooking, rather than butter, margarine, or other vegetable oils. Another option is to select eggs that are enriched with omega-3 fatty acids and vitamin E.

Aim to get at least 1,000 milligrams of omega-3 fatty acids per day. Here are tips to help you reach this goal:

- Have tuna salad for lunch.
- Choose a coldwater fish such as salmon or mackerel for dinner.
- Make a snack of shrimp cocktail.
- Order anchovies on your pizza.

- Use canola or flaxseed oil in your salad dressing.
- Use olive oil instead of margarine on your bread.
- Sauté poultry and vegetables in canola or safflower oil rather than butter.

By this stage of pregnancy, resting is far more important than cooking. Use the following easy menu suggestions to keep your meals and snacks simple yet satisfying. (An asterisk means the recipe appears at the back of this book.)

Menu Suggestions for the Third Trimester

BREAKFAST
Blueberry Muffins
*French Toast with Ham and Cheese
*Oatmeal-Almond Pancakes
*Weekend Hash Browns
Whole-wheat Toast with Peanut Butter

LUNCH OR DINNER
*Asparagus Quiche
Beef and Barley Soup
*Beef Stroganoff
*Beet Salad with Goat Cheese
Caesar Salad with Shrimp
*Chicken and Dumplings
*Chicken and Wild Rice Casserole
Grilled Pork Chops
Grilled Salmon
*Ham and Pumpkin Quiche
Manhattan Clam Chowder

*Maple Pork and Spinach Salad
*Pasta with Peas and Ham
*Salad Niçoise
*Salmon and Asparagus Salad
*Salmon Burgers
*Salsa Frittata
Shrimp Egg Foo Yung
*Spicy Shrimp Salad
*Spinach and Pumpkin Casserole
*Tuna Salad with White Beans

SNACKS
*Basic Fruit Smoothie
*Basic Vegetable Smoothie
Cottage Cheese and Fruit
*Golden Chicken Salad
*Pumpkin Custard
Vanilla Yogurt with Walnuts and
   Wheat Germ

Hopefully, you're feeling confident by now that you can nourish your unborn babies quite well by following the food plan in this book. Sure, there's a lot to learn—but the rewards are well worth it. As one reader reports, "Though I found some of the dietary guidelines challenging, they helped me to understand the needs of my developing twins, as well as to set goals for myself. After hitting 38 weeks, I delivered very healthy 7 lb., 5 oz. and 7 lb., 3 oz. boy/girl twins. Not bad for someone 5 feet, 1 inch tall."

Eat-Smart Strategies for Every Situation

You are much more likely to eat the right foods, in the right quantities, at the right times, if you plan ahead. To keep the foods you need at hand, wherever you are, try these tactics:

Stock your cupboards, refrigerator, and freezer with the basics.

"Right after our first appointment with Dr. Luke, my husband, Curt, went to the store and loaded up on meats, multigrain breads and cereals, frozen and low-sodium canned vegetables, and premium ice cream. He also shopped regularly for fresh produce and dairy products to make sure the cupboard was never bare," says Amy Maly, mother of identical twin girls.

If you have a large freezer, take a tip from Anne Seifert: "My husband had a meat delivery service stock our freezer with steaks, chops, chicken, and ground beef. It looked like a mountain of meat at first—but before the quads were born, I ate it all!"

Think takeout.

It's not always possible or practical to cook at home. Perhaps you and your partner both have busy schedules, or you've been put on bedrest, or you just don't feel like cooking. Yet that doesn't mean you can't eat well. Most grocery stores have a prepared-foods section, and delicatessens offer good-as-homemade lunch and dinner entrées and desserts. Depending on where you live, you may be able to place online orders for fresh fruits and vegetables or prepared meals, and have them delivered to your home. See what's available in your area. Judy Levy says, "I bought chopped liver in bulk from the best deli in town, and ate tons of it on crackers every night as a bedtime snack. At birth, Micah Marie weighed 7 lb. and Kayla weighed 6 lb., 4 oz. I took one look at my chubby, healthy twins and thought, '*That* is where all that chopped liver went.'"

On occasion, even fast-food restaurants can help you meet your dietary needs. Most offer hot breakfasts that provide plenty of calories and protein, like eggs and Canadian bacon on a biscuit. The hot sandwiches—cheeseburger, fish fillet, grilled chicken patty on a bun—are also good sources of calories and protein. Many fast-food restaurants offer extras like yogurt smoothies, baked potato bars, and hot chili. Look for a salad bar to round out the meal.

Practice on-the-job snacking savvy.

Remember, when you are pregnant with multiples, you should be eating *at least five times a day*—more often if you were slender before this pregnancy, or if you're expecting triplets or quads. This includes workdays. Because your schedule at work is likely to be less predictable than when you are at home, it's wise to bring food to the office. Stock your desk with nonperishables like whole-grain crackers, peanut butter, instant oatmeal, cup-of-soup mixes, canned puddings, and single-serving containers of applesauce.

If you have access to a refrigerator at work, bring in yogurt, cottage cheese, milk, and sandwiches. There's a microwave? A frozen prepared entrée can make a hearty, healthy lunch when paired with fruit or vegetables. You may want to explain your dietary needs to your supervisor or coworkers, but don't let their raised eyebrows keep you from eating whatever and whenever you should. "During business meetings, my boss would lose track of time and forget to break for lunch. I'd be *starving*, yet the conversation would go on and on," says Judy Levy. "Finally I had to throw politeness to the wind. I'd pack my pockets and purse with snacks—crackers, bananas, yogurt—and just dip in and eat whenever I got hungry. My boss would laugh and say to our clients, 'Don't mind her; she's expecting twins.' But he never got the hint that I needed real food."

Eat right, on the road and in the air.

If your work involves travel, whether around town or around the world, it's important to plan ahead for your diet. Keep beverages and snacks in your car, just in case you are running late or get caught in traffic. Stacy Moore says, "Since I sell advertising to car dealerships, I do most of my work from my car. To make sure I'd have plenty of food on hand during the workday, I packed a cooler with sandwiches, cheese, yogurt, and fruit, and ate between visits to clients."

When traveling by plane, you may not always know when or even if you'll be served a meal. Pack your carry-on bag with easy-to-eat snacks like peanut-butter crackers, mini-cheeses, and apples. The dry air of an airliner's pressurized cabin contributes to dehydration, so also purchase plenty of bottled water and juice boxes before boarding. Staying hydrated minimizes the uterine contractions that can lead to preterm labor. It also helps prevent the uncomfortable swelling that can result from sitting still too long, because all those fluids force you to get up and walk down the aisle to the bathroom.

Once you arrive at your destination, follow this strategy from Helen Armer: "Early in my triplet pregnancy, I had to travel on business several times a month. As soon as I got to the city where I was staying, I'd rent a car, find a grocery store, and buy whatever I needed to eat while at the hotel."

Additional tactics to try: Each morning, have a healthy and filling breakfast sent up by room service. If you are joining a client for lunch or dinner at a restaurant, order an appetizer, salad, soup, and entrée—even if your client is eating light, you and your babies need a complete meal.

Drink Water, Water Everywhere

Water is vital for every living creature. But when you're expecting multiples, it's particularly essential—for you and your babies. Here's why:

- Dehydration can trigger uterine contractions, which in turn can lead to premature birth. When you get dehydrated, your brain secretes the hormone vasopressin, which is almost identical to oxytocin—and oxytocin can be used to induce labor. "Anytime I slacked off on my water intake, I got dehydrated and started having contractions—sometimes as many as 12 an hour!" says quad mom Anne Seifert.
- The hormonal changes that occur during pregnancy make you more prone to urinary-tract infections, which also can trigger premature labor. Drinking plenty of water guards against this potential complication.
- During pregnancy, your metabolism revs up. In the first trimester, before your blood volume increases, an adequate intake of fluids helps to dissipate some of this additional body heat.
- Pregnancy hormones can leave you constipated. Drinking water improves regularity.
- Staying hydrated reduces your susceptibility to headaches, dry itchy skin, and complexion problems.

How much should you be drinking? Aim for at least *eight 16-ounce glasses* of water every day. Although taking in this much water every day may seem like a formidable task, with some forethought it can be integrated into your daily routine as easily as any other healthy habit.

"To keep track of my water intake and make sure I was getting enough, I developed a system," says triplet mom Ginny Seyler. "Each night, I filled up three jugs with Brita-filtered tap water and put them in the refrigerator. The following day, I made sure I finished one entire jug every few hours—for instance, one by lunchtime, the second by late afternoon, and the last one before bedtime."

For maximum convenience, plan to have water within easy reach at all times. Helen Armer, another mother of triplets, says, "At work, I kept a bottle of water on my desk constantly. After I went on bedrest, there was always a jug of water on the nightstand." In your car, keep a jumbo thermos of water and a travel mug (to reduce spills), or a cooler stocked with bottled water.

Some women have trouble developing a water-drinking habit because water just doesn't appeal to them. If that's true for you, experiment with the following ideas from other moms of multiples:

- "I like my water cold, so each night I froze several sports bottles full of water. That way they stayed refreshingly icy all through the next day while I was driving around in my car for work," says Stacy Moore.
- Lydia Greenwood, mother of boy/girl twins, had the opposite preference. "Ice water gave me stomach cramps. I preferred liter-size bottles of water served at room temperature."
- Some women find that a touch of flavor helps. "Getting all that water down was easier if I added a lemon slice or splash of fruit juice to it," says twin mom Marcy Bugajski.

There is one downside: "Drinking so much water every day made me have to go to the bathroom every 15 minutes," Marcy says. "I learned to finish it all by dinnertime so that I'd have a chance to urinate it all out before I went to sleep."

You can use those bathroom breaks as a means of double-checking your hydration level. "Dr. Luke told me to monitor myself. If I wasn't urinating at least once every two hours, or if my urine wasn't almost colorless, it meant I needed to drink more water," explains Judy Levy.

Understand that this prescription for fluids means mostly H_2O. Other beverages, if consumed in excess, have disadvantages:

- Milk is low in iron, and filling up on too much may decrease your appetite for iron-rich foods like beef and pork. A quart or two of milk per day is great for providing calcium and protein, but don't overdo it.
- Fruit juices can cause wide swings in your blood sugar levels. Limit juice to no more than 8 ounces per day.
- Carbonated beverages may make your stomach uncomfortably bloated, leaving little room for the food you and your babies need.
- Coffee and many types of tea contain caffeine, which can lead to unstable blood sugar levels as well as irritability, nervousness, and fatigue. They also act as a diuretic and thereby contribute to dehydration, which can in turn trigger contractions. What's more, caffeine can interfere with the absorption of minerals,

particularly calcium. Your best bet is to avoid caffeine during pregnancy, or at least to limit coffee and tea to no more than one or two cups daily.

So stick to water. You'll soon develop a taste for it, if you haven't already. To inspire you, here is one reader's success story: "My nurse said I was one of the most hydrated people she had ever seen. I told her that I had read about how important it was to drink, drink, drink as much water as possible—and so I did. The nurse said it was probably a factor in having such a lengthy twin pregnancy. My girls were 7 lb., 6 oz. and 6 lb., 11 oz. They left the hospital with me after three days."

Another bonus? Keeping up the water habit after you deliver will help you get your figure back more quickly.

Stay Motivated

Some expectant mothers of multiples find it fairly easy to eat the right foods in sufficient quantity to nourish their unborn babies. "When I got pregnant with my triplets, I was already accustomed to eating healthily, so I didn't have to make a lot of changes other than to eat more often and in greater quantity. And it's not like I had to force myself to eat, because I felt hungry," says Allison MacDonald. "I ended up gaining 60 pounds and carrying my babies for 36 full weeks. At birth, they were big for triplets—Drew weighed 5 lb., 8 oz., Cooper weighed 5 lb., 1 oz., and Shelby weighed 4 lb., 11 oz."

If moments do arise when it feels difficult to eat yet another snack or drink yet another glass of water, you may find it inspirational to have a graphic illustration of how your babies grow as the weeks of pregnancy pass. So imagine for a moment your babies' heads. What size are they now? What size will they be next month? What size will they be the first time you hold your newborns in your arms? Provided they are properly nourished, here's what you can expect:

- At 12 weeks into the pregnancy, your babies' heads are each about the size of a grape.
- At 16 weeks, the size of an apricot.
- At 20 weeks, the size of an egg.
- At 24 weeks, the size of a tangerine.
- At 28 weeks, the size of a lemon.

- At 32 weeks, the size of a large orange.
- At 36 weeks, the size of a grapefruit.
- At 40 weeks, the size of a small cantaloupe.

Given the proper guidance about diet and hydration, most expectant mothers of multiples are happy for the opportunity to have such a direct and positive influence on their pregnancy. Stacy Moore states it simply and eloquently when she says, "I was told that the bigger my twins were at birth, the more likely it was I'd be able to bring them home with me when I left the hospital. So I ate and ate and ate. And guess what? My boys did come home with me, just three days after their birth. For me, that was the ultimate goal—and the ultimate reward."

Chapter Five

Smart Dietary Strategies: Supplements and Special Situations

Even though you now know how much weight to gain and what to eat, you may still have questions about your own unique situation. For instance, should you take dietary supplements, and if so, which ones? What should you do if morning sickness makes it hard to get the nourishment you need? What are the particular dietary needs of women who are accustomed to following a vegetarian diet, or who develop gestational diabetes, or who have a history of bariatric surgery? In addition, you need to know about the ingestibles your babies want you to avoid.

Do You Need Vitamin or Mineral Pills?

With all the good food you're getting by following the dietary recommendations in this book, you're already a long way toward fulfilling your babies' nutritional needs as well as your own. Yet some supplements are still recommended.

Many pregnant women are told to take prenatal multivitamins. However, these may cause several problems:

- They can suppress your appetite, so you take in fewer of the calories your babies need. This is especially problematic with a multiple pregnancy, since your caloric needs are higher than those of a woman who needs to nourish just one baby.

- Because prenatal vitamins often contain too high a level of certain nutrients, they may make you feel nauseated, further affecting your ability to eat needed foods.
- These supplements often increase constipation.
- Prenatal formulas frequently include minerals that can interfere with your body's ability to absorb all the vitamins included in these pills.

So what should you do? Surprising as this may sound, your best bet is to skip traditional prenatal vitamins and, instead, incorporate the following supplements (all sold over the counter in drugstores, health-food stores, and online) into your daily routine.

A MULTIVITAMIN

The latest *Guidelines for Perinatal Care* (7th edition, 2012), issued jointly by the American College of Obstetricians and Gynecologists and the American Academy of Pediatrics, recommends taking a daily multivitamin. Choose a brand that contains only vitamins, not minerals, and that does not exceed the recommended dietary allowances (RDAs) or daily recommended intakes (DRIs) for pregnant women, as shown in Table 5.1. (The RDAs for lactating women are also shown for your future reference.)

Take a single daily dose of a multivitamin with these levels of nutrients during the first trimester of your multiple pregnancy. Increase to a double dose during the second and third trimesters.

Recommended Dietary Allowance (RDA) for Vitamins for Pregnant and Lactating Women

	Pregnant	Lactating
FAT-SOLUBLE VITAMINS		
Vitamin A (mcg/day)	770	1,200
Vitamin D (mcg/day)	15	15
Vitamin E (mcg/day)	15	19
Vitamin K (mcg/day)	90	90

	Pregnant	*Lactating*
WATER-SOLUBLE VITAMINS		
Folic Acid (mcg/day)	600	500
Niacin (mg/day)	18	17
Riboflavin (mg/day)	1.4	1.6
Thiamin (mg/day)	1.4	1.4
Vitamin B_6 (mg/day)	2.6	2.8
Vitamin C (mg/day)	85	120

Table 5.1

FOLIC ACID

Folate and folic acid are forms of vitamin B_9. Folate, the form that occurs naturally in food, is found in green leafy vegetables, beans, tomatoes, various fruits (oranges, melons, bananas), and some meats (including beef liver and kidney). Folic acid is the synthetic form of this vitamin. Since 1998, as required by federal law, folic acid has been added to cold cereals, flour, breads, pasta, and bakery items.

Research has shown that taking folic acid greatly reduces the risk of neural tube defects (such as spina bifida), which occur when a baby's spine does not close properly during development.[1] Studies have also reported that adequate folic acid intake may help control inflammation as well as prolong pregnancy.[2]

Here are the recommendations on dosage:

- All women of childbearing age should get at least 400 micrograms of folic acid per day from supplements or fortified food.[3, 4]

1. Wald N. Prevention of neural tube defects: Results of the Medical Research Council Vitamin Study. Lancet 1991; 338:131–7.
2. Kim H, Hwang J-Y, Ha E-H, et al. Association of maternal folate nutrition and serum C-reactive protein concentrations with gestational age at delivery. European Journal of Clinical Nutrition 2011; 65:350–6.
3. Centers for Disease Control and Prevention. Recommendations for the use of folic acid to reduce the number of cases of spina bifida and other neural tube defects. Morbidity and Mortality Weekly Reports 1992; 41 (no. RR-14).
4. Institute of Medicine. Dietary reference intakes for thiamin, riboflavin, niacin, vitamin B_6, folate, vitamin B_{12}, pantothenic acid, biotin, and choline. Washington, DC: National Academy Press; 1998.

- Women who are pregnant with multiples should supplement with 800 to 1,000 micrograms of folic acid per day.
- Women with a history of a previous pregnancy affected by a neural tube defect should take 4 milligrams (4,000 micrograms) of folic acid per day beginning one month before conception and continuing for at least the first three months of pregnancy.[5]

Check the label on your multivitamin to see how much folic acid it provides. Then take an additional folic acid supplement if necessary to reach the level that is appropriate for you, as outlined above.

CALCIUM, MAGNESIUM, AND ZINC COMBINATION

The World Health Organization has identified calcium, magnesium, and zinc as the nutrients with the most potential for reducing pregnancy complications and improving newborn health—yet these vital minerals are the ones most often lacking in women's diets.[6, 7, 8, 9]

It is most convenient to take a formulation that combines these three minerals in one pill. Look for a brand that contains, per tablet, 333 milligrams of calcium, 133 milligrams of magnesium, and 5 milligrams of zinc. Take three tablets twice daily, for a total daily dose of about 2 grams of calcium, 800 milligrams of magnesium, and 30 milligrams of zinc. Do not take the entire day's dose of minerals all at the same time—your body cannot absorb that much all at once. For the same reason, you should not take your minerals at the same time as you take your multivitamin, because the minerals would reduce your absorption of the vitamins.

Here's what each of these three important minerals can do for your own health, as well as for the health of your babies.

5. Centers for Disease Control and Prevention. Effectiveness in disease and injury prevention: Use of folic acid for prevention of spina bifida and other neural tube defects, 1983–1991. Morbidity and Mortality Weekly Reports 1991; 40:513–6.
6. Gülmezoglu AM, de Onis M, Villar J. Effectiveness of interventions to prevent or treat impaired fetal growth. Obstetrical and Gynecological Survey 1997; 6:139–49.
7. Ramakrishnan U, Manjrekar R, Rivera J, Gonzales-Cossio T, Martorell R. Micronutrients and pregnancy outcome: A review of the literature. Nutrition Research 1998; 19:103–59.
8. Kulier R, de Onis M, Gülmezoglu AM, Villar J. Nutritional interventions for the prevention of maternal morbidity. International Journal of Gynecology & Obstetrics 1998; 63:231–46.
9. Villar J, Gülmezoglu AM, de Onis M. Nutritional and antimicrobial interventions to prevent preterm birth: A review of randomized controlled trials. Obstetrical and Gynecological Survey 1998; 53:575–85.

Calcium: This mineral helps reduce your risk of developing pregnancy complications—primarily pregnancy-induced hypertension (high blood pressure) and preeclampsia. A review of 12 major studies published in the *Cochrane Database of Systematic Reviews*[10] and the *British Journal of Obstetrics and Gynaecology*[11] concluded that supplementing with calcium during pregnancy reduced the risk of preeclampsia by *one-half*. A large World Health Organization study of calcium supplementation at the level of 1.5 grams per day among women pregnant with singletons showed a significant reduction in severe gestational hypertension and maternal morbidity, as well as lower rates of prematurity and neonatal mortality.[12] In addition, studies show that children born to mothers who took calcium during pregnancy generally have lower blood pressure in childhood.[13]

Another important function of calcium supplementation during pregnancy and breast-feeding is to minimize the mobilization of calcium from a mother's bones. Here's what happens: If the woman's intake of dietary calcium is insufficient, the mineral from her own bones is used to meet the body's other needs. This weakens her bones. In addition, as the calcium is mobilized from the mother's bones, lead stored in the bones is released. Because lead is toxic, particularly to the brain and nervous system, this presents a hazard for the developing fetus and the nursing infant. Studies show that increased maternal blood lead levels (particularly those above 10 micrograms per deciliter during the first trimester) are associated with adverse effects on neurodevelopment,[14, 15] as well as greater risks for fetal growth restriction and prematurity. Calcium supplementation (along with higher dairy intake) can protect against the mobilization of both calcium and lead from the mother's bones, as indicated by lower lead levels in umbilical cord blood and breast

10. Hofmeyr GJ, Atallah AN, Duley L. Calcium supplementation during pregnancy for preventing hypertensive disorders and related problems. Cochrane Database of Systematic Reviews 2006; 3:CD00159.
11. Hofmeyr GJ, Duley L, Atallah AN. Dietary calcium supplementation for prevention of pre-eclampsia and related problems: A systematic review and commentary. British Journal of Obstetrics and Gynaecology 2007; 114:933–43.
12. Villar J, Abdel-Aleem H, Merialdi M, et al. World Health Organization Calcium Supplementation for the Prevention of Preeclampsia Trial Group. American Journal of Obstetrics & Gynecology 2006; 194:639–49.
13. Atalla AN, Hofmeyr GJ, Duley L. Calcium supplementation during pregnancy for preventing hypertensive disorders and related problems. Cochrane Database of Systematic Reviews 2000; 3:CD001059.
14. Jelliffe-Pawlowsk LL, Miles SQ, Courtney JG, Materna B, Charlton V. Effect of magnitude and timing of maternal pregnancy blood lead (Pb) levels on birth outcomes. Journal of Perinatology 2006; 26:154–62.
15. Hu H, Téllez-Rojo MM, Bellinger D, et al. Fetal lead exposure at each stage of pregnancy as a predictor of infant mental development. Environmental Health Perspectives 2006; 115:1730–5.

milk.[16, 17, 18, 19, 20] In addition, other studies have shown that maternal calcium supplementation results in better fetal bone mineralization[21]—which means the babies' bones benefit, too.

And there's an added bonus: Calcium supplements also help relieve heartburn, a common discomfort of pregnancy.

Magnesium: This essential mineral lowers your risk for premature labor by relaxing the smooth muscle of the uterus. It also has been shown to be effective in treating preeclampsia and preventing the progression to *eclampsia,* a potentially life-threatening condition that includes seizures. Magnesium also helps minimize heartburn.

Your babies benefit from this mineral, too. Magnesium helps protect unborn babies' developing nervous systems, so even if they are born early, their neurodevelopmental problems may be less severe.[22] In fact, if you are at risk for delivery prior to 32 weeks' gestation, and there is sufficient time, you may be given intravenous magnesium for 12 hours[23] because studies have shown that this helps reduce the risk of cerebral palsy in children born prematurely.[24, 25]

Zinc: During pregnancy, a mother's blood levels of zinc drop by 20 to 30 percent. Low di-

16. Ettinger AS, Téllez-Rojo MM, Amarasiriwardena C, et al. Influence of maternal bone lead burden and calcium intake on levels of lead in breast milk over the course of lactation. American Journal of Epidemiology 2006; 163:48–56.

17. Ettinger AS, Lamadrid-Figueroa H, Téllez-Rojo MM, et al. Effect of calcium supplementation on blood lead levels in pregnancy: A randomized placebo-controlled trial. Environmental Health Perspectives 2009; 117:26–31.

18. Hernández-Avila M, Gonzalez-Cossio T, Hernández-Avila JE, et al. Dietary calcium supplements to lower blood lead levels in lactating women: A randomized placebo-controlled trial. Epidemiology 2003; 14:206–12.

19. Ettinger AS, Hu H, Hernández-Avila M. Dietary calcium supplementation to lower blood lead levels in pregnancy and lactation. Journal of Nutritional Biochemistry 2007; 18:172–8.

20. Hernández-Avila M, Sanin LH, Romieu I, et al. Higher milk intake during pregnancy is associated with lower maternal and umbilical cord lead levels in postpartum women. Environmental Research 1997; 74:116–21.

21. Koo WW, Walters JC, Esterlitz J, Levine RJ, Bush AJ, Sibai B. Maternal calcium supplementation and fetal bone mineralization. Obstetrics & Gynecology 1999; 94:577–82.

22. Crowther CA, Middleton PF, Wilkinson D, et al. Magnesium sulphate at 30 to 34 weeks' gestational age: neuroprotection trial (MAGENTA)-study protocol. BMC Pregnancy and Childbirth 2013; 13:91.

23. Rouse DJ, Hirtz DG, Thom E, et al.; for the Eunice Kennedy Shriver NICHD Maternal-Fetal Medicine Units Network. A randomized, controlled trial of magnesium sulfate for the prevention of cerebral palsy. New England Journal of Medicine 2008; 359:895–905.

24. Doyle LW, Crowther CA, Middleton P, Marret S, Rouse D. Magnesium sulphate for women at risk of preterm birth for neuroprotection of the fetus. Cochrane Database of Systematic Reviews 2009; CD004661.

25. Conde-Agudelo A, Romero R. Antenatal magnesium sulfate for the prevention of cerebral palsy in preterm infants less than 34 weeks' gestation: A systematic review and meta-analysis. American Journal of Obstetrics & Gynecology 2009; 200:595–609.

etary intake of zinc has been linked to a twofold increased risk of low birthweight and preterm delivery, and a threefold increased risk of early preterm birth (less than 33 weeks' gestation).[26] Conversely, zinc supplementation has been shown to improve fetal growth as well as nervous system development.[27] Zinc also is essential for the normal functioning of the immune system. Other studies have shown that zinc supplementation lowers the risk of infection during pregnancy, which is helpful because infection is linked to preterm delivery.

VITAMINS C AND E

These nutrients are *antioxidants,* meaning that they protect cells against harmful molecules called free radicals. The DRI for these nutrients during a singleton pregnancy is 85 milligrams for vitamin C and 15 milligrams for vitamin E. (Vitamin E is sometimes measured in international units, or IU, in which case the DRI is 22 IU.)

In some studies, much higher intakes—1,000 milligrams of vitamin C and 268 milligrams (or 400 IU) of vitamin E[28, 29]—were shown to reduce the risk of preeclampsia, particularly among women who developed this complication in a previous pregnancy. Unfortunately, the encouraging results of these early studies have not been confirmed in larger follow-up trials.[30] Still, the use of these higher therapeutic dosages remains an option, particularly for women with a history of severe or early-onset preeclampsia. So while the type of multivitamin recommended earlier in this chapter would contain the DRI for vitamins C and E, it's worth checking with your physician to see whether higher daily dosages might be appropriate for you.

---

26. Scholl TO, Hediger ML, Schall JI, et al. Low zinc intake during pregnancy: Its association with preterm and very preterm delivery. American Journal of Epidemiology 1993; 137:1115–24.
27. Merialdi M, Caulfield LE, Zavaleta N, Figueroa A, DiPietro JA. Adding zinc to prenatal iron and folate tablets improves fetal neurobehavioral development. American Journal of Obstetrics & Gynecology 1998; 180:483–90.
28. Chappell LC, Seed PT, Briley AL, et al. Effect of antioxidants on the occurrence of pre-eclampsia in women at increased risk: A randomized trial. Lancet 1999; 354:810–16.
29. Chappell LC, Seed PT, Kelly FJ, et al. Vitamin C and E supplementation in women at risk of preeclampsia is associated with changes in indices of oxidative stress and placental function. American Journal of Obstetrics & Gynecology 2002; 187:777–84.
30. Spinnato JA, Freire S, Pinto E, et al. Antioxidant therapy to prevent preeclampsia: a randomized controlled trial. Obstetrics & Gynecology 2007; 110: 1311–18.

Vitamin D

This essential nutrient helps the body absorb and retain other minerals, including calcium. It also activates the immune system[31] and protects against prematurity,[32] preeclampsia,[33] and infections such as bacterial vaginosis.[34] (Adequate vitamin D levels have also been associated with better pregnancy rates among women treated for infertility.[35]) When a mother has adequate vitamin D intake during pregnancy, her baby is born with higher blood levels of this nutrient, and also has the benefit of better bone mineralization as well as improved bone mass in later childhood.[36] In addition, research suggests that the mother's vitamin D status during pregnancy may affect the child's susceptibility to asthma and other chronic disease in later life.[37, 38]

Vitamin D is known as the sunshine vitamin because it is synthesized when skin is exposed to sunlight. In fact, about 90 percent of vitamin D is obtained through sunlight exposure; only about 10 percent comes from food. That's why vitamin D deficiency is more common, especially during winter months, among people who:

- Live in cloudy or smoggy areas.
- Spend less than 30 minutes per week outside (without sunscreen).
- Have dark skin (because dark skin pigment reduces formation of the vitamin).
- Live at northern latitudes. Latitude lines run horizontally on the world map. Degrees of latitude are numbered from 0° at the equator to 90° North at the North Pole and 90° South at the South Pole. If you live north of the 38° North latitude—about the level of a line from San Francisco to Washington, DC—you

31. Liu PT, Stenger S, Li H, et al. Toll-like receptor triggering of a vitamin D–mediated human antimicrobial response. Science 2006; 311:1770–3.
32. Bodnar LM, Rouse DJ, Momirova V, et al. Maternal 25-hydroxyvitamin D and preterm birth in twin gestations. Obstetrics & Gynecology 2013; 122:91–8.
33. Bodnar LM, Catov JM, Simhan HN, et al. Maternal vitamin D deficiency increases the risk of preeclampsia. Journal of Clinical Endocrinology & Metabolism 2007; 92:3517–22.
34. Bodnar LM, Krohn MA, Simhan HN. Maternal vitamin D deficiency is associated with bacterial vaginosis in the first trimester of pregnancy. Journal of Nutrition 2009; 139:1157–61.
35. Polyzos NP, Anckaert E, Guzman L, et al. Vitamin D deficiency and pregnancy rates in women undergoing single embryo, blastocyst stage, transfer (SET) for IVF/ICSI. Human Reproduction 2014; 29:2032–40.
36. Javaid M, Crozier S, Harvey N, et al. Maternal vitamin D status during pregnancy and childhood bone mass at 9 years: A longitudinal study. Lancet 2006; 367:36–43.
37. Hypponen E, Laara F, Reunanen A, Jarvelin MR, Virtanen SM. Intake of vitamin D and risk of type 1 diabetes: A birth-cohort study. Lancet 2001; 358:1500–3.
38. McGrath, J. Does "Imprinting" with low prenatal vitamin D contribute to the risk of various adult disorders? Medical Hypotheses 2001; 56:367–71.

(and your babies) are at increased risk for low vitamin D. To find the latitude where you live, visit www.satsig.net/maps/lat-long-finder.htm.

Your need for vitamin D increases during pregnancy, especially if you had a prepregnancy body mass index (BMI) of 30 or greater. Supplementing can provide the extra vitamin D you need—but there is much debate regarding the appropriate dosage. In 2010, the Food and Nutrition Board of the Institute of Medicine recommended a daily supplement dosage of 15 micrograms (equal to 600 IU) for pregnant or breast-feeding women.[39] However, this recommendation has been challenged by leading nutrition authorities, who maintain that the Institute of Medicine recommendation was miscalculated and that the optimal intake is much higher. Many experts suggest a range of 1,000 to 4,000 IU (25 to 100 micrograms), while others suggest as much as 7,000 to 9,000 IU (175 to 225 micrograms) per day.[40, 41, 42, 43]

DR. NEWMAN: Investigators at the Medical University of South Carolina have been actively studying vitamin D levels in our obstetrical population in Charleston. Based on our review, it appears that the best pregnancy outcomes are associated with a maternal blood level of *25-hydroxy vitamin D* between 40 and 60 ng/ml. One of the most promising benefits appears to be a significant reduction in the risk of preterm birth among women with these vitamin D levels.[44, 45] However, even in Charleston, South Carolina, where there is no shortage of sunshine, more than 80 percent of white women and virtually all black and Hispanic women had vitamin D levels below this threshold—in many cases substantially below, in the range of severe deficiency.

39. Food and Nutrition Board, Institute of Medicine. Dietary reference intakes for calcium and vitamin D. National Academies Press: Washington, DC; 2011.
40. Veugelers PJ, Ekwaru JP. A statistical error in the estimation of the recommended dietary allowance for vitamin D. Nutrients 2014; 6:4472–5.
41. Heaney R, Garland C, Baggerly C, French C, Gorham E. Letter to Veugelers PJ, Ekwaru JP. A statistical error in the estimation of the recommended dietary allowance for vitamin D. Nutrients 2014; 6:4472–5. Nutrients 2015; 7:1688–90.
42. Hollis BW, Wagner CL. Vitamin D requirements during lactation: High-dose maternal supplementation as therapy to prevent hypovitaminosis D for both the mother and the nursing infant. American Journal of Clinical Nutrition 2004; 80(Suppl):1752S–8S.
43. American College of Obstetricians and Gynecologists. Committee opinion. Vitamin D: screening and supplementation during pregnancy. No. 495, July 2011.
44. Wagner CL, McNeil R, Hamilton SA, et al. A randomized trial of vitamin D supplementation in 2 community health center networks in South Carolina. American Journal of Obstetrics & Gynecology 2013; 137: 137–44.
45. Bodnar LM, Platt RW, Simhan HN. Early-pregnancy Vitamin D deficiency and risk of preterm birth subgroups. Obstetrics & Gynecology 2015; 125: 439–47.

It takes about 1,000 IU per day of vitamin D supplementation to raise a person's blood level of vitamin D by 5 ng/ml. This means, for instance, if your blood test shows that your level is only 20 ng/ml and your goal is 40 ng/ml, you need to supplement with 4,000 IU per day.

Table 5.2 has been adapted from information provided by GrassrootsHealth (www.grassrootshealth.net), a public health promotion organization. It can help you and your doctor calculate how much supplemental vitamin D (in the form of vitamin D₃, also called cholecalciferol) you need to take to raise your blood vitamin D level to the optimal range of 40 to 60 ng/ml.

Average Change in Vitamin D Blood Level
Based on Intake (IU per pound of body weight)

Target Level of Vitamin D (ng/ml)	40	50	60
CURRENT LEVEL (NG/ML)			
10	24	35	49
15	21	33	47
20	17	29	43
25	13	25	39
30	9	21	35
35	5	17	31
40		11	25
45		6	20
50			14

Table 5.2

Using Table 5.2 requires some simple math. First, find your current vitamin D blood level (as determined by your blood test) in the left-hand column. Then look to the right to find the number listed under the Target Level column headed with 40. (For instance, if your current level is 20 ng/ml, you will see the number 17.) Now multiply that number by your current body weight. The result is the number of IU of vitamin D_3 that you would need to take daily to increase your blood level to 40 ng/ml. (For example, suppose you weigh 153 pounds. Since $17 \times 153 = 2,601$, taking a daily dose of about 2,600 IU of vitamin D_3 would be expected to raise your blood D level from 20 ng/ml to 40 ng/ml. If your doctor recommends a higher target level of 50 or 60 ng/ml, multiply your body weight by the number listed under the corresponding Target Level.

DR. NEWMAN: Many different vitamin D supplements are available over the counter. A very popular one with our patients is Simply Vitamin D3 produced by Olly. It is a bit more expensive than some other supplements ($14 for 70), but many people enjoy these lemon-flavored chewable gummies. Each gummy provides 2,000 IU of vitamin D_3. Our expectant mothers typically take one, two, or three gummies per day, depending on the severity of their vitamin D deficiency.

FISH OIL

Like fish, fish oil supplements are an excellent source of long-chain omega-3 essential fatty acids, such as *docosahexaenoic acid* (DHA). Omega-3s play an important role in reducing both inflammation and the risk for prematurity.[46] When mothers supplement with fish oil during pregnancy, babies are born with higher blood levels of omega-3s[47]—and may have better visual acuity, cognition, and verbal and motor development.[48, 49]

Fish oil supplementation helps moms, too, by protecting their own stores of omega-3s, reducing postpartum depression, and improving cardiovascular health. For instance, DHA lowers blood levels of artery-clogging triglycerides (a type of blood fat), while another essential long-chain fatty acid called *eicosapentaenoic acid* (EPA) increases high-density lipoproteins

---

46. Roman AS, Schreher J, Mackenzie AP, Nathaniels PW. Omega-3 fatty acids and decidual cell prostaglandin production in response to the inflammatory cytokine Il-1. American Journal of Obstetrics & Gynecology 2006; 195:1693–9.

47. Krauss-Etschmann S, Shadid R, Campoy C, et al. Nutrition and Health Lifestyle (NUHEAL) Study Group. Effects of fish-oil and folate supplementation of pregnant women on maternal and fetal plasma concentrations of docosahexaenoic acid and eicosapentaenoic acid: A European randomized multicenter trial. American Journal of Clinical Nutrition 2007; 85:1392–1400.

48. Jacobson JL, Jacobson SW, Muckle G, et al. Beneficial effects of a polyunsaturated fatty acid on infant development: Evidence from the Inuit of Artic Quebec. Journal of Pediatrics 2008; 152:356–64.

49. Strain JJ, Davidson PW, Thurston SW, et al. Maternal PUFA status but not prenatal methylmercury exposure is associated with children's language functions at age five years in the Seychelles. Journal of Nutrition 2012; 142:1943–9.

(HDL), the good cholesterol. In addition, DHA may protect against age-related macular degeneration (a leading cause of blindness) and Alzheimer's disease, as well as combating prostate cancer in men.

American, Canadian, and European expert groups have all recommended an intake of at least 200 milligrams per day of DHA during a singleton pregnancy and lactation,[50, 51] while other researchers have suggested even higher dosages.[52] For a multiple pregnancy, supplements of 1,000 milligrams per day or more would be ideal, since the drain is greater with more than one baby.[53] Although eating fish is the optimal way to get omega-3s, most women do not consume enough fish or other DHA-rich foods to reach the target. Therefore, taking fish oil supplements is a good way to increase intake. For people who prefer a vegetarian source of omega-3s, algal oil is a reasonable alternative.

Nutritional Supplement Drinks: Turbo-Boosters for Your Diet

TAMARA: During the 18th week of my twin pregnancy, I lunched at a restaurant with seven coworkers—and five of us wound up with salmonella food poisoning. After nearly two weeks of nonstop vomiting and diarrhea, for which I was hospitalized, I had lost 16 pounds—everything I'd gained during my pregnancy, and then some. My already slender frame became spindly and my face looked almost skeletal.

As soon as I felt better, I worked hard to put the weight back on (and to persuade the local Department of Health to investigate that restaurant!). But for the twins growing inside me, the lost ground was never regained. At birth, they were *small for gestational age* (SGA)—the term doctors use to describe babies who are born weighing less than the 10th percentile for their gestational age. And because my babies were born nine weeks early, their SGA status compounded the problems associated with their prematurity.

50. American Dietetic Association and Dietitians of Canada. Position paper. Dietary fatty acids. Journal of the American Dietetic Association 2007; 107:1599–1611.
51. Koletzko B, Cetin I, Brenna JT; for the Perinatal Lipid Intake Working Group. Consensus statement: Dietary fat intakes for pregnant and lactating women. British Journal of Nutrition 2007; 98:873–7.
52. Jacobson JL, Jacobson SW, Muckle G, Kaplan-Estrin M, Ayotte P, Dewailly E. Beneficial effects of a polyunsaturated fatty acid on infant development: Evidence from the Inuit of Arctic Quebec. Journal of Pediatrics 2008; 152:356–64.
53. Foreman-van Drongelen, MMHP, Zeijdner EE, Houwelingen AC, et al. Essential fatty acid status measured in umbilical vessel walls of infants born after a multiple pregnancy. Early Human Development 1996; 46:205–15.

DR. LUKE: I wish I'd known Tamara when she was pregnant, because I'd have recommended that she immediately add nutritional supplement drinks to her daily diet. Any woman who loses weight while carrying multiples—whether from the nausea and vomiting of severe morning sickness, the flu, food poisoning, or any other illness—can benefit from these special products. I also recommend nutritional supplement drinks for pregnant women who begin pregnancy underweight, for ex-smokers (whose nutritional status is often compromised), and for anyone expecting three or more babies.

Nutritional supplement drinks are specially formulated beverages, available in ready-to-drink and powder form. They are nutritionally balanced, calorically concentrated, and easy to digest. Taken between meals and before bed—*not* as a replacement for meals—they can be a key factor in helping you achieve the early, rapid weight gain you need. One reader reports, "I can't always get enough calories from food alone because there simply is not enough space inside me. But it's very easy to drink these beverages throughout the day to make sure my little ones are getting enough nourishment."

There are three basic types of nutritional supplement drinks. Here's how they compare to a glass of whole milk:

- *Regular supplement drinks*: These provide one-third to two-thirds more calories than does the same-size serving of milk. They also contain 50 percent more protein and three times the carbohydrate. Two or three servings a day increase your caloric intake by 400 to 750 calories.
- *High-calorie or high-protein supplement drinks*: This type supplies about twice as much protein and four times as much carbohydrate as a glass of whole milk. These supplements also contain double the calories, so two or three servings daily can add 500 to 1,000 calories to your diet. These are often your best choice, because they're available in a wide range of flavors, which keeps your taste buds from getting bored, and because you can buy them in most supermarkets and drugstores.
- *High-calorie and high-protein supplement drinks*: Ounce for ounce, these pack the biggest nutritional punch. They're most useful for improving your nutritional status as quickly as possible, and with the smallest quantity of food. Compared to a glass of whole milk, these supplements provide more than three times as many calories, two to three times as much protein and fat, and more than four times the carbohydrate. Two to three servings per day add 900 to 1,400 calories to your

diet. In addition, they provide as much as 60 grams of high-quality protein—the equivalent of 20 ounces of steak! Although they cost about the same as high-calorie or high-protein supplement drinks, they are not as readily available in local stores, so ask your pharmacist to order them for you. Check with your health insurer, too, since these special supplements may be covered under your plan if your obstetrician writes you a prescription.

These types of nutritional supplement drinks also can be ordered online or by phone directly from manufacturers and delivered to your door. For maximum economy and convenience, buy several cans in your local store to see if you like the taste, then order them in quantity from these manufacturers:

- Carnation: Telephone 800-289-7313; website www.carnationbreakfastessentials .com. *Carnation Instant Breakfast brand.*
- Nestlé HealthCare Nutrition: Consumer & Product Support, 445 State Street, Fremont MI 49412. Telephone 800-247-7893 or 888-240-2713; website www .boost.com or www.nestlenutritionstore.com. *Boost brand nutritional drinks.*
- Ross/Abbott Nutrition: 625 Cleveland Avenue, Columbus, OH 43215-1724. Telephone 800-227-5767 or 800-986-8501; website www.abbottnutrition.com or www.ensure.com. *Ensure, Promote, and TwoCalHN brands.*

Nutritional supplement drinks are not for everyone. Because these beverages are sweet and rich, some women find that drinking them can trigger nausea, depress the appetite, or lead to diarrhea. However, for many moms-to-be of multiples, these high-powered dietary products are a boon. Anne Seifert says, "I drank two cans of supplements daily from my ninth week of pregnancy until the day I delivered my quads. Because they are really thick, like sweetened condensed milk, I thought they tasted best when served ice cold or diluted with water. For variety, I mixed in chocolate powder or blended in some fresh fruit. Especially considering the trouble I had eating much food in the final weeks, I think these drinks helped my babies to be born bigger than they otherwise would have been." Other women report that blending the supplement drink with ice cream to make a milkshake enhances the nutritional value as well as the flavor.

Comparison of Nutritional Supplement Drinks

(Per 8-ounce serving)

	Calories	Protein (g)	Carbs (g)	Fat (g)	Flavors
Whole Milk	150	8	12	8	Plain
Regular Supplements					
Ensure	250	9	41	6	Vanilla, Milk Chocolate, Dark Chocolate, Strawberry, Butter Pecan, Coffee Latte
Ensure High Calcium	220	10	31	6	Vanilla, Milk Chocolate
Ensure Fiber	250	9	42	6	Vanilla, Milk Chocolate
Boost Drink	240	10	41	4	Vanilla, Chocolate, Strawberry, Butter Pecan
High-Protein Supplements					
Ensure Plus	350	13	50	11	Vanilla, Milk Chocolate, Dark Chocolate, Strawberry, Butter Pecan
Ensure High Protein	230	12	31	6	Vanilla, Milk Chocolate, Wild Berry, Banana Cream
Promote Vanilla	240	15	31	6	Vanilla
Promote with Fiber	240	15	33	7	Vanilla
Boost Plus	360	14	45	14	Vanilla, Chocolate, Strawberry
Boost High Protein	240	15	33	6	Vanilla, Chocolate, Strawberry

	Calories	Protein (g)	Carbs (g)	Fat (g)	Flavors
High-Protein Supplements					
Carnation Instant Breakfast Original Ready-to-Drink	250	14	34	5	Vanilla, Milk Chocolate
Carnation Instant Breakfast No Sugar Added Ready-to-Drink	150	13	16	5	Milk Chocolate
Carnation Instant Breakfast Powder added to skim milk	220	13	39	1	Vanilla, Milk Chocolate, Chocolate Malt, Strawberry
Carnation Instant Breakfast No Sugar Added Powder added to skim milk	150	13	24	0	Vanilla, Chocolate
High-Protein, High-Calorie Supplements					
TwoCalHN	475	20	52	21.5	Vanilla, Butter Pecan

Table 5.3

Managing Morning Sickness

If you are lucky, you won't ever feel sick to your stomach during your pregnancy—some women don't. But, sorry to say, many expectant mothers of multiples do experience nausea and vomiting—and the more babies you're expecting, the worse it's likely to be. That's because these symptoms are triggered by pregnancy hormones, which, of course, are present in much higher amounts when you're expecting more than one baby. In this regard, that queasy feeling is a positive sign: It indicates that the placenta or placentas are growing and producing sufficient hormones for the pregnancy to continue.

Morning sickness is in fact an inaccurate name. "I felt nauseous almost all the time. For me, it was morning-noon-and-night sickness," says Marcy Bugajski, mother of fraternal twin boys. "It's hard to work up an appetite when you're constantly vomiting."

Finding successful ways to cope with queasiness is important, not only because you want to feel better, but also because you need to eat (and keep it down) if your babies are to thrive. Fortunately, there are many techniques for overcoming morning sickness. Use trial and error to find the ones that are most effective for you.

- The current thinking in the treatment of nausea and vomiting is the salty-and-sweet approach. Try eating some pretzels and lemonade, or some potato chips and cola. Though these foods are not very nutritious, they are often easier to keep down—and that's important during this difficult stage of pregnancy. Says Judy Levy, "This tactic really worked for me. The combination of lemonade and potato chips eased my nausea pretty quickly. Once I was feeling better, I could go on to eat healthier foods the rest of the day."
- Some women find it helpful to suck on sour candy or chew gum. "Lemonheads candy and Big Red chewing gum were my secret weapons. I could count on them to quell the nausea, at least for a while. This was especially important if I was out of the house," says Kelly McDaniel, mother of boy/girl twins.
- Going too long without eating or drinking causes your blood sugar to drop, which in turn can trigger nausea. So eat frequently—at least every two hours. In your purse or briefcase, carry portable snacks such as peanut-butter crackers and a juice box.
- Take advantage of any lulls in the nausea. Megan Ryerson, mother of boy/girl twins, says, "Whenever my nausea let up, I ate as much as I could because I knew the opportunity would be fleeting. I carried around bagels with almond butter and other simple but flavorful foods, so I'd be ready the instant the moment came that I'd be able to stomach them."
- It's a myth that eating only fruit will ease morning sickness. Though fruit triggers a rapid rise in blood sugar that makes you feel better for a short while, soon your blood sugar falls again, leaving you even more nauseated than before. To keep blood sugar on a more even keel, be sure to eat protein along with a carbohydrate snack.
- Be aware that foods you normally enjoy may be completely unappealing to you now. "I had always loved sweets, but during my quadruplet pregnancy, they made me sick. Yet here was the one time I needed such high-calorie foods!" says Anne Seifert. "Fortunately, I found that ice cream didn't upset my stomach the way candy or chocolate did."
- Some women find that dairy products stay down most easily. If that's true for you, when nausea strikes, reach for milk, yogurt, cottage cheese, ice cream, or a milkshake. Other women report that they do better with carbs. "Sweet potatoes,

baked potatoes, bread and biscuits—these were the foods that I could keep down best. I knew that I needed protein, too, so during those early months, I ate a lot of egg-and-muffin sandwiches," says Kelly McDaniel.

- If you tend to vomit even when your stomach is empty, try sucking on a Popsicle. "I ate a lot of Popsicles for breakfast," says Karen Danke, mother of fraternal twin boys. "Vomiting up a Popsicle was a lot less unpleasant than having the dry heaves."

- If mornings are your worst time, set your alarm for 2 A.M. (unless you can already count on a full bladder to awaken you in the middle of the night). Get up and have a bowl of cereal with milk, then go back to bed. When you wake up in the morning, your blood sugar won't be as low as it otherwise would have been. For many women, this reduces early-morning nausea.

- If you can't stand the thought of getting out of bed at night (after all, you'll be doing that often enough after the babies are born), keep a pack of dry crackers on your nightstand. Munch a few as soon as you wake up in the morning, even before climbing out from under the covers. Or ask your partner to provide a few bites of breakfast in bed. Karen Danke says, "It helped to have my husband bring me some dry toast to eat before I even tried to get up."

- Keep a queasiness diary. For a few days, write down the foods you eat and try to find a pattern to your nausea. You may notice, for example, that eating fried foods sends you running for the bathroom. Skip the French fries in favor of a more nutritious and digestible baked potato.

- In your diary, also make note of any smells that upset your stomach, then take steps to avoid these odors. Common offenders include cigarette smoke, perfume, coffee, and fish. "The odor of my cat's canned food never failed to make me throw up," says Karen Danke. If you feel nauseated while preparing a meal, it could be that cooking smells are setting you off. The fix: Get takeout, have your partner handle the cooking, or eat in a breezy, well-ventilated area away from the kitchen—or have an outdoor picnic, weather permitting.

- According to Eastern medicine traditions, ginger has a great ability to ease digestion and prevent nausea and vomiting. So try this recipe to see whether sipping ginger tea settles your stomach: Peel and finely dice a knuckle-size piece of fresh ginger. Place in a mug and fill with boiling water; steep for five to eight minutes. Add brown sugar to taste.

- Try herbal infusions and green and black teas by Tazo. Ones that may be particularly helpful for nausea during pregnancy include:

Calm herbal infusion (with chamomile)

Citron black tea (with orange and lemon)

Green Ginger green tea (with ginger)

Lemon Maté herbal infusion (with green yerba maté, lemon myrtle, ginger, and cardamom)

Organic Spicy Ginger herbal infusion (with ginger, green rooibos, citrus, chamomile, and licorice root)

Refresh herbal infusion (with peppermint, spearmint, and tarragon)

Wild Sweet Orange herbal infusion (with lemongrass, citrus, licorice root, and orange essence)

Zen green tea (with lemongrass, spearmint, and lemon essence)

- Whip up a Ginger Smoothie, included in the recipe section of this book (Appendix A). It is specifically designed to ease nausea, and it tastes delicious.
- Try the ginger beverages and ginger candies by the Ginger People (www.gingerpeople .com), available in many supermarkets. Nonalcoholic *Ginger Beer* and *Lemon Ginger Beer*, as well as *Ginger 'Gizer* and *Ginger Soother*, pack a healthy dose of ginger to soothe your stomach and reduce nausea. The Ginger People also make delicious *Ginger Chews*, *Gin Gins*, and *Gin Gins Boost* ginger candies—great to keep on hand at home, in the car, and in your purse for whenever an upset stomach strikes.
- You'd rather swallow a pill than sip tea or smoothies? Studies show that, in dosages of 1 gram per day, capsules containing ginger significantly reduce nausea and vomiting in pregnancy.
- Dress for comfort. Clothing that's too snug around the waist or neck can trigger the gag reflex. Skip the turtlenecks and buttoned-up collars in favor of crewnecks and V-necks. Hit the stores for loose-fitting maternity skirts and slacks, rather than squeezing into your prepregnancy wardrobe. Wear belts around the hips rather than the waist. Switch from briefs to bikini underpants.
- Try acupressure. Look in pharmacies or health food stores for a pair of antinausea wristbands called Sea-Bands or Psi Bands (typically advertised as a remedy for motion sickness). Each elasticized band has a plastic button that presses on the acupressure point P6 on the wrist, which is known to ease queasiness. The P6 point is located on the palm side of the wrist. To locate the point, place the middle three fingers of one hand on the inside of the opposite wrist, with the edge of the ring finger on the wrist crease. The P6 point is under the edge of the index finger, about 1½ to 2 inches from the wrist crease, in the midline. Repeat on the opposite side to

find the P6 point on the other wrist. For best results, the P6 point should be pressed and released repeatedly, for about 5 seconds at a time, continuing until nausea eases.

- Consider an over-the-counter mild sleep aid called Unisom SleepTabs. Each tablet contains a low dose (25 milligrams) of doxylamine succinate, an antihistamine that has proven effective in reducing nausea and vomiting during pregnancy. (Make sure that you purchase the Unisom SleepTabs—not other Unisom products, such as Unisom SleepMinis or Unisom SleepGels, that contain Benadryl instead of doxylamine.) Take one Unisom SleepTab at bedtime along with a 30-milligram dose of a vitamin B_6 supplement to see if it helps prevent morning nausea and vomiting.
- Ask your doctor about the prescription oral medication Diclegis, which contains 10 milligrams of doxylamine and 10 milligrams of vitamin B_6 (pyridoxine) combined into one pill. The usual dose is two pills at bedtime and two more the following morning if needed. Four tablets per day is the maximum dose. Diclegis was recently approved by the FDA for preventing nausea and vomiting and, according to the FDA, is considered safe for use during pregnancy.

None of these strategies relieves your morning sickness? Don't cajole yourself into putting up and shutting up. Instead, call your obstetrician right away if:

- You haven't been able to keep any food or water down for 24 hours or more.
- Your mouth, eyes, and skin feel dry.
- You are becoming increasingly weak and fatigued.
- Your ability to think clearly and to concentrate is decreasing.

These are signs of serious dehydration. You may need to be admitted to the hospital to receive fluids, nutrients, and medications intravenously. In fact, about 42,000 pregnant women in the United States are hospitalized every year for severe nausea and vomiting, also called *hyperemesis gravidarum*. The treatment you receive in the hospital should help you feel better fast—and that's exactly what your unborn babies need most.

Rest assured, though, that for most expectant mothers of multiples, symptoms subside by the end of the first trimester. Even though the placental hormones that contribute to morning sickness rise faster and higher with multiples than with a singleton, they will fall back around week 12 to week 14 of your pregnancy. Says Karen Danke, "The most encouraging thing I can say about morning sickness is that it does eventually come to an end. Hang in there! And in the meantime, try all the tips anyone offers for easing the nausea. You never know what might work for you."

Guidelines for Vegetarians

DR. LUKE: Normally, a vegetarian diet can be very healthful if you are knowledgeable about nutrition, conscientious about getting enough protein, and careful to combine foods properly to ensure that you get all the essential amino acids. Remember, though, that a multiple pregnancy places extra demands on your body, including a greatly increased need for calories and protein. Satisfying these demands can make a significant difference in the size and health of your babies at birth. These nutritional needs can be met most easily and reliably through a diet that includes animal-based proteins, particularly red meat.

However, if you are strongly committed to vegetarianism and are willing to monitor your food intake carefully, the following section can help you satisfy your own and your babies' nutritional needs. Be sure to check out the many vegetarian recipes at the back of this book. I've designed each one for maximum nutrition—plus great taste.

There are several different types of vegetarian diets. As shown in Table 5.4, some vegetarian diets are far more restrictive than others.

Types of Vegetarian Diets

Vegan	Eliminates all animal products, including eggs and cheese, concentrating solely on vegetables, legumes, fruits, grains, nuts, and seeds.
Macrobiotic	Emphasizes cooked foods, especially whole grains, with moderate amounts of vegetables and beans, minimal amounts of fruits, little if any dairy foods or eggs, and occasional small servings of mild white fish.
Lacto-vegetarian	Includes dairy products along with vegetables, fruits, and grains, but eliminates eggs.
Ovo-vegetarian	Includes eggs along with vegetables, fruits, and grains, but eliminates dairy products.
Lacto-ovo-vegetarian	Includes dairy products and eggs along with vegetables, fruits, and grains.

Table 5.4

Protein is critical to a healthy pregnancy because it provides the body's basic building blocks. In fact, protein is the single most vital nutrient for your babies' growth. That's why the focus of this section is on a lacto-ovo-vegetarian diet, which includes both eggs and dairy products. Omitting these vital components makes it extremely difficult to meet the nutritional demands of a multiple pregnancy (or even a singleton pregnancy).

If you currently follow a vegan, macrobiotic, or other more restrictive diet, it is extremely important that you add eggs and dairy to your diet starting today. In fact, every meal or snack you eat should include milk, cheese, or yogurt. Eat plenty of eggs, too. Egg whites contain the highest-quality protein, while egg yolks are an excellent source of iron.

The chief components of protein are 20 amino acids that are needed for protein synthesis (see Table 5.5). Of these acids, 10 are considered nonessential because the body can synthesize them. However, the remaining 10 cannot be formed by the body and must be supplied from food. These 10 are termed *essential amino acids*.

The Amino Acids

Nonessential Amino Acids	*Essential Amino Acids*
Alanine	Arginine
Asparagine	Histidine
Aspartic acid	Isoleucine
Cysteine	Leucine
Glutamic acid	Lysine
Glutamine	Methionine
Glycine	Phenylalanine
Proline	Threonine
Serine	Tryptophan
Tyrosine	Valine

Table 5.5

Foods that provide all of the essential amino acids include milk, yogurt, cheese, and eggs (as well as beef, poultry, and fish). Many other foods contain protein, but are missing one or more of the essential amino acids, or provide them only in very small amounts.

In planning your pregnancy diet, consult Table 5.6 and Table 5.7. They will help you identify the foods that can best provide the essential amino acids. Table 5.6 compares the amino acid content (in grams) of a typical-size serving for each type of food—for instance, 8 ounces of milk versus 3.5 ounces of fish versus 1 ounce of cheese. *Important*: When referring to Tables 5.6 and 5.7, note that the boldface numbers in each column represent the six foods with the highest content of each of the essential amino acids.

For the sake of comparison, these foods can be ranked according to the number of boldface figures each food merits, per serving. (Remember, a boldface figure indicates that the food is one of the top six providers of a given amino acid.) Awarding one point for each figure, here's how these foods stack up:

- Beef, chicken, and fish: 10 points.
- Eggs: 10 points.
- Cottage cheese: 9 points.
- Yogurt: 8 points.
- Milk: 1 point.
- Peanut butter: 1 point.
- Lentils: 1 point.

Some vegetarian readers may be more accustomed to analyzing food choices in terms of equal amounts of food, rather than by the typical serving sizes used in Table 5.6. For that reason, Table 5.7 provides a comparison of the amino acid content of various protein-rich foods, based on equal weight—in this case, 100 grams, or about 3.5 ounces. Again, the boldface numbers in each column represent the six foods with the highest content (per 100 grams) of each of the essential amino acids.

The foods can also be compared according to the number of boldface figures each earns, per 100 grams. Awarding one point for each boldface figure, here's how they rank:

- Beef, chicken, and fish: 10 points.
- Cheese: 10 points.
- Peanut butter: 9 points.
- Cottage cheese: 7 points.
- Eggs: 4 points.

Essential Amino Acid Content (in Grams) of Protein-Rich Foods, per Serving

Food	Serving Size	Arginine	Histidine	Isoleucine	Leucine	Lysine	Methionine
Beef	3.5 oz.	**1.87**	**1.01**	**1.33**	**2.34**	**2.46**	**0.76**
Chicken	3.5 oz.	**1.71**	**0.80**	**1.36**	**1.99**	**2.22**	**0.73**
Fish	3.5 oz.	**1.48**	**0.73**	**1.14**	**2.00**	**2.27**	**0.73**
Cheese	1 oz.	0.27	0.25	0.44	0.68	0.59	0.19
Peanut butter	2 tbsp.	**0.97**	0.20	0.28	0.52	0.29	0.10
Cottage cheese	3.5 oz.	0.57	**0.42**	**0.73**	**1.28**	**1.01**	**0.38**
Eggs	2 jumbo (130 g)	**0.98**	0.38	0.88	1.38	1.16	**0.50**
Lentils	3.5 oz.	**0.70**	0.25	0.39	0.65	0.63	0.08
Yogurt	8 oz.	0.42	**0.35**	**0.77**	**1.41**	**1.26**	**0.41**
Tofu	3.5 oz.	0.44	0.19	0.32	0.50	0.43	0.08
Bread	2 slices (60 g)	0.18	0.10	0.20	0.34	0.14	0.08
Milk	8 oz.	0.29	0.22	0.49	0.79	0.64	0.20

Phenylalanine	Threonine	Tryptophan (kcal)	Valine (g)	Calories (g)	Protein (g)	Carbohydrate	Fat
1.16	**1.29**	**0.33**	**1.44**	222	29.6	0	10.7
1.06	**1.13**	**0.31**	**1.33**	239	27.3	0	13.6
0.96	**1.08**	**0.28**	**1.27**	113	24.7	0	0.9
0.37	0.25	0.09	0.47	114	7.1	0	9.4
0.42	0.28	0.08	0.34	190	8.1	6.2	16.3
0.67	**0.55**	**0.14**	**0.77**	103	12.5	2.7	4.5
0.86	**0.78**	**0.20**	**1.00**	194	16.2	0	13.0
0.45	0.32	0.08	0.45	116	9.0	20.0	0.5
0.77	**0.58**	0.08	**1.16**	137	14.0	18.8	0.4
0.32	0.27	0.10	0.33	68	6.6	2.0	3.7
0.24	0.14	0.06	0.22	160	5.0	30.0	2.2
0.39	0.36	**0.11**	0.54	149	8.0	11.4	8.2

Table 5.6

Essential Amino Acid Content (in Grams) of Protein-Rich Foods, per 100 Grams (3.5 Ounces)

Food	Arginine	Histidine	Isoleucine	Leucine	Lysine	Methionine	Phenylalanine
Beef	**1.87**	**1.01**	**1.33**	**2.34**	**2.46**	**0.76**	**1.16**
Chicken	**1.71**	**0.80**	**1.36**	**1.99**	**2.22**	**0.73**	**1.06**
Fish	**1.48**	**0.73**	**1.14**	**2.0**	**2.27**	**0.73**	**0.96**
Cheese	**0.94**	**0.87**	**1.55**	**2.39**	**2.07**	**0.65**	**1.31**
Peanut butter	**3.01**	**0.64**	**0.89**	**1.64**	**0.90**	0.31	**1.31**
Cottage cheese	0.57	**0.42**	**0.73**	**1.28**	**1.01**	**0.38**	**0.67**
Eggs	**0.75**	0.30	0.68	1.06	0.89	**0.39**	0.66
Lentils	0.70	0.25	0.39	0.65	0.63	0.08	0.45
Yogurt	0.17	0.14	0.31	0.58	0.51	0.17	0.31
Tofu	0.44	0.19	0.32	0.50	0.43	0.08	0.32
Bread	0.32	0.18	0.32	0.58	0.22	0.14	0.40
Milk	0.12	0.09	0.20	0.32	0.26	0.08	0.16

Threonine	Tryptophan	Valine (kcal)	Calories (g)	Protein (g)	Carbohydrate (g)	Fat
1.29	**0.33**	**1.44**	222	29.6	0	10.7
1.13	**0.31**	**1.33**	239	27.3	0	13.6
1.08	**0.28**	**1.27**	113	24.7	0	0.9
0.89	**0.32**	**1.66**	403	25.0	1.3	33.0
0.86	**0.25**	**1.06**	593	25.2	19.3	51.0
0.55	0.14	**0.77**	103	12.5	2.7	4.5
0.60	**0.15**	0.76	149	12.4	1	10
0.32	0.08	0.45	116	9.0	20.0	0.5
0.24	0.03	0.47	56	5.7	7.7	0.2
0.27	0.10	0.33	68	6.6	2.0	3.7
0.24	0.10	0.36	267	8.2	50.0	3.6
0.15	0.05	0.22	257	31.0	0.58	0.51

Table 5.7

In selecting your meals and snacks, remember the basic rule about combining grains either with dairy products or with legumes. This pairing of foods ensures that you are getting enough of all the amino acids at each meal or snack—both the essential and the nonessential—and that your intake of protein is sufficient. Good combinations include:

- Cereal with milk.
- Macaroni and cheese.
- Peanut butter with whole-grain bread.
- Rice with beans.

For more ideas, refer to the recipes at the back of the book. You'll find many vegetarian entrées, plus side dishes, snacks, and smoothies.

DR. NEWMAN: Whenever an expectant mother of multiples tells me that she is a vegetarian, I am concerned about her intake of essential amino acids. I ask about her willingness to consume eggs, dairy, fish, and poultry—and if the answer to each of these questions is no, I honestly share my concern that she will not be able to take in an adequate amount of protein and other nutrients to optimally nourish her babies.

In my practice, I have found that most pregnant vegetarians strongly resist the suggestion to eat red meat. For those women, close attention must be paid to their iron levels and the likely need for iron supplementation. In my experience, however, many vegetarians are willing to temporarily resume eating eggs and dairy, and sometimes fish and/or poultry, in order to meet the increased nutritional requirements of a multiple pregnancy.

For Megan Ryerson, the desire to provide optimal nourishment for her twins motivated her to temporarily modify her vegetarian diet. Megan explains: "I had been a vegetarian for 15 years before I got pregnant with twins. My doctor said that I could keep on being a vegetarian, but I would have to be a *great* vegetarian—always vigilant about getting plenty of high-quality protein and calories. That challenge, plus those eye-opening weight-gain guidelines, convinced me that it would be best for my babies if I started eating chicken and turkey as well as some fish. To feel better about it, I chose organic and sustainable products. It wasn't a perfect solution, but I knew it didn't have to last forever. And it worked! I gained 55 pounds overall, and my babies were big and healthy at birth—my son weighed 7 lb., 7 oz., and my daughter weighed 6 lb., 7 oz."

If You Develop Gestational Diabetes

Gestational diabetes is a temporary form of diabetes that resolves after delivery. It occurs when the mother's production of the hormone insulin—which is needed to pull glucose into the cells for use as energy—is not sufficient to keep up with the body's demands. As a result, the mother's blood sugar levels soar. Uncontrolled gestational diabetes increases the risk for stillbirth. It can also cause newborn babies to develop low blood sugar and other metabolic problems that have the potential to compromise their health, not only after delivery but in the long term as well.

Women pregnant with multiples are two to three times more likely than their singleton counterparts to develop this complication. The risk increases further among expectant mothers of multiples who also are over age 30 or are overweight, or who have a family history of diabetes.

Gestational diabetes can usually be controlled through diet. In that regard, you are already one step ahead—because the diet program described in Chapter 4 is basically a diabetic diet. The best thing you can do is to continue to follow the guidelines. To help stabilize your blood sugar levels, it is especially important for you to:

- Make sure that every meal and every snack has a combination of protein and carbohydrate.
- Eliminate all concentrated sweets—such as candy, pastries, regular soda, and added sugar—from your diet. Instead, focus on high-fiber, complex carbohydrates.
- Eat three meals plus two or three healthy snacks each day.
- Eat every three to four hours if you are expecting twins. Eat every two to three hours if you are pregnant with triplets or quads or if you were underweight when you began your twin pregnancy.
- Include a dairy bedtime snack, such as a small bowl of cereal and milk, or cheese and crackers, or even ice cream. Dairy is digested slowly and will help maintain your blood sugar levels throughout the night.

DR. LUKE: I want to clarify one point—that eating the types and amounts of foods recommended in this book will *not* cause or exacerbate gestational diabetes. Unfortunately, even many health care professionals are confused about this.

For instance, one expectant mother of twins wrote to me after being hospitalized for preterm labor. Because she had developed gestational diabetes, the hospital staff restricted her to less than 2,000 calories per day. She reported, "The nurses even take food off my tray. I feel like I'm starving all the time. I see stars, and I have lost 3 pounds in the two weeks that I've been in the hospital."

I was appalled. I recommended that this woman immediately speak to the hospital dietitian and request double servings of protein-rich foods—eggs, meat, poultry, cheese—which would provide the calories and nutrients she and her babies needed, without making her blood sugar rise. In addition, I suggested that her husband bring such high-protein foods to her every day, to make up for what the hospital was not providing.

If you have gestational diabetes and your doctor or dietitian does not seem knowledgeable about the special needs of expectant mothers of multiples, find a health care provider who is. If you need additional personalized advice, please visit my website at www.drbarbaraluke.com.

Pregnancy After Bariatric Surgery

In the United States in recent decades, the incidence of bariatric surgery has increased more than eightfold, with women in their childbearing years accounting for 83 percent of procedures.[54] In obese patients, bariatric surgery produces rapid and significant weight loss by making the stomach smaller, limiting the amount of food that can be eaten, and increasing feelings of satiety. The most rapid period of weight loss is during the first 6 to 12 months after surgery, during which time women are advised against becoming pregnant.

Research indicates that women who get pregnant after bariatric surgery are less likely than obese women to experience obesity-related pregnancy complications, such as gestational diabetes, preeclampsia, and cesarean delivery. However, bariatric surgery does increase the risk for nutritional deficiencies, which in turn can lead to fetal growth restriction. In addition, a mother's history of bariatric surgery increases her baby's risks for prematurity and small-for-gestational age birthweights.[55]

Another uncommon but serious concern for expectant mothers who have had bariatric surgery is the increased risk of intestinal complications such as obstruction, erosions, and bleeding. These complications can arise at any time following bariatric surgery, but they are more com-

54. Maggard MA, Yermilov I, Li Z, et al. Pregnancy and fertility following bariatric surgery: A systematic review. Journal of the American Medical Association 2008; 300:2286–96.
55. Roos N, Neovius M, Cnattingius S, et al. Perinatal outcomes after bariatric surgery: Nationwide population based matched cohort study. British Medical Journal 2013; 347:f6460; doi: 10.1136/bmj.f6460.

mon during pregnancy—especially multiple pregnancy—due to increased abdominal pressure and displacement of the intestines by the enlarging uterus.

Common nutritional deficiencies among pregnant bariatric patients include low levels of vitamin A, vitamin B_{12}, vitamin K, folate, calcium, and iron.[56] There are also increased risks for poor absorption of fat, lactose intolerance (inability to digest milk sugars), and dehydration. Because the nutritional demands of a multiple pregnancy are greater than those of a singleton pregnancy, bariatric patients expecting multiples are particularly vulnerable to nutritional deficiencies.

The degree of risk depends in part on the type of bariatric surgery. A restrictive procedure (laparoscopic adjustable gastric banding) poses less of a risk for nutritional problems than a malabsorptive procedure (biliopancreatic diversion or Roux-en-Y gastric bypass). If you have had a restrictive procedure, it may be advisable to have the gastric band released during your pregnancy, so that you can eat adequately and absorb normally during your pregnancy.

If you had bariatric surgery prior to your multiple pregnancy, you should take steps to reduce your risk for such complications. Here's what to do:

- Consume at least four to six small meals a day.
- Liquids should be consumed either well before meals or no sooner than 30 minutes afterward.
- At each meal, eat your protein-rich foods before your fats and carbohydrates for better absorption.
- At least 30 grams of carbohydrate should be consumed at each meal to help maintain adequate blood sugar levels.
- Be sure that your bariatric surgeon or obstetrician performs testing early in your pregnancy to determine if you are experiencing baseline deficiencies of one or more vital nutrients, such as iron, calcium, folate, or vitamin B_{12}. If any deficiencies are found, they should be corrected as soon as possible either by dietary adjustments or by specific supplementation.
- Work with a registered dietitian who specializes in bariatric surgery. Discuss with her the weight-gain and nutrition guidelines for expectant mothers of multiples, as outlined in Chapters 3 and 4, so she can customize a dietary program suited to your situation.

---

56. Guelinckx I, Devlieger R, Vansant G. Reproductive outcome after bariatric surgery: A critical review. Human Reproduction Update 2009; 15:189–201.

Dietary supplements are particularly important for expectant mothers of multiples who have had bariatric surgery. The appropriate supplementation regimen depends on the type of surgery and your nutritional status. All pregnant women who have had bariatric surgery should have their nutritional status monitored throughout pregnancy, and their supplement regimens should be tailored by their health professionals according to individual need.[57]

If ultrasounds reveal that your babies' growth is too slow despite your best dietary efforts, to protect your babies' health, you may need to receive nutrition intravenously, bypassing the gastrointestinal tract. This type of therapy is called total parenteral nutrition.

Ingestibles Your Babies Want You to Avoid

Along with all the things you should be eating and drinking, there are several things you should *not* be ingesting while pregnant:

Bacteria-Prone Foods

Certain foods are particularly likely to harbor bacteria that can lead to food poisoning. While you are pregnant, be sure to avoid the following: fish, meat, or poultry that is rare or raw (such as sushi or steak tartare); undercooked or uncooked eggs; certain cheeses (Brie, Camembert, queso blanco, queso fresco, Roquefort); or anything that has mold or has passed its expiration date. Do not consume unpasteurized dairy products. These may contain listeria bacteria, which can spread from your bloodstream to your babies and result in premature birth or stillbirth.

Medications

Before you became pregnant, you probably didn't worry too much if you had to take aspirin for a headache or antibiotics for an infection. But now that you're expecting, you must be more mindful of the medications you take.

That's not to say you have to suffer stoically through whatever symptoms might develop. Some over-the-counter drugs are generally considered safe during pregnancy. These include acetaminophen (Tylenol) for headache and other pain, and vaginal creams that contain

---

57. American Society for Metabolic and Bariatric Surgery Guidelines. ASMBS Allied Health Nutritional Guidelines for the Surgical Weight Loss Patient. Surgery for Obesity and Related Diseases 2008; 4:S73–S108.

clotrimazole (Gyne-Lotrimin) or miconazole (Monistat 7, Monistat 3) for yeast infections. Of course, it is important to realize that even when a drug is considered safe to use during pregnancy, it must be used correctly. For instance, if acetaminophen is taken in excess (more than eight 500-milligram capsules per day), it can result in irreversible liver damage.

Many other drugs, whether available over the counter or by prescription, can have serious negative effects on your babies' growth and development. Aspirin, for example, may cause bleeding problems. The common antibiotic tetracycline can permanently stain your children's teeth and may slow bone growth. The acne drug Accutane can cause major birth defects, as can some tranquilizers and psoriasis medications. Common blood pressure drugs called ACE inhibitors and blood-thinners such as Coumadin must be discontinued during pregnancy (or, ideally, prior to pregnancy) and replaced with medications that are safer for the babies.

Be sure that *all* of your health care providers—not just your obstetrician, but also your allergist, internist, dentist, etc.—are aware that you are pregnant. That information is crucial in determining whether or not the benefits outweigh the risks in prescribing a particular medication.

Also, review with your doctors the list of medications you normally take, whether occasionally or regularly, by prescription or over the counter. If you have a chronic condition such as allergies, your doctor may switch you from one type of medication to another type that is safer during pregnancy. Do not, however, suddenly stop taking important medications, such as those for asthma, lupus, or seizures, without your doctor's approval. Be aware that certain herbal remedies and supplements can also have negative effects—so do not take any such products without your doctor's okay.

ALCOHOL

Many women report that they develop an aversion to alcoholic beverages during pregnancy, even if they had enjoyed an occasional drink before conceiving. This is no mere coincidence. It is Mother Nature's way of protecting unborn babies. "Normally I enjoy a glass of wine with dinner, but once I got pregnant, alcohol didn't appeal to me at all. The smell alone turned me off," says Lydia Greenwood, mother of boy/girl twins.

The fact is that alcohol is poison to your unborn babies, for several reasons:

- Alcohol can alter levels of at least seven vital nutrients. These nutritional deficits contribute to the increase in birth defects. For instance, drinking during pregnancy more than doubles the risk of having a baby with cleft lip.

- The amniotic fluid surrounding the babies acts as a reservoir for alcohol. Because the babies lack the necessary enzymes to metabolize alcohol, they continue to be exposed to it long after your body has cleared it from your own blood supply.
- Alcohol interferes with protein synthesis, a critical process in your babies' development. Potential consequences for your unborn babies include stunted growth, birth defects, and mental retardation. In the United States, alcohol use during pregnancy is the major cause of mental retardation and learning and behavioral problems.
- Alcohol may also be directly toxic to the placenta, resulting in reduced ability to transport nutrients to your unborn babies.

The effects of alcohol are dose-related, meaning that the more a woman drinks, the more profoundly damaged her babies are likely to be. The term *fetal alcohol spectrum disorders* (FASDs) refers to the whole range of physical, neurological, and/or behavioral problems that can affect an individual whose mother drank alcohol during pregnancy.

FASDs include:

- *Fetal alcohol syndrome* (FAS), the most serious end of the FASD spectrum. Some FAS babies die. Those who survive often have abnormal facial features, neurological problems, growth problems, difficulty with vision and hearing, mental retardation, and/or problems with attention, learning, communication, and behavior.
- *Alcohol-related neurodevelopmental disorder* (ARND). Individuals with ARND often have intellectual disabilities and problems with learning, behavior, attention, judgment, and impulse control.
- *Alcohol-related birth defects* (ARBD). Babies born with ARBD have problems with their heart, kidneys, bones, and/or hearing.

In the United States, FAS is thought to affect as many as 5,000 babies per year—that's one in every 700 births. Even when a pregnant woman's alcohol consumption is significantly less than that of chronic alcohol abusers, her babies are still at risk. For instance, experts estimate that the full range of FASDs may affect as many as 5 percent of young school-age children in the United States and some Western European countries.[58]

How about moderate drinking? For nonpregnant women, moderate alcohol consumption

---

58. http://www.cdc.gov/ncbddd/fasd.

is defined as no more than one drink per day. Yet even as little as three drinks per week can more than *double* your babies' risk for being born weighing less than 5½ pounds. This greatly compounds the potential problems, given that multiples are already at higher risk for low birthweight.

The message is clear: When you are pregnant, total abstinence is the only prudent course. There is no safe amount of alcohol that you can have during pregnancy.

Did you have a few drinks before you realized you were expecting? Don't panic—they're not likely to have done your babies harm. But if you continue to use alcohol now, you are endangering all your babies. The wisest course of action is to stop drinking immediately. If you find that you cannot stop, tell your doctor at once. You have a serious medical problem that is adversely affecting both you and your unborn babies—but effective medical treatment is available.

CIGARETTES

Smoking is one of the worst habits you can possibly have when you're pregnant. You already know all the hazardous long-term effects cigarettes can have on your own body, such as cancer, heart disease, and emphysema. But you may not be aware of the harm it can do in the relatively short period of time you are pregnant—with very serious consequences for your children's health.

With each cigarette, you expose your unborn multiples to many toxic substances. Your body must then divert some of its stores of vitamins to detoxify these substances, thereby reducing the amount of essential nutrients available for fetal growth. One of these toxic substances is carbon monoxide, which binds to hemoglobin and lowers the amount of oxygen in your blood. This is turn reduces the oxygen to the placenta, the vital middleman in your babies' growth and development. The result is an increase in placental infarcts, or areas where the placental tissue dies due to lack of oxygen. Consider these facts:

- Miscarriages occur significantly more frequently among smokers.
- Your babies are already at risk for preterm birth by virtue of being multiples. If their prenatal environment is polluted, the danger rises even higher. For instance, even if you smoke fewer than 10 cigarettes a day, you increase your risk of delivering your twins before 37 weeks' gestation by 30 percent; 10 or more cigarettes daily increases that risk by 40 percent. Delivering your twins before 35 weeks is three times more likely if you smoke. Delivering extremely prematurely, before 33 weeks, is four times more likely for smokers.

- Low birthweight is also an inherent hazard for twins, triplets, and quads. Maternal smoking doubles twins' risk of being born weighing less than 5½ pounds and increases *more than sevenfold* their risk of weighing less than 3⅓ pounds (very low birthweight) at birth.
- Mental retardation occurs 60 percent more often among children whose mothers smoked during pregnancy. The more you smoke, the greater the risk.
- Cleft lip is nearly 80 percent more common among babies born to smokers.
- Neural tube defects such as spina bifida occur more often among children exposed to cigarette smoke before birth. In part, this may be due to the fact that cigarettes deplete the mother's levels of folic acid.
- A serious digestive disorder called pyloric stenosis occurs twice as often in infants born to smokers. The condition causes projectile vomiting and requires surgical correction.
- Children whose mothers smoked during pregnancy have a threefold increased risk of experiencing problems with motor control, attention, and perception.

Even after delivery, your smoking—or smoking by anyone in your household—can present serious hazards to the health of your babies. Here is why:

- Sudden infant death syndrome (SIDS) occurs significantly more often among infants exposed to secondhand smoke.
- Children of smokers are more prone to respiratory illnesses, including asthma, bronchitis, and colds.

Don't fool yourself: There is no safe level of smoking or secondhand smoke exposure. Even the lightest smokers—those who have only one to five cigarettes per day—are 56 percent more likely than nonsmokers to have babies with low birthweights. In fact, mere exposure to smoke from a household member or coworker has been associated with reductions in birthweight.

The use of smokeless tobacco products (chewing tobacco, snuff, dissolvable tobacco) during pregnancy is also extremely dangerous, as they have been associated with stillbirth, preterm birth, and infant apnea.

What about e-cigarettes? They are not considered safe to use during pregnancy, either. E-cigs (also known as e-liquid, vaping, and tailpiping) are battery-operated devices that turn chemicals including nicotine—one of the main toxins implicated in the harmful effects of smoking during pregnancy—into a water vapor that is inhaled. Many e-cigarettes contain even more nicotine than a regular cigarette. Since e-cigarettes are sometimes touted as a safer alternative to smoking, and their use may be permitted in some places where smoking is prohibited, many people use e-cigarettes even more times per day than they would actually smoke. If this is your habit, you may in fact be exposing your unborn children to even more risk than if you were smoking.

Make no mistake about this—there are no studies establishing the safety of e-cigarettes during pregnancy, and the FDA has not approved them as a cessation aid for smokers trying to quit.

You may be wondering whether it's a good idea for a pregnant woman to use nicotine replacement products such as nicotine gum, patches, inhalers, nasal sprays, and lozenges. The answer is probably no. First, there is virtually no evidence that these products are superior to willpower in achieving smoking cessation during pregnancy, a time when women generally are already quite motivated to stop smoking. Second, while it is true that nicotine replacement products are less hazardous than smoking, some people start using the replacement products but then continue to smoke anyway—which only increases their risk even further.

There are some studies suggesting that nicotine patches are safe to use in pregnancy. However, their use probably should be limited to cases in which women have tried and failed to stop on their own and are still smoking more than 15 cigarettes per day. For women who smoke fewer than 15 cigarettes per day, the patch probably exposes the unborn babies to more nicotine than the smoking does.

There are no data establishing the safety of smoking cessation drugs such as Zyban or Chantix for pregnant women. These drugs should not be used during pregnancy.

If you are among the 15 to 20 percent of pregnant women who still smoke, today is the day to stop. Consider joining a support group, either a local face-to-face group or an online option such as www.quitnet.com. Because such groups provide encouragement and moral support, plus practical advice on handling cravings, they—coupled with your motivation to do what's best for your babies—can be the key to successfully kicking the cigarette habit.

Chapter Six

Your Body: How to Look Good, Feel Great, Work Smart, and Play It Safe

When you're expecting multiples, you're likely to experience the physical changes of pregnancy sooner and more intensely than do women carrying a singleton. There are two main reasons for this. The first is hormonal: During a multiple pregnancy, your body produces much higher levels of the various pregnancy hormones, including estrogen and progesterone. The second reason has to do with sheer size—your belly will grow far larger than that of a woman pregnant with just one baby. Consider these comparisons:

- With twins, your uterus is the same size as that of a singleton mom who is 6 to 8 weeks further along in her pregnancy.
- With triplets, your uterus is the same size as that of a singleton mom who is 10 to 12 weeks further along in her pregnancy.
- With quadruplets, your uterus is the same size as that of a singleton mom who is 14 to 16 weeks further along in her pregnancy.

Some of the changes in your body you may regard as delightful. Others can cause discomfort, so you'll want to find safe and effective ways to minimize the symptoms. Most important, certain physical changes that accompany a multiple pregnancy require significant—but temporary—modifications in your lifestyle. Do your best to follow the guidelines in this chapter, and you'll be taking important steps toward safeguarding your own health and that of your unborn babies.

Beauty and the Belly

You're expecting your figure to be transformed, of course. But did you know that your hair and skin might look different, too? A revved-up circulation and those pregnancy hormones (which for you are present in such abundance) are responsible. "My hair got very thick and luxurious. It was enormous! I loved that," says Stacy Moore, mother of fraternal twin boys. It's common during pregnancy for your hair to thicken noticeably and to grow more quickly. Enjoy it while it lasts! Soon after delivery, it will return to normal as you shed those extra strands.

What about coloring your hair? Most experts believe this to be safe because so little dye is absorbed through the skin. If you are concerned that the dye might potentially be harmful to your babies, however, hold off on hair coloring until after you deliver. Or consider getting highlights or lowlights instead of allover color—with these processes, only a minimal amount of dye comes in contact with the scalp.

Certain changes are also taking place in your skin, many of which you'll welcome. "The whole time I was expecting, my complexion was peaches-and-cream—soft, rosy, and clear, with no blemishes. Maybe it was the glow of pregnancy times two," says Lydia Greenwood, mother of boy/girl twins.

Other skin conditions brought on by hormonal changes are, however, less pleasing. Some women develop a brownish discoloration around their eyes and over their noses, called chloasma or the mask of pregnancy. Also commonly making an appearance is a brownish line, the *linea nigra,* which runs from the center of the abdomen to the top of the pubic bone. On your legs, little spider veins may surface. There's not a lot you can do about these skin conditions other than to apply moisturizer, if it makes you feel better, and to take heart in knowing that, because these changes are primarily due to increased estrogen during pregnancy, they will disappear shortly after delivery.

What about stretch marks—those reddish, slightly indented striations that often spring up on the bellies of pregnant women? It's the luck of the draw. Some mothers-to-be of multiples don't get stretch marks, even after gaining 60 pounds or more. This trait tends to run in families, so to get a hint of what might be in store for you, ask your own mother how she fared.

Don't be too surprised or dismayed if stretch marks do develop, however. The phenomenon is common enough among mothers of multiples that it has a special name: *twin skin.* Stacy Moore confides, "At about six months, bright red stretch marks sprouted all over my belly. They faded to silver after the boys were born, yet still I'm left with twin skin. Bikinis are a thing of the past, I guess. But I try to look at those marks as a badge of motherhood."

DR. NEWMAN: Many women notice drier skin and increased itching during pregnancy. To soothe itchy skin, I recommend the use of unscented moisturizers and mild, unscented soap because added fragrances in toiletries can cause additional irritation. Be sure to thoroughly rinse off any soap after your bath or shower. It also helps to avoid taking long, hot showers or baths, because these further dry out skin. Instead, take warm oatmeal baths, using a product such as Aveeno Soothing Bath Treatment. Apply cool, wet compresses to itchy areas as needed. Avoid going out in the heat because perspiration can intensify itching. Another good strategy is to wear loose, smooth, cotton clothing.

Has your skin not only started to itch but also broken out in hives? You may have a pregnancy-related skin condition called pruritic urticarial papules and plaques of pregnancy (PUPPP), which affects about 1 percent of pregnant women. It is characterized by a hive-like rash that usually begins on the belly (typically within the abdominal stretch marks) before spreading to the thighs, buttocks, back, and chest, and is accompanied by itchy red bumps. The onset of PUPPP is usually in the third trimester, when the abdominal skin is stretched the most, but it can develop earlier—particularly when a woman is carrying twins, triplets, or quads. Fortunately, PUPPP is not dangerous to mother or babies, so treatment is directed simply at controlling the itchiness with antihistamines, topical hydrocortisone, and, in severe cases, oral steroids. Symptoms disappear within a few days after delivery.

If you develop extremely intense itching (without a rash) that initially affects the palms of the hands and the soles of the feet before spreading over the entire body, see Chapter 7 for information on how to handle a potentially serious complication called intrahepatic cholestasis of pregnancy (ICP).

What to Wear When Expecting a Pair (or More)

Many women who are pregnant with twins, triplets, or quads are dismayed to discover how poorly regular maternity clothes fit. Garments that fit well through the shoulders and hips are too tight in the tummy, while those that have enough room at the waist are way too big everywhere else.

DR. LUKE: Pregnancy clothes are a special challenge for expectant mothers of multiples—clothing needs to be stylish enough for work and evenings out, but practical enough for everyday life. The type of fabric used is critical. Since women who are expecting have an increase in both body temperature and skin sensitivity, a natural fabric that allows the skin to breathe is best. Fit is also an important consideration—you want pregnancy clothes that are going to fit well at the neckline, shoulders, and sleeves, and be roomy where you need it most—at the waist. And you want quality and value—clothes that will hold up well with frequent washings, keep their color and shape throughout your pregnancy, and be a good value for the cost. I searched for maternity clothes that would meet the needs of my mothers-to-be of multiples, but they just weren't available anywhere.

It was with all of these factors in mind that I designed my line of pregnancy clothes, *Barbara Luke Maternity-for-Multiples*. Each style has been designed based on input from real women expecting twins, triplets, or quads. I worked closely with a major U.S. manufacturer to choose the best-quality fabric—a buttery-soft blend of modal (a natural fiber) and spandex—and to ensure that the garments are well constructed. My pregnant moms gave me lots of feedback on fit, color, style, and quality—and I listened. The result: Clothes that are comfortable, stylish, easy-care, beautiful, and economical. All of the pieces work well together, so it is simple to put together a whole pregnancy wardrobe with clothing that will last from your first trimester through to delivery and beyond. Take a look on my website, www.drbarbaraluke.com.

"Most of my regular maternity tops rode up at the stomach, exposing the bottom of my belly, which felt indecent. And even the clothes that fit okay at first never fit for long, considering the way my abdomen seemed to grow by the hour," says Katy Lederer, mother of boy/girl twins. "It was such a relief to find a line of maternity clothing designed especially for mothers of multiples, with all the necessary room in front, good coverage for the cleavage and belly, and pretty pleats in back—all in comfortable fabrics that didn't make me sweat."

Do plan on needing a maternity wardrobe much sooner than the mother of a singleton might. "When I was pregnant with my firstborn, I was five and a half months along before I started to wear maternity clothes. With the twins, though, I had to break out the maternity wardrobe at eight weeks," says Judy Levy. "Because I'm normally petite, all my old maternity clothes were size small. I grew out of most of them halfway through the twin pregnancy and had to buy a whole new maternity wardrobe in much larger sizes."

Considering that your feet must now bear a lot more weight than they're accustomed to, it's no surprise that they may ache. Choose shoes that provide good support, with nonskid soles and extra cushioning. "I stuck primarily to sneakers. They were the most comfortable, and with those deep treads and rubber soles, I didn't have to worry about slipping," says Stacy Moore.

You may need to buy a few pairs of shoes in a larger size than you normally wear. During pregnancy, the hormones that loosen up your pelvis in anticipation of delivery also loosen the ligaments around your other joints, including those in the feet. Coupled with a tendency for the lower extremities to swell during pregnancy, it's no wonder that your regular shoes may feel too snug.

As for high heels, leave them in the closet until after delivery. Your center of balance shifts forward during pregnancy, and even more so with multiples, making you less steady on your feet and more prone to twisting an ankle or tripping on an uneven sidewalk. Any heel higher than an inch or two leaves you at risk for a fall, which can increase your risk of bleeding early in pregnancy, or trigger contractions and preterm labor later on.

Unless you're sure you'll need it, you can hold off on buying a maternity coat. Judy Levy, mother of fraternal twin girls and an older daughter, explains, "Even though it was winter, I was so warm all the time that I could just wear my regular coat, leaving it unbuttoned."

Common Discomforts of Pregnancy ... Multiplied

With all those babies inside, your extra-large belly can lead to some extra aches and pains. Here's how to ease those uncomfortable physical symptoms:

BACKACHES

With each passing month, the curve in your lower back becomes more exaggerated due to the increasing weight of your belly and a shifting center of gravity. This can trigger back pain, particularly in the lower (lumbar) region.

- Limit standing to no more than an hour at a time up until the 20th week of pregnancy, and to a maximum of half an hour at a time after that point. If you have been diagnosed with cervical changes, feel uterine contractions, or have had an episode of preterm labor, limit on-your-feet time even more strictly. When you must stand, place one foot on a low stool; every few minutes, switch around and elevate the other foot.
- Weigh your purse and try to limit its contents to no more than 2 pounds. Carrying a too-heavy handbag throws your posture out of alignment and can cause spasms in the muscles of your back and neck. Place the strap of your purse diagonally across your chest, use a messenger-style bag or backpack, or switch

the shoulder holding your bag every few minutes. Lighten the load by removing nonessential items, such as loose change and seldom-used keys.

- When you sit, choose a chair with a straight back, armrests, and a firm cushion; elevate your legs on a footstool whenever possible. To protect your back (and your balance) as you rise to a standing position, place one foot about 6 to 8 inches farther forward than the other, then push off from that foot as you lean forward, keeping your back and neck straight.

- Check your mattress for firmness. If it seems overly soft, ask your partner to place a board between the mattress and box spring. Then take advantage of every opportunity to get horizontal. "For back pain, what helped me the most was rest," says twin mom Judy Levy. When it's time to get up, start from a side-lying position and gently push yourself up sideways.

- A gentle massage relieves backache and other pains. Marcy Bugajski, mother of fraternal twin boys, says, "My husband, Dave, often gave me a back rub while I lay on my side. That was heaven! And if I woke up with leg cramps in the middle of the night, he'd gently straighten my legs, flex my feet, and rub my calves till the ache went away." You might also look for a professional masseuse with experience in providing massage for pregnant women. She should use a special chair that allows you to lean forward with full-body support and a perfectly aligned spine, or an arrangement of pillows that offers support in a side-lying position. Call local spas and ask if they have special programs for pregnant women, or get a recommendation from your health care professional.

- Warm water soothes tired muscles, but it can be risky to climb in and out of the tub when a multiple pregnancy diminishes your sense of balance. Invest in a shower stool so you can sit in your shower stall and enjoy the pulsating water on your neck and back.

- Another useful but often forgotten treatment is the old-fashioned hot water bottle or hot wheat bag applied to your lower back while resting or sleeping. A more expensive approach is to use heat-wrap products such as ThermaCare. These are essentially large bandages that can be placed on the lower back to deliver heat to the area for six to eight hours.

- The typical stance of a pregnant woman—with fingers clasped under her belly— provides support for your growing uterus. But it's hard to carry groceries, open doors, work at a keyboard, or wash the dishes with your hands holding up your belly. A more practical solution is a harness-like maternity garment, such as the

Prenatal Cradle, that supports your abdomen while helping to keep your shoulders back and posture erect. Anne Seifert, the mother of quadruplets, explains, "It has straps that go over your shoulders and crisscross on your back, and a band that winds around your middle and hooks down under your belly. It does look funny—the first time my husband saw me wearing it, he said, 'What in the world is that contraption?'—but it really does keep pressure off your back and bladder. Was it worth the money? You bet." Simpler support garments (such as Prenatal Cradle Mini Cradle and other belly bands) as well as the Prenatal Cradle are available online from Amazon.com and various other sites.

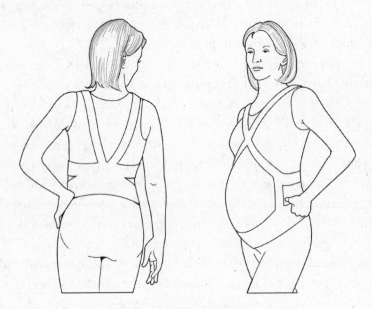

Prenatal Cradle supportive maternity garment

- Like your belly, your breasts are growing, too, and the increased weight up top also contributes to backache. A good bra eases discomfort by providing proper support. If you're full-figured, wear a bra to bed at night, too.
- A safe and soothing home remedy for backache is a glass of warm milk with a spoonful of honey. Before taking anything stronger, such as Extra-Strength Tylenol, get the go-ahead from your obstetrician. It is important to remember that nonsteroidal anti-inflammatory pain relievers like ibuprofen (Motrin, Advil, etc.) and naproxen (Aleve, Naprosyn) should not be taken during pregnancy due to potentially harmful fetal effects.

- If back pain persists, consider seeing a physical therapist or chiropractor, who can help restore the normal alignment of your spine. For a referral to a physical therapist, call the American Physical Therapy Association at 800-999-2782 or 703-684-2782 or visit the website at www.apta.org. For a referral to a chiropractor, call the American Chiropractic Association at 703-276-8800 or visit the website at www.acatoday.org.

SIDE ACHES

Toward the end of your pregnancy, growth in the height of the uterus slows down and the babies begin to spread out. Your doctor doesn't measure this sideways growth the way she measures fundal height, but the increased width will be obvious to you. For one thing, your maternity clothes will suddenly feel snug. What's more, this rapid growth causes the ligaments that suspend your uterus within your pelvis to stretch. This can cause discomfort—a dull ache at times, or perhaps a sharp pain—along your side. It's likely to be more pronounced if you've never been pregnant before. To ease the sensation, take a warm shower or lie down with some pillows supporting the weight of your belly.

SWELLING

A common complaint among pregnant women is swelling (also called edema), particularly in the legs and ankles. In large part this is caused by the fact that the growing uterus blocks the return of blood to the heart—an effect compounded in a multiple pregnancy because the uterus is so much bigger.

The best remedy for swelling is down time—meaning time spent lying down on your side. A prone position improves circulation to your kidneys and allows excess fluid to be eliminated. Your heart will not have to work as hard either, so you'll feel better all around. Want proof? Measure your ankles before and after a nap, or in the morning and again in the evening on a day when you didn't take a nap, and note the significant difference in the amount of swelling you experience.

If you have access to a swimming pool, simply getting into the water can help with uncomfortable swelling. When your lower body is submerged, water pressure exerts an external force on the soft tissues of your feet and lower legs, temporarily encouraging edema fluid to mobilize back into the blood vessels.

Swelling can also cause pressure on nerves, particularly in your arms and legs. Some pregnant women develop *carpal tunnel syndrome*, a painful disorder caused by compression of the nerves and ligaments of the wrists. This will subside after delivery, but in the meantime, wrist splints may help ease the discomfort. Lydia Greenwood says, "Dozens of times a day and throughout the night, I was getting that uncomfortable pins-and-needles feeling in my hands. But as soon as I started wearing wrist splints to bed, the tingling disappeared."

Another cause of swelling is dietary. Every gram of carbohydrate holds two grams of water—hence the philosophy of carbohydrate-loading (eating a pasta dinner) practiced by many runners before a big race to help with hydration. To minimize excess fluid, cut back on your carbohydrate consumption at dinner. For instance, eat a steak and salad, but pass on the rice or potatoes, and see how your hands and feet feel in the morning.

Heartburn or Gastroesophageal Reflux Disease (GERD)

Heartburn—also called gastroesophageal reflux disease (GERD)—that develops during pregnancy is caused primarily by a reflux of acid secretions from the stomach into the lower part of the esophagus. This occurs for several reasons. First, your growing uterus pushes aside the stomach and intestines, and this crowding triggers reflux. Second, the hormones of pregnancy cause changes in the gastrointestinal tract, including a slowing down of digestion and elimination. This is Mother Nature's way of allowing you to absorb more nutrients from the foods you eat—but it contributes to heartburn, too. Progesterone also relaxes the hiatal valve that separates the stomach from the esophagus. This valve is normally closed except when swallowing, but when relaxed can allow gastric acids to reflux from the stomach into the esophagus. This creates the characteristic burning sensation underneath the breastbone or in the throat.

With a singleton pregnancy, symptoms typically begin at about 31 to 34 weeks. But because the uterus grows faster and hormone levels are higher with a multiple pregnancy, heartburn occurs sooner and can be much more severe, depending in part on the position of the babies. With a twin pregnancy, heartburn may begin around weeks 23 to 28; with triplets, by weeks 19 to 24; and with quadruplets, as early as weeks 16 to 21. "I had excruciating heartburn, particularly after week 26. I think that was the worst part of the whole pregnancy," says quad mom Anne Seifert.

While you may be tempted to try an over-the-counter remedy such as Tums, Mylanta, or Maalox, you're better off with the calcium/magnesium/zinc supplements recommended in Chapter 5. These provide needed nutrients while doubling as effective therapy for heartburn, with fewer side effects such as gas or diarrhea. Remember to avoid antacids that contain aluminum or are high in sodium.

It also may help to cut down on high-fat foods, fried foods, spicy foods, onions, and chocolate, all of which can exacerbate heartburn. You may also find that you need to avoid acidic foods such as citrus fruits and juices, tomatoes and tomato sauces, mustard, and vinegar. In addition, avoid drinking large quantities of fluid during meals, which increases the slushiness of the stomach contents and predisposes you to reflux.

Additionally, increase your consumption of foods that contain beneficial digestive bacteria called probiotics. These may reduce the harmful effects of acid in the esophagus. Look for yogurt or kefir with a label specifying that the product contains live and active cultures.

Large meals may trigger symptoms, so try eating smaller but more frequent meals throughout the day. Take time to chew thoroughly.

For maximum comfort, wear loose clothing. Avoid any garment that is tight around your waist.

If symptoms are so severe that you can't sleep or get comfortable, ask your doctor about prescription medication. Says Anne, "Oral medicine helped for a while, but toward the end, the only thing that relieved the discomfort was IV medication."

DR. NEWMAN: Many pregnant women find that heartburn is particularly troublesome at night, which further disrupts efforts to get a good night's sleep and thus makes the problem even more frustrating and irritating. A common mistake is to pile up a bunch of pillows to elevate your sleeping position—but all this accomplishes is to flex you at the waist, pushing your uterus up against your stomach and making the problem worse.

A better strategy is to place a couple of bricks or a pair of 6- to 8-inch wood blocks underneath the two head bedposts. This puts the bed on a mildly elevated slope, allowing you to sleep relatively flat while still enlisting the aid of gravity to keep stomach acids down where they belong.

Be selective about the foods you choose for a bedtime snack, avoiding anything acidic, spicy, or highly seasoned. If nighttime heartburn continues, have your bedtime snack earlier—no less than one hour before you lie down. Also, chew a stick of gum just before going to bed; this stimulates salivary secretions that can help neutralize stomach acids.

It is important to realize that severe heartburn is not merely a trivial discomfort, particularly in a multiple pregnancy, because it can interfere with your ability to eat—which means that you may not take in adequate nutrients to meet your weight-gain goals and provide for your babies' growth. So don't hesitate to inform your doctor if you are experiencing heartburn that is not significantly relieved by the strategies described above.

FULL BLADDER

Has the bathroom suddenly become the most popular room in your house? As you may have realized for yourself, increased urinary frequency is one of the earliest signs of pregnancy, often being noticed four to six weeks into the first trimester. Blame your frequent need to urinate on the same two factors that contribute to heartburn: a growing uterus and elevated hormones.

The bigger your babies get, and the more of them you're carrying, the more pressure your uterus exerts on your bladder. This sensation can be particularly strong if the baby closest to your cervix is positioned deep in your pelvis.

Hormonal changes of pregnancy also play a role, as does the fact that pregnancy involves a dramatic increase in circulating blood volume, including blood flow to the kidneys. This is particularly true in a multiple pregnancy. The amniotic fluid around the babies is changed many times a day to eliminate their urine and discarded cells. Your kidneys and bladder must therefore do double duty now, to expel not only your own wastes but also those of your unborn babies. With a multiple pregnancy, there is more amniotic fluid to process and higher levels of hormones acting on the kidneys. The result is a near-constant need to urinate.

This can be a real problem when you don't have easy access to a bathroom. "My drive to work takes about an hour. By the time I arrived each morning, I'd have to urinate so badly! Sometimes I couldn't imagine how I'd make it to my office building, which was two blocks away from the parking lot," says twin mom Judy Levy. To avoid that bursting-bladder sensation, check out your commuting route and find a restaurant or service station midway where you can stop to use the bathroom facilities. Whenever you enter a building where you'll be for some time, ask for directions to a restroom—so you'll know where to go when you need to go.

The urge to urinate may also wake you in the middle of the night. Don't attempt to resolve this by cutting back on your intake of water. Remember, you need to drink eight 16-ounce glasses of water daily (as discussed in Chapter 4) in order to stay hydrated, avoid constipation, and reduce the risk of urinary-tract infection. But do take in your fluid before 8 P.M. so that most of it has time to pass through before you go to bed. It also helps to put your feet up for a few hours or to wear support stockings after dinner. This allows fluids that have pooled in your legs during the day to be reabsorbed into your bloodstream and processed as urine before bedtime.

Are those nightly bathroom visits continuing despite these strategies? Here's how Judy Levy looks at it: "I woke up to urinate at least three times a night. I kept telling myself it was good practice because, once the twins were born, I'd need to get up for all those nighttime feedings."

If you're expecting triplets or quads, the bladder problem can seriously interfere with sleep toward the end of your pregnancy. Helen Armer, mother of triplets, explains: "By week 30, sleeping for more than two hours at a stretch was almost impossible because my bladder would wake me up. So all day and all night, I'd nap briefly, get up to use the bathroom, then read awhile or watch a video with my preschooler before dozing off again for another hour or two." There's little more you can do to improve the situation at this point other than feel glad that your delivery date is getting closer with each passing day.

Some women experience slight incontinence during pregnancy, leaking a little urine with every sneeze or laugh. If you share this problem, you might want to wear an absorbent pad or try a supportive undergarment called the V2 Supporter, which looks similar to a jockstrap. It is available online from Amazon.com and various other sites.

Also, practice Kegel exercises, which strengthen the muscles around the urethra (the outside opening of the urinary tract). Unfortunately, many women who think they are doing Kegels correctly—contracting the muscles of the pelvic floor—are instead clenching the abdominal or buttocks muscles. To learn the proper technique, contract or squeeze the muscles you normally use to halt the flow of urine, hold for 10 seconds, then release. Repeat 10 to 20 times. Do three complete sets of these exercises daily, and in a short time you will see significant improvement in your ability to hold your urine. If the problem persists, consult your doctor.

Using the bathroom may also present a problem you hadn't anticipated: joint pain. Judy Levy explains: "Every time I went to the bathroom and had to squat down to reach the toilet seat, my knees ached. I wish I had thought to rent one of those toilet seats for the handicapped, which have handrails and a higher seat. That would make life easier for an expectant mother of multiples."

CONSTIPATION

Many expectant mothers develop constipation, particularly if they are taking iron supplements to combat anemia. To promote regularity, stay well hydrated by drinking at least eight 16-ounce glasses of water each day. Also have several dried plums or a glass of prune juice daily. Be sure your diet includes foods high in fiber, such as raw fruits and vegetables, bran cereal, and beans. Also consider a wheat-bran fiber supplement, which causes less gassiness than other fiber-rich foods. And, provided your doctor has not instructed you to avoid exercise, you can help your digestive system work more efficiently by walking or swimming for 30 minutes a day.

If these measures are not enough to prevent constipation, ask your doctor about taking an over-the-counter stool softener such as Colace, a fiber preparation such as Metamucil, or a gentle laxative such as Senokot.

SHORTNESS OF BREATH

Like your other internal organs, your lungs can be compressed by the growing uterus. The rib cage widens to adapt, but not enough to compensate fully for the reduced lung volume as pregnancy progresses. As the uterus grows, it pushes up on the abdominal contents and the diaphragm (a large, flat muscle separating the chest and abdominal cavities), making it harder for your lungs to fully expand. That means you won't be able to breathe as deeply as you normally do—so you won't be able to do things that require full, deep breaths, such as walking up a flight of stairs or hurrying for a bus. Even carrying on a conversation may leave you winded. This shallower breathing leads to the sensation of shortness of breath. The good news is that, although the sensation may be uncomfortable, it is harmless and does not adversely affect your babies. The symptoms are simply manifestations of your body's adaptation to provide ample oxygen to your twins, triplets, or quads.

You may find some relief from practicing deep-breathing techniques. These increase your lung capacity and breath control, and ease the anxiety that often accompanies shortness of breath. The simplest technique is to slowly inhale through your nose as fully as possible, hold for a moment, then exhale through your mouth as slowly and completely as you can. Continue for several minutes. It's also helpful to raise your arms over your head to relieve some of the pressure on the diaphragm and rib cage.

If you're uncomfortable even when lying down, try a semi-seated position instead. "Gradually it became harder and harder to breathe in bed. The triplets took up so much space inside me that there was little room left for my lungs," says Helen Armer. "It helped to stay propped up with lots of pillows instead of reclining all the way."

OVERHEATING

Pregnant women are like portable heaters: They're hot all the time, regardless of the season or thermostat reading. This is largely due to the high metabolism of the unborn baby—or babies, in the case of a multiple pregnancy—and the amount of heat they generate.

To help dissipate the extra heat, the mother's blood volume increases—by about 50 percent for a singleton pregnancy, by nearly 100 percent for twins, and even more for triplets or quads. One sign of this increase is when you feel your heart beating faster and stronger, and perhaps hear the blood pounding in your ears. Even with the increased blood volume, however, you're likely to find yourself perspiring while others around you are shivering. "I got overheated much more easily during the twin pregnancy than in my previous singleton pregnancy. I had to sleep on top of the covers, even when my partner was huddled beneath several blankets trying to stay warm," says Judy Levy.

To minimize discomfort, dress in layers so you can peel off some clothes when overheated and put them back on when the hot flash passes. Keep a jug of ice water handy. Put a small electric fan on your desk and your bedside table. To avoid arguments over the bedroom thermostat setting, try an electric blanket with dual controls.

SLEEP DISCOMFORTS

When you are pregnant with two or more babies, it is absolutely critical for your physical and emotional well-being that you get enough rest. During the first three months, as your body adjusts to pregnancy, you may feel unusually tired, owing to rising hormones. By the second trimester, most women feel more energetic. But as your pregnancy progresses into the third trimester, you tire quickly. Ironically, it's at this point that the high metabolism of your growing babies, as well as their constant drain on your own metabolism, may be giving you the most trouble with sleeping.

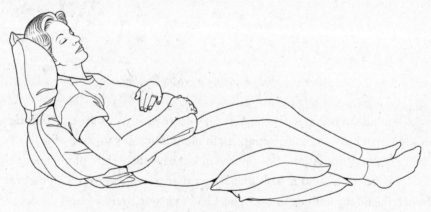

Suggested position for getting comfortable

A primary problem is finding a comfortable position for sleep. You can't lie on your stomach for obvious reasons. You shouldn't lie on your back because the weight of the babies would press on blood vessels supplying the uterus, causing your blood pressure to increase and possibly triggering contractions.

That leaves one option: lying on your side. The right arrangement of pillows maximizes comfort. A wedge-shaped cushion, for example, tucks in right under your tummy to provide support where it's needed most. Place another pillow between your knees, to keep the weight of your belly from pulling you too far forward and straining your back muscles. If you tend to roll onto your back while you sleep, use pillows behind your shoulders and buttocks to keep you on your side. Try a contoured pillow that is thicker along one or two edges than in the center—the thick edge supports your neck while keeping your head and spine aligned. Or simplify matters with this strategy from twin mom Stacy Moore: "I bought a wonderful head-to-toe pillow that was stuffed with feathers, so it molded to my body everywhere. It made lying on my side much more comfortable. In fact, it was the best investment I made during my entire pregnancy."

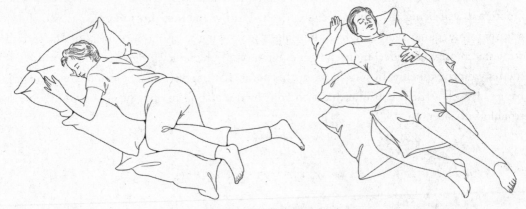

More suggested positions for getting comfortable

Rolling from side to side may also be difficult—increasingly so with each passing week and with each additional baby you're expecting. Twin mom Judy Levy says, "By the third trimester, rolling over in bed was impossible. I couldn't stand to have the weight of my huge belly on top of me even for a moment—and it took a lot longer than a moment to roll all the way over. To change from lying on my left side to my right, I had to get up, walk around the bed, and climb back in on the other side of the bed. Of course, this would wake up my partner. We ended up sleeping in separate beds for the last few months. I needed space to get comfortable." If you, too, end up temporarily evicting your mate, don't feel guilty. Expectant moms of multiples need to spread out when they sleep—and counting all those babies, there are already a lot of people sharing your bed.

Surprisingly, quad mom Anne Seifert had less trouble with sleep discomfort than did many mothers of twins or triplets. The credit, she says, goes to her waterbed. "It was wonderfully comfortable when I was pregnant. Waterbeds provide excellent support and don't cause any painful pressure points. You definitely need the motionless kind, though, because otherwise the waves bounce you around too much."

DR. NEWMAN: Other tips that can help mothers of multiples get better rest include taking a warm bath or shower at bedtime and avoiding any arguments or stressful situations prior to going to bed. Also, try to use the bed only for sleeping, not for watching television, reading, or using the computer. You may find that playing relaxing music or natural background sounds may help make you sleepy.

If your sleep is interrupted by nighttime leg cramps, you can gently stretch your leg muscles before bedtime, or have your partner give you a leg massage. Some women advocate the application of topical heating rubs like Bengay, Atomic Balm, or Tiger Balm to the legs to help increase circulation and reduce cramps.

Also, use nightlights to illuminate the path from your bed to the bathroom. That way, when you get up to use the toilet in the middle of the night, you won't have to turn on the bathroom light. Avoiding exposure to any bright light will make it easier to get back to sleep.

What About Sex?

Sleep isn't the only bedroom activity that tends to change during pregnancy. Chances are, you've got some questions and concerns about sex, too.

In most uncomplicated singleton pregnancies, couples can continue to have intercourse until the woman goes into labor or her membranes break. But with a multiple pregnancy, there's a greater chance that your doctor will tell you to limit or avoid sexual activity. This is particularly likely if you've had more than one miscarriage or if you've experienced any complications such as an incompetent cervix, placenta previa, infection, bleeding, leaking of amniotic fluid, uterine contractions, a very short cervical length, or a history of preterm labor. Why is sex considered risky in such cases? It's because both a woman's orgasm and the prostaglandins in semen can trigger uterine contractions.

DR. NEWMAN: It is normal and common for a pregnant woman to be aware of some mild uterine contractions after orgasmic sex. However, if those contractions are painful or last more than a minute, I would consider that a warning sign and advise you to discuss the matter with your obstetrician. Your doctor may want to do a transvaginal ultrasound and/or digital exam to confirm that your cervix remains long and closed, and provide reassurance that continued sexual relations are okay.

In addition, if any pain, bleeding, or loss of fluid from the vagina occurs during or after lovemaking, it is vital to contact your health professional immediately, and to follow whatever instructions he or she may give you.

Your doctor has given sex a green light? You may find that lovemaking is more satisfying and exciting than ever, owing to the higher levels of hormones, increased sensitivity of the breasts and genital area, and freedom from any concerns about contraception.

For some women, though, libido takes a nosedive during pregnancy. In the first trimester, nausea may interfere with desire. By the third trimester, your big belly and aching back may make it tough just to get comfortable in bed, much less get amorous. "My sister adored sex while she was pregnant. She even had intercourse just hours before labor began! But with two babies inside me, I felt clumsy, achy, and exhausted," says Lydia Greenwood. The more babies you're expecting, the earlier that too-big-for-comfort feeling is likely to kick in.

Not all the loss of libido stems from physical factors. Emotions come into play, too. For instance, some women feel so baby-focused during pregnancy that having sex simply doesn't cross their minds very often. "My doctor never prohibited sex, but I admit that while I was pregnant, it was the last thing on my mind. This was tough on my husband, because sex is usually the first thing on his mind, all day, every day," says Miriam Silverstein, mother of fraternal twin boys. "As I headed into my 38th week, though, I was eager for this pregnancy to be over. I had read that sex could bring on labor, so I started jumping on my husband every night. It wasn't really the sex I wanted—I was just eager to meet my babies. And he knew it!"

Other expectant mothers of multiples may feel strange about their growing bodies. "I've always taken pride in my slender, sexy figure. But once I was pregnant with twins, my bigger body seemed unfamiliar. It's not that I felt unattractive—I just didn't feel like myself," Lydia Greenwood admits. You may also be concerned about how your husband views your very pregnant body. Be honest about your concerns, and he's likely to reassure you that he finds you more appealingly feminine than ever. "Ed told me again and again that he thought my big belly was beautiful. That helped me to feel more alluring," says Lydia.

Fear for the babies can also interfere with sexual desire. "Early on, the obstetrician had told us that it was okay to have sex whenever and however we wanted. But when an ultrasound done midway through the pregnancy showed that our babies might have a physical abnormality, we were too afraid to do anything that might hurt them," explains one mother of twins. "Within a month it was determined that the twins were going to be fine, and bedroom activity immediately picked up again."

With your doctor's okay, try these tips for enhancing sex during pregnancy:

- Experiment with positions. "Because I wasn't able to lie on my back, my husband and I were inspired to find some new and interesting positions for sex," Miriam Silverstein says. Side-lying and woman-on-top positions are best, as they do not place undue pressure on your abdomen.
- Don't play the martyr. Tell your partner what feels good and what doesn't.
- If you don't feel like having intercourse, or if your doctor has cautioned against it, explore other ways of sharing sensual pleasure. Give each other a massage, take a shower together, or read a sexy novel aloud.

Physical Activity: What's Safe, What's Not

TAMARA: During my twin pregnancy, I was constantly on the go—attending prenatal exercise classes, working late many evenings, remodeling my kitchen, planning a last romantic getaway with my husband. Maybe it's because I was in New York City, where people rush to do as much as possible, as quickly as possible. Maybe it's because I'd read a book that urged expectant mothers of twins to "make a double effort to stay in shape" and to challenge any doctor who tried to impose "unnecessary restrictions" on activities. Maybe it's because I'm a type A person by nature.

Whatever my reasons, they were misguided. In hindsight, I realize that my body was sending me signals about the need to slow down. Such as? The light-headed sensation that sometimes came over me when I went to my prenatal exercise class during lunch hour instead of putting my feet up and relaxing. The vaginal pressure I sometimes experienced when I hurried to catch the train home. The throbbing in my back as I walked through stores, searching for kitchen cabinets. The exhaustion I felt on vacation as my husband and I explored Key West.

My motto was "Everybody's uncomfortable when they're pregnant, so just do what needs to be done without whining." Not a bad philosophy—except that my interpretation of what needed to be done was way off the mark. My body was not telling me to be stoic and strong; it was trying to tell me that I needed to rest, relax, and limit my activities.

DR. LUKE: All pregnant women must be more cautious when it comes to physical activity—the day-to-day kind like climbing stairs and carrying groceries as well as recreational choices like running or bicycling. But as a mother-to-be of multiples, you need to be especially careful because you're challenging your body to do something extraordinary.

Physical exertion, particularly when it involves the large muscles of the back or legs, shunts blood away from your uterus. This in turn can trigger preterm contractions through the actions of the stress hormones called catecholamines. The effect: An increased risk of having your pregnancy cut short by days, weeks, or even months. That means if your babies are to have the time they need to grow and get strong, it's important for you to slow down.

It's not always easy to alter the pace of your life. You've got a lot going on, and you hate to neglect any of it. When you see your friends who are pregnant with singletons carrying on pretty much as they normally do, you're tempted to behave likewise. "When I was pregnant with my first daughter, I didn't cut back on my activity at all. I was a full-time law student, worked part-time, and went to the gym regularly, too," says Judy Levy. "During my twin pregnancy, though, I really had to take it easy. Dr. Luke was like a mother hen, reminding me to cut back on my activities. But that was good, because I needed the extra prodding."

Could you use some extra prodding, too? It's at your fingertips, as one reader of an earlier edition of this book reports: "This book, more than anything else I read, made me realize that I wasn't just pregnant, but responsible for the future of two other human beings. I credit following the advice in this book for the health and size of my twins."

Here are the specific guidelines to follow:

Get as much rest—lying down—as possible.

Studies show a strong connection between fatigue and preterm labor. Lying down, on the other hand, decreases the catecholamines that can trigger uterine contractions. A prone position also improves circulation to the kidneys, thus helping to eliminate excess fluids.

Blood flow to your babies is better when you're horizontal and better for you, too, since your body doesn't have to work against gravity to pump blood back to your heart. Judy Levy says, "I felt woozy several times a day during the second half of the pregnancy. At first I tried to push through it and just keep on doing whatever I was doing. But then Dr. Luke explained, 'What you're experiencing is called *circulatory stress*. When you feel like you're going to pass out, it means your brain isn't getting enough oxygen. That means your babies aren't getting enough oxygen either.' Once I realized that, I started lying down at the first hint of dizziness."

There's no need to wait until you're exhausted to lie down. Instead, schedule regular rests into your daily routine. If you're a stay-at-home mom, lie down during your toddler's naptime, or take a rest while your older children are in school or at a play date. If you work outside the home, try to arrange for some horizontal time at lunchtime—for instance, if there is a couch in the ladies' room at work, or if you can close your office door and rest on a cot in private. If these options aren't possible, then be sure to lie down as soon as you get home from work—it will make a difference.

And don't let anyone tease you about being lazy. While you are resting, you're not doing nothing. You're *gestating*—helping your babies grow bigger and stronger, and keeping yourself healthier, too.

Don't stand when you can sit.

Women who stand for more than six hours at a time triple their risk of preterm birth, a national study of nurses found.[1] When you stand, blood vessels outside the uterus get compressed against the pelvis. In an attempt to restore circulation, the uterus contracts.[2] "Going into the sixth month, I started to feel a lot of vaginal pressure. That motivated me to look for creative ways to sit down more often," says Marcy Bugajski. Set the ironing board to its lowest position and pull up a chair. Place stools by the stove and sink. If you are stuck in a long line, at a theater or bank, for instance, ask the person behind you to hold your spot while you go sit on a nearby bench until it's your turn at the head of the line.

Limit stair-climbing, stooping, and bending.

Strenuous activity that involves the large muscles of the back or legs is particularly likely to trigger contractions. To prevent this, organize household tasks to minimize trips up the stairs. On errands, take the elevator. Instead of stooping, sit on the floor to pick up clutter or use one of those grabbing devices designed to extend your reach. Recruit someone else to vacuum rugs, mop floors, and scrub the tub. "Once we learned that vacuuming and other household chores could bring on contractions, my husband took over the housework. That was okay with me!" says Stacy Moore, mother of fraternal twin boys.

---

1. Luke B, Mamelle N, Keith L, Munoz F, Minogue J, Papiernik E, et al. The association between occupational factors and preterm birth: A United States nurses' survey. American Journal of Obstetrics & Gynecology 1995; 173:849–62.
2. Schneider KTM, Bollinger A, Huch A, Huch R. 1984. The oscillating "vena cava syndrome" during quiet standing—An unexpected observation in late pregnancy. British Journal of Obstetrics and Gynaecology 1984; 91:766–80.

Avoid lifting and carrying.

Weight bearing causes abdominal muscles to tighten, increasing pressure on the uterus and possibly setting off contractions. Don't lift anything heavy. In lifting even a lightweight object, keep your spine straight and bend your knees in order to protect your back. To maintain your balance, never lift anything from overhead or carry anything so large as to make your gait awkward. The alternatives? Use a rolling basket to transport clothes to the laundry room. Find a grocery store that delivers or that has a motorized cart you can ride. Put your toddler in a stroller, not a backpack.

Keep air travel to a minimum.

Though restrictions vary among airlines, most U.S. carriers allow pregnant women to fly up to 36 weeks' gestation on domestic flights, and up to 35 weeks' gestation on international flights. However, these guidelines pertain to uncomplicated singleton pregnancies, not to pregnancies in which there's an increased risk of premature labor. As an expectant mother of multiples, you'd be well advised to fly only prior to week 24, only if absolutely necessary, and only with your doctor's approval. After the 24th week, it's best to resign yourself to staying home.

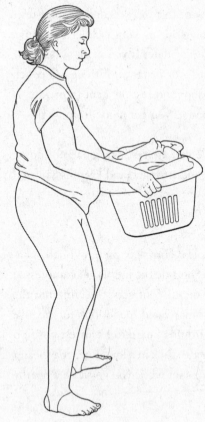

If you must lift something, keep it close to your body and use your knees, not your back.

Why this restriction? Because long-distance travel can trigger contractions. Flying often involves standing in long lines, rushing to make connections, carrying luggage, missing meals, sitting in one cramped position for extended periods of time, and experiencing changes in cabin pressure. The consequences include fatigue, hunger, dehydration, poor circulation, and stress, all of which increase the risk of preterm labor.

If you absolutely must fly during your multiple pregnancy, follow these recommendations:

- Allow sufficient time for checking in and making connections, so you won't have to rush.
- Have a companion or porter handle all luggage.

- If you're tired, don't be shy about requesting a wheelchair or the shuttle cart to get to and from your gate.
- Carry aboard plenty of healthful snacks, but avoid gas-producing foods that might increase in-flight discomfort. If you are not allowed to bring your own bottled water onto the airplane, ask the flight attendant for several bottles as soon as possible after boarding.
- Wear support stockings to improve blood flow.
- Keep your seat belt on continuously while seated in the plane, since air turbulence cannot be predicted, and you don't want to risk a fall.
- Walk around the cabin for a few minutes at least every two hours to improve circulation in your legs. While you're up, visit the bathroom—an overfull bladder is uncomfortable and can trigger contractions.

Get help caring for your older children.

"My daughter was only 18 months old when I got pregnant with the twins, which meant she was still in diapers. By my sixth month, I couldn't change her anymore. I wasn't supposed to lift anything heavy, so I couldn't place her on a changing table. If I sat on the floor to deal with the diaper, I could barely get back on my feet again. I also wasn't able to lift her into or out of her crib or car seat," recalls Judy Levy. "This meant that I simply could not be home alone with my toddler. Someone else had to be available to handle all the 'heavy work.'"

As Judy discovered, reducing daily physical activity can be especially challenging when you have one or more older children. The best solution is to make arrangements for others to help you with their physical care. Enroll children in day care, hire a caregiver to come to your house, or line up a network of friends to provide assistance whenever your partner is not at home. If you are new to your neighborhood, contact a local community organization or house of worship for help.

Another smart option is to find a local club for parents of multiples. Join even before your babies are born, and you'll benefit greatly from the practical advice and moral support of women who've already been down the road you're traveling now. Options include:

- Multiples of America (also known as the National Organization of Mothers of Twins Clubs): 2000 Mallory Lane, Suite 130-600, Franklin, TN 37067-8231. Email Info@MultiplesofAmerica.org; website www.multiplesofamerica.org.
- Raising Multiples (formerly Mothers of Supertwins): P.O. Box 306, East Islip, NY 11730. Telephone 631-859-1110; website www.raisingmultiples.org.

Easy-Does-It Exercise

DR. LUKE: As a swimmer since my teens, I can appreciate that many women today have made a firm commitment to fitness. That's why we've included guidelines on working out safely during pregnancy, as well as a chapter on regaining your figure after your babies are born. We've drawn on the expertise of physical therapist Elaine Anderson, P.T., M.P.H., research associate in the Department of Obstetrics and Gynecology at the University of Michigan. In this section and in Chapter 7, you'll find exercises specifically designed for expectant mothers of multiples.

You've heard hundreds of times how essential exercise is to good health—and in general that's true. The American College of Obstetricians and Gynecologists (ACOG) recommends that pregnant women engage in regular, moderate physical activity in order to achieve a variety of health benefits, including a decreased risk of gestational diabetes.[3]

When you're pregnant with multiples, however, heavy-duty workouts can do much more harm than good. As with other types of physical activity, intense or prolonged exercise drives blood toward muscles and away from your uterus. It also increases blood levels of catecholamines, the hormones that can trigger contractions. So if you weren't very physically active before this pregnancy, now is *not* the time to become an athlete. Even if you have been accustomed to regular workouts, you still should modify your routine significantly.

Meredith Alcott learned that lesson the hard way. "I had always worked out before I got pregnant, so I figured I could keep it up—especially since my obstetrician didn't say anything to me about cutting back on physical activity. I'd go to work, come home exhausted, nap for two hours, then get up and hit the StairMaster," says Meredith, mother of identical twin girls. "Afterward I'd be so tired that it was all I could do just to eat dinner before collapsing back in bed. At the time, I didn't realize I was overdoing it, though looking back, that seems obvious."

Are you expecting triplets or quads? No matter how fit you are, you should avoid vigorous exercise entirely. After all, carrying triplets or quads is enough of a workout in itself! Starting the day her multiples are diagnosed, a woman pregnant with three or more babies should limit exercise to short walks and slow, relaxed swimming.

What if you're expecting twins? Provided you have no pregnancy complications or other risk factors for preterm labor, exercise within the following limits is generally safe:

---

3. American Academy of Pediatrics; American College of Obstetricians and Gynecologists. Guidelines for Perinatal Care. 7th edition. Elk Grove, IL, 2012; 137–8.

- Get your doctor's go-ahead before doing any exercise program, even if it's a workout routine you've done for years. Don't start any new exercise programs.
- Do not overexert yourself. Warning signs such as perspiration, rapid heartbeat, breathlessness, or fatigue mean you need to slow down or stop.
- Scale back to a less intense type of workout. Examples include walking instead of running; taking a leisurely swim instead of doing race-the-clock laps; switching from Zumba to a stretching class.
- Shorten your workouts. The 75-minute classes you used to take are too rigorous right now. Limit each exercise session to no more than 30 to 45 minutes.
- Look for gentle yoga classes that focus on easy postures, breathing techniques, and deep relaxation. Save the more challenging ashtanga and anusara yoga styles—and especially the hot yoga or Bikram classes—until after your babies are born. If at any point even gentle yoga seems like too much, stop. "My doctor told me that I could keep doing yoga until week 20, but I ended up stopping at week 19. It just felt like it was time," says Arlene McAndrew, mother of fraternal boy/boy/girl triplets and an older son.
- Avoid maneuvers that require you to lie on your back. The weight of your uterus compresses major blood vessels, restricting circulation and possibly triggering contractions. If you're devoted to Pilates, stick to the seated exercises for now. You can resume those back rolls and bridges after the babies are born.
- Weight-training workouts should include absolutely *no heavy lifting*. Instead, maintain muscle strength safely by following the exercise routine called Muscle-Tone Maintenance in Chapter 7.
- Avoid activities that challenge balance, such as bicycling. An expanding uterus alters your center of gravity and leaves you more prone to falling. Love to cycle? Go for a leisurely spin on a stationary bike.
- Many fitness centers offer easy-does-it prenatal exercise classes. These can be a good option—but don't assume that a program is safe simply because it's marketed toward pregnant women. If the instructor urges participants to exceed the guidelines in this section, don't enroll.
- Dehydration can set off contractions, so drink plenty of fluids before, during, and after exercising.
- Consider wearing a belly band or Prenatal Cradle Mini Cradle to provide extra support and to lift the uterus off the bladder.
- When the weather is hot or humid, exercise indoors to avoid becoming overheated.
- Listen to your body—it is telling you to slow down. "I had been accustomed to

running 40 to 60 miles a week, but once I was pregnant with the twins, my body just didn't feel like running. Walking and swimming and just living life felt like exertion enough," says Megan Ryerson, mother of boy/girl twins.

- Immediately halt your workout and call your doctor if you experience pain, dizziness, palpitations, or bleeding or leaking of fluids from the vagina.
- When you reach your 24th week of your twin pregnancy, cut your cardio exercise routine to daily short walks and leisurely swimming only.

Is your prepregnancy workout partner teasing you about turning into a couch potato? She's misinformed. Share with her this reader's articulate words: "There is a perception, especially among younger, college-educated women, that any doctor who advises a pregnant mother to slow down and limit her physical activities is a neo-Victorian throwback who thinks pregnancy is a disease. As the first among my girlfriends to get pregnant, I heard a lot of this sort of talk. My (childless) workout buddy even tried to convince me to ignore my obstetrician's orders and exercise anyway! The fact remains that even for a healthy, fit woman, a multiple pregnancy carries higher risks for mother and babies than a singleton pregnancy does."

Remember, a few months away from the gym will not turn your muscles to mush. The body-building routine to follow now is the one that best builds your *babies'* bodies—in other words, rest and relaxation. You'll have plenty of time to regain your shape after your multiples are born—and when that time comes, Chapter 12, "A Better Body after Babies," will help you do just that.

A Word to Working Mothers-to-Be

DR. LUKE: Approximately eight out of ten women of childbearing age work outside the home.[4] Pregnant women who work in physically and/or mentally stressful jobs, studies show, are two to three times as likely to deliver prematurely. They are also more prone to pregnancy complications such as preeclampsia.

Most at risk are women in physically demanding occupations such as nurses, doctors, saleswomen, cleaning staff, assembly-line workers, and military personnel; those in occupations that involve a lot of standing, working with chemicals or vibrating machines, or in a noisy, cold, or wet environment; those who work a non-daytime shift; those who put in more than 45 hours per week; and those who retain responsibility

---

4. US Bureau of Labor Statistics, Bulletin 2217 and Basic Tabulations, Table 12.

for the majority of household chores in addition to working outside the home.[5] Mix any one or more of these risk factors with a multiple gestation, and you've got a potent recipe for trouble.

Does your work involve strenuous physical activity, exposure to hazardous substances (for instance, harsh cleaning products, pesticides, or paint fumes), or high levels of stress? Are you experiencing any pregnancy complications? If so, speak to your doctor about being temporarily reassigned to a position that does not involve these hazards.

Otherwise, an expectant mother of multiples can probably continue to work safely for several months by sticking to the guidelines below. True, following some of these guidelines will require a significant restructuring of your usual workday—but please remember that the limitations are only temporary, and that your babies stand to benefit greatly.

Rest during and after work.

In the course of an eight-hour shift, an expectant mother of multiples ideally should lie down and rest for a minimum of 20 to 30 minutes. Use a cot or sofa in the ladies' room, employee lounge, a spare office, or your company's occupational health office, if possible. Or simply shut your office door, spread a thick blanket on the floor, and rest there. Twin mom Amy Maly suggests another option: "Since I live close to where I work, I was able to come home at lunchtime each day and lie down for an hour."

Make it an inviolable part of your weekday routine to rest again the minute you get home from work. Lie down for at least 20 to 30 minutes. What about dinner? Let your partner fix the meal or order takeout, so you don't have to stand in the kitchen and cook.

Reduce the physical demands of your job.

Extraneous physical activity can be avoided once you set your mind to the task. "To keep from overexerting myself, I made a conscious decision not to get up from my chair unless absolutely necessary," says Amy Maly, who works in the field of marketing. "Instead of walking to a coworker's office to give her a message, I emailed everything. Whenever someone stopped by my desk, they would ask if I needed anything—photocopies, paper clips, a refill of my water carafe. People were always happy to help. It was amazing how much this conserved my energy."

Figure out how to arrange your office to keep everything within easy reach, so you don't have to get up from your chair. Then ask coworkers or maintenance personnel to do the heavy

---

5. Mozurkewich EL, Luke B, Avni M, Wolfe FM. Working conditions and adverse pregnancy outcomes: A meta-analysis. Obstetrics & Gynecology 2000; 95(4):623–35.

work in rearranging furniture as needed. Be sure to place a footstool beneath your desk, so you can elevate your feet.

If your job is inherently physically demanding, ask to be temporarily reassigned. "I'm an occupational therapist, so mine is not a sit-down type of job. At first, I wasn't sure how I would cope with the restrictions on physical activity that Dr. Luke suggested," says Heather Nicholas, mother of boy/girl twins. "My supervisor was very understanding, though. We agreed that whenever one of my patients needed to be lifted from the bed into a wheelchair, I would ask someone else to handle it. Any patient who required a lot of lifting was transferred to a different therapist. We even figured out ways that I could sit rather than stand while doing most of the therapy."

Cut back on work hours.

If you are experiencing complications in your pregnancy, such as preterm labor, cervical shortening, episodes of bleeding, or other problems (detailed in Chapter 7, "Pregnancy Complications: How to Lower Your Risk"), it is strongly advisable that you arrange to limit the number of hours you work per day and the number of days you work per week. Yes, this might be challenging, and, unfortunately, it may require financial sacrifices or a temporary slowdown of your career—but your babies stand to benefit greatly from your commitment to making such changes. Here are some points to consider:

- If you get your health insurance through your job, ask your benefits manager if there is a minimum number of hours you must work—for instance, 25 hours per week—to retain your insurance.
- With your boss, discuss the option of telecommuting—doing a portion or even all of your job from home. This cuts down on the stress of commuting, lets you rest when you feel tired, and may even allow you to get more done in less time since you won't have to deal with constant interruptions from coworkers. "I was so exhausted during the first trimester that it was clear to my boss that something was affecting my productivity. When I explained that I was pregnant with twins, my boss said I could work from home whenever I needed to, coming to the office only when I felt up to it. I realize not everyone is fortunate enough to have this option, but for those who do, it is such a gift," says Megan Ryerson.
- If you normally work a rotating shift, ask to be temporarily reassigned to more regular hours. Research shows that shift rotations are especially fatiguing, since the body must constantly adjust to different schedules of sleep and wakefulness.

- Once you have cut down on your hours, set realistic goals for what you can achieve in that amount of time. Resist the urge to try to accomplish in 10 hours what normally takes 20 hours to do. If your supervisor sets impossible deadlines, renegotiate your duties. Do not let yourself be pushed into doing the extra work from home.
- Do not fill the time you used to spend at work by doing extra household chores. Research has shown that when a pregnant woman reduces her work schedule but then assumes a larger share of household responsibilities, it undermines the very reason for cutting back on work hours and results in more emergency room visits and hospitalizations.[6]

Stress-proof your commute.

Leave home early enough to catch your ride without rushing. If the bus or train is crowded, ask a fellow commuter to give up his seat for you.

Going by car? Always remember to use your seat belt and shoulder harness, fastening the lap strap below your abdomen. Stop the car and walk around for a few minutes if your legs start to swell or cramp.

Judy Levy, an attorney, learned the importance of taking safety precautions. "My commute required an hour's drive each way. One morning in the 24th week of my twin pregnancy, as I was zooming down the middle of a 12-lane expressway, my tire blew out. I pulled over onto the center strip and sat there watching the 18-wheel trucks zoom by so fast that my car quivered. As I imagined myself trying to waddle across six lanes of high-speed traffic, I started to sob. Thank goodness I had my cell phone and membership in an automobile association—two things no pregnant woman should be without. Help arrived about a half hour later, and pretty soon I was on my way again, shaken but unharmed. This experience woke me up to the fact that I couldn't just keep up with my normal life. I had to be careful in everything I did. Step one was to buy new tires!"

If parking is a problem at your workplace, don't be shy about asking your doctor to authorize a temporary handicapped parking permit (check with your state's department of motor vehicles for details). Megan Ryerson, mother of boy/girl twins, says, "I was reluctant when my doctor first suggested this. But it turned out to be a huge help because I no longer needed to arrive at work two or three hours early just to get a decent parking spot."

---

6. Luke B, Avni M, Min L, Misiunas R. Work and pregnancy: The role of fatigue and the "second shift" on antenatal morbidity. American Journal of Obstetrics & Gynecology 1999; 181(5):1172–9.

DR. LUKE: We prescribed handicapped parking permits for all our mothers in the Multiples Clinic, and designated that they be valid for a full year. Not only did the permits make parking easier during pregnancy—for prenatal appointments, grocery shopping, and parking at work—but they also helped after delivery, when our moms of multiples were loading and unloading strollers and equipment for two, three, or four babies at a time.

Leave the air travel to coworkers until after your babies are born.

As discussed earlier in this chapter, flying involves a number of risks for women pregnant with multiples. The fatigue, dehydration, poor circulation, and stress associated with long-distance travel can all trigger contractions. Yes, you may have to miss a business conference or skip the customary face-to-face contact with a faraway client. But those scenarios are infinitely preferable to finding yourself at an out-of-town hospital in preterm labor—or, worse, giving birth before your babies are ready.

PLANNING AND NEGOTIATING A WORK LEAVE

TAMARA: At my 24-week prenatal checkup, my obstetrician casually suggested that I go on medical leave from work when I hit week 28. I was stunned. Most of my friends had worked right up to their due dates, and it had never occurred to me that I might need to stop sooner.

"I just started a new job, and I had planned to work until 36 weeks or so," I said. "Are you sure I have to go on leave so soon?"

"Well, how about if we compromise on 32 weeks?" my easygoing doctor suggested. That seemed like a reasonable plan—until my twins shocked us both by being born at week 31.

DR. LUKE: When you're carrying multiples, please do *not* expect to work past your 28th week. In fact, we urged our patients at the Multiples Clinic to go on leave at 24 weeks, because that's when they needed to begin getting off their feet for at least a few hours each day. If a woman develops complications, or if she's expecting triplets or quads, it's likely that she'll have to stop working even sooner. Quad mom Anne Seifert, for example, left her job as a dental hygienist at 16 weeks.

There's a good chance that you're dismayed by what I've just said. Truly, my coauthors and I understand that it may be a shock to learn that you should begin your work leave long before you expected to. We understand that this may involve financial difficulties or career setbacks for you. We understand that you're reluctant to use up your paid maternity leave before your babies are even born.

We wish that the family leave laws in the United States were more enlightened, so that every mother-to-be could have as much time off, with pay, as she needed. And we wish that we could tell you exactly how to overcome every single challenge created by taking an earlier-than-anticipated work leave. Unfortunately, we cannot do that for you—but we can offer some suggestions to help you strike the right balance between protecting your job and protecting your unborn babies.

Whatever date your doctor gives you for beginning your leave of absence, don't argue or try to bargain for a later date.

In some cases, your work may be able to wait until you return. If it can't wait, someone else can take care of it while you're out.

"It did hurt to hear that I should stop working at 28 weeks, especially since I had just transitioned into a new position. I could tell that my boss thought it was bad timing, and I knew that I could lose a big professional opportunity," says Michelle Brow, mother of fraternal twin girls. "But I decided not to push. I went on short-term disability leave right at 28 weeks because I didn't want to have any regrets when it came to doing what was best for my kids."

Before you break the news to your boss about the date your work leave will begin, find out what you're entitled to under the law and company policy.

Many workers are covered under the federal Family and Medical Leave Act (FMLA). This guarantees an employee the right to take up to 12 weeks of unpaid leave per year to care for a newborn, newly adopted baby, or seriously ill relative, or if the employee has a serious health condition. The physical limitations imposed by a multiple pregnancy qualify under this last category, provided your doctor submits a written statement to this effect to your employer. During the leave time, the person's job or an equivalent one must be held for her, and health insurance provided through the employer must remain in effect (though the employee may need to make arrangements to pay her usual portion of the health insurance premiums during her unpaid leave). The law applies to companies with 50 or more employees within a 75-mile radius. To qualify, an employee must work more than 25 hours per week and have been on the job for a minimum of 12 months.

The Pregnancy Discrimination Act requires employers with more than 15 employees to guarantee job security and paid leave to pregnant women if and to the same extent that they guarantee those benefits to workers with other medical conditions, such as broken legs or heart attacks. In other words, if your company gives male employees longer leaves for other health conditions, female employees may not be limited to 12 weeks for pregnancy- or childbirth-related health conditions. Likewise, if Joe in the next office got six months off for a sabbatical or midcareer training program, you should be able to command a similar deal—meaning that if you stop working at 28 weeks and your multiples are born at 36 weeks, you'd still have more than four months at home with your babies before you'd have to return to work.

A number of states also have temporary disability insurance (TDI) laws that provide partial salary replacement for non-work-related disabilities, including pregnancy- and childbirth-related conditions. The percentage of salary paid under TDI varies from state to state, as does the duration of the disability period allowed. To check on your state, call the regional office of the Department of Labor's Wage and Hour Division (listed in the U.S. Government Offices section of the phone book's blue pages).

Many companies offer their employees benefits that go beyond what's required by law. You can investigate your company's policy through an employee manual, a company website, an in-house online benefits file, or the human resources department's anonymous hotline. You might also contact the following organizations:

- The Women's Bureau at the Department of Labor: www.dol.gov/wb/.
- 9to5, National Association of Working Women: www.9to5.org.
- Your state's labor department.

Talk to your health professional about your work situation. She can prepare whatever documentation is necessary to help you obtain all the benefits to which you are entitled.

Make your announcement in the most professional way possible.
Conventional wisdom says not to announce a pregnancy until you're well into the second trimester, when the risk of miscarriage decreases. With multiples, though, you may want to break the news sooner. You will need to begin your leave much earlier in your pregnancy than the average mother of a singleton would, and you don't want your supervisor to feel that you've left her with inadequate time to prepare for your absence.

Be sure your boss is the first one in the office to learn the news. Keep your announcement professional in tone: "I'm pleased to announce that I'm expecting twins in mid-May." Don't sound apologetic ("Sorry to inconvenience you . . ."), pleading ("I need a favor . . ."), or overly personal ("I've been trying for years to get pregnant . . ."). Then present a plan for how your work could be covered in your absence. A clear-cut strategy sets a collaborative tone—so that when your boss learns that you'll need an extra-long maternity leave, she'll think, "This sounds doable," rather than, "Argh, we can't possibly cope."

Next, outline the schedule you anticipate: "My obstetrician has advised me to begin my leave at 28 weeks, which will be February 15." Do prepare your supervisor for the possibility of an earlier departure: "Should complications with my pregnancy arise, my doctor may tell me to stop working sooner, perhaps without advance notice. I'll keep you apprised of any developments."

Karen Danke, mother of fraternal twin boys, says, "In hindsight, the best advice I can offer is to warn your boss ahead of time that you may need to stop working abruptly and go on immediate bedrest. That's what happened to me—but I wasn't prepared for it. I couldn't go into the office even for a day to tie up loose ends, so nobody knew what to do when all of a sudden I wasn't available. My boss and I both wish we had set up a contingency plan well ahead of time."

Note that under FMLA, you must give your employer 30 days' notice that you intend to take a leave—but only if your medical condition allows this advance notice. If you go into premature labor or have complications that require you to stop working immediately, you are not bound by this 30-day rule.

Be honest about your physical limitations and how they affect your job.

But don't make your special needs the central focus of every staff meeting or conversation around the watercooler. To maintain your professional image, refrain from complaining about morning sickness and swollen ankles. Use your cell phone or home phone, not the office line, to research Lamaze classes. Schedule prenatal checkups well in advance, to claim those hard-to-get 8 A.M. or 6 P.M. appointments.

If you've proven yourself to be a valuable employee, chances are your boss and coworkers will be thrilled for you and happy to help in whatever way they can. "When I told my boss that I'd have to stop working almost immediately, he was wonderfully supportive," recalls Anne Seifert. "He said, 'I know all that you've been through to have children. You take as much time off as you need—now and after you deliver—and take care of yourself and those quadruplets. When you're ready to come back, your job will be here waiting for you.'"

DR. LUKE: Though you may at first be dismayed at the idea of leaving your job, even temporarily, look on the bright side. Without exception, women say that they feel much less stressed, and much more relaxed and well rested, once they go on hiatus from their jobs. If these precautions seem excessive, remember that old adage—*an ounce of prevention is worth a pound of cure*. Every day, every week that your babies can continue to grow and mature before their birth will help them to be that much stronger and healthier whenever they are born—even if that birthday comes sooner than expected. So try to implement as many of these recommendations as you can, without berating yourself if you cannot always follow them 100 percent. You and your babies will all benefit from your efforts.

A few days after her leave began, for instance, one expectant mother of twins called me up and said, "That last week at the office, I was so exhausted and felt such intense vaginal pressure that I could hardly concentrate on work. Now that I don't have to set my alarm for 6 A.M., I can sleep late every morning. And it's great to be able to eat whenever I want, to read or relax all afternoon, and to take a nap when the mood strikes. I wish I hadn't resisted your suggestion to quit working even sooner, because I'm infinitely more comfortable here at home—and I think my babies are, too."

Chapter Seven

Pregnancy Complications: How to Lower Your Risk

Here's good news: Many mothers-to-be of multiples sail through all three trimesters with no complications at all. "I didn't have any problems whatsoever with my twin pregnancy, not even morning sickness," says Stacy Moore, mother of fraternal twin boys.

Still, it's smart to be familiar with the warning signs of trouble—because this will help you spot problems as early as possible, greatly increasing the chances that timely medical intervention will bring the situation under control before any serious consequences develop.

Amy Maly, mother of identical twin girls, knows firsthand the importance of staying vigilant. "Everything was fine until my 31st week of pregnancy, when suddenly something just didn't feel right. There were no obvious symptoms—no pain, no bleeding—but I was suspicious enough that I called my doctor anyway. Thank goodness I did, because it turned out I was in preterm labor," says Amy. Prompt medical intervention halted the contractions and allowed Amy's pregnancy to continue for another five weeks. At that point, she developed preeclampsia—but by then, her twins were big enough to be born safely.

In some cases, despite taking precautions, reporting symptoms early, and receiving appropriate care, complications simply are not preventable. However, even when problems do develop in a multiple pregnancy, it still may be possible to minimize the severity of those complications and to have babies who are born healthy and strong. Heather Nicholas, for example, had a very difficult pregnancy—vaginal bleeding, cervical complications, anemia, digestive problems, frequent contractions—and had to stay on strict bedrest for many months. Nonetheless, she carried her twins to 38½ weeks, ultimately delivering a daughter who weighed 7 lb., 3 oz. and a son who weighed 6 lb., 15 oz.!

Knowledge is power, and you can use it to your advantage. As one reader of an earlier edition of this book explains, "My doctor later told me that, overall, I had one of the healthiest twin pregnancies she had ever seen—normal blood pressure, no anemia, very few preterm contractions, no bedrest, and two healthy babies who were discharged to go home with me. I think the crash course in high-risk obstetrics that I got from reading this chapter is one of the chief reasons why."

So as you read this chapter on pregnancy complications, try not to become unduly alarmed. The goal is to familiarize yourself with the warning signs. That way, if trouble develops, you will recognize it and can alert your doctor immediately—and you will have a sense of some of the treatment options available. "I understand why some people find this information upsetting. But my wife and I appreciated the opportunity to go through our triplet pregnancy with our eyes wide open. It was comforting to know that there were steps we could take to lower the risk of developing certain complications, and to have guidelines on what to do if problems did arise," says Kevin McAndrew, father of fraternal boy/boy/girl triplets and an older son.

Remember the old adage, forewarned is forearmed. Early detection and appropriate treatment are the best safeguards for your own health and that of your multiples.

Signs to Watch for and Steps to Take

DR. LUKE: When patients from the Multiples Clinic call with a question, they sometimes begin the conversation with an apology: "I'm so sorry to bother you with this trivial concern, because it's probably nothing." This stems from the fact that many women tend to be stoic and self-sufficient, giving of themselves to others without taking time to meet or even take notice of their own needs.

This generosity of spirit is admirable in many areas of life. But when you're pregnant with twins, triplets, or quads, stoicism can be problematic. Right now, you need to give top priority to your own needs and those of your babies, so don't hesitate to bring up any concerns you may have. Informed, open, and two-way doctor-patient communication is a vital component of good medical care, so discuss the following conditions with your doctor.

BLEEDING PROBLEMS

Early Vaginal Bleeding

Some women experience slight bleeding within the first week to 10 days after conception, when the fertilized egg or eggs implant in the lining of the uterus. This bleeding is perfectly normal and relatively common. Yet because women who have conceived multiples are likely to experience heavier implantation bleeding than mothers of singletons, you may initially mistake it for a menstrual period.

"I had been trying to get pregnant for almost a year, with no success. So when I got my period in the middle of my sister's baby shower, I could hardly keep from crying. I didn't realize until weeks later that the bleeding I had thought to be a light period was in fact caused by *twins* implanting in my uterus," says Lydia Greenwood, mother of boy/girl twins.

More serious is bleeding later in pregnancy, which may signal a miscarriage. With multiples, the risk of miscarriage before the 20th week of pregnancy is slightly higher than with a singleton. Miscarriage risk is also greater for monochorionic twins (who are always identical) than for dichorionic twins (who are usually fraternal).

There is also the possibility that one or more babies may be lost, while the remaining baby or babies continue to grow and develop normally. When this occurs early in a multiple pregnancy, it is called *vanishing twin syndrome*—a reference to a situation in which a yolk sac or fetus was identified on an earlier ultrasound, then found to be gone on later ultrasounds.[1]

DR. NEWMAN: You may be surprised to learn that an estimated 10 to 15 percent of all live births begin as a twin conception. In other words, for every live-born twin pair, there are as many as 10 to 12 gestations that start as a multiple pregnancy but result in a singleton birth. We were unaware of this vanishing twin phenomenon until the use of ultrasound became common, especially following pregnancies conceived through assisted reproductive technologies.

The spontaneous loss of one or more multiples with the retention of a surviving fetus is most common early in the first trimester. It is often, but not always, accompanied by some vaginal spotting that may be mistakenly dismissed as implantation bleeding.

Approximately 30 percent of implantations identified after in-vitro fertilization but before the identification of fetal heart activity are spontaneously lost. After the point at which a beating fetal heart can be visualized (typically around 5 to 6 weeks'

---

1. Landy H, Keith LG, Keith D. The vanishing twin. Acta Geneticae Medicae et Gemellologiae 1982; 31:179–94.

gestation) but prior to 9 weeks' gestation, there is still a 5 percent to 6 percent vanishing twin rate. Triplets also experience high rates of spontaneous reduction, to either twins or singletons, ranging from 15 to 30 percent. Fortunately, these early vanishing twins do not appear to have an adverse effect on the surviving fetus or fetuses, and no specific treatment is needed or recommended.

I urge my fellow physicians to be careful with the overdiagnosis of vanishing twin syndrome. Lots of things, like small collections of blood or fluid, may be seen by ultrasound and misidentified as a gestational sac. A vanished twin should not be diagnosed unless the doctor identifies embryonic parts, including the yolk sac. A careless misdiagnosis or offhanded comment can have adverse psychological effects on the mother, who may feel as if she lost a baby (even though a second baby had not in fact existed), and potentially on the child, who may someday feel as if he or she lost a sibling.

Cervical Insufficiency

Another reason for bleeding early in pregnancy is *cervical insufficiency,* or CI (sometimes called an *incompetent cervix*), a condition in which the cervix spontaneously and painlessly opens early in pregnancy. CI is believed to be the cause of many miscarriages that occur in the second trimester between 13 and 24 weeks, especially in multiple gestations.

It was previously believed that CI resulted from a genetic weakness of the cervix, or from trauma to the cervix during a previous delivery or other medical procedure. While these factors could be the cause in some cases, many experts now believe that CI is an early extreme in a continuum of premature cervical ripening (cervical softening, loss of strength, increased elasticity, shortening of the cervix, and ultimately dilation). This cervical ripening is a continuous process that can contribute to both early pregnancy loss and, later, to preterm labor or premature rupture of the membranes.

CI is more common in multiple pregnancies, possibly due to an altered hormonal environment or more rapid distension of the uterine cavity. It also seems to be more common in multiple gestations arising from ovulation induction or in-vitro fertilization (IVF), and may be related to multiple ovarian follicles being stimulated and some of the peptide hormones (such as relaxin) those follicles produce.

Other possible symptoms of CI may include an increase in mucus or jelly-like vaginal discharge and/or a feeling of increasing heaviness or pressure in the pelvis. These signs can occur even in the absence of bleeding—so any such symptom warrants an immediate call to your doctor.

If detected early enough, the cervix may be sutured closed. In a procedure called *cerclage,* a stitch is placed around the cervix and tied tightly like a purse string. "At 15 weeks, I started to bleed. It wasn't as heavy as a period, but it did last for two days. A vaginal ultrasound showed that my cervix was shortening," says twin mom Heather Nicholas. "My obstetrician said we could wait a week and see what happened, or we could put in a cerclage the next day. I opted for the cerclage, after which I had to go on bedrest for a week." Typically the cerclage is removed at about 36 to 37 weeks' gestation, or just prior to delivery.

Rarely, the procedure may need to be repeated. Karen Danke, mother of fraternal twin boys, recalls: "My doctor put in a cerclage at 17 weeks. But at 21 weeks, the membranes started to bulge through the opening of my cervix. My obstetrician did a second cerclage, then had me spend the next 24 hours in a special inclined bed that kept my lower body elevated above my head. This was kind of uncomfortable, but it did keep pressure off my cervix. Fortunately, the second cerclage held."

Placental Problems

Complications involving the placenta or placentas are the most common causes of bleeding after the 20th week of pregnancy.

With a condition known as *placenta previa,* the placenta implants low in the uterus, partially or completely covering the cervix. This is more common in multiple gestations, owing to the increased number and/or size of the placentas present. As the cervix begins to open toward the end of the pregnancy, vaginal bleeding or spotting can occur. Most bleeding with placenta previa occurs after 35 weeks' gestation, but it can occur earlier. The bleeding is bright red and generally is painless.

A condition called *abruptio placenta* or *placental abruption* occurs when the placenta partially detaches from the uterus before delivery. This can result in moderate to severe abdominal pain. In addition, there usually is moderate to heavy vaginal bleeding, with the blood typically appearing dark red—however, in 10 to 20 percent of placental abruptions, there is no obvious vaginal bleeding. Mild abruptions (sometimes called *marginal sinus abruptions*) are the most common type and are a frequent cause of preterm labor and preterm birth. Moderate to severe placental abruptions can jeopardize the lives of the unborn babies.

What You Can Do

Immediately report any vaginal bleeding to your obstetrician. He or she will need to determine the cause of the bleeding and suggest appropriate treatment. Be prepared to go on bedrest if instructed to do so. (See "All About Bedrest" later in this chapter.)

Placenta previa occurs fairly randomly, though increased risk may be related to the number of prior pregnancies and, more important, prior cesarean deliveries. For those reasons, not much can be done to prevent it. However, the risks associated with the condition can be minimized by careful monitoring of the pregnancy and by abstaining from strenuous activities and/

or sexual intercourse if so instructed by your doctor. Bleeding is most likely late in pregnancy as contractions increase. This risk can be minimized by scheduling an elective cesarean delivery for between 34 and 36 weeks of gestation.

There *are* several ways to reduce your risk for placental abruption. These include not smoking, not using cocaine or amphetamines, and avoiding contact sports and other activities that could lead to trauma to the abdomen. It is also very important to get treatment if you have hypertension—prevention of placental abruption is one of the most important benefits of controlling your blood pressure during pregnancy.

IRON DEFICIENCY ANEMIA

The majority of women pregnant with multiples eventually develop iron-deficiency anemia, a condition characterized by low levels of iron in the red blood cells that carry oxygen to the tissues. Your risk increases with each additional baby you're carrying, particularly if you had low or borderline iron reserves before becoming pregnant.

Symptoms include fatigue, light-headedness, dull headache, pallor, and shortness of breath. Admittedly, these signs are difficult to differentiate from the signs of pregnancy itself. "Toward the end of the pregnancy, my anemia was so bad that I felt tired all the time, even though all I was doing was lying in bed. It took every bit of my energy just to breathe," says Helen Armer, mother of triplets.

If untreated, anemia can adversely affect the unborn babies' growth, increase the risk of preterm birth, and increase your likelihood of needing a blood transfusion at the time of delivery. That's why your doctor routinely tests your hemoglobin and hematocrit (the iron-carrying components of your blood) several times during pregnancy—typically when you begin prenatal care, again at about 26 weeks, and again just before you deliver.

What You Can Do
To boost your iron stores, increase your intake of iron-rich foods, particularly red meats, liver, liver pâté, and dishes that include bone marrow. Leafy green vegetables also contain iron, but not nearly as much as red meat, and the iron in vegetables is not as readily absorbed.

Your physician may also recommend iron supplements. Judy Levy, mother of fraternal twin girls, says, "Despite all the liver and beef I was eating, I became anemic. My doctor told me to take blood-building medications that included iron along with vitamins B_6, B_{12}, and C, and were specially coated to minimize stomach irritation and maximize absorption. The supplements didn't completely fix the anemia, but they did keep it from getting worse." (Iron supplements are notorious for causing constipation, so see Chapter 6 for treatment strategies.)

GESTATIONAL DIABETES

Gestational diabetes (also called gestational diabetes mellitus, or GDM) is more common in women who are over age 30, are overweight or obese at the start of their pregnancy, or have a family history of diabetes. It is also more common among expectant mothers of multiples, who develop the disorder two to three times more often than singleton moms do, perhaps due to the increased levels and effects of placental hormones, especially human placental lactogen (HPL).

Here's how it occurs: The body requires insulin, a hormone produced by the pancreas, to pull glucose into the cells for use as energy. By about the sixth month of pregnancy, the baby or babies are growing fast, so the mother must make extra insulin. Yet at the same time, the placenta is producing hormones that interfere with the action of insulin. When the insulin supply cannot keep up with the demand, the mother's blood sugar levels soar and she becomes temporarily diabetic.

If gestational diabetes is poorly controlled, the babies are at increased risk for stillbirth. Gestational diabetes also can cause newborn infants to develop hypoglycemia (low blood sugar) and other metabolic problems that have the potential to compromise their health, not only after delivery but in the long term as well.

To check for gestational diabetes, your urine should be tested for the presence of glucose at each prenatal checkup. In addition, all women are routinely screened at about 24 to 28 weeks of pregnancy—though you may be screened earlier and more frequently because you're expecting multiples. One hour after drinking a special beverage that contains 50 grams of glucose, your blood is drawn to determine your blood glucose level. If this reading is elevated (usually defined as a glucose level above 140 mg/dl, although some medical centers use slightly lower values), you undergo a second test in which blood is drawn hourly for three hours. If the results of this second test are also abnormal, gestational diabetes is diagnosed.

What You Can Do
Be alert for the warning signs of gestational diabetes—excessive thirst, increased frequency and volume of urination, constant fatigue, and recurrent vaginal yeast infections. Also, find out whether any members of your extended family have diabetes or developed gestational diabetes during pregnancy, and if so, alert your doctor to this fact.

If you are diagnosed with this disorder, your obstetrician may have two new members join your health care team: a physician and a dietitian who specialize in diabetes. You need to follow a diet in which carbohydrates are evenly distributed throughout the day. It should be possible to stay on the diet described in Chapters 4 and 5 with few, if any, changes—because it is basically a diabetic diet. In many cases, diet therapy is effective in controlling blood glucose levels, though some women may require insulin injections to normalize the elevated blood sugars. It also is likely that you will need to monitor your blood sugar levels at home, typically upon awakening in the morning and again one to two hours after each meal, and to record those results in a log to be reviewed during each visit with your health care providers.

If you have gestational diabetes, close adherence to your diet, medication schedule, and blood glucose self-monitoring regimen will be essential to a successful pregnancy outcome. This may be hard to accept at first. "I had been so tired that I felt like a zombie. That's when I was diagnosed with gestational diabetes. Then I felt betrayed by my body. It seemed like pregnancy should be the one time when I could eat what I wanted, but suddenly I could barely have any carbs at all, or my blood sugar would go wild. It also was a big adjustment to have to test my blood sugar levels throughout the day," says Michelle Brow, mother of fraternal twin girls. "But I kept reminding myself that the stakes were high and I was doing this for my babies. It was easier after the first couple of weeks on insulin, because my energy came back and I started feeling so much better physically."

The severity of gestational diabetes usually worsens as pregnancy progresses due to the growing placentas and higher concentration of anti-insulin placental hormones. So keep in mind that changes in treatment are frequently necessary—and those changes are best determined with a full knowledge of your blood sugar values as reflected in your daily log.

After delivery, gestational diabetes resolves. However, women who experienced this disorder during pregnancy have up to a 30 percent chance of developing type 2 diabetes during the next 10 to 20 years. After you deliver, make sure that your doctor checks you for diabetes at your postpartum visit and during each of your annual checkups in the future.

Intrauterine Growth Restriction (IUGR) and Selective Intrauterine Growth Restriction (sIUGR)

Multiples are at increased risk for *intrauterine growth restriction* (IUGR). This is assessed by comparing the estimated fetal weight to the expected fetal weight at a given gestational age. If the babies' estimated weight is below the 10th percentile, they are considered to potentially be experiencing intrauterine growth restriction. By late pregnancy, up to 30 percent of twins and a higher percentage of triplets and quads are IUGR. In the absence of other medical or obstetrical conditions complicating the pregnancy, much of this IUGR is due to an inadequate nutrient supply—not surprising, considering the increased demands of a multiple pregnancy.

Another type of growth restriction among multiples is known as *selective intrauterine growth restriction* (sIUGR), sometimes called *growth discordance*. Here's what happens: Multiples don't always grow at the same rate *in utero*. One baby may receive a disproportionate share of nutrients if the placental structure favors that baby more than the other or others. A sibling who gets a smaller portion of nutrients ends up growing more slowly and being significantly smaller than its co-twin or co-triplets. Some discrepancy between multiples is expected, but at the extremes, sIUGR can reflect a dangerous situation. This discrepancy is usually revealed through ultrasound and may be evident even early in the pregnancy. Discordance is calculated as the difference in the estimated weights of the largest and smallest baby divided by the weight of the larger baby multiplied by 100.

"The doctor discovered at about 24 weeks that one twin was growing much more slowly than the other was," recalls Marcy Bugajski, mother of fraternal twin boys. "That baby ended up being a lot smaller at birth—3 lb., 11 oz., compared to his brother's birthweight of 5 lb., 8 oz."

What You Can Do

Meeting the nutritional challenges of a multiple pregnancy, as discussed in prior chapters, is key to minimizing the risk for intrauterine growth restriction. If all your babies show signs of IUGR, or if it's determined that one baby has begun to lag behind his or her siblings and shows signs of sIUGR, your doctor will want to keep a close eye on the situation. You may be asked to come in for additional checkups, weekly or twice-weekly testing of fetal well-being using electronic fetal heart rate monitoring (the nonstress test), and/or ultrasound assessment of fetal behavior and amniotic fluid volume (the biophysical profile). Careful attention to your diet, of course, becomes more crucial than ever.

In the case of serious sIUGR, it may become necessary at some point to deliver all your multiples in order to give the smallest baby the best possible chance for survival. "At 20 weeks, my ultrasound showed that all three of my babies were growing well. But by week 25, one baby's growth was about a week behind the others. Another ultrasound at 29 weeks showed that this baby had scarcely grown at all in the previous month," says Ginny Seyler, mother of triplets. "By 30 weeks, it was clear to my doctor that this child needed to be delivered, so I ended up having a cesarean section that day. We went through some rough weeks after their birth, but now all three children are fine."

PERIPARTUM CARDIOMYOPATHY

This is a rare form of congestive heart failure that some women develop in late pregnancy or during the first year after delivery. It usually involves the left ventricle of the heart, which has dilated and is not pumping efficiently. The compromised function of the left side of the heart allows fluid to back up into the lungs and to leak into the breathing spaces. This is referred to as *pulmonary edema*. Most cases are diagnosed among women of African descent, but this complication has been reported among women of all races and ethnicities.

Symptoms include difficulty breathing, particularly when lying down and at night; fatigue and palpitations; chest and abdominal pain; and a cough with or without blood. Risk factors for developing peripartum cardiomyopathy include multiple pregnancy (accounting for about 10 percent of reported cases), history of preeclampsia, family history of peripartum cardiomyopathy, and Guillain-Barré neuropathy. This complication is diagnosed with an echocardiogram (an ultrasound of the heart) and a chest X-ray, and treated with medications to increase the contraction strength of the heart and to eliminate extra fluid.

What You Can Do

Fortunately, this is a rare pregnancy complication. However, if you develop any symptoms that might be indicative of peripartum cardiomyopathy, report them to your physician at once. Early detection and treatment are critical. Depending on the extent of heart damage, some women are advised against becoming pregnant again.

PREECLAMPSIA

This condition is characterized by a rapid rise in blood pressure, the presence of protein in the urine, sudden weight gain, and swelling of the hands and face from fluid retention. The cause of preeclampsia is unknown, but it is more common among women who have a prior pregnancy complicated by preeclampsia, or preexisting high blood pressure or diabetes. Preeclampsia occurs in about 1 out of 20 singleton pregnancies, but in nearly 1 in 5 multiple gestations—particularly among mothers who are older or overweight, or for whom this is their first pregnancy. (If you've previously delivered a baby at full term without preeclampsia, your risk for developing preeclampsia during your multiple pregnancy is greatly reduced.)

Preeclampsia typically occurs during the second half of pregnancy. However, in multiple gestations, preeclampsia generally occurs earlier and can be more severe than in singleton pregnancies. Particularly when a woman is carrying triplets or quads, preeclampsia tends to be atypical, meaning that hypertension is not always the initial sign, nor is protein always present in the urine.

Bedrest is usually the recommended treatment if the symptoms and blood pressure elevation are mild. If your condition becomes severe, you are admitted to the hospital and given medications to lower your blood pressure. You also receive magnesium sulfate to prevent *eclampsia* (the onset of seizures). Other tests are done to determine if your preeclampsia is having adverse effects on your liver or kidneys or on your blood's ability to clot.

Because preeclampsia resolves after delivery, the ultimate cure is to give birth. However, the seriousness of the mother's condition must be balanced against the babies' readiness to face life outside the womb. "One Tuesday when I was getting close to 36 weeks, Dr. Luke called me to see how I was doing. I told her I felt puffy and my feet looked like blocks, and my legs were so swollen that they measured two full inches larger than normal. When Dr. Luke heard that, she said, 'I'm coming to get you right now. You're going to the hospital.' Sure enough, I had developed preeclampsia," recalls Amy Maly. "Because my blood pressure was so high, and because the doctor knew that both babies were already over 5 pounds, we decided not to postpone labor any longer. My identical twin girls were born early Thursday morning."

What You Can Do
Reduce your risk of developing this condition by increasing your intake of foods and/or supplements that provide certain nutrients:

- Omega-3, an essential fatty acid found in all seafood.
- Calcium, an essential mineral found in dairy products.
- Vitamin C, an antioxidant available in citrus fruits and juices, kiwi, strawberries, red peppers, sweet potatoes, broccoli, and tomatoes.
- Vitamin E, another antioxidant found in vegetable oils, nuts, seeds, wheat germ, mangoes, and asparagus.

DR. NEWMAN: Although taking a low-dose of baby aspirin (81 milligrams per day) has been extensively studied as a possible approach to preventing preeclampsia, the results of these studies have been contradictory. When tested specifically in women carrying multiples, low-dose aspirin did not significantly reduce the risk of preeclampsia or improve pregnancy outcomes. However, analysis of all available studies suggests that baby aspirin may reduce the risk of preeclampsia by a modest 10 to 15 percent among women who are at increased risk. And the therapy has been determined to be entirely safe during pregnancy.

My advice? I do not routinely recommend baby aspirin for healthy expectant mothers of twins who have had a prior uncomplicated pregnancy. However, I do start baby aspirin as early as possible for women whose multiple pregnancy is their first pregnancy, for women with a history of chronic hypertension or prior preeclampsia, and for women expecting triplets or quads.

Prevention strategies aside, it is vital that you learn the warning signs of preeclampsia: swelling, particularly of the face; severe or constant headaches; abdominal pain in the upper right quadrant; blurred vision or a sensation of seeing flashing lights or exploding fireworks; and/or rapid weight gain (a pound or more per day). This is particularly important if you began this pregnancy overweight, as excess pounds appear to increase a woman's risk of preeclampsia.

Don't make the mistake of passing off these symptoms as normal discomforts of pregnancy. "I got so incredibly bloated that my weight jumped up 18 pounds in two weeks—but it was all due to water retention. Then I started seeing little silver spots in front of my eyes. Yet even though I'm a nurse, I didn't put two and two together," admits twin mom Marcy Bugajski. "I guess I tended to brush off the warnings. The doctors would talk about symptoms to watch for, but the words never really penetrated. You always think, 'This will never happen to me.' But I'm living proof that complications can develop even when you're sure they won't."

Intrahepatic Cholestasis of Pregnancy (ICP)

This liver disorder, which develops in the late second trimester or the third trimester, affects about 1 percent of pregnant women—and a higher percentage of women carrying multiples. When the bile doesn't flow normally in the small bile ducts of the liver, bile salts accumulate in the skin, leading to severe itching. Usually ICP first affects the hands or feet, classically between the fingers or between the toes, but it can occur anywhere and may spread all over the body. The itchiness can be intense and is typically worse at night. While ICP does not cause a rash, you can end up with red, irritated abrasions from scratching.

ICP can have serious pregnancy-related consequences. Women with ICP have higher rates of preterm labor and delivery. Their babies also are at increased risk for unexpected stillbirth, meaning stillbirth that is not anticipated either by changes in fetal growth or by abnormalities on fetal heart rate testing due to hypoxia. One theory is that the accumulation of bile acids has an adverse effect on the conduction system of the fetal heart, predisposing a fetus to a lethal arrhythmia.

What You Can Do

If you develop symptoms that might suggest ICP, it is very important to alert your doctor immediately. There are several treatments, such as the medication ursodiol, that help bind the bile salts and relieve the symptoms. It is believed, but not proven, that lowering the maternal bile acids also lowers the risk of stillbirth. You also may undergo increased fetal testing. However, due to the risk of unexpected stillbirth, doctors often recommend early induction of labor or a cesarean (if appropriate) when patients develop ICP.

The symptoms of ICP usually disappear within one to seven days following delivery. However, there is an increased risk of recurrence in future pregnancies—so if you developed ICP during a previous pregnancy, be sure to share that information with the doctor who is caring for you during your multiple pregnancy.

Complications Unique to Monozygotic Pregnancies

If twin-type testing, as discussed in Chapter 1, has determined that your multiples are dizygotic (fraternal), you can skip this next section and move ahead in this chapter to the section called "Preterm Labor: The Major Problem in Multiple Pregnancies." That's because the pregnancy complications covered next occur only among monozygotic (identical) multiples—and specifically, only among those who are also monochorionic, meaning that they share a single placenta and outer fetal membrane called the chorion.

Some of these complications affect only those multiples who also share a single amnion or inner membrane—the monoamniotic, monochorionic (mo/mo) twins. Other complications can affect both mo/mo and diamniotic, monochorionic (di/mo) twins who share a chorion but have their own amnions. So if you are carrying monozygotic twins who are diamniotic, dichorionic (di/di), you too can skip this section.

Fortunately, the complications associated with di/mo or mo/mo pregnancies are fairly rare and, in many cases, can be effectively treated. But, unfortunately, these complications are typically serious, and usually there is nothing that can be done to prevent them.

So if your multiples are di/mo or mo/mo, the choice of what to do with the information presented here is yours. You may want to skip this section for now, looking up the relevant section later only if you are diagnosed with a particular complication. Or if you're the type of person who prefers to know about potential problems before they arise, even though the likelihood of ever having to face them is small, you may want to review the information below in advance.

It's also a good idea to share Appendix E of this book with your obstetrician. Titled "Doctor to Doctor: A Research Update," this appendix includes more detailed and research-oriented information geared toward physicians whose patients are carrying multiples, with an emphasis on di/mo and mo/mo gestations. Your doctor can review this appendix and then discuss the information with you directly, explaining in detail anything that is specifically relevant to your situation.

STRUCTURAL ANOMALIES IN MONOCHORIONIC PREGNANCIES

Fetal structural defects occur approximately twice as often in multiple gestations compared to singletons.[2] Although monochorionic twins account for the majority of this increase, it is

2. Kohl SG, Casey G. Twin gestation. Mt. Sinai Journal of Medicine 1975; 42:523–9.

relatively rare for both twins to be affected by the same anomaly. The most common structural defects are cardiac malformations, spina bifida, facial clefts, gastrointestinal anomalies, anterior abdominal wall defects, and bladder defects. Many of these anomalies are considered midline defects, which are probably a consequence of errors in the underlying process of zygote splitting in monozygotic twins.

Another cause of fetal malformations in monochorionic twins is ischemic injury (meaning injury related to inadequate blood supply) to the brain, bowel, or kidneys that occurs due to placental vascular abnormalities. These are covered later in this section, in the discussions on twin-twin transfusion syndrome and acute intertwin transfusion.

Optimizing outcomes when pregnancies are complicated by fetal anomalies requires that those anomalies be detected. That is one reason why all women who are carrying multiples should undergo a fetal anatomic survey, usually between 18 and 22 weeks of gestation. Done via ultrasound (as described in Chapter 2), this involves a very thorough evaluation of the internal and external organs of each baby as well as the structure of the placenta or placentas. Though the anatomic survey is not guaranteed to reveal whether or not a structural anomaly exists, it is highly likely to do so. At the Twin Clinic at MUSC, for instance, Dr. Newman's staffers have identified 85 percent of fetal anomalies in their multiple gestations, with no false-positive diagnoses.

What is the value of knowing whether malformations are present before the babies are born? Prenatal diagnosis often allows for medical interventions, such as increased fetal testing to help prevent stillbirth of the affected twin; fetal therapy or surgery prior to delivery; a change in the timing, location, or route of delivery; and advance consultation with neonatal and pediatric subspecialists who may provide immediate or long-term care after the birth. Prenatal diagnosis of severe malformations also provides an opportunity for parents to consider the option of *selective multifetal reduction* (eliminating a nonviable fetus in order to improve the outcome for the remaining fetus) or pregnancy termination. And even in cases in which nothing can be done, many parents prefer to be forewarned about possible problems with any of their unborn children.

Acardiac Twin (TRAP Sequence)

Acardiac twin, also known as *twin reversed arterial perfusion* (TRAP) sequence, is an extremely rare defect that occurs in only about 1 percent of monozygotic twin pregnancies, and only in di/mo or mo/mo gestations. Acardia means that one baby is only partially developed and has no heart of its own. The acardiac twin relies on an abnormal vascular connection across the shared placenta, so that the normal twin (called the *pump twin*) is actually providing the blood supply to the acardiac twin. This responsibility puts tremendous strain on the normal twin.

The acardiac twin cannot survive. The goal of treatment is to protect the life and health of the normal twin, who is at risk for congestive heart failure, polyhydramnios (excessive amniotic fluid, which can lead to premature rupture of the membranes and maternal respiratory problems), and preterm birth. The normal twin's prognosis depends in part on the size of the acardiac twin—the smaller the acardiac twin is relative to the normal twin, the less stress there is on the normal twin and the better the outcome is likely to be.

When the acardiac twin is small (less than 50 percent the size of the normal twin), the pregnancy should be carefully monitored but no immediate action may be necessary. However, if the acardiac twin is relatively large or if the normal twin develops signs of heart failure, an attempt can be made to interrupt the abnormal vascular connection and halt the blood flow between the two fetuses. This can be accomplished either by ultrasound-guided injection of a substance into the acardiac twin's umbilical artery or by performing prenatal surgery with laser ablation of the vascular connection or direct umbilical cord ligation. These sorts of interventions generally require a referral to a facility that performs fetal surgery. Your doctor can provide a referral, or you can contact the North American Fetal Therapy Network, an association of medical centers in the United States and Canada that perform advanced in utero fetal therapeutic procedures (website www.naftnet.org; email information@NAFTNet.org).

Conjoined Twins

Conjoined twinning, which is also exceedingly rare, occurs only in mo/mo monozygotic gestations. It means that the fetuses are fused and share certain organs or body parts.

Conjoined twins can be reliably diagnosed using ultrasonography, usually by the end of the first trimester. The combination of ultrasonography and MRI can identify the extent of organ sharing. Sadly, a substantial percentage of conjoined twins are stillborn and another large percentage do not survive past 48 hours after birth. Among the survivors, the prognosis depends on the degree of shared organs, the vital nature of those organs, and their amenability to surgical separation.

Twins joined at the belly (omphalopagus twins) usually have the best chance for surgical separation and survival, especially if they share no organs and there is only a skin or muscle bridge connecting them. Twins joined at the chest (thoracopagus) have the poorest prognosis because of the high frequency of a shared and abnormal heart. With twins joined at the head (craniopagus), the prognosis generally can be predicted only after birth because it's difficult to assess the degree of intracranial fusion and vascular connections before delivery.

If there is a possibility of survival, conjoined twins should be delivered by elective cesarean at a center capable of the complex postdelivery evaluation and care that will be required. Even if the conjoined twins are not expected to survive, cesarean delivery is usually needed to avoid maternal trauma. When the diagnosis of conjoined twins is made in the first or early second trimester, particularly if the prognosis is poor, parents may consider the option of pregnancy termination.

Conjoined twinning is believed to be a random event associated with delayed splitting of the single fertilized egg, and the risk of recurrence is negligible. There has never been a reported case of a conjoined twin giving birth to conjoined offspring.

Twin-Twin Transfusion Syndrome (TTTS)

Probably the most common serious complication in monochorionic twin pregnancies is twin-twin transfusion syndrome (TTTS). It can occur in both di/mo and mo/mo twins, but is more common in di/mo gestations. TTTS is a consequence of unbalanced blood flow in the shared monochorionic placenta.

Specifically, TTTS is caused by large vascular abnormalities (called arteriovenous malformations) that are not balanced out by connections between blood vessels that allow blood to flow in the opposite direction. This results in one twin, the *arterial donor,* receiving too little blood—while the co-twin, the *venous recipient,* gets too much blood.

The donor twin may develop anemia, low blood volume, low blood pressure, and growth restriction. Reduced blood flow to the kidneys leads to reduced fetal urination, which in turn causes a dangerous drop in the amount of amniotic fluid. As a result, the amniotic membranes can stick to the donor fetus like plastic food wrap, pasting the fetus to the side of the uterine wall in a phenomenon referred to as a *stuck twin.* The donor twin also may suffer injury to the brain, kidneys, and intestines due to poor blood flow.

Meanwhile, for the recipient twin, the increased blood flow from the placenta causes excessive circulating blood volume, straining that fetus's heart and increasing the risk of congestive heart failure. Increased urination leads to excessive amniotic fluid, which contributes to uterine overdistension and increases the risk of premature rupture of the membranes and preterm labor.

TTTS can be clinically categorized as mild, moderate, or severe based on the gestational age at onset and on the anticipated outcome:

- Mild TTTS is the most common form and is the least dangerous. The diagnosis is usually made in the third trimester based on discrepancies in fetal weights (with the donor twin being smaller and the recipient twin being larger) and in amniotic fluid volumes. The anticipated outcome of mild TTTS is reasonably good, similar to that of other twin pregnancies with selective growth restriction.
- Moderate TTTS is usually diagnosed after 20 weeks, in the late second or early third trimester. Without medical intervention, the mortality rate ranges between 50 and 70 percent.

- Severe TTTS is usually identified before 20 weeks' gestation. Without intervention, delivery usually occurs before 30 weeks and, sadly, neither twin is likely to survive.

Because of the severity of early-onset TTTS and its tendency to progress rapidly, it is recommended that monochorionic twins undergo ultrasound scanning every two weeks after 16 weeks of gestation to measure the amniotic fluid in each sac and to assess the condition of each fetus's bladder. In addition, umbilical artery Doppler studies should be performed to evaluate placental dysfunction. The donor twin also should be checked for anemia using ultrasound Doppler flow velocities.

TTTS often can be successfully treated, allowing one or both twins to survive. For moderate to severe cases, a therapy called placental laser photocoagulation is now the standard of care before 26 weeks' gestation. With this technique, a device known as a fetoscopic laser is inserted into the uterus and gestational sac, and used to identify and block off the abnormal placental vascular connections between the two fetuses. The effectiveness of this treatment has continually improved since its introduction more than two decades ago. However, risks remain considerable in severe cases. While survival of at least one fetus occurs in 80 to 90 percent of cases, survival of both fetuses occurs only 50 to 60 percent of the time. Studies are under way to determine whether or not laser photocoagulation is beneficial in mild cases of TTTS.

Another therapy for TTTS is amniocentesis to remove the excess amniotic fluid from around the recipient twin. Though not as effective as laser photocoagulation,[3, 4] reduction amniocentesis can be helpful beyond 26 weeks' gestation in certain cases, especially when the mother is experiencing respiratory difficulty or shows signs of preterm labor.

For more information, emotional support, and a list of medical centers that perform laser surgery for TTTS, contact the Twin to Twin Transfusion Syndrome Foundation (website www.tttsfoundation.org; email info@tttsfoundation.org).

Acute Intertwin Transfusion

Sadly, it sometimes happens that one unborn multiple dies in utero. When this happens during the second or third trimester, it potentially can lead to complications that pose risks to the

---

3. Rossi AC, Vanderbilt D, Chamit RH. Neurodevelopmental outcomes after laser therapy for twin-twin transfusion syndrome. Obstetrics & Gynecology 2011; 118:1145–50.
4. Salomon LJ, Örtqvist L, Aegerter P, et al. Long-term developmental followup of infants who participated in a RCT of amniocentesis vs. laser photo-coagulation for treatment of TTTS. American Journal of Obstetrics & Gynecology 2010; 203:444–51.

surviving fetus or fetuses. Monochorionic twins are at higher risk than dichorionic twins. In twin pregnancies complicated by the demise of one twin, intrauterine death of the co-twin occurs in 12 to 15 percent of monochorionic gestations but in only 3 to 4 percent of dichorionic gestations.[5, 6]

In a monochorionic twin pair, following the death of the first twin, the resulting low pressure in that twin's circulatory system results in blood from the survivor rapidly back-bleeding into the demised fetus. If the resulting low blood pressure is severe, the surviving twin is at risk for damage to vital organs, including the kidneys and bowel. The brain of the surviving twin also may be adversely affected by the lack of blood flow and low oxygen supply. To check this, some doctors offer ultrasound and/or MRI to women with monochorionic placentas approximately three to four weeks after the demise of one twin has been detected. Although a normal ultrasound or MRI does not definitively rule out any brain abnormalities in the surviving twin, it is certainly an encouraging finding.

Additional surveillance also can be done to assess the surviving fetus's growth and well-being. Ultimately, 10 to 25 percent of monochorionic twin survivors will demonstrate evidence of neurodevelopmental delay after the loss of its co-twin in utero.

If the demise of one twin occurs at 34 weeks' gestation or later, delivery should be considered. If there are no other complications, however, a single fetal demise in a twin pregnancy at less than 34 weeks should not necessitate immediate delivery. In the absence of acute intertwin transfusion, careful surveillance offers the advantage of allowing the surviving twin to reach a greater gestational age prior to delivery.

Monoamniotic Gestations and the Need for Extra Monitoring

Less than 1 percent of monozygotic twin gestations are monoamniotic. Mo/mo twinning occurs approximately once in every 25,000 to 30,000 pregnancies. Since both fetuses are in the same amniotic sac, umbilical cord entanglement is present in virtually all monoamniotic twin sets. Tight knotting of the cords can result in sudden, unexpected fetal demise. Fortunately, there has been a substantial reduction in stillbirths among mo/mo twins since the advent of imaging technologies that allow for prenatal identification and monitoring of monoamniotic gestations.

In early pregnancy, it is easy to differentiate dichorionic from monochorionic twins using

---

5. Ong S, Zamora J, Khan K, Kilby M. Prognosis for the co-twin following single-twin death: A systematic review. British Journal of Obstetrics and Gynaecology 2006; 113:992–8.
6. Hillman SC, Morris RK, Kilby MD. Co-twin prognosis after single fetal death: A systematic review and meta-analysis. Obstetrics & Gynecology 2011; 118:928–40.

ultrasound. But it is more difficult to differentiate diamniotic from monoamniotic twins, as both of these conditions are associated with only a single placenta and fetuses of the same gender. The key ultrasound findings that your doctor looks for to help diagnose monoamniocity are the presence of a single yolk sac and the absence of a thin amniotic membrane separating the two fetuses. Because it is hard to identify the thin dividing amniotic membrane before 12 to 13 weeks' gestation, the diagnosis of monoamniotic twins generally cannot be certain until at least 14 to 16 weeks. Even after that time, efforts to identify the dividing amniotic membrane should continue, given that diamniotic/monochorionic twins are 30 times more common than monoamniotic/monochorionic twins.

If you do have monoamniotic twins, an essential point to discuss with your doctor concerns fetal monitoring. Because of the unpredictable risk of dual fetal loss due to constriction of umbilical cord blood flow, monoamniotic twin pregnancies need increased fetal surveillance. There are two options: frequent outpatient fetal monitoring (usually three times per week) or admission to the hospital for daily fetal monitoring.

Although the number of cases studied is small, the available data suggest that inpatient monitoring is best. In studies, among monoamniotic twins whose mothers were admitted to the hospital, there were no stillbirths, whereas there was a 15 percent loss rate when the pregnancy was managed on an outpatient basis.[7]

If inpatient management is chosen, the next decision concerns when to enter the hospital. Some physicians advise hospital admission at the point of viability, which is approximately 24 weeks of gestation, while others favor 26 weeks or even later, when the survivability rate is higher and the risk for long-term health problems is lower. You should discuss this with your doctor, but ultimately the decision is up to you and your partner.

During your hospital stay, you undergo fetal monitoring on a set schedule, typically three hour-long sessions per day. In addition, you probably will be given injections of antenatal corticosteroids to enhance the babies' lung development, which is very important in case an emergency delivery becomes necessary.

If you and your doctor opt for outpatient monitoring, you will probably have frequent fetal nonstress testing, typically three times per week. This testing can reveal evidence of umbilical cord constriction or fetal hypoxia (lack of adequate oxygen supply).[8]

No matter what type of monitoring you undergo, you should be aware that most obstetri-

---

7. Heyborne KD, Porreco RP, Garite TJ, Phair K, Abril D; Obstetrix/Pediatrix Research Study Group. Improved perinatal survival of monoamniotic twins with intensive inpatient monitoring. American Journal of Obstetrics & Gynecology 2005; 192:96–101.

8. Rodis JF, McIlveen PF, Egan JFX, et al. Monoamniotic twins: Improved perinatal survival with accurate prenatal diagnosis and antenatal fetal surveillance. American Journal of Obstetrics & Gynecology 1997; 177:10469.

cians recommend delivery of mo/mo twins between 32 and 34 weeks' gestation to minimize the risk of stillbirth while balancing that against the risk of serious newborn complications. The optimal timing of delivery is discussed in more detail in Chapter 9.

Preterm Labor: The Major Problem in Multiple Pregnancies

Of all the potential complications that might develop during a dizygotic or monozygotic multiple gestation, preterm labor—characterized by the presence of regular uterine contractions and cervical changes that occur prior to 37 weeks of gestation—is probably the most common. It is also potentially one of the most dangerous for your babies because preterm labor can lead to preterm birth.

Approximately 11 percent of singletons, 60 percent of twins, 93 percent of triplets, and virtually all quadruplets are preterm or premature, meaning that they are born prior to 37 completed weeks of pregnancy. Among infants born prematurely, nearly one in 10 does not live. In fact, preterm birth is the leading cause of neonatal and infant death in this country. Preemies who do survive are at higher risk for various physical and cognitive difficulties, such as hearing loss, vision problems, developmental disabilities and delays, cerebral palsy, and perhaps autism.[9, 10] The earlier in pregnancy the babies are born, the more serious the consequences are likely to be.

Sometimes there is a medical reason why multiples need to be delivered early—for instance, because the mother develops severe preeclampsia or because one or more of the babies have a serious medical complication that cannot be addressed in utero. But approximately 70 percent of preterm births are unintended and spontaneous, resulting from early rupture of the membranes or early onset of labor.

Many experts believe that uterine overdistension plays the greatest role in causing spontaneous preterm birth among multiples; the increasing stretch on the uterine wall triggers a number of biochemical and physiologic changes. These in turn result in increased uterine contractions and inflammatory changes in the cervix and fetal membranes, all contributing to premature onset of the delivery process.

---

9. Wadhawan R, Oh W, Perritt RL, et al. Twin gestation and neurodevelopmental outcome in extremely low birth weight infants. Pediatrics 2009; 123:e220–e7.
10. Wadhawan R, Oh W, Vohr BR, et al. Neurodevelopmental outcomes of triplets or higher-order extremely low birth weight infants. Pediatrics 2011; 127:e654–e60.

Poor growth of one or more infants can also be a significant factor for preterm labor.[11] In addition, in vitro fertilization and other forms of assisted reproduction may be an independent risk factor for preterm delivery of multiples, compared with multiples who are spontaneously conceived.

And, of course, the more babies there are, the greater the risk for preterm birth—and the more premature the babies are likely to be. Here's how the average gestational age at delivery decreases as the fetal number increases:

- Twins, on average, are born at 35.4 weeks' gestation.
- Triplets, on average, arrive at 31.8 weeks.
- Quadruplets, on average, are born at 29.7 weeks.

CRITICAL TIME PERIODS

Think of your multiple pregnancy as divided into six time periods, each with differing implications for babies born during that period. Here's how it breaks down:

Conception to week 20: Any pregnancy (singleton as well as multiple) involves some possibility of ending during this period. At this stage, the fetus or fetuses are not yet viable, and the pregnancy loss is called miscarriage.

Weeks 20 to 24—the border of viability: Most babies born in this time period do not survive. Those who do must remain hospitalized for many months. Their chances of experiencing permanent adverse health effects are high.

Weeks 25 to 28—very early preterm: The odds of survival are better, but babies born during this period must still spend weeks or months in the neonatal intensive care unit. They are at substantial risk for long-term medical consequences.

Weeks 29 to 32—early preterm: Many triplets and quadruplets and some twins are born during this time period. Although the babies typically remain in the hospital for several weeks or more, depending on their medical condition, the outlook is generally good. If the mother receives steroids to hasten the babies' lung development prior to delivery, the infants have a distinct advantage.

Weeks 33 to 36—late preterm: Many twins are born during this time period. If they are well-grown, they generally spend a week or two in the hospital. Although most end up

---

11. Hediger ML, Luke B, Gonzalez-Quintero VH, Witter FR, Mauldin J, Newman RB. Fetal growth rates and very preterm birth of twins. American Journal of Obstetrics & Gynecology 2005; 193:1498–507.

doing fine, research suggests that babies born during this period may be at increased risk for long-term adverse health effects.[12]

Weeks 37 to 39—term for twins: This is the ideal time for twins to arrive.[13, 14] Babies born during this period, if well-grown and healthy, tend to be as robust as the average newborn singleton. Usually they are able to leave the hospital soon after birth, at the same time the mother is discharged.

An infographic from the *British Medical Journal* (*BMJ*) illustrates the level of risk for various neurodevelopmental consequences, such as cerebral palsy, vision and hearing impairment, and motor dysfunction, based on the degree of prematurity. This infographic, titled "Neurodevelopmental Consequences of Preterm Birth," can be viewed online at www.bmj.com/content/350/bmj.g6661/infographic.

DR. LUKE: I like to use a football metaphor, thinking of each of the time periods described previously as a potential touchdown. The goal is to make your pregnancy last all the way through whatever time period you're in now, add another touchdown to your score, and then *stay in the game*. The more touchdowns you get before you deliver, the more likely you are to win big in the end—by taking a full team of healthy babies home with you when you are discharged from the hospital.

Another way to view the health of babies at birth is to look at the length of their hospital stay and their hospital bill. In 2005, we conducted a study with the four university centers in our twin consortium to evaluate the optimal gestational period for twins to be born. We looked at length of stay and costs at birth, adjusted to 2002 dollars. The results of the study are shown in Table 7.1.[15] (To adjust these dollar figures to 2017, multiply the figures by about 35 percent.)

12. Petrini JR, Dias T, McCormick MC, Massolo ML, Green ES, Escobar GJ. Increased risk of adverse neurological development for late preterm infants. Journal of Pediatrics 2009; 154:169–76.
13. Hartley RS, Emanuel I, Hitti J. Perinatal mortality and neonatal morbidity rates among twin pairs at different gestational ages: Optimal delivery timing at 37 to 38 weeks' gestation. American Journal of Obstetrics & Gynecology 2001; 184:451–8.
14. Luke B, Brown MB, Alexandre PK, Kinoshi T, O'Sullivan MJ, Martin D, et al. The cost of twin pregnancy: maternal and neonatal factors. American Journal of Obstetrics & Gynecology 2005; 192:909–15.
15. Ibid.

Duration and Cost of Hospital Stay for Newborns

Weeks Gestation	<28	28–29	30–31	32–33	34–35	36	37	38	39	40+
Cost per Infant	$295,231	$216,013	$92,684	$43,071	$23,936	$15,623	$9,352	$6,166	$5,383	$7,624
Days in Hospital	68	60	36	20	11	7	6	5	5	6

Table 7.1

CERVICAL LENGTH: ASSESSING THE RISK FOR PRETERM BIRTH

DR. NEWMAN: Far and away, the best test we have to predict the likelihood of preterm birth in a multiple gestation is a mid-trimester transvaginal ultrasound measurement of cervical length, done between 20 and 24 weeks' gestation. This measurement is called a *transvaginal cervical length,* or TVCL. Funneling of the internal cervical opening with shortening of the overall cervical length (less than 25 millimeters) predicts the occurrence of early preterm birth better than the mother's obstetrical history, a digital cervical examination, the presence or absence of contractions, the mother's height or weight, or any other factors.

The shorter the cervical length becomes and the earlier in the pregnancy that the shortening occurs, the greater the risk of preterm birth. For instance, a woman with a TVCL of less than 10 millimeters at 22 to 24 weeks' gestation has a 60 to 70 percent risk of a spontaneous preterm birth before 32 weeks.[16] That risk rises to approximately 80 percent if the TVCL is less than 10 millimeters at 16 to 20 weeks' gestation.

Some health care providers do not obtain TVCL measurements for patients pregnant with multiples because they're not convinced that anything can be done to help prevent or delay preterm delivery. I disagree with that. At MUSC, we routinely perform TVCL measurements on all patients carrying twins, triplets, or higher-order multiples during their routine ultrasound examinations between weeks 18 and 24.

---

16. Souka AP, Heath V, Flint S, et al. Cervical length at 23 weeks in twins in predicting spontaneous preterm delivery. Obstetrics & Gynecology 1999; 94:450–4.

One reason we do so is that when a woman is found to have a long mid-trimester TVCL (greater than 35 millimeters), it is highly reassuring—she is at very low risk of early delivery. In my opinion, this information frequently allows for the avoidance of unnecessary limitations on activity, travel, work, or sexual relations.

The most important question, of course, is what to do when a shortened mid-trimester TVCL is identified. Although it is true that there are no therapies *guaranteed* to prevent preterm birth of twins or triplets, there are several management options that can help prolong pregnancy. These include the following:

Reduced activity and increased rest. These are among the most commonly recommended interventions for expectant mothers of multiples at risk for preterm birth. Based on several studies, it is now clear that routinely hospitalizing women for bedrest in the absence of other complications does not improve outcomes in twin or triplet pregnancies. However, many obstetricians—myself included—do recommend increased rest and the restriction of strenuous activity (as described in Chapter 6) for their patients carrying multiples, especially those with a shortened cervical length. After 30 years of practicing obstetrics and caring for thousands of women pregnant with multiples, I am certain that increased time on your feet, increased physical exertion, and increased stress all add to the risk of preterm delivery. Expectant mothers of multiples who have a shortened TVCL, or who have a history of a prior preterm birth, or who are carrying three or more babies are at the highest risk for an early premature birth—and those are the pregnancies where we would most encourage rest and activity restriction.

At MUSC, our studies on uterine activity prior to labor showed that maternal rest is associated with a reduction in uterine contraction frequency. Dr. Luke and others have done research on occupational fatigue and have demonstrated a significantly increased risk of preterm birth associated with physically demanding work, prolonged standing, shift work, and night work.[17, 18, 19, 20] While studies addressing occupational

17. Luke B, Mamelle N, Keith L, Munoz F, Minogue J, Papiernik E, et al. The association between occupational factors and preterm birth: A United States nurses' survey. American Journal of Obstetrics & Gynecology 1995; 173:849–62.
18. Mozurkewich EL, Luke B, Avni M, Wolfe FM. Working conditions and adverse pregnancy outcomes: A meta-analysis. Obstetrics & Gynecology 2000; 95:623–35.
19. Schneider KTM, Bollinger A, Huch A, Huch R. The oscillating "vena cava syndrome" during quiet standing—An unexpected observation in late pregnancy. British Journal of Obstetrics and Gynaecology 1984; 91:766–80.
20. Naeye RL, Peters EC. Working during pregnancy: Effects on the fetus. Pediatrics 1982; 69:724–7.

fatigue involved singleton gestations, it would be naïve to assume that a similar, if not magnified, effect did not occur in multiple gestations.

Vaginal progesterone. When an expectant mother of multiples is found to have a short mid-trimester TVCL (less than 25 millimeters), we at MUSC also recommend daily treatment with vaginal progesterone in suppository or gel form. A recent analysis of all available high-quality studies demonstrated a 50 percent reduction in adverse newborn outcomes and a 30 percent reduction in delivery prior to 33 weeks' gestation for those twins whose mothers were treated with vaginal progesterone.[21] Most of these studies were performed using a 200-milligram progesterone vaginal suppository called Prometrium, although a 90-milligram progesterone vaginal gel called Crinone also has been used.

Another progesterone medication you may have heard of is called 17-alpha hydroxyprogesterone caproate (17P). For women who are pregnant with singletons *and* have a history of a prior preterm delivery, weekly injections of 17P between 16 and 36 weeks' gestation can help prevent preterm birth. However, there is no evidence that 17P helps in either twin or triplet pregnancies—in fact, one study found that 17P was associated with an *increased* rate of delivery before 32 weeks' gestation. My position? I do not give 17P to my patients who are expecting multiples even if they have a shortened TVCL or a prior preterm birth.

Vaginal pessary. This is a removable device made of soft plastic, typically shaped like a shallow cup or a doughnut, which fits over the cervix. It is designed to relieve direct pressure on the cervix and to redistribute the weight of the growing fetus(es) and uterus onto the muscles of the vaginal floor.

There has been a resurgence of interest in the use of the vaginal pessary to reduce the risk of preterm birth in multiple gestations, particularly in Europe. A large study performed at 40 hospitals in the Netherlands recruited more than 800 women pregnant with twins and compared outcomes for those who used pessaries and those who did not. While the researchers found no significant differences in outcomes overall, among the women with a shortened cervix (TVCL at or below the 25th percentile), both maternal and newborn outcomes were significantly im-

21. Romero R, Nicolaides K, Conde-Aqudelo A, et al. Vaginal progesterone in women with an asymptomatic sonographic short cervix in the mid-trimester decreases preterm delivery and neonatal morbidity: A systematic review and meta-analysis of individual patient data. American Journal of Obstetrics & Gynecology 2012; 206:124–39.

proved in the subgroup of women who did receive pessaries.[22] These results need to be confirmed in future studies. However, the findings are promising enough that at MUSC we are introducing pessary use when the cervical length is significantly shortened and continues to shorten despite maternal rest and the use of vaginal progesterone.

Cerclage. Suturing the cervix closed has been shown to be beneficial in singleton pregnancies in which the mother has a history of two or more prior mid-trimester pregnancy losses consistent with a diagnosis of cervical insufficiency (described earlier in this chapter). Cerclage has also recently been shown to be beneficial for women with a singleton pregnancy, a short cervix, and a prior preterm birth.

Unfortunately, cerclage generally has not proven beneficial in preventing preterm birth in twin or triplet gestations, even if the mother has a shortened cervix. In my practice, I advise a cerclage in multiple gestations if the mother has a classic history of cervical insufficiency or if, despite bedrest and vaginal progesterone, the cervix dilates and exposes the amniotic membranes when the fetuses are still at a previable gestational age.

Improved nutrition. It bears repeating what has been said in previous chapters— that good nutrition is one of the simplest and most personally empowering options to reduce the risk of preterm birth. Poor fetal growth in utero is clearly associated with an increase in both spontaneous and medically indicated preterm delivery, and the early onset of restricted fetal growth is strongly associated with dangerously early preterm deliveries. There are a wealth of data demonstrating the benefits of a comprehensive nutritional program in prolonging pregnancy, reducing the risks of preterm birth, and improving infant outcomes for twins, triplets, and higher-order multiples. Whether or not you have a shortened TVCL, it is strongly recommended that you follow the weight-gain and nutrition guidelines presented in Chapters 3, 4, and 5.

In Appendix E, which is geared toward physicians, I provide additional detailed information about the research on the topics above. I invite you to share this appendix with your obstetrician or maternal-fetal medicine specialist.

If at some point you are diagnosed with actual preterm labor (and not just a shortened TVCL), there are other interventions that can help reduce the risk for preterm birth and im-

---

22. Liem S, Schuit E, Hegeman M, et al. Cervical pessaries for the prevention of preterm birth in women with a multiple pregnancy (ProTwin): A multi-centre open label randomized controlled trial. Lancet 2013; 382: 1341–9.

prove newborn outcomes. These are described later in this chapter. But first, it is important to learn the warning signs of preterm labor—so you will be better equipped to recognize them if they do develop.

WARNING SIGNS OF PRETERM LABOR

TAMARA: It's easy to miss the vague signs of premature labor, particularly if this is your first pregnancy. That's what happened to me.

Those frequent yet painless contractions that began around my 28th week I assumed to be the harmless Braxton-Hicks contractions I'd read about in pregnancy books. That pelvic pressure I experienced (particularly when tired) I interpreted as a normal discomfort of pregnancy. My persistent lower backache I attributed to the muscle strain that naturally went along with carrying twins.

Had I recognized these symptoms for what they really were—warnings that my babies would soon be born—I might have received medical attention in time to halt preterm labor. My babies might have had the benefits of an additional few days or even weeks to grow, before confronting the challenges of life outside the womb.

Study the following list and memorize the warning signs. If you experience contractions or *any* of the other possible symptoms of preterm labor, first drink a big glass of water and empty your bladder—dehydration and a full bladder can trigger contractions. If any symptoms continue, *call your doctor, day or night.* It is far better to be told that it's a false alarm than to ignore an alarm that's real. Here are the warning signs to watch for:

- Contractions occurring at a rate of six or more per hour.
- Painful contractions.
- Rhythmic or persistent pelvic pressure.
- Menstrual-like cramps, with or without diarrhea.
- Sudden or persistent low backache.
- Vaginal discharge, particularly discharge that has changed in color, consistency, or amount.

DR. LUKE: To this list (which your obstetrician should discuss with you in detail), I want to add one more symptom. If you have any intuition, premonition, or funny feeling that something just isn't right, let your doctor know without delay. Sometimes a vague impression is the only warning.

I'm reminded of the day a patient at the Multiples Clinic came in for a routine checkup at 30 weeks. She said, "I've been feeling kind of down lately—achy and depressed, nothing more. I wasn't even going to bother mentioning it, but my mother insisted I tell you." We did a pelvic exam and also monitored her contractions, and, sure enough, she was experiencing preterm labor. We immediately took steps to stop the labor and succeeded in postponing delivery for an additional seven weeks. Yet if that woman hadn't mentioned the way she'd been feeling, her preterm labor probably would have progressed and her babies been born much sooner.

Her story is not at all unusual. Over and over, readers tell me of similar experiences. For instance, one woman writes, "My obstetrician gave me this book, and it undoubtedly saved my pregnancy. At 23 weeks, when I was feeling a subtle abdominal tightening, I looked up that sign and learned that I was experiencing labor symptoms. Without this advice, I probably would have been too embarrassed to call my doctor or to go to the hospital so early in my pregnancy. I probably would have discounted my feelings as stress or indigestion. My preterm labor was stopped because this book helped me to identify the early signs and validated my feelings that something was not right."

How to Monitor for Uterine Contractions

Occasional contractions are a normal part of pregnancy. But excessive ones—more than five or six in an hour—increase your risk of preterm labor. The longer the contractions continue and the stronger they become, the more difficult they are to stop.

That's why one of the most important things you can do during your multiple pregnancy is to monitor yourself for uterine contractions daily. There are three beneficial aspects to this:

- You learn what a contraction feels like.
- You identify the activities that trigger contractions.
- You realize when contractions are occurring too frequently.

Women experience contractions through the entirety of pregnancy, but the majority of these contractions are of such low intensity that they cannot be perceived or palpated (felt by touching the abdomen with the fingertips). As contractions get somewhat stronger in the prelabor period, they can be palpated, but they still are not painful or easy to perceive unless a woman is really paying attention. Contractions generally have to become significantly stronger before they are recognized as painful. The stronger and more uncomfortable contractions are, the more likely they are to be causing cervical changes and possibly preterm labor. However, even mild and painless contractions can cause cervical changes if they are frequent enough.

If this is your first pregnancy, you may have difficulty identifying the sensation of a uterine contraction. If you've given birth before, it should be easier to recognize contractions—but it is very important to realize that *preterm contractions are much less intense* than the contractions you experienced during labor in a previous pregnancy.

Try this: Lie on your side and press your fingers gently over your abdomen. Normally your belly feels soft. But during a contraction, your uterus tightens painlessly for 20 seconds to two minutes and feels hard, like your biceps when you make a muscle. You may also feel a heaviness or squeezing sensation in the abdomen, or an ache in the mid to lower back, as the uterus tightens. Some women report that they often feel their babies balling up—though, in fact, this sensation usually does not signal a change in fetal position but, rather, a uterine contraction.

It is a good idea to build a session of uterine monitoring into your daily routine, beginning in your 20th week of pregnancy. It doesn't matter what time of day you monitor, but ideally you should do it for one hour each day. Again, lie on your side and use your fingertips to detect the abdominal tightening that signals a uterine contraction. Use a watch with a second hand or the stopwatch app on your phone to time the duration of each contraction, then write down the exact time the sensation begins and when it subsides.

Also write down what you were doing before you lay down to monitor yourself. Were you cleaning the house? Standing in line at the bank? Carrying a toddler in from the car? Handling some crisis at work? Arguing with your mother over what to name the babies? Your notes help you identify the specific physical activities and emotional stresses that tend to trigger an increase in the number or frequency of contractions—so you can take steps to avoid these in the future.

At the end of each hour-long monitoring session, look over your records to see how many contractions occurred and how far apart they were. Then follow these guidelines:

- If you had *fewer than four contractions* in an hour, you're doing well. Plan to monitor again tomorrow.
- If you had *four or five contractions* in an hour, but no other symptoms of preterm labor, drink several glasses of water to combat the dehydration that can bring on contractions. Then lie on your side and monitor again for another 30 to 60

minutes. If the contractions have slowed, you can get up—but be sure to avoid any activities you suspect may have triggered the earlier contractions.

- If you have *six or more contractions* in an hour, call your doctor immediately. Be prepared to go to the hospital's labor and delivery unit for evaluation if instructed to do so.

DIAGNOSING PRETERM LABOR

If your doctor suspects preterm labor, he or she is likely to instruct you to go directly to the hospital's labor and delivery unit for evaluation. There, a monitor is placed around your abdomen to record the frequency and intensity of your uterine contractions. An internal examination determines if you are experiencing cervical changes such as effacement (when the cervix thins out and gets shorter) or dilation (when the cervix begins to open).

You doctor may also perform a vaginal swab to determine if fetal fibronectin is present or absent. (As discussed in Chapter 2, fetal fibronectin is protein that attaches the fetal sac to the uterine lining.) After about 22 weeks' gestation, significant amounts of fetal fibronectin normally are not detectable in the cervical or vaginal secretions until a pregnancy is near full term—so if the fetal fibronectin test is positive, there is an increased likelihood that your symptoms do indicate true preterm labor.

Next, you lie on your side and receive fluids, usually intravenously, since dehydration is a frequent cause of preterm labor. Then, unless there are major changes requiring immediate action, you are likely to be observed for several hours. During this period of observation, one of the following occurs:

- You have no cervical changes, and the contractions decrease or stop. This would be strongly supported by negative results on the fetal fibronectin test. You are likely to be sent home to rest and advised to monitor for other episodes of preterm contractions.
- You have no cervical changes, but the contractions continue. You may be given additional fluids and medication to relax the uterus in an attempt to reduce the number of contractions. You may stay in the hospital a few more hours or even overnight until the contractions have subsided. This course of action would be supported by positive results on the fetal fibronectin test.
- You do have cervical changes and the contractions continue and become regular. If this occurs, your doctor may give you medications called tocolytics, which are used in an attempt to stop preterm labor.

Tocolytic Medications

Commonly used tocolytics include magnesium sulfate, terbutaline (Brethine), indomethacin (Indocin), and nifedipine (Procardia). Typically, tocolytics are given intravenously or by injection to try to stop an episode of preterm labor.

Unfortunately, tocolytics are far from a perfect solution. Most studies suggest that tocolytics are effective for delaying preterm birth for the short term (for 48 hours to 7 days) but are not effective in ultimately preventing preterm birth. And depending on the type of medication used, they may cause various side effects. For example:

- Indomethacin side effects may include stomach irritation and heartburn.
- Magnesium sulfate side effects may include nausea, vomiting, diarrhea, constipation, flushing, sleepiness, fatigue, muscle weakness, blurred vision, slurred speech, and reduced blood levels of calcium.
- Nifedipine side effects may include increased heart rate, lowered blood pressure, and feelings of warmth due to blood vessel dilation.
- Terbutaline side effects may include increased heart rate, fluid retention, nausea, vomiting, constipation, high blood sugar, feelings of warmth due to blood vessel dilation, nervousness, trembling, and trouble concentrating.

DR. NEWMAN: The way obstetricians use tocolytics has changed in recent years. For instance, terbutaline was once commonly prescribed. However, in 2011 the FDA warned that injectable terbutaline should not be used in pregnant women for prolonged treatment (beyond 48 to 72 hours) of preterm labor due to concerns over maternal cardiovascular complications and potential fetal effects. In addition, the FDA said that oral terbutaline should not be used at all to prevent or treat preterm labor because it had not been shown to be effective and had similar safety concerns.

Another recent change has to do with the long-term use of tocolytics. Previously, it was common practice, after an acute episode of preterm labor had passed, to prescribe oral tocolytics for weeks or months in an attempt to keep preterm labor from starting again. However, most well-designed studies have not found such treatment to be helpful in preventing recurrent preterm labor or preterm birth. If your doctor does recommend long-term tocolytic use, it would be wise to ask for a detailed explanation as to why, and perhaps to seek a second opinion.

On the positive side, several recent studies have demonstrated that giving magnesium sulfate to pregnant women at risk of early preterm delivery can help protect babies against several neurodevelopmental conditions including cerebral palsy, a disabling condition that affects about 10 percent of infants born before 28 weeks' gestation.[23] It is currently recommended that women at risk for imminent delivery prior to 32 weeks' gestation, regardless of the number of fetuses they are carrying, should receive 12 hours of intravenous magnesium sulfate to help protect their babies against neurological problems.

Amy Maly's experience with preterm labor is fairly typical. She tells her story: "I was 31 weeks pregnant with my twins. Suddenly my belly started to look really contorted—so tight that it seemed I could see the shapes of the babies right through the skin. It was confusing, because there wasn't any pain. But still, I figured something wasn't as it should be, so I called my doctor. I was told to drink a big glass of water and then come straight to the labor and delivery unit.

"At the hospital, an internal exam showed that my cervix had not dilated. Yet because I was having erratic contractions, I was admitted and given intravenous magnesium sulfate. The nurse explained that this smooth-muscle relaxant could help to halt my contractions. The 'mag sulfate,' as it's called, sapped my energy so severely that it was all I could do to blink! I couldn't even walk to the bathroom by myself. But it worked—the contractions stopped. After four days I was allowed to go home, but I had to stay on strict bedrest. That lasted for five weeks. Thank goodness for my two wonderful sisters, who came in from out of state to take care of me."

Like Amy, many expectant mothers of multiples are able to return home once their preterm labor has been stopped. However, if rest and tocolytic therapy aren't enough to control your contractions, you need to stay in the hospital.

If you are hospitalized for preterm labor, it is very important that you receive injections of antenatal corticosteroids (betamethasone or dexamethasone). These will hasten the maturation of your unborn babies' lungs and reduce the likelihood or severity of prematurity-related respiratory distress syndrome, as well as the risk of intraventricular hemorrhage.[24] Typically, a woman at risk for preterm delivery is given four injections of dexamethasone or two injections of betamethasone, 12 to 24 hours apart, between 24 and 34 weeks' gestation. (There is no current evidence that steroids are beneficial after 34 weeks.) Such a course of antenatal corticoste-

---

23. Doyle LW, Crowther CA, Middleton P, Marret S, and Rouse D. 2009. Magnesium sulphate for women at risk of preterm birth for neuroprotection of the fetus. Cochrane Database of Systematic Reviews, Issue 1. Art. No.: CD004661. DOI: 10.1002/14651858.CD004661.pub3.

24. National Institutes of Health. Consensus statement. Antenatal corticosteroids revisited: Repeat courses. 2000, August 17–18; 17(2):1–18.

roids has not been associated with any significant risk to the babies. For the mother, the only concern is if she has diabetes, as these injections may cause a spike in blood sugar.

All About Bedrest

As you've probably noticed, many complications of pregnancy share a common treatment: bedrest. Staying horizontal can do lots of positive things for your pregnancy. For example, bedrest can:

- Reduce the strain on your heart.
- Improve blood flow to your kidneys, which helps to eliminate excess fluids.
- Increase circulation to the uterus, thus providing additional oxygen and nutrients to your unborn babies.
- Minimize blood levels of catecholamines, the stress hormones that can trigger contractions.
- Take pressure off your cervix.
- Limit your physical activity, thereby reducing contractions.
- Conserve your energy so that more of what you eat goes directly to promoting your babies' growth.

DR. LUKE: There's no denying that it can be boring, frustrating, and inconvenient to stay in bed for days, weeks, or even months. But if your obstetrician puts you on bedrest, try to think of it as a positive force—something concrete you can do to benefit your babies. It's been said that attitude is nine-tenths of any job, and that's particularly true when it comes to bedrest. The first and most important step is to accept that this is the best therapy for the situation.

In our Multiples Clinic, we've tried to devise ways to show patients how big their unborn babies are at any given time, because it's hard to translate the fuzzy black-and-white images on an ultrasound screen into an accurate mind's-eye picture of real babies. We came up with the idea of using paper measuring tapes to show the measurements—head circumference, abdominal circumference, and femur (thigh bone) length—from the patient's most recent ultrasound. When we show these measurements, the mom-to-be has a very strong sense of just how tiny babies born at 25 or 28 weeks really are—and how much her babies benefit, week to week, by staying snug in her womb.

This idea is taken one step further in the drawing that follows. The circles show an average baby's head circumference at various weeks of gestation. Imagine if your babies were born at your current stage of pregnancy, and you were cupping a little newborn's head in your hand. Then imagine your pregnancy continuing for another week, another two weeks, another two months—and see how much bigger your babies would be at birth.

Each day, each week that your babies spend growing stronger and healthier inside you is one less day, one less week that they are likely to spend in the hospital after their birth. Let this drawing inspire you to follow to the letter your doctor's instructions about bedrest.

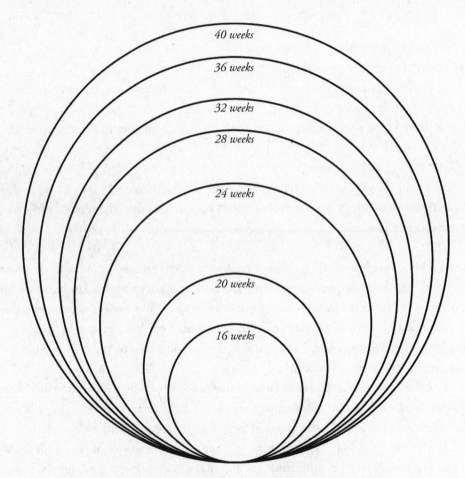

40 weeks

36 weeks

32 weeks

28 weeks

24 weeks

20 weeks

16 weeks

Average baby's head circumference at various weeks of gestation.

In fact, thinking in these terms makes it easier to accept not only bedrest, but also any other inconveniences or restrictions your pregnancy may bring. Judy Levy put it eloquently:

"It all came down to evaluating everything I did in terms of its potential effect on my unborn twins. Should I eat this steak, even though I wasn't eager for another serving of meat? Yes, that would be good for the babies—so I ate it. Should I try to talk my doctor into letting me work an extra week? No, that might be bad for the babies—so I quit when he told me to. I did this even with little things like washing the dishes. Were the benefits of having a clean kitchen worth the risk of overexerting myself and perhaps triggering contractions? Of course not! When I looked at activities in that light, the answer was crystal clear."

EXACTLY WHAT IS MEANT BY BEDREST?

There are three basic levels of bedrest. If your obstetrician orders you into bed, be sure to clarify exactly what she means.

Modified Bedrest or House Arrest

This is the least restrictive form of bedrest. It means staying at home, avoiding any strenuous housework, lifting nothing heavier than 10 to 15 pounds, and being on your feet for no more than 30 minutes at a time. Triplet mom Helen Armer explains, "I was told to stay in bed for two hours every morning and again every afternoon, as well as all evening and all night. This of course meant I could spend very little time away from home! I also had to strictly avoid any lifting, carrying, or housework, and to limit myself to one trip up and down the stairs daily."

In some cases, brief excursions out of the house are permitted, provided you take steps to avoid overexertion. Judy Levy recalls, "I hated the thought of missing out on all the fun of shopping for the twins' baby equipment. So with my doctor's permission and help, I got a handicapped parking sticker and a wheelchair, which allowed me to navigate through the stores. At first, I felt embarrassed. What if I was spotted by someone who knew I wasn't really disabled? But after the first time, I knew there was no other way I could handle any shopping without placing the babies at risk."

Your doctor cautions against such trips to the outside world? Then stay home. Violating your house arrest may well bump you up to the next level of bedrest.

Strict Bedrest

This generally means you must spend almost all your time lying down on a bed, couch, or recliner. You may be placed on strict bedrest if modified bedrest proves inadequate. "I was diagnosed with a short cervix around the end of my second trimester, so my doctor put me on modified bedrest. But my cervix kept getting shorter, so I was placed on strict bedrest instead. For two months, I barely ever even sat up because I didn't want to put any pressure on my cervix. It worked—I ended up carrying my twins to 37 weeks," says Katy Lederer, mother of boy/girl twins.

For some women, strict bedrest begins much earlier in the pregnancy. Heather Nicholas describes her experience: "At 19 weeks into my twin pregnancy, I started to feel lots of contractions. Because I'd already had a cerclage for an incompetent cervix, I immediately had to go on strict bedrest. I was allowed to shower once a day and to use the toilet as necessary. But that was it for the next four months, until I hit 36 weeks and the risk of preterm birth was past."

For many women on strict bedrest, a shower becomes the highlight of the day. "My daily shower made me feel so much more human," says twin mom Amy Maly. "For extra safety and comfort, my husband put a chair in the tub so I could sit down while I showered. He also asked me to shower only when he was home, in case I needed help." (Please note: Bathroom privileges do *not* include doing a load of laundry or other household chores on your way to the bathroom.)[25]

There are potential risks associated with strict bedrest. Chief among them is an increased risk for blood clots, such as deep vein thrombosis (DVT) or pulmonary embolism. That's why women with a history of blood clots are likely to require additional therapies to reduce their risk for a recurrent thrombosis while on bedrest. This may include drugs, such as prophylactic subcutaneous heparin, and/or sequential calf compression devices.

Other potential risks associated with strict bedrest include loss of muscle mass, bone demineralization, social disruption, and stress. Ways to minimize these problems are discussed later in this chapter.

Hospital Bedrest

At some point in your pregnancy, complications such as recurrent preterm labor or preeclampsia may make it necessary for you to be admitted to the hospital. Routine hospitalization for bedrest is no longer recommended for twin or triplet gestations, as there is no evidence that it improves outcomes if these pregnancies are otherwise uncomplicated. Depending on your situation, you may stay in the hospital just overnight, or for several days, or for many weeks. Karen Danke says, "Because I had a history of preterm birth, my doctor was very concerned when, despite a cerclage, the membranes started to bulge through my cervix 21 weeks into my twin pregnancy. He put in a second cerclage, and then had me on the strictest hospital bedrest. I was not even allowed to use the bathroom—it was bedpans and sponge baths only. After a

25. Luke B, Avni M, Min L, Misiunas R. Work and pregnancy: The role of fatigue and the "second shift" on antenatal morbidity. American Journal of Obstetrics & Gynecology 1999; 181:1172–9.

week, I was allowed to shower and use the toilet but still had to stay in the hospital for another seven weeks."

DAY-TO-DAY LIFE: THE VIEW FROM THE BEDROOM

When you're spending the vast majority of your time in a horizontal position, you obviously have lots of practical concerns to address. First, you need to know how to get up safely. When you rise from bed after being prone a long time, you may feel light-headed—and that could lead to a fall. To minimize the risk, follow these tips:

- Make sure your partner has cleared a path from bedroom to bathroom, removing all obstacles you could trip over, such as throw rugs, toys, and knickknacks.
- Never sit straight up from lying on your back. Instead, come first to a side-lying position, then slowly use your arms to push yourself up.
- Once you are sitting, remain seated in bed for a few minutes to allow any dizziness to subside.
- Slowly ease over to the edge of the bed and push yourself up with your arms and legs.
- Once standing, keep your tummy tucked under and your chin tucked in, to maintain proper posture.
- Walk slowly and carefully to and from the bathroom.

Another immediate concern is how to manage meals while on bedrest. Remember that it is extremely important to meet all your nutritional needs. Start by writing out a very thorough grocery list and reviewing it with your partner, friend, or other person handling your shopping. Next, figure out how you'll keep that good food accessible. Here are some tips from women who've met the challenge:

- "Each morning, my husband packed a cooler full of food for me and put it near the bed, so I could eat without getting up," says Heather Nicholas.
- "We got a mini refrigerator and put it upstairs, so I'd always have plenty to eat," Ginny Seyler explains.
- A husband who's handy in the kitchen can make sure that each day gets off to a nutritious start and that each evening includes an appetizing and balanced dinner. Amy Maly recalls, "Each morning before he left for work, Curt cooked breakfast for me. And he always cooked a great dinner when he got home."

- Find a nearby friend or relative who can make a midday meal. "My dad often came by to fix my lunch," says Heather Nicholas.
- Set a schedule for eating. "I seldom felt truly hungry, but I knew that I had to eat almost around the clock in order to take in enough calories. So I created a schedule of when to eat, and I stuck with it, day in and day out. I thought of it as my job," says Katy Lederer.
- Many large and medium-size cities have grocery stores, caterers, or other companies that offer convenient meal delivery services. As one mother says, "When I was on bedrest, I could call a local specialty food distributor and order dinner from any of the many restaurants that they had partnered with. They would deliver the meals hot and delicious soon after my husband arrived home from work. He was happy not to have to cook after a long day at work, and I got to enjoy some really good food. It took a lot of stress off both of us and allowed us to spend more time together."
- If you're on hospital bedrest, get your doctor's okay to bring in favorite foods from the outside. "I got pretty tired of the food from the hospital cafeteria, so it was hard to work up an appetite," admits Karen Danke. "To make sure I was getting the calories I needed, Dr. Luke brought me breakfast every morning—an egg sandwich with Canadian bacon and cheese, and orange juice. For snacks, my husband, Chris, brought my favorite muffins and big cartons of milk. And my family often delivered take-out dinners. All that went down a lot more easily than the institutional food."

You may need to arrange for professionals to handle certain tasks you are not able to manage from bed. For instance:

- A cleaning service can take over any household chores your partner doesn't have time for.
- Unless friends or relatives can manage the full-time care of your older children, a babysitter is a must. "Bedrest would have been impossible without my nanny," says Helen Armer. "Three-year-old Caroline was pretty cooperative about letting me rest, and we enjoyed watching videos, reading storybooks, and coloring together. But when she needed active play, it was vital to have the sitter on hand to take her bike riding or to the playground. And, of course, the nanny gave Caroline her meals and baths."

- Medical services may be available through your hospital, so ask your obstetrician. Says Ginny Seyler, "The hospital runs a home-nursing program. Through this, I received visits from a childbirth educator and a lactation consultant, as well as visiting nurses who came to draw blood for lab tests."
- For personal needs—haircuts, massages—call local salons and day spas to ask if they provide at-home services.

BATTLING BOREDOM

Once you have the practical matters ironed out, you may confront another common concern that bedrest brings—boredom. Ginny Seyler admits, "It was hard to switch from being on the go all day to suddenly being confined to bed with nothing to do. I missed my work, my exercise routine, my friends, everything." To combat boredom, consider these suggestions:

- Begin each day by changing out of your pajamas. You'll feel less like an invalid when wearing real clothes, even if just an oversized T-shirt and maternity leggings.
- Put a television in your bedroom, and keep the remote on your night table. Watch mind-expanding programs to learn more about history, nature, and the arts. Also ask friends to suggest favorite movies and shows.
- Keep a laptop computer or notebook and pen handy. Then write a pregnancy blog or journal, thank-you notes, holiday cards, a novel, a note to a faraway friend, a business plan for that home-based company you've always dreamed of starting.
- If your job is completely sedentary and low stress, your doctor may give you the go-ahead to do some work from bed. "I had my own home-based business as a headhunter. After I went on bedrest, I hired someone to come to my house and handle my email and other computer tasks. For instance, she read each email out loud to me, and I dictated my responses to her," says Katy Lederer.
- Catch up on all the reading you've never had time to do. Go for variety— newspapers, magazines, professional journals, classics, romances, parenting books.
- Listen to audio books when your eyes are tired. Most libraries have a selection on CDs, or you can download audio books onto your tablet or e-reader.
- For a change of scenery, set up a second bedrest area in the spare bedroom or on the living room sofa. Spend mornings in one room and afternoons in the other. If you're in the hospital, follow Karen Danke's suggestion: "When I needed a new

venue, my husband took me for gurney rides around the hospital building and grounds."

- Try Sudoku, crossword puzzles, jigsaw puzzles, word searches, and other brainteasers.
- Do volunteer work over the phone or online. Raise funds for charity, chat with elderly shut-ins or other expectant moms on bedrest, or gather information for an environmental group. To get connected, contact a local house of worship, the American Red Cross, nearby community service agencies, or local public schools.
- Use an online program, DVDs, or CDs to develop a skill—learning a language, studying a cooking technique, or planning a garden.
- Earn continuing-education credits or take an online college course. Says Anne Seifert, "I used my months on bedrest to take several courses I needed to maintain my professional accreditation. Having a home-study project made me feel like my time was well spent."
- Organize your collections of photographs, coins, stamps, or seashells.
- Use catalogs or websites to shop for baby equipment and household items. Get a jump on birthday and holiday shopping, too.
- If you have a talent for art, use this quiet time to sketch or paint. Need a model? Find inspiration in photographs. Create a masterpiece to hang in the nursery, or design your babies' birth announcement.
- Learn a craft or art like crocheting, knitting, crewelwork, rug-hooking, or scrapbooking. "I had never done crafts before, but I did enjoy cross-stitching some little baby bibs," Karen Danke says.
- Establish a daily routine for these various activities. Boredom is more easily kept at bay when you have a schedule and a sense of purpose.

KEEP YOUR SPIRITS UP

Emotional support is vital for a woman on bedrest. As one reader reports, "My doctor put me on bedrest at 24 weeks. Knowing what to do to get emotional support really helped me, especially because some family members were less than supportive about all the extra care my husband and I took to make sure we got these babies here safely." To keep your spirits high, try these ideas:

- Contact with the outside world is vital, so set up standing phone dates or text-messaging or Skype times with your husband, friends, relatives, and coworkers.

"I loved that my husband called me two or three times each day, just to check on me and offer moral support," says Amy Maly.

- Join a support group for moms-to-be on bedrest, such as Sidelines High Risk Pregnancy Support: P.O. Box 1808, Laguna Beach, CA 92652. Telephone 888-447-4754; email sidelines@sidelines.org; website www.sidelines.org.

- Ask your doctor or childbirth educator for names and telephone numbers of local women in your situation, and set up your own phone support group. Says Karen Danke, "It was so helpful to be able to share my frustrations with other people who were in the same boat as I was. Some of the women Dr. Luke put me in touch with are still my good friends today." If you're in the hospital, chances are you'll find moral support right there in the obstetrics wing. "My six weeks on hospital bedrest went by surprisingly fast. I became friends with the other patients, and we all gave each other encouragement and support," says quad mom Anne Seifert. "The nursing staff was wonderfully compassionate, too. They pampered me so much that I didn't have anything to whine about."

- Devise a countdown system. Karen Danke explains, "To make my hospital bedrest seem less interminable and more finite, Dr. Luke made me a huge wall calendar that I could see from across the room. It had 100 squares—one for each day from the time I began my bedrest until my 34th week, when it would be safe for me to go home—and special stickers for all the holidays. Each morning, Dr. Luke came to see me and we'd cross off the previous day. Those big red Xs helped me focus on how far I had come already, and how each day was taking my twins one step closer to a healthy start in life." That calendar is now in Karen's home—hanging on the wall in her boys' bedroom.

MUSCLE-TONE MAINTENANCE

Another excellent way to combat boredom and discouragement while staying in bed is to do some *very gentle* exercises. A bedrest workout also helps to alleviate stiffness in the joints, maintain muscle strength, prevent circulation problems, and prevent constipation. The moves described here, specifically designed for pregnant women on bedrest, have been developed by Elaine Anderson, P.T., M.P.H., a physical therapist and research associate in the Department of Obstetrics and Gynecology at the University of Michigan.

Before you begin this exercise program, show your doctor the bedrest exercises in Tables 7.2 and 7.3, and have him or her check off the exercises that will be beneficial for you. Ask your doctor to fill in the appropriate number of repetitions (usually 12) for each movement, as well as the proper weight for dumbbells (typically 3 pounds), if using. Also ask if you should do the entire workout every day, or if you should alternate between the lower-body workout and the upper-body workout.

Whenever you exercise, observe these general guidelines:

- Drink a glass of water before and after your workout.
- Empty your bladder before exercising. A full bladder may stimulate contractions.
- Do *not* hold your breath. Inhale through your nose, then exhale through your mouth during the active part of the movement (i.e., exhale on the exertion). Breathe in again as you return to the starting position.
- All exercises should be performed smoothly and slowly, with no jerking. Your level of exertion should be low.
- Do not skip the stretching movements. Stretching promotes flexibility and helps prevent muscle soreness.
- If any exercise is uncomfortable, triggers contractions, or causes bleeding or an increase in vaginal discharge, immediately stop the workout and call your doctor without delay.

Lower-Body Bedrest Workout

Ankle Pumps

POSITION: Sitting or side-lying

MOTION: Begin with legs straight. Flex foot to bring toes toward you as far as possible, then point toes away from you to make an arch. Switch to other leg.

REPETITIONS: _____

Ankle Circles

POSITION: Sitting or side-lying

MOTION: Rotate foot in circles, first clockwise and then counterclockwise. (Only foot should move, not entire leg.) Switch to other leg.

REPETITIONS: _____

Buttocks Tightening

POSITION: Sitting or side-lying

MOTION: Tighten the muscles in your buttocks; hold 5 to 10 seconds; relax.

REPETITIONS: _____

Pelvic Tilt

POSITION: Semi-sitting (propped up with pillows)

MOTION: Bend both knees up toward chest and place feet flat on bed. Tighten abdominal muscles while pressing lower back against the pillows to flatten the arch. Hold 5 to 10 seconds; relax.

REPETITIONS: _____

Inner Thigh Stretch

POSITION: Semi-sitting

MOTION: Begin by doing a pelvic tilt (described above). While holding the tilt, let knees fall open to feel a stretch along inner thighs; then bring knees back together.

REPETITIONS: _____

Leg Rolls

POSITION: Semi-sitting

MOTION: Straighten legs on bed, keeping feet shoulder-width apart. Roll knees inward toward each other, then outward away from each other.

REPETITIONS: _____

Leg Slides

POSITION: Semi-sitting

MOTION: Bend right knee toward chest and place right foot flat on bed. Straighten left leg, then slowly bend left knee and slide left heel toward you, bringing heel as close to buttocks as possible. Hold for a count of 3; slowly slide left leg back out until straight. Repeat on opposite side.

REPETITIONS: _____

Inner/Outer Thigh Toner

POSITION: Semi-sitting

MOTION: Keeping legs straight, slide right leg out to the right side until you feel a stretch; then slide leg back to the center. Repeat with left leg.

REPETITIONS: _____

Thigh Tightening

POSITION: Semi-sitting or side-lying

MOTION: With legs straight, consciously tighten quadriceps muscle on top of right thigh. Hold for a count of 5; relax. Repeat with left leg.

REPETITIONS: _____

Leg Lifts

POSITION: Semi-sitting

MOTION: Bend right knee toward chest and place right foot flat on bed. Straighten left leg, then raise it off bed 4 inches. Hold for a count of 3; lower leg. After finishing a complete set of repetitions, switch to other leg.

REPETITIONS: _____

Table 7.2

Upper-Body Bedrest Workout

Chin Tuck

POSITION: Sitting

MOTION: Pull chin in toward chest; at the same time, lift back of the head up, elongating the neck. Done correctly, you should feel a stretch along the back of the neck and the upper back.

REPETITIONS: _____

Neck Side Bend

POSITION: Sitting

MOTION: Keeping shoulders down, gently tilt head sideways to the right, as if trying to place right ear on right shoulder. Repeat on left side. (Do not tilt head backward.)

REPETITIONS: _____

Reverse Shoulder Circles

POSITION: Sitting

MOTION: Raise both shoulders toward ears, then ease them toward the rear while squeezing shoulder blades together. Hold for a count of 3; relax.

REPETITIONS: _____

Front Arm Raises

POSITION: Sitting

MOTION: Begin with arms at sides, elbows straight. Slowly raise both arms out in front of you, then overhead, reaching as high as possible. Hold for a count of 3; slowly lower back to starting position. (If using handheld weights, you can alternate arms instead of doing both together.)

REPETITIONS: _____

HANDHELD WEIGHTS: _____ pounds

Side Arm Raises

POSITION: Sitting

MOTION: Begin with arms at sides, elbows straight. Slowly raise both arms out to the side, lifting until arms are at shoulder level. Hold for a count of 3; slowly lower arms to starting position. (If using handheld weights, you can alternate arms instead of doing both together.)

REPETITIONS: _____

HANDHELD WEIGHTS: _____ pounds

Biceps Curl

POSITION: Sitting

MOTION: Begin with arms at sides, elbows very slightly bent and pressed against your sides. With palms facing up, slowly bend elbows and raise hands toward shoulders. Tighten upper-arm muscles and hold for a count of 5; slowly straighten arms while lowering to the starting position. (If using handheld weights, you can alternate arms instead of doing both together.)

REPETITIONS: _____

HANDHELD WEIGHTS: _____ pounds

Shoulder Stretch

POSITION: Sitting

MOTION: Gently clasp hands behind head. Move elbows forward, toward each other; then move elbows backward, so they point out to the side. Squeeze shoulder blades together; hold for a count of 5; relax.

REPETITIONS: _____

Table 7.3

You may need to spend only a few days or a few weeks in bed before your doctor determines that a potential crisis has been averted and allows you to return to your usual activities. In other cases, a woman may stay on bedrest until she delivers. If you complete your 36th week of pregnancy without going into labor, chances are you'll be released from bedrest. By that point, your multiples are big enough to be born safely, and no further attempts to delay delivery are needed.

"After spending 20 weeks on bedrest, I was finally allowed out of bed at 36 weeks when the cerclage was removed. The doctor expected me to go into labor almost immediately, but nothing happened," says Heather Nicholas. "I was allowed to resume some activity, but I'd get winded just walking across the room. I was huge and uncomfortable, but I took a lot of satisfaction in knowing that I'd made it to the point where my babies would be delivered at good birthweights. Two weeks later, they were born—with my son just an ounce shy of 7 pounds, and my daughter 3 ounces over. I was so proud when Dr. Luke said my multiples were about the same size as the average *singleton!*"

Selective Multifetal Reduction: A Difficult Decision

Eighty percent of all triplets, and nearly all quadruplets and other higher-order multiples, are conceived through infertility treatments, also known as assisted reproductive technologies (ART). In some cases, doctors prescribe medication that causes a woman to release more than one egg during a single cycle. In other cases, doctors transfer several fertilized eggs into a woman's uterus or fallopian tubes, in the hope that at least one will implant successfully. The purpose of such techniques is to boost the chances that the woman will get pregnant at all—yet the result is often a multiple gestation.

This occurs because, with ART, it can be difficult to determine the exact number of embryos that will actually implant. The problem is that the more fetuses there are, the lower the chances that any of them will survive.

That's why the technique of selective multifetal reduction was devised. The rationale is straightforward: Eliminating one or more fetuses may improve the pregnancy outcome for those that remain. It is usually presented as an option to women carrying quadruplets or more, and it may be used in triplet pregnancies if requested. Typically the goal is to leave behind twins. Selective multifetal reduction does not completely eliminate the risk of preterm labor, given that there appears to be a slightly greater rate of preterm delivery among higher-order multiples reduced to twins than among unreduced twins conceived through ART. Still, particularly when four or more fetuses are present, reduction to twins could be an option that some parents may want to consider.

The procedure is done toward the end of the first trimester. The doctor passes a needle through the woman's abdomen (using ultrasound guidance) and injects potassium chloride into the fetal heart, which then stops beating. The fetal tissue is reabsorbed, and the pregnancy can continue uneventfully.

The chorionicity of the multiples must be well established before fetal reduction is performed. Monochorionic twins or triplets share the placental circulation, so the potassium chloride injected into the heart of one twin would also cause the unintentional demise of the monochorionic co-twin or co-triplet.

Even when multiples are not monochorionic, the advisability of reduction is not always clear-cut. The procedure does carry a risk of causing miscarriage of all the fetuses. One large study showed that the greater the number of starting fetuses, the higher the risk of miscarrying all. For instance, when starting with three fetuses, the rate of full miscarriage from reduction is 4 percent; when starting with four fetuses, the rate is 7 percent; when starting with six, the rate is 15 percent. Also, reducing to triplets involves a higher risk of losing all the fetuses than does reducing to twins.

Further complicating the issue, doctors may offer conflicting opinions. "Because I had undergone fertility treatments, I knew it was a possibility that I would conceive multiples. So I wasn't all that shocked to find out several weeks into the pregnancy that three embryos had implanted. That's when my reproductive endocrinologist counseled me to strongly consider reducing to twins," says Hannah-Beth Rhodes. "Yet my obstetrician disagreed. He doesn't recommend reduction unless there are four or more fetuses because, he said, the outcome for triplets generally isn't much worse than for twins. I was prepared to do whatever the medical experts advised, but with two opposing opinions, I felt confused."

Ginny Seyler had a similar experience. "At seven weeks, my fertility doctor did an ultrasound. When she saw the second baby, my husband and I were thrilled. But when she saw the third, we got scared. Right away, the doctor started talking about selective reduction," Ginny recalls. "Yet when I later phoned a friend who is an obstetrician and asked if she recommended reducing from triplets to twins, she said, 'You can carry three. Go for it.'"

DR. LUKE: Complicating the issue is the absence of any national criteria for determining the advisability of selective reduction. That's why when patients would come to the Multiples Clinic seeking guidance, our approach was to evaluate her individual situation with regard to a number of factors:

- Placentation: When each fetus has a separate placenta, the risks for growth restriction and early preterm birth are lower.
- The woman's height: Just as an individual who is 6 feet tall has a larger heart and greater lung capacity than someone who's 5 feet, a taller woman has a larger uterus and more room for her babies to grow before birth than does a shorter woman.
- Prepregnancy weight: A woman's weight before conception is an indirect measure of her nutrient reserves, which is an important consideration for fetal development. Being more than 10 percent below the ideal weight-for-height is associated with an increased risk for miscarriage, poor fetal growth, and premature birth. Conversely, women who prior to pregnancy were at a normal weight—or even as much as 20 percent above ideal weight—generally have more favorable pregnancy outcomes and are likely to carry higher-order multiples longer.
- Lifestyle: Habits that can be harmful during any pregnancy—smoking, drinking, strenuous physical activity, and so on—are particularly dangerous during a triplet or quad gestation.
- Obstetric history: A woman who has given birth previously has an advantage. Because her uterus has already been stretched, she is likely to carry her higher-order multiples about two weeks longer than a first-time mother will. On the other hand, a history of preterm birth in a prior singleton gestation would be very concerning, as it suggests that a subsequent triplet or quad pregnancy would be extremely high risk.

For example, when Hannah-Beth Rhodes came to the Multiples Clinic and asked about reduction, we used these criteria to counsel her. She had a trichorionic, triamniotic placenta (meaning that each fetus was in a separate sac and had a separate placenta). She was 5 feet, 6 inches tall—well above the minimum we hope for in a triplet pregnancy. Her preconception weight of 146 pounds was optimal, and she had been eating well and gaining appropriately from the very beginning of her pregnancy. She didn't smoke or drink alcohol. There were no preexisting health problems. She had a sedentary job and was willing to take a leave of absence whenever it should become advisable. Her health care team was excellent, she lived close to the hospital, and she was committed to following all instructions from her doctors. Best of all, Hannah-Beth had an excellent obstetric history: Her first pregnancy had gone to 42 weeks and resulted in a healthy 9 lb., 2 oz. baby. In short, there was every reason to believe she could handle a triplet pregnancy.

And she did, beautifully. When Hannah-Beth's babies were born at almost 36 weeks' gestation, the largest weighed nearly 6 pounds—a whopping size for a triplet. Even the smallest weighed well over 4½ pounds, which is 25 percent heavier than the national average for triplets.

Since the publication of the first edition of this book in 1999, the national rates of triplets, quadruplets, and quintuplets have dropped significantly—from 1 in 540 births (for a total of 7,321 infants) to 1 in 881 births in 2014 (for a total of 4,526 infants). This decline is due in large part to the effect of national guidelines issued by the Society for Assisted Reproductive Technologies (SART). These guidelines recommend limits on the number of embryos to transfer during a cycle of IVF based on a woman's age and the characteristics and quality of her embryos. Since ART is responsible for the majority of triplet and quadruplet pregnancies, these guidelines have reduced their frequency—and as a result, multifetal reduction has decreased dramatically.

MAKING YOUR CHOICE

What if the odds of a successful pregnancy with higher-order multiples seem *not* to be in your favor? In some cases, it may be prudent to consider reduction. "Because I was taking the fertility drug Pergonal, I had two multiple-gestation pregnancies. First I conceived quadruplets, and we reduced to twins. But in the second trimester, I lost both those babies," says Karen Danke. "A year later, I conceived again—quintuplets this time. Given that even a twin pregnancy had failed the first time, we knew there was no way I could ever carry quints. So again we opted to reduce, and this time I was able to hang on to 34 weeks. We have healthy twin boys now, and we're thrilled to be parents at last."

In some cases, the toughest part of the selective reduction decision is not the analysis of the physical criteria that affect a woman's chances of carrying triplets or quads. Rather, it is the emotional element involved that requires the most serious soul-searching on the part of the pregnant woman and her partner.

"For years, we had longed to be parents, and we underwent a series of infertility treatments in our quest for children. Finally I conceived, only to be faced with this wrenching decision—to risk losing all my babies by continuing a quadruplet pregnancy or to purposely sacrifice two so that the others might have a better chance to live," says Joni Quinn. "We knew we could love our quads no matter how disabled they might be. But it didn't seem fair to doom them all to living with severe handicaps—or worse, to dying at birth—when it was probably within our power to give two of them normal lives. It was the most difficult choice we ever had to make."

If you, like Joni, must struggle with a decision about selective reduction, seek help from a psychologist or social worker familiar with fertility issues. Don't rush; you have some time to make your choice, and there's a chance that Mother Nature will make it for you. "My husband and I were told that if we opted to reduce from quads to twins, the procedure would be done around the 10th week of pregnancy. We were also told that one or more of the fetuses might spontaneously miscarry before that," says Anne Seifert. "We decided that the best short-term policy was just to wait and see what would happen."

Should you ultimately choose reduction, don't let outsiders question or criticize your decision. One mother explains it this way: "I conceived quadruplets from taking Pergonal. After weeks of introspection, advice from doctors, and support from our families, my husband and I together decided to have the selective reduction. It was not easy, but we did what we felt was appropriate for us. I firmly believe it was the wisest choice, because even with 'just twins,' my pregnancy was very difficult—cervical problems, placenta previa, and preeclampsia. After eight months, though, we finally became the parents of healthy twins. No one should criticize our choice unless they have walked a mile in our shoes." Some women who undergo selective reduction do experience regret for variable periods of time, but the majority ultimately decide that they would make the same choice again.

If you do decide to reduce to twins, keep one point in mind: Your unborn babies are still at greater risk for slowed growth than other twins are. To promote optimal fetal growth after reduction, be vigilant about fulfilling your dietary needs and limiting physical activity.

What if you do opt to continue a triplet or quad pregnancy? Some couples say they find strength in turning the decision over to a higher power. "I spent 24 hours thinking of nothing except whether or not to do the selective reduction, then finally told my husband that this could not be an option for us," says Ginny Seyler. "I figured God had put these babies here for a purpose, and he would see us through this. Once the decision was made, I felt much more at peace."

For Anne Seifert, the wait-and-see approach brought her to 12 weeks—and still all the quads were growing fine. At that point, her decision came down to two simple questions. "Dr. Luke asked me, 'Do you want four children? And if so, are you willing to drastically change your lifestyle for many months in order to help them be born as healthy as possible?' My answer to both questions was an emphatic *yes*! In the end, it was that simple." Anne ended up carrying her quads to 31 weeks. At birth, Andrew and Sarah weighed just over 2 pounds each; Lindsey and Mason topped 3 pounds. All four ended up doing fine.

Chapter Eight

The Emotional Ups and Downs of Pregnancy . . . Multiplied

Many women fantasize about the perfect pregnancy. Most often the ideal includes a nine-month glow that leads to a healthy, full-term singleton, born vaginally with no complications and minimal discomfort, successfully breast-fed, and discharged to go home right along with Mommy.

With the diagnosis of a multiple pregnancy, however, each aspect of this cherished dream may be altered. Yes, some parents-to-be are delighted right from the start to learn that more than one baby is on the way, and everything goes smoothly—but even when that's the case, the parents still must come to terms with the fact that their family situation is not a typical one. For other expectant parents, though, the news of a multiple pregnancy takes quite a bit of getting used to. And, of course, the ideal image is shaken up even more when a pregnancy complication or crisis arises—which happens more frequently when twins, triplets, or quads are on the way.

So it's no wonder that these months before your multiples are born may prove to be one of the most emotionally charged periods of your life. Understanding the typical psychological patterns of this time can help you cope in ways that are both emotionally and physically healthy.

Your Inner World: An Emotional Journey from Shock to Joy

DR. LUKE: Every patient I encounter in my work is in the midst of an emotional journey. It began the day she learned she was pregnant, but it intensified markedly the moment she was told that multiples were expected.

Because I follow patients for many months, from the diagnosis of twins, triplets, or quads to the day of delivery and beyond, I've seen many women confront the myriad and mixed feelings that often accompany this unique kind of pregnancy. From my observations, I've concluded that this psychological journey typically consists of five fairly predictable stages: shock, denial, anxiety/anger/depression, bargaining, and acceptance/adaptation. These are basically the same five stages first described by Dr. Elisabeth Kübler-Ross (herself a triplet) as the stages of grieving.

If you are surprised to hear that grief could have anything in common with a happy event like pregnancy, consider this: any major life event—even a positive one—can trigger a series of emotions, and these emotions often follow a similar pattern. After all, when a significant change ushers in a new era in your life, no matter how excited you are about what's to come, you still experience some sense of loss over the old life being left behind. And few events are more profoundly life-altering than having a baby—except, of course, having several babies at once.

What's more, parents who have just been told that they're expecting multiples do in a sense grieve for the loss of the typical pregnancy and typical family they had imagined would be theirs. Ginny Seyler, mother of triplets, explains it this way: "It took me some time to come to terms with the fact that this was going to be a high-risk pregnancy and not the nice, normal, nine-month pregnancy I had always dreamed of. And because few people expect to have three children at once, I also had to get used to the idea that I would never have a 'normal' family. It was disturbing to realize that forevermore I'd be thought of as 'the person with the triplets.'"

Not everyone reacts in exactly the same way, of course. Some individuals may get stuck at one stage, while others may even skip a stage. And any new significant development or problem in the pregnancy can spark the sequence anew, sending the parents-to-be back to Stage 1 to start over. Being familiar with these patterns can help you and your partner understand your emotions, ease your confusion, and inspire you to do whatever is in your babies' best interests.

STAGE 1: SHOCK

Even when a couple has been trying to conceive, a positive pregnancy test can come as a shock. The sensation is then repeated, but more intensely, with the news that you're carrying twins, triplets, or quadruplets. This is particularly true when multiples are conceived spontaneously rather than through infertility treatments. "The possibility of having twins had never even crossed my mind, so I simply could not believe it at first when the doctor showed us two heads on the ultrasound. I was sure the image on the screen must be coming from someone else and not from me," says Stacy Moore, mother of fraternal twin boys.

The shock can be compounded if the entire pregnancy was a surprise, or if you had reason to believe that the pregnancy would be lost. "Midway through the first trimester, I had an episode of pretty severe bleeding. I went in for an ultrasound, expecting to be told that I was miscarrying my baby. Instead, we learned that there were *three* babies. My husband and I were in complete shock—there is no other way to describe it," says Ginny Seyler.

The more babies you're carrying, the more of a jolt you're likely to feel—especially if you had nearly lost hope of ever getting pregnant at all. Sarah Turner shares her experience: "I had endured 13 years of infertility. I lost both my fallopian tubes after ectopic pregnancies, had many attempts at IVF, and had one triplet pregnancy that ended at seven weeks. Then we tried IVF using four donor eggs that had been fertilized by my husband's sperm. Twelve days later, I went to the lab for a blood test to check my blood hormone level. It showed that not only was I pregnant, but my hormone level was much higher than you'd expect in a singleton pregnancy. I was thrilled, because I figured it meant I was carrying twins. Then five weeks into the pregnancy, I had my first ultrasound. Everyone was in total shock when we discovered *four* babies."

It is also normal to experience renewed shock if a pregnancy complication arises. For instance, a diagnosis of an incompetent cervix, the detection of a birth defect, the news that a cesarean delivery will be necessary, or the onset of preterm labor can spark a resurgence of that sense of shocked disbelief.

STAGE 2: DENIAL

The second stage of adjusting to a crisis involves temporarily blocking out reality. For some women, denial takes the form of a restrained or muted reaction to the multiple pregnancy. Triplet mom Hannah-Beth Rhodes explains, "Initially I was rather unresponsive to the news that I had conceived triplets. I told myself it was probable I'd lose one fetus, if not all three, and would never need to deal with the reality of having three babies at once. That feeling lasted for several weeks."

Even moms-to-be who readily embrace the news of an impending multiple birth can still experience denial as the pregnancy progresses, in that they may ignore any information that seems too alarming. Meredith Alcott, mother of identical twin girls, admits, "I started to read some books about twins, but they stressed all the things that could go wrong during the pregnancy. I was too freaked out to finish reading them. Instead, I tried to block any scary stuff from my mind."

Denial can also involve an automatic assumption that all the babies will be born big and healthy. "In whatever pregnancy books I read, I always skipped over the sections about the NICU. I just assumed all three of my babies would be coming home from the hospital with me a few days after delivery. I was in total denial of the fact that most triplets do need NICU care," says Ginny Seyler.

Because denial serves as a shock absorber, allowing a more gradual emotional adjustment to surprising news or a sudden crisis, it does have a useful purpose. But if the denial stage persists too long, it can interfere with expectant parents' judgment as to what might be best for their unborn babies.

TAMARA: I've come to believe that denial was a factor in my unrealistically optimistic attitude during my twin pregnancy, and that the stage had been set many years before. I was in kindergarten when my fascination with twins first took hold. Perhaps it was because my best friends, Penny and Paula, were twins, and my second-best friend had *two sets* of twin siblings. It seemed that everyone in the neighborhood was a twin, and I wanted to be one, too.

My mother explained that she could not manufacture a twin for me out of thin air; if a person had not been born with a twin, the opportunity was forever lost. I settled on the next best thing: Someday, I vowed, I would have 12 children, and they would all be twins or triplets.

As I grew up, of course, I realized that my chances of ever having twins of my own were slim. So when the radiologist told me he saw two babies on my ultrasound, I sang out in exultation, "Twins! I can't believe it! I'm having twins!"

The radiologist was taken aback. "You're . . . you're happy about this?" he asked. "I'm ecstatic!" I said. "This is the most thrilling moment of my life!"

The doctor squinted at me skeptically. "Most women are pretty shaken up when they first get the news. I think you're the only one who has ever danced on the examining table. Well, hang on to that positive attitude. You're going to need it."

I took his advice *too* literally perhaps, and spent the next months in a state of high glee. I was certain that my dream was coming true at last and that nothing could possibly go wrong. In this state of euphoric denial, I mistook the subtle warning signs of preterm labor as normal discomforts of pregnancy.

DR. NEWMAN: In my practice, whenever I start seeing a woman who is pregnant with twins or triplets, I make a point of spending a substantial amount of time at our first appointment reviewing the challenges and risks presented by a multiple pregnancy. It's necessary—but it's almost never fun. If the parents-to-be are thrilled about having multiples, like Tamara was, I feel like I am raining on their parade and ruining their excitement. If the expectant parents are experiencing shock or fear over the disruption of the ideal pregnancy they had imagined, I feel like I am piling on the bad news and making them feel even worse.

What I have learned over time, however, is that most patients don't recall much of what we discuss at that first prenatal visit. Maybe it is shock, maybe denial, or maybe both, but couples are frequently emotionally unprepared to deal with the planning and preparation that a multiple pregnancy requires, at least at first. That's why, during subsequent appointments, I review the information again and again. As couples move past their initial shock and denial, they are better able to assimilate what we've talked about and follow the guidelines we've suggested.

DR. LUKE: One effective way to help expectant parents move past denial is to make their unborn babies seem more real to them. Naming the children is a good first step. Health professionals refer to individual multiples as Baby A, Baby B, Baby C, Baby D, and so on, typically counting clockwise by position in the womb, with Baby A being the one closest to the cervix. But there's no reason you can't name your children long before you look into their eyes for the first time.

Joanie Stevens, mother of fraternal twin boys, explains: "I didn't want to find out the babies' genders before birth, so during the whole pregnancy I called them Peter-Louise and Amy-Jamie. It started as a joke, but as soon as I began using these names, I felt much closer to my unborn babies. They became real children to me, not merely a positive pregnancy test or a pair of fetuses."

You're not yet ready to settle on names that will stick after birth? An affectionate nickname can serve the same loving purpose.

Another boon to parents who are working through the denial stage are ultrasounds. Years ago, before this technology was in common use, it was much more difficult for parents to conceptualize their unborn babies as real little people. They could see the mother's belly getting bigger, and they could listen to the babies' heartbeats, but still it was hard to imagine what their children looked like.

Today ultrasound is an integral part of prenatal care, particularly in multiple pregnancies, since it offers a means by which to monitor fetal growth and well-being. At the same time, it has the marvelous effect of demonstrating how each child is unique in temperament from the earliest stages of life. Many studies have documented the impact of prenatal ultrasound on both maternal and paternal bonding with the unborn babies. For the mother-to-be, it can be the single greatest motivator for keeping up positive health behaviors, like staying off her feet and eating well. For the father-to-be, it can bring the message home: "These are your children, your responsibility."

> **DR. LUKE:** I remember one instance when we were looking at triplets on the ultrasound monitor, and the expectant mom said to her husband, "See how big they are getting, honey! Joshua is really the busy one, but I think Amanda is going to be the boss." I looked over toward her husband, whose color had drained from his face and who had backed up against the wall. Clearly, the experience of visiting their triplets via ultrasound was very different for each partner!

STAGE 3: ANXIETY/ANGER/DEPRESSION

Moving beyond the numbness of shock and denial, an expectant mother of multiples often finds herself flooded with emotion—especially anxiety. She experiences all the worries any pregnant woman may feel, only more so, because her pregnancy involves additional risks and she has concerns about several children rather than just one.

Judy Levy, who conceived fraternal twin girls when her older daughter was two years old, explains, "My twin pregnancy was such a different emotional experience compared to my first. Instead of sheer excitement and joy mixed with a bit of apprehension, the balance was reversed—with the heaviest emphasis being on the apprehension."

Worry is even more pronounced when pregnancy complications arise. "For the first few weeks after I was ordered onto bedrest, I was an emotional wreck. I was terrified every moment that I'd lose the triplets," recalls Ginny Seyler.

If you had problems in an earlier pregnancy, the sad memories can compound your present fear, making it difficult for you to take pleasure in this pregnancy or to plan for the babies' arrival. Karen Danke, mother of fraternal twin boys, explains: "My husband and I were scared the whole time, because we had previously lost twins at 21 weeks. This time, we were afraid to buy any baby clothes or furniture until we had passed the 30th week."

During this overwhelmed stage, it's common to feel like you are no longer in control of your own life. "First I had preterm labor, then weeks of bedrest, then preeclampsia. I'm the kind of person who likes to be in charge, but once all these complications developed, I felt helpless. Nothing seemed to be under my control—not my job, or my babies' health, or even my own body," says Benita Moreno, mother of fraternal twin boys. That feeling can trigger resentment. "Nothing was normal. I couldn't keep on with my regular life, nor could I enjoy this new experience of being pregnant. I felt cheated," Benita adds. You don't have to be a Type A personality to be disturbed by the sense of lost control. It is one of the most common sentiments expressed by expectant mothers of multiples who develop complications or are hospitalized.

At that point, the guilt typically kicks in. One mother of twins explains it this way: "It was a chain of uncomfortable emotions. First I felt overwhelmed with worry about the babies. Then I felt angry about being forced to worry. Then I felt guilty for feeling angry, because anger seemed so unmaternal."

For other women, guilt arises from a sense (however undeserved) that they themselves are to blame for the high-risk status of their pregnancy. "I carried a real burden of guilt because I believed that by taking Clomid and conceiving triplets, I had put all my babies in danger," Ginny Seyler confides. Many women who undergo IVF express the same guilt over their decision to transfer multiple embryos.

From self-blame to depression can be just a short hop. "I got really down for a while, feeling like I was a bad mother and I didn't deserve these sweet babies," admits one twin mom. "Fortunately, that let up after about a week, and I was able to let go of the guilt and develop a healthier, more productive attitude."

If you find yourself stuck in anxiety, anger, guilt, or depression, it's important to take steps to regain a sense of control—not only for your own sake, but also for your babies' sake. Why? Because emotional stress can trigger the same type of physiological reaction as can physical stress or overexertion. The body releases catecholamines, the stress hormones that can bring on uterine contractions. In fact, a study from Kaiser Permanente found that pregnant women with severe depressive symptoms had more than twice the risk of preterm delivery as women without depression.

Fortunately, there are a number of ways to lower your stress level and brighten your outlook:

- Remind yourself that pregnancy hormones can launch any woman on a mood-swing roller coaster. And since you've got higher levels of virtually every pregnancy hormone than does a singleton mom, your hormonal upheaval may be significantly greater. Before you start feeling bad about yourself, realize that your mixed feelings are in part physiologically based. As your body adjusts physically, you'll regain your emotional equilibrium.
- Accept your anxieties, without obsessing about them. Instead of berating yourself for feeling worried, try to acknowledge that anxiety is simply part of your life for now. Judy Levy explains, "I called a friend who had recently delivered triplets after a series of pregnancy difficulties, and I asked her, 'When you were pregnant, how did you get rid of the anxiety?' She answered, 'I didn't. I *was* anxious, and there

was no getting around that.' Somehow her words made me feel better, as though she had given me permission to be nervous. After that, I was better able to relax."

- Fight fear with information. Another key to coping with overwhelming emotions is to empower yourself through education. As you learn how to minimize risk by taking sensible steps to protect your own health and that of your babies, your sense of alarm diminishes. Your obstetrician and other health care providers are excellent sources of information, so talk candidly with them. Make lists of your questions, and bring them to each prenatal appointment. If you don't understand the answers, ask to have things explained again.

- Practice relaxation techniques. When you feel anxious or upset, try some deep breathing. Inhale slowly and deeply for a count of four, hold for four, then exhale slowly for a count of four, and hold for four more. Continue for several minutes. A meditative approach is to repeatedly recite a mantra, such as "I am filled with peace."

- Empower yourself. The purpose of this book is to provide you with information that can help prevent pregnancy complications, prepare you in case problems do arise, and offer potential solutions. The goal is not to be scary or pessimistic, but rather to forearm you by forewarning you. When you're feeling anxious, review the chapters on nutrition and weight gain, and the guidelines on physical activity—these help put power in your hands to prolong your pregnancy and grow bigger, healthier babies.

- Seek moral support. It's normal to feel ambivalent about having multiples, so share your emotions with someone who truly understands your negative feelings as well as your positive ones. The best candidate for that unique type of empathy: another mother of multiples. "What helped most in handling my fear and guilt was to connect with other moms-to-be of triplets who were also on bedrest, and with women who had already given birth to multiples. We wrote emails and talked on the phone for hours. They gave me the information and support I needed, and helped me to feel less alone," Ginny Seyler says. "How did I find them? Through the Internet and Mothers of Supertwins." Also inquire whether your local Mothers of Multiples club has a support group for expectant dads—your partner may find it helpful to speak with other fathers of multiples. (For information on support groups, see Appendix D.)

Your obstetrician may be able to provide emotional support as well. "One thing I loved about my doctor was how tuned in he was to the psychological challenges of a high-risk pregnancy," says Ginny Seyler. "For instance, by my third day on bedrest, I was despondent. I paged my obstetrician, and he spent 45 minutes on the phone with me—helping me face the reality that I might lose them, yet reassuring me that my chances of delivering three healthy babies were good. It was so important to know that he was there for me when I needed him."

If you should continue to feel very upset about the pregnancy for more than a few weeks, seek professional help in working through these feelings. While the support of a loving friend or dedicated obstetrician is important, sometimes a person needs the extra measure of insight and objectivity that a mental health professional can provide.

STAGE 4: BARGAINING

The bargaining stage of dealing with a pregnancy crisis represents an advance from the help-lessly overwhelmed emotions that preceded it, in that you now may feel a greater sense of calm and control over your situation. The problem is, if you push the bargaining too hard, your pregnancy may be jeopardized. Attempts at negotiation are especially common among two categories of expectant mothers of multiples: those who want or need to keep on working and do not understand the connection between long hours, stressful conditions, and preterm labor, and those on bedrest who feel frustrated by the lack of freedom and mobility.

"As an oncology nurse, I was working about 50 hours a week. Twenty weeks into my pregnancy, I was advised to quit and go on modified bedrest, but I had just started a new job and didn't think I was eligible for a leave of absence. Besides, I felt sure I'd be able to take this pregnancy to 37 weeks at least, and I wanted to work as long as possible. So I kept negotiating. 'What if I cut back my hours? What if I promise to elevate my feet whenever I'm at my desk? What if I lie down as soon as I get home from work?'" says Marcy Bugajski, mother of fraternal twin boys.

"Then, in my 28th week, an internal exam of my cervix revealed that I was already fully effaced and slightly dilated. When she discovered that, Dr. Luke said, 'Marcy, you are off work and onto strict bedrest as of this moment.' But I replied, 'I can't just up and quit. I've got a job to do.' Dr. Luke looked at me sternly and said, 'If you don't get into bed right now and stay there, you are endangering your twins.' Suddenly the message got through to me, and I felt really scared. I realized the job could go on without me, but these little babies could not. My priorities had to change—and fast."

DR. LUKE: Too often I've seen mothers-to-be of multiples bargain with their doctors, bend the rules, or insist on taking over major decisions about their care. "Why should I stop working now? I feel fine. How about if I continue for another six weeks? Okay, four weeks?" Or "I can't stand being on bedrest. I'll just pop this load of laundry in, then run to the grocery store. I'll be back in half an hour, and no one will even know I was out." Or even "I'm determined not to have a cesarean section. Doctor, promise me that you'll let me deliver vaginally."

It's understandable that patients want to be informed and involved. Particularly for women who by personality or profession are accustomed to wielding authority, it can be hard to let someone else take charge. But now that you're pregnant with multiples, you really do need to hand over control to the people best qualified to make the decisions about your care: your obstetrician and other health care team members. Try to understand that the limitations they may place on your activities are not punishments but precautions. Attempting to plea-bargain for a reduced sentence—to change strict bedrest to house arrest, for example—may only lead to deeper trouble.

Your doctor and the other members of your health care team have years and years of training and experience upon which to base their decisions and the judgment needed to determine what is in your babies' best interests. Chances are, you do not have this training—and even if you are a physician, you are not in a position to view your own case with the open-mindedness and objectivity that are required for optimal care.

Regardless of your role in the everyday world, your most essential role for the next few months is as a patient. Do some of our recommendations—to rest, relax, relinquish responsibilities and activities—make an expectant mother's job seem annoyingly passive? Try not to look at it that way. You're not doing nothing; you're *gestating*.

No one is suggesting that you're nothing more than a baby-making machine, or that your other interests and concerns don't matter. Yet right now, you are the *only* person in the world who can do the vitally important job of gestating these babies—doing whatever you can to allow your pregnancy to continue as long as possible, to help your babies develop as well as possible, and to keep yourself as healthy as possible.

So go ahead and ask for information and explanations; communicate your concerns and preferences. But don't argue with your doctor or try to cut a deal. Instead, let him guide your care. Take careful note of his advice, and that of any other member of your health care team, and follow it as best you can.

DR. NEWMAN: Obstetrics is much more about prevention than it is about treatment. In fact, effective treatment options are limited for many of the major complications of pregnancy, especially when one of those complications is a multiple pregnancy. We can predict the risk of preterm birth with mid-trimester cervical length measurements, the risk of fetal growth restriction with ultrasound, or the risk of gestational hypertension with Doppler studies and blood pressure readings.

Unfortunately, most such warning signs appear at a time when the mother is feeling well and is energetic, and still has much that she wants to accomplish before the arrival of the babies. So it's understandable that an expectant mother would be tempted to bargain for a loosening of restrictions. It's understandable—but it's *not* advisable.

One of the most difficult things for any human being to do is to delay immediate gratification in favor of a future benefit that may be weeks or months away, as is the case during pregnancy. Under these circumstances, trust between you and your obstetrician is vitally important. Remember, your doctor's advice regarding rest, stress reduction, nutrition, lifestyle, and work activities represents years of accumulated experience in helping other expectant mothers of multiples prevent or deal with complications affecting their pregnancies.

Stage 5: Acceptance/Adaptation

The fifth and final stage of coming to terms with a pregnancy crisis involves finding ways to cope that are healthy for both mind and body. Acceptance means developing a new attitude—finding within yourself the willpower and maturity to see what needs to be done. Adaptation means translating your acceptance into appropriate actions—modifying your behavior to give your babies the best chance to be as healthy as possible.

Below, women who have achieved this acceptance/adaptation share the secrets of their success:

- Figure out how to alleviate your frustrations without increasing your risk, Ginny Seyler urges. "One of the most aggravating aspects of bedrest was not being able to get our home ready for the triplets. Friends had given us tons of equipment and clothes, and I was dying to go down to the basement and sort through everything, but of course that wasn't allowed. Finally I found the perfect solution. I hired a teenager to come over, lug the stuff upstairs, unpack everything, organize it with me, and arrange it all according to my instructions. Not only was this an entertaining way to pass the long hours of bedrest, but it also helped me to feel more prepared for the babies' arrival."
- Focus on the ultimate reward, says Amy Maly, mother of identical twin girls. "Sure, I missed being able to just jump in the car and go wherever I wanted, whenever I wanted to. But I realized that this was hard and serious work, growing

two babies at once. To keep on track, I concentrated on the incredible payback we were aiming for—a pair of healthy newborn twins."

- Find creative ways to motivate yourself, advises Helen Armer, mother of triplets. "Because I'm an engineer, I am used to working with graphs and numbers. I'm also very goal-oriented, and I was determined that all of my triplets would have healthy birthweights. I designed a chart to track fetal size and weight as estimated by monthly ultrasounds, and then extrapolated to calculate the babies' growth with each passing week. Whenever I needed a motivational boost to drink yet another quart of milk or stay in bed for that extra hour, I looked at my chart and got inspired."

- Take comfort in the fact that you are not alone in what you're experiencing. "I realize that some expectant mothers feel scared when they hear about possible problems during a multiple pregnancy. But I appreciated the chance to read about women who did develop complications. It made me feel less alone—like I had a friend who'd already been through what I was going through—and that was comforting," says Michelle Brow, mother of fraternal twin girls.

- Think of other challenges you have faced, and draw on the lessons you learned from those. For instance, some years before she conceived her identical twin boys, Erin Justice was diagnosed with multiple sclerosis, a chronic disease of the central nervous system. Erin says, "What advice would I offer to other expectant mothers of multiples who also have chronic health problems? I'd encourage them to recognize that they may be better prepared to create a great pregnancy than women who've never had to consider their health before. When you have a chronic disease, you learn to listen to your body, pay attention to your diet, rest when you need to, and set appropriate priorities. The 'work' we assign ourselves when we're pregnant is to grow healthy babies, which is much more fun and fulfilling than just managing an illness. And we get a wonderful prize at the end—our beautiful babies."

- Cultivate cautious optimism, suggests Heather Nicholas, mother of boy/girl twins. "There is no need to have a gloomy outlook, because not all multiple pregnancies are complicated. Even if you do have problems, some aspects of your pregnancy will be perfect. For instance, I had a lot of difficulties, including a weak cervix, tons of contractions, and 20 weeks on bedrest. But my delivery was a wonderful experience—painful of course, but beautiful, too—and my babies were born huge and healthy."

- Look for the silver lining, Judy Levy advises. "If I hadn't conceived twins in my second pregnancy, I probably would have had only one more child. So despite the challenges of a difficult pregnancy, I really do feel multiply blessed because I'm finding that it's wonderful to have three children."

The World at Home: You, Your Partner, and Your Multiples

"This pregnancy wasn't the best timing, because my wife had just begun a new job. Benita and I had been talking about starting a family, but we hadn't planned to begin trying for at least a year. So when she conceived accidentally, it was quite a surprise for both of us. Then she went in for her first ultrasound at 16 weeks. Immediately after that appointment, she called me from the car and told me that we were going to have twins. I was so freaked out that I had to leave work and come straight home. My stomach was in knots for a week," confesses Donald Moreno, father of fraternal twin boys.

Expectant fathers, just like expectant mothers, typically react with shock to the startling news that multiples are on the way. From there, they progress through essentially the same emotional stages described above as they come to terms with the implications of a high-risk pregnancy.

As the initial shock subsides, denial may set in. Telling himself that his own life won't change much until after the children are born, a man may wrongly assume that for the duration of the pregnancy, it will be business as usual. That naïveté can set the stage for extreme dismay when his partner no longer joins him for martinis after work or a scuba-diving expedition—or when complications force the mom-to-be onto bedrest and the dad must suddenly assume the role of caretaker for her and for the household.

Any partner who is in a denial rut needs to learn more about the risks and precautions associated with a multiple pregnancy. One mother of twins reports, "My husband kept asking me to go to the gym with him as we always used to do. Then I convinced him to come with me to a prenatal checkup, where my obstetrician explained why it was so important for me to limit my activity. After that, my husband was much more understanding."

Moving on to the next stage, a man may experience the same level of overwhelming anxiety that his wife feels over a multiple pregnancy. Yet for him, the worry may center primarily on his role as a provider and protector. Because twins, triplets, or quads magnify these responsibilities, an expectant father of multiples may be especially anxious about his ability to meet these challenges.

Fiscal concerns may come to the fore now. Ed Greenwood, father of boy/girl twins, explains, "I had been planning to leave a corporate job I found stifling and start my own business, but then I learned that Lydia was expecting twins. She encouraged me to follow my dream anyway, but I felt that with two babies to support, we would need the security of a steady paycheck. For a few weeks, it seemed that all I could think about was money."

Worries about the health of his wife and unborn babies can also overwhelm an expectant dad, triggering his protective instincts. If he takes his role as guardian to extremes—obsessively counting every calorie you eat, telling dinner guests it's your bedtime and hustling them out of the house if you so much as yawn—you may feel smothered. Try to appreciate the loving concern behind his actions, and encourage him to balance his instinct to protect with your need to be treated like a responsible adult.

Once that balance is achieved, chances are you'll enjoy being taken care of. "It was sweet to see how protective my husband became once I was pregnant with the twins," says Amy Maly. "He'd remind me to eat, get whatever I needed so I wouldn't overexert myself, and call me several times a day just to make sure I was okay. When I was on hospital bedrest, he even brought me milkshakes because I had complained about the hospital food."

Once your partner reaches the bargaining stage, there may be some temptation to negotiate with the obstetrician on your behalf—"Come on, doctor, she really wants to work another few weeks, and I support her in that. Don't you think the leave of absence could be postponed a bit longer?" Or your partner may try bargaining with you, when his desires conflict with your own—"I know you're not up for a big vacation, honey, but a romantic weekend getaway could do us a lot of good." Your partner is in bargaining mode? Gently remind him that it's vital to the babies' well-being that you adhere to your doctor's instructions and listen to your body's signals about the need for a low-key lifestyle right now.

There are several other important steps you can take to help your partner accept and adapt to a multiple pregnancy. Consider these suggestions:

Make communication a top priority.

"I think husbands often keep their feelings hidden, because they want to be the great protectors for their wives. They try to be strong and macho, so as not to add to whatever worries the women may have," says twin mom Karen Danke. "But knowing the risks associated with a multiple pregnancy, it's too hard for a guy to handle all those emotions on his own. You've got to get him to open up and talk about his fears, or eventually the pressure inside him will build to the point where he just blows up." Keep in mind that, although you and your partner are likely to pass through the same five emotional stages as you cope with a life crisis, you won't necessarily be at the same stage at the same time. Often (but not always) expectant fathers move through the stages more quickly than expectant mothers do. In addition, your response at each stage may be different, making communication even more difficult. Try to remain patient and supportive, to honestly discuss your feelings, and to be mutually respectful of where the other person is in the process.

Encourage your partner's involvement in the pregnancy.

Conflict can also stem from the fact that men and women experience pregnancy very differently, physically and emotionally. No matter how focused on your partner you may have been previously, bodily changes now cause you to shift attention inward. You track your babies' every movement—you know when they're all asleep, when one has hiccups, and when they are jostling each other—and you are aware of them at every moment. Your most important world becomes the world within, and your introspective mood is a normal part of protecting and nurturing your children.

Your partner, however, not having the constant physical reminders, can forget about the pregnancy for hours on end. Your single-minded focus on the babies can therefore make your partner feel left out of the loop. One father of triplets says plaintively, "My wife was so tuned in to what the babies were doing inside her belly—each kick, each hiccup—I felt like a fifth wheel." A man's sense of isolation is compounded when the outside world lavishes attention on the expectant mother of multiples and more or less ignores him.

To help your partner feel like a vital part of the action, encourage him to participate in the pregnancy as much as possible. Tell him when a baby is kicking, and place his hand on your belly so he can feel that miracle, too. Let him assign silly or affectionate nicknames to each baby—"Pelican," "Kicky Feet," "Sweet Pea"—and then refer to the babies by those names. If he wants to play Mozart to your tummy to share his love of music with his progeny, go along with it. And bring him to your doctor appointments so that he can hear firsthand all the news of the pregnancy. "My husband came to every single one of my prenatal checkups, taking time off from work when necessary," says Stacy Moore. "It made us feel closer to each other and helped him feel closer to the twins. I let him know how happy his involvement and moral support made me."

Show your appreciation for all he does.

Given the physical limitations imposed by a multiple pregnancy, your partner will have to take over a number of responsibilities that you two used to share. The shopping, cooking, cleaning, gardening, and errand running may all fall on his shoulders for now, and he probably misses your contribution in those areas. Hearing a word of thanks from you helps him to handle these chores with good grace.

"I worried that my husband might feel unappreciated for all of the work he had to do taking care of me and our unborn babies," says twin mom Meredith Alcott. "So I told him, and often, that I recognized and appreciated his many efforts." Keeping it out in the open this way helps to alleviate any resentment that otherwise might fester. Tell your partner how proud you are of him for all he's doing to help your babies grow healthy and strong, and he'll feel proud, too.

The Outside World: Everyone Wants in on the Action

Stacy Moore loves to tell the story of how she first shared the news of her twin pregnancy with the outside world. "Our families knew we were scheduled for our first ultrasound that day, and we had invited people to come over in the evening and see the videotape of the baby that the radiologist had promised to make for us," Stacy explains. "Everyone was sitting in our living room—my mom, Tim's parents, his grandmother, his sister, and her boyfriend. As I turned on the video, I said, 'Now watch carefully to see what the technician types.' Then on the screen appeared the letters, one by one: 'H-E-A-D-S.' Everyone said, 'Heads? Heads! Two heads! Oh, my God, it's twins!' Then they all started jumping up and down and hugging us. That was the most wonderful moment."

The world is fascinated by multiples, and as an expectant mother of multiples, you become an instant source of fascination to everyone around you. It's like being a movie star—the spotlight can be a thrill, but on occasion, it's an annoyance. You're likely to experience the positives as well as the negatives almost as soon as you break the news that multiples are on the way.

A FAMILY AFFAIR

You're probably noticing a shift in your relationship with your own parents and in-laws, particularly if this is your first pregnancy. Getting pregnant can be a rite of passage that makes you truly adult in their eyes, and your special status as the mother-to-be of multiples may lead the previous generation to treat you with new respect.

At the same time, though, your high-risk pregnancy may trigger a resurgence of protective parental instincts in them. As a result, they may bombard you with advice. "As soon as they learned I was expecting twins, both my mother and my mother-in-law started to tell me what to do all the time—stop driving, drink more milk, don't dye my hair. It was sweet in a way, because I knew they were thrilled about becoming grandparents. But sometimes it drove me crazy," admits Lydia Greenwood, mother of boy/girl twins.

You may feel like saying, "Back off! These are *my* babies." But everyone benefits if you can practice diplomacy, so keep these suggestions in mind:

- Grin and bear it, if you can. Your parents and in-laws want what's best for you and your multiples, and offering advice is their way of trying to help. Listen politely, but don't feel compelled to comply with every edict.
- Try not to get defensive. Your own subconscious concerns about your ability to cope with multiples may make you extra sensitive, even when no criticism is intended.
- If you feel you must speak up, say, "I know your advice is well meant. But please rest assured that I have an excellent health care team, and I need to follow *their* instructions." Then be generous about sharing less sensitive aspects of your pregnancy experience, such as your ideas for decorating the nursery. Parents are less pushy when they feel less shut out.
- Remind yourself that your parents' and in-laws' willingness to get involved may prove to be vitally important if you end up going on bedrest or being hospitalized—especially if you have other children who will need supervision and care.

FRIENDS AND ACQUAINTANCES: THE HELPFUL AND THE NOT-SO-HELPFUL

Close friends, casual acquaintances, coworkers, and even complete strangers may all want to feel that they are a part of the excitement of your multiple pregnancy. Sometimes that can be a lot of fun. "I was one of the first among my friends to get pregnant, so to have it be twins cranked up the thrill factor for everyone. I really enjoyed all the extra attention and excitement that went along with being an expectant mother of multiples," says Stacy Moore.

That spotlight can be a boon, because people are more likely to lend a hand when they know that two or more babies are on the way. Judy Levy says, "Everyone was extra supportive because I was expecting twins. For instance, our neighbors threw a baby shower for me, even though this wasn't a first baby. It was nice to know people cared and wanted to help."

Unfortunately, not everyone offers help that is truly helpful. Due to the publicity that frequently surrounds multiple-birth babies born in sets of six or more, many people have become blasé about twins and even triplets. "I constantly heard remarks like, 'Oh, you're having twins? Well, just be glad it's not a half-dozen babies.' I didn't consider such comments to be particularly useful," says Judy Levy.

You may find yourself the target of thoughtless or impolite remarks. "Toward the end of my pregnancy, I was admittedly huge," says Kelly McDaniel, whose twins had a combined birthweight of almost 17 pounds. "But I thought it was rude when one shopkeeper told me he hoped I'd finish my shopping and leave his store soon because he didn't want me to go into labor there."

Even worse are the horror stories. "It seemed that every week there was another news show about the dangers of multiple births—complete with video footage of minuscule infants on respirators. But it was hardest to handle the personal stories people told me. For instance, one woman revealed that she had lost a twin pregnancy at 24 weeks. Why would anyone think I needed to hear this?" Judy says. She coped by putting such stories in perspective. "I reminded myself that my situation was different from theirs. For example, the woman whose twins didn't make it had gained only 8 pounds during her pregnancy, whereas I had gained 40 pounds by my 24th week."

TAMARA: Just as people don't always know where to draw the line between helpful and hurtful remarks, they don't always recognize the difference between enthusiasm and intrusiveness. In our society, pregnant women are sometimes viewed as public property. And the more obviously pregnant you are, the more liberties people tend to take—touching your belly, guessing at your weight, and asking the nosiest of questions.

I can't begin to count the number of times that casual acquaintances and even complete strangers asked, "Did you take fertility drugs?" or "Will you be able to deliver vaginally?" or "Do you plan to breast-feed?" I'm no prude, but I didn't feel particularly comfortable discussing my sex life, my vagina, or my breasts with people I scarcely knew!

At first, I'd give some vague answer, then try to change the subject. But after a number of embarrassing episodes, I came up with several stock phrases that helped to nip the nosiness in the bud. Give it some thought, and you'll be able to come up with appropriate ready responses to impertinent questions. For instance:

Did you take fertility drugs?
Why do you ask?

Will you be able to deliver vaginally?
We'll see when the time comes.

How can you even think about breast-feeding twins? You'll feel like a cow.
I'm having babies, not calves, and I'm looking forward to nursing.

Twins are double trouble.
Actually, they're twice as nice.

Do multiples run in your family?
I expect it won't be long before they run all around the house.

Pregnant with twins? Oh, you poor thing. The workload! I'm glad they're yours and not mine.
I'm glad they're mine, too.

BODY-IMAGE BLUES

DR. LUKE: Another insensitive comment our patients too often hear, particularly if they are petite, is, "But you're so small, you can't possibly carry multiples!" I recall that one of the first women to attend our Multiples Clinic arrived at several appointments in tears. She felt discouraged because friends, neighbors, and even strangers in the supermarket frequently told her that she didn't look big enough to be pregnant with twins. Because her unborn babies were growing beautifully, we suggested that she respond by saying, "My multiples experts assure me that we're all doing just fine," but our encouragement was not enough to ease her distress.

Finally, two days before her due date, she walked into the Multiples Clinic radiant with joy. She was very large. As she stood sideways, nearly filling the doorframe, she said, "At last, everyone who sees me believes that I'm going to have twins!" Her babies ended up being two of the biggest multiples we've ever had in our program.

So if you find yourself feeling overly frightened by the insensitive remarks of every Tom, Dick, or Harriet, put your anxiety to good purpose. Use those comments as further motivation to eat right, get enough rest, and monitor yourself for contractions. If you do, chances are good that you will ultimately prove the naysayers wrong.

As aggravating as it is to be told that you're too small to carry multiples, to be teased about getting too big is also hurtful—and potentially more harmful, if you let it affect your diet. Yet if you're following the recommendations to gain 40, 50, even 65 pounds or more (depending on your prepregnancy weight and the number of babies you're expecting), chances are that someone will say, "Lady, you are getting *fat*." You need to disregard such comments if your babies are to thrive.

Admittedly, this is not always easy to do in our body-conscious society where slenderness is the ideal. You've probably been on a weight-watching vigil for much of your adult life, with the goal of taking off rather than putting on pounds. Slender women in particular may need to significantly alter their attitude about weight. "I'd always been proud of my slim figure, so it was a shock to think of gaining 50 pounds," confesses Lydia Greenwood. "I knew my twins needed the nourishment, but I couldn't keep from feeling upset the day a coworker teased, 'So much for miniskirts! You'll never be skinny again.' I had to remind myself that when you're pregnant with twins, big is beautiful. And guess what? Within three months of delivering my twins, I was back down to my prepregnancy weight and back into my miniskirts. All the weight I gained during my pregnancy really *did* go toward nourishing my babies."

Women who are overweight prior to conceiving may confront a public unsympathetic to the need to gain additional weight during a multiple pregnancy. "When you're heavy to start with, there is such a stigma about eating. Even when you're expecting, you hear people whispering, 'Oh, my gosh, do you see how enormous she is getting?'" says Marcy Bugajski. "I even read a pregnancy guide that warned overweight women like me against gaining more than 25 pounds. Dr. Luke told me, 'Throw out that book! You can lose weight later. Right now, your babies need every mouthful.' Once I had permission to gain, it was easier to ignore the snide remarks from uninformed outsiders."

While rude remarks from strangers may not be too hard to disregard, your partner's reaction may be more worrisome to you. Fortunately, most expectant fathers of multiples are very supportive. "My husband, Curt, made it his personal mission to be sure I was gaining enough weight. For instance, each morning he'd cook me two English muffins with eggs, cheese, and Canadian bacon—and he wouldn't leave for work until I'd eaten them both," says Amy Maly.

You may find it helpful if your obstetrician or dietitian explains to your partner the importance of adequate nutrition. Marcy Bugajski reports, "After Dr. Luke talked to my husband about the effect my diet would have on our unborn babies, he would constantly encourage me to eat. For instance, if I was too tired to get up and fix myself a snack, David would do it for me."

For additional moral support, your partner may even modify his own diet to more closely match your nutritional needs. "Fred knew that I wasn't happy about having to add red meat to my diet. So even though he didn't care for beef either, he started to cook it for dinner and eat it with me every night," says Heather Nicholas. "I appreciated that gesture. It made me feel like we were really in this together."

You're still feeling panicked as you see the scale climb toward 150, 175, or 200? Remind yourself that the extra weight is temporary. The pounds you put on are accounted for by the babies themselves and the adaptations your body is making to accommodate them—a larger uterus, multiple placentas, extra amniotic fluid, expanded blood volume, and stored calories for later in pregnancy. Research has shown that if you return to your prepregnancy eating habits (provided you were eating well and wisely before you conceived), you will get back to your former weight within three to six months—even quicker if you breast-feed.

Megan Ryerson, mother of boy/girl twins, cultivated a very helpful attitude. "At first I was intimidated by the thought of gaining so much, but I recognized all the research that had gone into establishing the weight-gain guidelines. So I reminded myself that there are seasons to life, and this was not my season to be my slimmest and fittest—it was the season to make my babies' well-being the top priority," says Megan. "I ended up putting on 55 pounds overall, and my belly was so big that I looked like a cartoon of a pregnant woman! Yet despite that, after the babies were born, the pounds just dropped off me."

DR. LUKE: Keep in mind that this may be one of the most emotional times of your life. Because not all the news you receive during your multiple pregnancy is guaranteed to be good news, you need to stay aware of how you and your partner are coping with any crises.

In the course of these few months, you may have to deal with a barrage of physical and psychological issues. Although these trials may take a short-term toll, if you and your partner can stay on a healthy track, the long-term results will be great personal growth and a stronger partnership. Those are wonderful qualities to bring to your new role as parents of multiples.

Chapter Nine

Giving Birth to All Those Babies

The countdown is near. You've been eating right, resting as much as possible, going to your prenatal checkups, and visiting your unborn children via ultrasound to watch them grow with each passing month. It won't be much longer now before your multiples are born—and that knowledge may leave you with a mix of emotions, from exhilarated anticipation to high anxiety. Delivery is undeniably easier when you're prepared, both mentally and physically. Childbirth preparation classes (as discussed in Chapter 2) can provide valuable information and emotional support, as well as training in specific exercises and techniques to use during labor. But because most of these courses are designed for expectant parents of singletons, you will want to study this chapter to ready yourself for the unique experience of giving birth to multiples.

Share this information with your partner, too. Today most expectant partners are eager to participate in childbirth by offering comfort and coaching. This not only makes labor more manageable for the mother, but also enhances a father's emotional bond to the children. Make sure that your partner keeps his cell phone charged and on, so you can reach him if you go into labor unexpectedly.

Well in advance of your due date, you should review with your doctor the plan for exactly what to do once labor begins. Be sure you know the best phone number to call, especially if it's after hours. And discuss where to go—some doctors practice at several different hospitals, but one will be the preferred hospital for delivering multiples. You don't want to wind up at the Level I community hospital where your prenatal office visits have been, for instance, only to learn that your doctor is waiting for you at the Level III hospital across town.

How to Recognize When Labor Has Begun

Although women have been giving birth since time immemorial, scientists still are not completely sure what triggers the onset of labor. Various physical changes or signs occur in concert to prepare your body for childbirth, beginning several days or even weeks before you actually deliver. When you notice the following developments, you'll know that labor is not far off.

LIGHTENING

Toward the end of pregnancy, a woman typically senses that the baby's head has settled deep into her pelvis. This event, known as lightening or dropping, is evident owing to the lower position of the belly. The mother-to-be is now able to breathe more easily and eat more comfortably—but the trade-off is additional pressure on the bladder and increased awkwardness while walking. Lightening is often a sign that delivery will occur within a few weeks, a few days, or even a few hours, as the pressure of the baby's head encourages the cervix to thin and dilate.

As an expectant mother of multiples, however, you may have felt this deep-down pressure for a prolonged period of time. Owing to the crowded conditions inside the uterus, the baby closest to the cervix may nestle down into your pelvis much earlier than a singleton would. If this is a new sensation for you, though, it indicates that delivery will probably occur soon.

BLOODY SHOW

The next sign of impending labor is when the mucous plug—the blood-tinged, jellylike substance that has filled the opening of the cervix—is dislodged by changes in the cervix: dilation and effacement. Measurements of dilation—the opening up of the cervix—range from undilated or closed (0 centimeters) to fully dilated (10 centimeters). Effacement is the thinning that occurs before and during labor, ranging from no effacement to 100 percent thinned out.

RUPTURE OF MEMBRANES

Your babies have been growing inside a membranous sac, sometimes called the bag of waters. If this sac ruptures, you will feel fluid coming from your vagina, in anything from a slow trickle to a sudden gush. Although you may often hear comments like "My water broke, so I knew that labor had begun," this will not necessarily be what happens in your case. Some women, in fact, deliver their babies with the membranes intact. For others, the membranes rupture days or even weeks before delivery—a dangerous complication called *preterm premature rupture of membranes* (PPROM) that increases the risk of infection. For that reason, as soon as you realize or even suspect that your water has broken, it's vital to call your obstetrician and then go to the hospital immediately.

STRONGER, MORE FREQUENT UTERINE CONTRACTIONS

Chances are that you've been feeling some contractions throughout your pregnancy. Called Braxton-Hicks contractions, these are normal. They differ from true labor contractions in that they are irregular; though noticeable, they are not typically painful; they are brought on by fatigue, dehydration, or physical activity; and they disappear with rest and hydration. True labor contractions, on the other hand, occur at regular intervals of about 5 to 15 minutes, with each contraction lasting about 30 to 60 seconds, and they continue regardless of what you do. Table 9.1 presents a comparison of true and false labor.

True Versus False Labor

Signs and Symptoms	False Labor	True Labor
Frequency of contractions	Irregular intervals	Regular intervals (5–15 minutes apart)
Change in contractions	Disappear with rest	Continue despite rest
Location of contractions	Usually felt in the abdomen	Usually felt in the back and abdomen
Strength of contractions	Decrease in strength	Increase in strength
Effect of pain medicines	Pain is eliminated	Pain is less affected
Cervical changes	No change	Progressive effacement and dilation

Table 9.1

DR. LUKE: For women pregnant with one baby, the signs of true labor typically occur at term, or about 38 to 41 weeks of pregnancy. But with two or more babies, labor usually comes earlier—sometimes much earlier. While the average singleton is born at 38.8 weeks, the average twins are born at 35.4 weeks, triplets at 31.8 weeks, and quadruplets 29.7 weeks.

The difficulty may be in recognizing symptoms of labor, particularly when they occur sooner than anticipated. Compounding this problem is that some women do not trust their own intuitive feeling that something is going on and therefore fail to act on it. So remember, at whatever point in your pregnancy you experience any symptoms of labor, *call your physician.* He will most likely instruct you to come to the office or the hospital for further evaluation.

TAMARA: If you're close to your due date, you probably won't have any qualms about calling your doctor, day or night, at the first possible indication of labor. But when labor begins well before the 37th week of pregnancy, the symptoms can be much milder and therefore more difficult to recognize. You may also be in a psychological state of denial: "It's way too early for the babies to be born, so these signs probably mean nothing at all. I'll just wait and see if they go away."

That's what happened to me. Just 31 weeks into my pregnancy, asleep in bed at 1 A.M., I was awakened by a moist feeling between my legs. "Better go to the bathroom," I thought sleepily, and made my way to the toilet. Back in bed, though, I gradually realized that there was still a slight, slow trickle. I had heard that when a woman's water broke, fluid could come gushing out, so I doubted that this tiny trickle could have the same significance. And I was reluctant to wake my doctor in the middle of the night just because my bladder was acting up.

After a while, I nudged my husband and told him what was happening. Groggily he murmured, "Based on my experience, I'd say everything is fine. We should both go back to sleep." And he did.

His words were not reassuring. "Based on his experience? *What* experience? *He* has never been pregnant before either." Finally, around 2:30 A.M., I called my obstetrician. "No contractions? Then you're probably just leaking a little amniotic fluid," he said reassuringly. "You may need to go on bedrest for a while. Meet me at the hospital, and we'll see what's going on."

Arriving at the labor and delivery unit, I said to the nurse on duty, "I guess I might be in labor." She laughed and said, "Honey, if you're not sure, you aren't." But as her fingers reached inside to check my cervix, her expression changed. "You're 9 centimeters dilated! Don't you feel any contractions?" Numbly I shook my head. The vague discomfort in my abdomen was nothing like what I had imagined labor to be. Moments later, my doctor entered the room. Labor had progressed too far to attempt to stop it now, he said. My babies were born vaginally about 45 minutes later, at 4 A.M.— just three hours after my water had broken.

If I had called my obstetrician as soon as I felt that first little leak of fluid, could anything have been done to delay my twins' birth for another few days or weeks? Perhaps not, given how quickly my cervix had dilated. But who knows? All that's certain is that with every moment of hesitation, opportunity had slipped away.

So please don't second-guess any symptoms you may have. Whether you're preterm or full term, when there is even the slightest suspicion that labor has begun, instantly alert your doctor.

DR. NEWMAN: I agree entirely with both Dr. Luke and Tamara. You should err on the side of caution because the risks of early delivery and rapid delivery are both higher with multiples.

Tamara's experience is not unusual. It can be surprisingly difficult to tell when you are in labor—and it's even harder with a multiple gestation. Compared to a singleton pregnancy, the uterus that is carrying two or more babies is overdistended, and it has enlarged faster. Women carrying multiples have more contractions throughout the latter half of pregnancy, and they are significantly worse at perceiving them.[1, 2] There are several reasons why:

- The overdistended uterus contracts more frequently but with lesser intensity. Since the uterine muscles are spread thinner, many of these contractions generate only low pressures (in the range of 10 to 20 mmHg) that are simply below the threshold at which a woman can perceive them.
- Women carrying multiples have a higher baseline intrauterine pressure, which makes it harder for them to recognize mild uterine contractions superimposed on a background of greater baseline discomfort.
- The increased fetal movement that occurs with multiples also can impede the recognition of contractions.
- Even though prelabor contractions are milder with multiples than with just one baby, their incessant nature can lead to early cervical ripening—which in turn allows cervical changes to progress more rapidly when labor intensity begins to pick up.

1. Newman RB, Gill PJ, Katz M. Uterine activity during pregnancy in ambulatory patients: Comparison of singleton and twin gestations. American Journal of Obstetrics & Gynecology 1986; 154:530–1.
2. Newman RB, Gill PJ, Wittreich P, Katz M. Maternal perception of prelabor uterine activity. Obstetrics & Gynecology 1986; 68:765–9.

One consequence of following our recommendation not to dismiss subtle labor symptoms is that you could experience false alarms. That's okay! Your doctor wants to be alerted to whatever is going on. It is not uncommon for women to experience flurries of contractions, sometimes painful, that last 30 minutes to an hour before dissipating. You don't have to decide whether or not your contractions mean labor has actually begun—that's your doctor's job, and it is likely to require an examination of your cervix.

What to Expect at the Hospital

When labor is suspected, your doctor will probably instruct you to go to the labor and delivery unit of the hospital. There, you change into a hospital gown and a nurse takes your pulse, blood pressure, and temperature (your vital signs). The nurse or physician also performs a pelvic exam to determine if you are in labor and how far you have progressed.

Next, your contractions are monitored by a pressure gauge attached to a belt placed around your abdomen. An ultrasound device also attached to the belt monitors each baby's heartbeat. This is the same type of monitoring you may have received during the last few months or weeks of your pregnancy, referred to as nonstress testing (see Chapter 2). Also known as electronic fetal monitoring, these machines provide a record of the pattern of your contractions and your babies' heartbeats in response to the contractions, alerting the labor and delivery room staff to potential problems.

If your due date is still many weeks off, you may be given fluids orally or intravenously to combat dehydration and attempt to stop labor. You may also have a fetal fibronectin test if you are experiencing preterm labor. Fetal fibronectin, a protein produced during pregnancy, functions like biological glue attaching the fetal membranes to the uterine lining. Up to about 22 weeks' gestation, fetal fibronectin is present in the cervical and vaginal secretions. After 22 weeks, this substance is no longer detected until one to three weeks before delivery. The presence of fetal fibronectin between 24 and 34 weeks' gestation, along with other signs and symptoms of labor, indicates that you are experiencing preterm labor.

Tocolytic medications can also be given through an intravenous (IV) line, as described in Chapter 7. If it is determined that you are in labor but will not deliver for at least a day, and you're between 24 and 34 weeks' gestation, you will probably be given corticosteroid injections. These help your babies' lungs and cerebrovascular system to mature more rapidly, thereby reducing the severity of certain complications of prematurity.

Throughout these procedures and those to follow, you are cared for by a team of nurses and other hospital staff. They work under the direction of your obstetrician, who checks on you periodically. If this is a teaching hospital, you may also be seen by physicians in training, including medical students, interns, and obstetrical residents.

WHEN LABOR IS INDUCED

Sometimes it's advisable to deliver the babies promptly, even though labor has not spontaneously begun. In such cases, unless a cesarean delivery is being performed, labor must be induced. To achieve this, the doctor may rupture the membranes and/or administer prostaglandins or a drug called Pitocin (a form of the hormone oxytocin) via IV to stimulate uterine contractions.

One reason for inducing labor is that after a certain point in gestation, a fetus becomes what is called *postmature*. As the aging placenta begins to function less efficiently, the uterine environment is no longer the healthiest place for the baby. If the pregnancy continues, the baby is more likely to experience complications. With singletons, this postmature point is typically reached at 41 to 42 weeks. With multiples, however, this point comes earlier. "When I reached 37 weeks, my doctor said it was time to get the babies out. She was concerned that if we waited too long, the placentas would stop working as well. Since we knew from the ultrasound that the twins were each close to 6 pounds already, we scheduled the delivery for a few days later," says Michelle Brow, mother of fraternal twin girls.

Placentas are graded using ultrasound, with Grade III indicating the most aging and highest amount of calcification present, and the greatest loss of function. Placentas age more quickly with maternal smoking, diabetes, chronic hypertension, and in multiple pregnancies.

Take a look at Table 9.2. From the graph you can see that, in this study of twin versus singleton pregnancies, a higher percentage of twin pregnancies had Grade III placentas, beginning at 29 to 31 weeks (15 percent for twins versus 0 percent for singletons). This difference between the percent of Grade III placentas became greater as pregnancy progressed: By 35 to 37 weeks, 60 percent of twin pregnancies versus 25 percent of singleton pregnancies were Grade III; and by 38 to 40 weeks, 75 percent of twin pregnancies versus 35 percent of singleton pregnancies had Grade III placentas.

The optimal timing of delivery of multiples depends on various factors. Here's what the research shows:

- For **fraternal** twins and **dichorionic identical** twins, the optimal time for delivery is between 37 and 38 weeks' gestation.[3]

---

3. Luke B, Brown MB, Alexandre PK, Kinoshi T, et al. The cost of twin pregnancy: Maternal and neonatal factors. American Journal of Obstetrics & Gynecology 2005; 192:909–15.

Comparison of Distribution of Ultrasonic Placental Grade III in Twin Versus Singleton Gestations by Weeks of Gestation

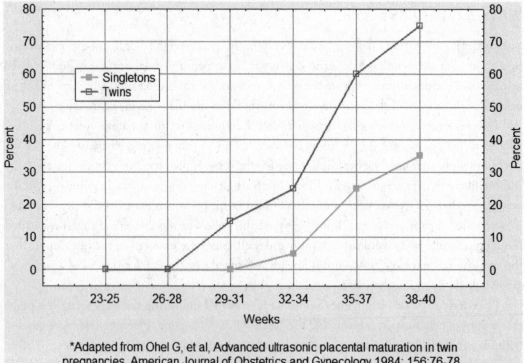

*Adapted from Ohel G, et al, Advanced ultrasonic placental maturation in twin pregnancies. American Journal of Obstetrics and Gynecology 1984; 156:76-78.

Table 9.2

- For **monochorionic identical** twins, the optimal time for delivery is between 36 and 37 weeks' gestation.[4, 5, 6, 7] While there are some published recommendations to deliver monochorionic twins as early as 34 weeks due to concerns about unexpected

---

4. Hartley RS, Emanuel I, Hitti J. Perinatal mortality and neonatal morbidity rates among twin pairs at different gestational ages: Optimal delivery timing at 37 to 38 weeks' gestation. American Journal of Obstetrics & Gynecology 2001; 184:451–8.
5. Jauniaux E, Kilby M. Minimizing perinatal mortality in twins: planned birth at 38 weeks of gestation for dichorionic and 36 weeks of gestation for monochorionic twins. British Journal of Obstetrics and Gynaecology 2014; 121:1284–90.
6. Burgess JL, Unal ER, Nietert PJ, Newman RB. Risk of late-preterm stillbirth and neonatal morbidity for monochorionic and dichorionic twins. American Journal of Obstetrics & Gynecology 2014; 210:578.e1.
7. Dias T, Akolekar R. Timing of birth in multiple pregnancy. Best Practice & Research, Clinical Obstetrics and Gynaecology 2014; 28:319–26.

stillbirth even in apparently uncomplicated pregnancies, most specialists agree that delivering this early is not necessary or advisable as long as careful fetal and maternal surveillance is being done to confirm that the pregnancy remains uncomplicated. The advantage of waiting is that newborn complications are significantly reduced when monochorionic twins are delivered between 36 and 37 weeks rather than at 34 weeks of gestation. "I was induced right at 37 weeks. Because my identical twin girls were monochorionic, we didn't want the pregnancy to go any longer. Fortunately, everything went fine—Kate weighed 5 lb., 9 oz., and Audrey weighed 5 lb., 0 oz. Neither one had any health problems, and both came home from the hospital with me two days later," says Hannah Steele.

- For **monoamniotic identical** twins, most obstetricians recommend delivery between 32 and 34 weeks of gestation. The final decision requires balancing the risks associated with prematurity against the increased risk for unexpected stillbirth in mo/mo gestations. With outpatient fetal monitoring, the risk of stillbirth between 32 and 34 weeks is approximately 5 percent, while the risk with inpatient monitoring is close to zero. So if you are undergoing inpatient monitoring of your mo/mo twins, your doctor may recommend trying to reach 33 or 34 weeks of gestation before advising delivery.

- For **triplets,** the best time to be born is between 34 and 36 weeks, depending on their weights and estimates of fetal well-being.

- For **quadruplets,** the optimal time for delivery is less well defined but is probably between 32 and 34 weeks of gestation. However, most quadruplets end up being born earlier than this, due to either preterm labor or maternal complications.

Even if you have not yet reached the optimal delivery time for your type of multiples, labor may be induced early if it is determined that one or more of your babies is in distress inside the womb—for instance, due to growth abnormality or a problem with the placenta or umbilical cord. "Not quite 34 weeks into my twin pregnancy, electronic fetal monitoring revealed that one baby's heart rate was fluctuating too much. My doctor told me this meant it was time to deliver. I was started on a Pitocin drip at noon, and shortly after 6 P.M., my babies were born," says Karen Danke, mother of fraternal twin boys.

In other cases, a concern about the mother's health may necessitate an earlier delivery than had been anticipated. For example, a complication such as preeclampsia may not be controllable with bedrest and medication. Marcy Bugajski says, "Because I developed preeclampsia, the doctor had to induce labor immediately, even though I was only at 34 weeks. I received IV magnesium to prevent seizures, as well as IV Pitocin to stimulate contractions. Still, nothing much happened until after the doctor broke my water. At that point, the contractions came quickly. My fraternal twin boys arrived five hours later."

Options for Pain Relief

Long before you go into labor, you should familiarize yourself with the options for managing the discomforts of labor. Knowing ahead of time the pros and cons of the various medications will help you to feel calmer and more in control as your babies are born.

For some women, the relaxation techniques and breathing exercises learned in childbirth education classes are sufficient for coping with labor pains. "I told my doctor that I didn't want any pain medication unless it became absolutely necessary. In the end, I managed without it because I didn't feel the contractions that much. The only really painful part was a stabbing sensation in my leg, because one of the twins was hitting on a nerve," says Marcy Bugajski.

Other women find medical hypnosis techniques to be helpful. "I was committed to having a drug-free delivery because I'd once had a lumbar puncture that led to a terrible spinal headache afterward. So I took a six-week class through Hypnobabies and also practiced at home every day for months. By the time labor came, the techniques were second nature to me. I certainly wouldn't say labor was painless, but I did get through it without drugs," says Erin Justice, mother of identical twin boys.

When additional relief is needed, two categories of medications can be used. The first type, called analgesia, lessens but does not eliminate pain. The second type, called anesthesia, produces numbness with or without a loss of consciousness. The most frequently used medications include the following.

Analgesics

A narcotic such as morphine or Nubain can be administered via the IV line or by intramuscular injection. One mother of twins says, "I appreciated the way the analgesic medication took the edge off my pain and eased my anxiety. It helped me regain my composure and focus without taking away all sensation." Some women, however, dislike the drowsiness this medication can bring on. "I was sorry I'd had the drug because not only did it make me nauseous, but it left me groggy at a time when I wanted to be fully alert," says another mother of twins.

Different patients respond differently to narcotic analgesics, so it is hard to predict the exact dose that will significantly reduce your pain without creating too much sedation. Nausea is a fairly common side effect of these drugs, which is why some physicians add a small amount of an antinausea medication like Phenergan to the analgesic. You should be aware that analgesic drugs do cross the placenta. That's why you may be encouraged to forgo analgesia in the last hour or two before delivery, so that the babies will not be born sedated or with respiratory depression.

With all that to consider, how can you know whether a narcotic analgesia is right for you? Your best bet is to discuss your concerns and preferences with your obstetrician well in advance of your due date—and be sure to describe any previous experience, positive or negative, that you may have had with this type of medication.

Epidural Block

This technique for administering analgesia is currently the most common method of pain management in labor. Medication is given via an epidural catheter (a small tube) inserted through a needle into the epidural space just outside the spinal cord. While an epidural is very effective at minimizing labor pain, it can interfere with the mother's urge to push once the cervix is fully dilated. For that reason, the drug may be decreased or stopped as the time for delivery nears, allowing the mother to have full control over pushing.

"I used no medication when I delivered my boy/girl twins. But two years later, when I gave birth to my singleton son, I asked for an epidural," says Lydia Greenwood. "Which would I recommend? Every woman has to make her own choice—but if I were doing it again, I'd opt for the epidural."

An epidural is also commonly used for certain cesarean deliveries, though for this, a higher dosage of medication is given. Oftentimes this just requires a redosing of the epidural used for labor. A distinct advantage of epidural anesthesia for cesarean delivery is that the mother can remain awake and alert during the birth of her babies.

Spinal Block

Spinal anesthesia is very similar in effect to epidural anesthesia and is used almost exclusively for cesarean deliveries. With a spinal block, the anesthesia medication is injected directly into the spinal canal in the lower lumbar region (rather than into the epidural space surrounding the spinal canal). A spinal block cannot be continuously infused the way an epidural can, so it is not very helpful for labor—however, its one- to two-hour duration of action is perfect for a cesarean birth. Many anesthesiologists prefer the spinal block for cesareans because of its greater reliability of effectiveness, its more rapid onset of action, and the opportunity to combine the anesthesia with an analgesic agent that will provide the patient with about 24 hours of postoperative pain relief.

Local Anesthesia

This type of medication is typically administered by injection at the opening of the vagina. It is given just before birth if the physician decides to perform an episiotomy, a small incision that widens the vaginal opening to allow the babies to fit through more easily. In the past, episiotomies were commonly done, primarily for larger babies, but these days they are fairly rare—especially for multiples, who tend to be smaller.

General Anesthesia

Because it produces unconsciousness, this category of medication is usually given only for emergency cesarean deliveries or in the case of an emergency vaginal delivery. A potential danger of general anesthesia is that food or stomach acid may be aspirated into the patient's lungs. For that reason, it's wise to limit your intake to clear fluids as soon as you think labor has begun, in case you end up needing general anesthesia. Your doctor or anesthesiologist may also give you antacid medication to reduce the amount of acid in your stomach.

Although every effort is made to accommodate a patient's wishes regarding pain relief, other considerations can come into play. Chief among these is the health of your babies. Most drugs can pass through the placentas and may slow the babies' heartbeats before birth. Pain medication taken by the mother also can affect the babies' ability to breathe after delivery, depending on the dosage and how soon before birth the drug was given.

Will You Deliver Vaginally?

Nearly every pregnant woman spends nine months wondering whether she'll deliver vaginally or by cesarean. Often this question cannot be answered until the woman is actually in labor, when the course of events determines which method of delivery would be most appropriate.

An expectant mother of multiples, however, may have her answer long in advance of her delivery date. That's because most triplets and virtually all quadruplets are delivered by cesarean (sometimes called a C-section). The surgery, which involves making an incision through the wall of the uterus, is scheduled in advance, and the woman does not actually go into labor at all.

For most twin pregnancies, however, the vaginal-versus-cesarean issue is part of an ongoing discussion between the mother-to-be and her obstetrician. A number of factors need to be considered when determining the route of delivery. These factors include the babies' positions in the uterus, their gestational age and estimated weights, whether they are monoamniotic, the mother's own obstetrical history, the availability of real-time ultrasound on the labor floor and in the delivery room, and the doctor's ability to monitor each twin independently during the entire labor process.

Careful consideration of all these factors is essential because the birth process is more prone to complications when more than one baby is being born. There is also a possibility that the first baby might be delivered vaginally while the second would end up needing to be delivered by cesarean, although this occurs in fewer than 5 percent of twin pregnancies.

Here's what you should know about the factors that affect the mode of delivery for multiples. (Additional information geared toward physicians is included in Appendix E, titled "Doctor to Doctor: A Research Update," which readers are encouraged to share with their obstetricians.)

The Babies' Presentation

In determining whether you are likely to deliver vaginally or will need a cesarean, a vital consideration is the babies' presentation, meaning their position in the uterus. As soon as you are admitted to the labor and delivery unit, the presentation of each of your babies should be confirmed by ultrasound. If the babies' weights have not been estimated via ultrasound within the past week or two, this should be done as well.

All combinations of twin presentation can be classified into one of three groups (with Baby A referring to the baby closest to the birth canal). Here is how these various combinations affect delivery options:

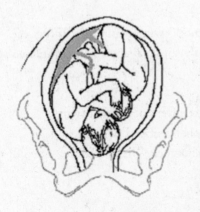

Both Baby A and Baby B cephalic (head-down).

The cephalic/cephalic presentation (also called vertex/vertex) occurs in about 40 percent of twin pregnancies. It is the most favorable scenario for a successful vaginal delivery, especially when the crown of Baby A's head (rather than the forehead or face) is closest to the birth canal. Most obstetricians believe that a trial of labor and vaginal delivery is appropriate for cephalic/cephalic twin pregnancies, regardless of gestational age or estimated fetal weight. Studies have found no benefit to routine cesarean delivery of cephalic/cephalic twins.

It's important to note, however, that in a small percentage of cases the presentation of the second twin may change after vaginal delivery of the first twin. When that happens, it sometimes necessitates that Baby B be delivered by cesarean. "Both of my twins were head-down when labor started, but I knew that the second baby might sprawl into a transverse position after the first was born. That's why I delivered in an operating room, so I'd already be where I would need to be if the second baby ended up having to be delivered by cesarean. But to my relief, everything went well and I was able to deliver both girls vaginally," says Hannah Steele.

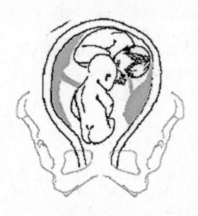

Baby A breech (buttocks or feet-first) or transverse (sideways) and Baby B in any position.

This presentation combination occurs in about 20 percent of twin gestations. It almost always leads to a recommendation for cesarean delivery.

A baby lying in a transverse position cannot deliver vaginally. With a breech presentation, the concerns are twofold. First is the fear of *interlocking,* in which the chin of the breech Baby A gets caught beneath the chin of the cephalic Baby B during the delivery process. This is very rare. More common and thus more concerning is the risk of extension of the fetal head of the breech Baby A, which can lead to injury of the cervical spine (neck) during delivery. With a breech singleton delivery, a baby's chin is kept safely tucked against the chest by the surrounding uterine muscle. However, when there is a second twin inside the uterus, there is no similar pressure keeping the first baby's chin tucked, so the risk of injury is greater. That's why cesarean delivery is generally considered safest for twin pregnancies in which Baby A has a noncephalic presentation.

Baby A cephalic and Baby B breech or transverse.

This presentation combination occurs in about 40 percent of twin pregnancies. If the second twin does not move into a head-down position after delivery of the first twin, there are two options for vaginal delivery:

- *External cephalic version (ECV).* Immediately after the delivery of the first twin, the doctor attempts to manually maneuver the noncephalic second twin into a head-down position by pressing against the mother's abdomen. The procedure,

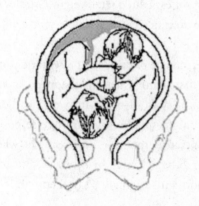

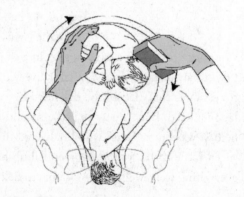

which is guided by ultrasound and sometimes aided by a uterine relaxant medication, is successful approximately 70 percent of the time.[8]

However, even if Baby B does move into the desired cephalic position, complications can arise that would preclude a vaginal delivery. For instance, if the placenta begins to separate from the uterine wall, or if the umbilical cord prolapses (descends into the birth canal) before Baby B does, an emergency cesarean will be needed to deliver the second baby. Thus it is wise, prior to going into labor, to have a discussion with your obstetrician about his or her experience with ECV.

- *Breech extraction.* Most of the recent study data on mode of delivery in twin gestations with a cephalic-presenting first twin and a noncephalic second twin show that a breech extraction can be a good option for achieving a safe vaginal delivery provided that certain conditions are met. These conditions include a gestation of at least 32 weeks' duration, estimated fetal weights of at least 3 lb., 5 oz. (1,500 grams), and an obstetrician and supporting staff with sufficient training and experience in this type of delivery. In such cases, there appears to be no conclusive safety advantage to a planned cesarean delivery rather than a vaginal delivery.

DR. NEWMAN: The importance of your obstetrician's training, experience, and usual practice cannot be underestimated as factors affecting the safe vaginal delivery of twins, particularly when the second twin is in a noncephalic presentation. In the past two decades, concerns about possible negative outcomes associated with singleton breech deliveries have led to the virtual abandonment of vaginal delivery for breech-presenting singletons. As a consequence, fewer obstetricians are acquiring or maintaining the skills needed to safely perform vaginal breech extractions of noncephalic second twins. That's why a frank discussion between you and your doctor is essential.

TRIPLET GESTATIONS

Although vaginal delivery is sometimes an option for triplets, there are no large studies establishing its safety. Adequate monitoring of all three babies throughout labor and delivery is very

---

8. Gocke SE, Nageotte MP, Garite T, Towers CV, Dorchester W. Management of the nonvertex second twin: Primary cesarean section, external version or primary breech extraction. American Journal of Obstetrics & Gynecology 1989; 161:111–4.

challenging. Also, with triplets there is a much higher rate of noncephalic presentation, as well as an increased likelihood of the triplets being very preterm or very low birthweight. As a result, a planned cesarean delivery is generally considered the optimal strategy.

If vaginal delivery of triplets is considered, it is best limited to cases in which each baby has an estimated weight of at least 3.5 pounds, there is a cephalic presentation of Baby A and Baby B (and preferably Baby C as well), and the obstetrician is experienced in such deliveries.

Monoamniotic Gestations

Many experts agree that the safest route of delivery for monoamniotic twins is by cesarean. This is based on concerns about entanglement of the umbilical cords, which occurs in nearly all monoamniotic twin pregnancies. This can lead to cord constriction as one twin is pushed down the birth canal, cutting off the fetal oxygen supply.

If a vaginal delivery is going to be attempted, it is optimal for both twins to be in a head-down presentation and well grown. Continuous fetal monitoring during labor is essential, because acute fetal distress can develop quite suddenly, particularly during the second stage of labor (when the cervix has fully dilated), necessitating immediate delivery by cesarean.

The Mother's Obstetrical History

Another important consideration in determining the method of delivery of your multiples is your own obstetrical history—specifically, whether you had a cesarean in a previous pregnancy. Years ago, it was believed that once a woman had given birth by cesarean, she had to deliver by cesarean for every pregnancy that followed. That's because the scar in the uterus—from the vertical type of incision commonly used in the past—was at risk for rupturing during a subsequent labor.

This practice has changed. Today surgeons generally make a transverse (side-to-side) incision across the lower part of the uterus. This heals with a stronger scar and does not disrupt the muscular portion of the womb, so it is far less likely to cause problems in a future labor.

Because a vaginal birth offers several advantages, including lower risk of infection, less bleeding, and quicker recovery, nowadays many women who previously had a cesarean are offered the option of attempting to deliver vaginally. This is called a trial of labor after cesarean, or TOLAC. When successful, the delivery is referred to as a vaginal birth after cesarean, or VBAC (pronounced *vee-back*).

In singleton gestations, a prior low transverse uterine incision is associated with a 0.5 percent to 1 percent risk of rupture during a future labor. The risk for rupture in a twin gestation is not as well defined as it is for singletons, but most obstetricians believe it to be similar, at about 1 percent. While this risk is low, the consequences are potentially severe. That's why any decision to attempt a trial of labor after a prior cesarean must undergo the same careful evaluation in a twin pregnancy as it does in a singleton pregnancy.

Keep in mind that, although the risk of uterine rupture is similar for twin gestations and for singleton gestations, the likelihood of ending up with a successful VBAC is lower for twins. That's primarily due to the fact that twins overall are at greater risk for cesarean delivery. If you had a cesarean in the past, your best bet is to discuss your situation and options with your obstetrician.

The Hospital's Capabilities

Whenever a trial of labor is attempted with a multiple gestation, there are several capabilities that the labor and delivery unit must have. Be sure to discuss these points with your doctor well in advance of delivery to confirm that the hospital where you plan to deliver is properly equipped.

First, the unit needs a portable ultrasound machine, which is used to estimate the babies' weights. The portable ultrasound also is needed to determine the babies' presentation during labor—and again in the delivery room, to assess the position of Baby B after Baby A has been delivered. There should be someone else in the room capable of performing the ultrasound, so that your obstetrician remains free to attend to you.

It is also important that the nursing staff be able to continuously monitor both twins—or all three triplets—during the first stage of labor (when the cervix is dilating) as well as the second stage (while you are pushing in the delivery room). The dual monitoring capability of almost all current fetal monitors makes this fairly easy to achieve. It is vital for the fetal monitor to go with you to the delivery room when delivery seems imminent.

The necessary staffing for a trial of labor with multiple gestation includes an experienced obstetrician, an anesthesiologist, newborn nursing or neonatology staff appropriate for the gestational age of the babies, and extra nursing staff to assist with delivery. At all times, the staff should be prepared to perform a cesarean without delay if this becomes necessary.

Vaginal Delivery of Multiples

Vaginal delivery involves three distinct stages of labor that last altogether about 12 to 14 hours, or somewhat longer for a first pregnancy. If you are having a scheduled cesarean delivery, you do not experience any of these stages because the surgery is performed before actual labor can begin. If you have a trial of labor but ultimately it's determined that you need a cesarean, you may proceed through part or all of the first stage, and possibly into the second, before a surgical delivery is performed. Here's what to expect during each stage.

First Stage

With each contraction, the normally thick cervix thins out and begins to dilate as it prepares to allow the first twin's head to pass from the uterus into the birth canal. A physician or nurse periodically places a few fingers inside your vagina to check the status of your cervix and, if necessary, to see whether your membranes have ruptured. This stage of labor is divided into three phases: early, active, and transition.

- During the early phase, contractions are mild, occurring at intervals of about 5 to 15 minutes, with each contraction lasting about 60 to 90 seconds. The cervix begins to dilate from 0 centimeters to about 4 centimeters.
- As you enter the active phase, contractions become stronger and more frequent until they are about 3 minutes apart. Each contraction lasts an average of 45 to 60

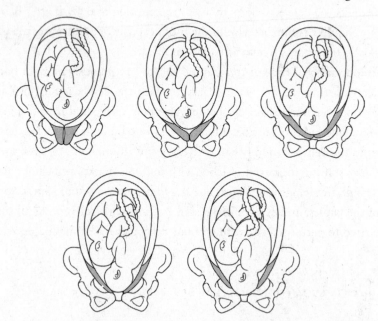

Dilation and effacement of the cervix during the first stage of labor

seconds. Your membranes may rupture during this phase if they have not done so earlier. The cervix continues to dilate to about 8 centimeters.

- Transition, the end of the first stage of labor, is typically the most uncomfortable phase of childbirth. During this time, the cervix dilates from 8 to 10 centimeters. Contractions occur every 2 to 3 minutes, with each contraction lasting about 60 seconds.

DR. LUKE: Depending on the position of the twin closest to your cervix, the transition phase of labor may involve a backache that gets progressively worse. Some women report feeling nauseated, chilled, and irritable. You're also likely to feel extremely tired. When I was in labor with my own son, I remember thinking, "I'm so exhausted, I don't know how I'm going to stay awake for the birth of this baby."

Many mothers laboring to deliver multiples find the physical and emotional sensations to be overpowering. You may completely lose track of time or even experience a kind of temporary amnesia. If you feel overwhelmed or panicked, rely on your partner or labor coach to help you cope.

SECOND STAGE

Once the cervix has fully dilated, the head of the first twin can begin moving down into the birth canal. Your contractions may slow down, occurring every 2 to 5 minutes, with each one lasting about 60 to 90 seconds. The second stage can last more than an hour, so try to rest and relax between contractions.

You may have an urge to push or bear down with each contraction. This is a basic instinct, and for most women the active participation feels gratifying. With an epidural analgesia, however, the urge to push may be delayed until the first twin's head has descended deeply into the birth canal.

As the first baby's head crowns, or becomes visible at the opening of the vagina, you may feel intense pressure and a burning sensation. This is due to the stretching of the perineum, the area between the vagina and the rectum. In a few moments, the stinging sensation abates as the pressure from the baby's head stretches the vaginal tissues, causing a natural numbing of the nerves. (It is relatively rare these days for an obstetrician to perform an episiotomy, or a surgical incision in the perineum to enlarge the vaginal opening, in an attempt to assist the delivery or prevent injury to the perineum.)

As the infant's head emerges, the physician checks to make sure the umbilical cord is not wrapped around the neck, wipes the baby's eyes, and removes any fluid from the nose and mouth. With the next contraction and a strong push from you, the first twin's shoulders are usually delivered, followed by the body. By convention, health care professionals refer to the firstborn twin as Baby A, regardless of how the twins may have been positioned in your uterus during pregnancy.

In some cases the second twin, Baby B, arrives just a minute or two later. "I pushed four times and out came Jacob. With the very next push, Zachary was born. It all happened so fast that the doctors didn't even have time to change their gloves between babies," Karen Danke recalls.

More commonly, the second twin follows after about 5 to 15 minutes, though it can take longer. During this interval, your health care team continues to monitor the unborn baby. Provided all is going well, they may encourage you to relax awhile before proceeding with the birth. There is no particular time limit during which the second twin needs to be delivered. Heather Nicholas says, "My first twin was born at 10:37 P.M. Then the doctor wanted me to rest, so the second twin wasn't born until 11:18. That was okay with me. I'd had an epidural, so although I could feel contractions, they weren't painful." After delivery of the first twin, it sometimes is necessary to give Pitocin to restart the contractions.

DR. NEWMAN: Obstetricians used to consider the time interval between delivery of the first and second twin to be an important factor affecting delivery outcome. Consequently, it was previously recommended that the interval between deliveries should ideally be 15 minutes or less, and certainly not more than 30 minutes. The worry was that, after delivery of the first twin, the uterine contractions might cease; the umbilical cord of the second twin might prolapse, cutting off the blood supply to that baby; or placental abruption might occur. Each of these would pose a risk to the undelivered second twin. In addition, the cervix could close up, making rapid delivery of the second twin impossible if problems developed with that baby.

While those are legitimate concerns, we now have more flexibility when it comes to the interval between the delivery of Baby A and Baby B. That's because of the advent of continuous and dual intrapartum fetal monitoring capability.

Studies published since the introduction of this type of fetal monitoring during labor have generally confirmed that the interval between deliveries is unimportant, as long as the fetal heart rate remains normal.[9, 10] When the second twin is not dem-

9. Rayburn WF, Lavin JP Jr., Miodovnik M, Varner MW. Multiple gestation: Time interval between delivery of the first and second twin. Obstetrics & Gynecology 1984; 63:502–6.

10. Chervenak FA. The controversy of mode of delivery in twins: The intrapartum management of twin gestation (part II). Seminars in Perinatology 1986; 10:44–9.

onstrating signs of distress, a less hurried approach appears to reduce the incidence of problems that can arise for mother or baby when a difficult delivery is rushed in order to meet an arbitrary deadline.

If the twins were in separate amniotic sacs, and the second twin's sac is intact, the doctor ruptures these membranes when it's time to get under way again. Take your cues for pushing from your body sensations, unless your health care team instructs you to do otherwise. If the second baby is in a breech position but your doctor determines that it is safe to try for a vaginal delivery, it is particularly important for you to push and to refrain from pushing as your doctor directs.

DR. LUKE: Women are always relieved to hear that labor is generally no more painful with twins than with a singleton baby. You need to go through the first stage of labor, including transition, only once, even though you are giving birth to two babies.

While you do go through the second stage twice, this usually proceeds more rapidly with baby number two, particularly if she is smaller than the firstborn twin. And most of our patients who also have an older child tell us afterward that delivering multiples is no more uncomfortable than pushing out a singleton.

THIRD STAGE

After both babies are born, you may continue to feel mild contractions as the placentas separate from the uterine wall and are delivered through the vagina. Usually the placentas are intact, but your doctor will examine them carefully to see whether any small fragments may have remained inside you. If so, these are removed manually. Otherwise, the uterus would not be able to contract completely and bleeding would continue.

You may also be given medication such as Pitocin to help the uterus stay firm and to further reduce bleeding. Women who deliver multiples are at increased risk of postpartum bleeding due to uterine exhaustion, in which the uterus fails to contract. If this occurs and Pitocin is not sufficient to correct the problem, there are several other medications that can be used. If you had an episiotomy or a tear in the perineum, it is repaired with stitches at this time.

After the hard work of labor, you may feel very hungry, shaky, or chilled. But the overriding sensation, provided all has gone well, is usually profound relief and a great sense of satisfaction.

Table 9.3 summarizes what is happening and how you may feel during each stage of labor.

Stages of Labor for Vaginal Birth of Twins

Stage of Labor	Contractions	Physical Changes	How You May Feel	What You Can Do
First Stage				
Early	Mild contractions, 5–15 minutes apart, lasting 60–90 seconds	Bloody show; cervix is 0–4 cm dilated	Relieved that labor has finally begun	Relax, sleep, practice relaxation techniques
Active	Stronger contractions, building to about 3 minutes apart, lasting about 45–60 seconds	Membranes may rupture; cervix is 5–8 cm dilated	Anxious, more tired; you may have a backache	Work with your labor coach; use your relaxation techniques; request pain relief if desired
Transition	Contractions are 2–3 minutes apart, lasting about 1 minute	Cervix finishes dilating to 10 cm	Nauseated, chilled, irritable, very tired; backache may worsen	Relax between contractions; pant or blow during contractions; do not push yet
Second Stage	2–5 minutes apart, lasting 60–90 seconds	First baby's head descends into the birth canal; first twin is born; then second baby descends and is born	Alert, in control	Push with your contractions
Third Stage	Contractions continue, but are less painful	Placentas separate from the uterine wall and are expelled	Exhilarated; perhaps shaky, hungry, chilled	Enjoy holding your newborns

Table 9.3

Important Information on Cesarean Birth

As they study their books on pregnancy, some expectant mothers skip over the chapters about cesarean birth. Attending childbirth classes, they tune out when the talk turns to surgical delivery. That's because most women dream of having a typical, natural childbirth experience that includes an uncomplicated vaginal delivery. And it's human nature to think, "Some people have problems, but *I* won't be one of them."

Yet the fact is that, as a mother-to-be of multiples, your chances of needing to deliver by cesarean are high. In the United States, the overall rate of cesarean delivery exceeds 30 percent. But for multiples, the rate is much higher: More than 70 percent of twins and nearly all triplets and quadruplets are delivered surgically. Chances are that you'll find greater satisfaction in giving birth if you accept the possibility of a cesarean before your delivery date arrives.

Why are so many multiples delivered by cesarean? For triplets or more, the answer is that it's not possible to adequately monitor all the babies during active labor. It would be exceedingly difficult to detect when a baby had developed a problem or even to identify which baby was in distress. Vaginal delivery of higher-order multiples also carries a high risk of excessive bleeding and other complications for the mother.

With twins, a number of factors can affect the decision. Situations in which twins would typically be delivered by cesarean include the following:

- Breech or transverse presentation of the presenting twin (the one closest to the cervix). This occurs in approximately 20 percent of twin sets.
- Breech or transverse presentation of the second twin, which occurs in approximately 40 percent of twin sets, and an obstetrical contraindication to breech extraction or an obstetrician inexperienced with breech extraction.
- A prior cesarean delivery and no interest in TOLAC.
- Failure of one of the babies to descend into the birth canal.
- A trial of labor that does not progress adequately, such as when the cervix does not dilate fully.
- Placenta previa: One of the placentas is blocking the birth canal.
- Abruptio placenta: A placenta separates from the uterine wall.
- Fetal distress due to a tangled or compressed umbilical cord or other problem that prevents one of the babies from getting sufficient oxygen.
- An umbilical cord or fetal limb that is prolapsed.
- A health problem in the mother—such as severe infection, preeclampsia, or gestational diabetes—that would be aggravated by the stress of labor.
- An active herpes infection in the mother, which could be passed on to the babies as they travel through the birth canal, with potentially life-threatening consequences.

Scheduled Versus Emergency Cesareans

In some cases (such as with twins in transverse or breech presentation, or with higher-order multiples), it is known well ahead of time that a cesarean will be performed. In that event, the surgery can be scheduled in advance. "By the 31st week of my quadruplet pregnancy, I was experiencing intense vaginal pressure, extreme nausea, and constant contractions despite the use of tocolytic medications. My body was clearly saying it couldn't take much more," says Anne Seifert. "My obstetrician told me, 'It's better to schedule the surgery for a time of day when the labor and delivery unit and the NICU will be fully staffed. We don't want to wait too long and have you go into labor at 1 A.M.' So we scheduled the cesarean for the following Friday morning."

In other cases, the expectant mother may be fully aware that she'll be having a C-section eventually, but early onset of labor or a sudden complication necessitates emergency surgery. "At 30 weeks, I was admitted to the hospital because the doctor feared that the smallest baby was not doing well in utero," says Ginny Seyler, mother of triplets. "An ultrasound revealed that blood flow to this baby was inadequate and his heart rate was not strong. Even though the other two babies would be better off staying inside me, this child clearly needed to come out. The doctors gave us 15 minutes to make a decision, and we opted to do the cesarean right away."

Sometimes a woman actually goes into labor and progresses up to a certain point before a vaginal delivery is finally ruled out. "My water broke at 8 P.M. the Friday of my 38th week, but I wasn't contracting. Pitocin did bring on contractions, yet still I didn't dilate. The doctor kept increasing the dosage of Pitocin, which made the contractions really hard—I remember one that lasted eight minutes! But my stubborn cervix stayed closed," says Stacy Moore, mother of fraternal twin boys. "Saturday night, my obstetrician suggested a C-section, but I asked to postpone it unless doing so would present a danger to the twins. The babies were fine, so we waited. By Sunday morning, though, I was still only 3 centimeters dilated. I hadn't slept or eaten in 36 hours. Dr. Luke came to see me, took my hand, and said, 'Stacy, you have put up a really good fight, but now it's time to see those babies.' I knew she was right, so we went ahead with the surgery. And guess what? The cesarean wasn't nearly as bad as I had feared."

Megan Ryerson had a similar experience. "By 38 weeks, my twins were plenty big enough, so my doctor decided to induce labor. Then, two days before the induction date, my water broke and labor started. Because both babies were head-down, it seemed like a vaginal delivery would be fine. But I labored from 3 P.M. until the following morning without making any progress—my cervix didn't dilate, Baby A didn't move down. I remembered reading that sometimes you need a course correction, and that helped me make the decision to go ahead with the cesarean," says Megan. "I felt sad not to have the experience of a vaginal delivery, but I also felt calm as I was being prepped for surgery because I focused on the fact that I would soon be holding my son and daughter. Then the doctor made the incision and cried out, 'These are *huge* babies!' That really was a glorious moment."

Because a cesarean is major abdominal surgery, it does involve some risks. For instance, any use of anesthesia can potentially cause adverse side effects. Any operation carries a risk of excess bleeding, blood clots, and infection. And uterine surgery leaves a scar that can weaken the womb and perhaps complicate a subsequent pregnancy. But because cesarean deliveries are performed so frequently in the United States and around the world, the risks associated with this type of surgery are minimal. When a cesarean delivery is clearly needed for the sake of the mother or the babies, the benefits certainly outweigh the risks.

WHAT TO EXPECT IN THE OPERATING ROOM

For a scheduled cesarean, you are admitted to the hospital the morning of the surgery or the day before, if you haven't already been admitted previously for observation or other treatment. "The morning of my scheduled C-section, my husband helped me to shower, massaged my feet with my favorite lotion, and got me into my hospital gown," says Anne Seifert. "Then we held hands as I was wheeled down to the operating room. I saw that it was room number 4—a good sign, I thought, when you're about to give birth to four babies."

First an IV line is put in to allow administration of fluids and medications. The anesthesiologist then performs a spinal block and injects the anesthesia needed for surgery, or inserts the catheter if you're having an epidural block. For an emergency delivery, general anesthesia may be used, in which case you will be asleep for the entire operation. Your abdomen is washed with antiseptic solution or covered with an antiseptic-coated film. A cloth or paper drape is placed over your abdomen and legs and vertically above your chest to block your view of the surgical field.

One big difference between a cesarean delivery of multiples versus a singleton is the number of people in or around the operating room. Along with your anesthesiologist and obstetrician and any doctors or nurses who will assist with the surgery, there is a team of neonatologists—one or more for each baby—as well as pediatric nurses. There are also usually extra circulating nurses. When triplets or quads are on the way, the room can get downright crowded. "There were about two dozen people in the operating room, including a camera crew from the University of Michigan, plus another two dozen people looking in from behind a huge window. Clearly, giving birth to quadruplets was not a private, intimate experience,"

Anne Seifert says. Most hospitals also allow your husband or other labor coach to remain in the operating room, usually seated by your head behind the screen that shields your view of the surgery.

The obstetrician makes an incision through the skin, then another incision into the uterus. Next, the amniotic fluid is suctioned away. Although you aren't able to see what's going on, if you're awake and alert, you can hear everything, and you may feel some tugging sensations. One mother of twins says, "There wasn't any discomfort, but I had the funniest sensation of being a bottle from which the doctor was attempting to extract two model ships."

For Kelly McDaniel, the primary physical sensation was one of relief—not surprising, given that her baby girl weighed 7 lb., 11 oz., and her baby boy weighed 9 lb., 4 oz. "My daughter was born first. Then when the doctor pulled out my son, right away I said, 'I can breathe!' It was the first deep breath I had been able to take in many months," says Kelly.

Unlike a vaginal delivery, where the baby closest to the cervix is, of course, born first, there is no set birth order for delivering babies surgically. The obstetrician removes the babies from the uterus in whatever order seems most expedient. Usually the lowest baby is delivered first, but not always. Again, the first to emerge is designated Baby A, the second is Baby B, the third is Baby C, and so on.

Anne Seifert describes the scene at the birth of her quadruplets: "Making the incision took a while, because I had lots of scars and adhesions from previous surgeries. I know the doctor was pushing my belly all over, but I couldn't feel a thing. Then he reached in on the left side and pulled out Lindsey. I heard her cry loud and strong, and everyone said, 'Oh, what a big baby!' She *was* pretty big for a quadruplet born at 31 weeks—3 lb., 2 oz.

"Next to arrive was Mason, weighing 3 lb., 1 oz. It took the doctor a minute to get him out because he was up high, under my heart, and his foot was hooked around somebody's umbilical cord. He gave a good loud yell, too. Then the doctor moved over to the right side of my uterus and lifted out Sarah. She was smaller—2 lb., 2 oz.—and her cry was softer. Finally it was time for Andrew, but the obstetrician couldn't seem to get him out. So a female doctor reached in with her smaller hands, and she was able to get hold of him. He was the littlest, at 2 lb., 1 oz., but he screamed the loudest.

"It was like tag teams. After a baby was born, a nurse would rush that infant over to a side door where a group of neonatologists was waiting. Then another baby would be pulled out of me, and he'd be whisked over to a neonatologist. The first baby was born at 11:10, and the last arrived at 11:14, so the whole thing happened amazingly fast."

After all your babies are delivered, the obstetrician removes the placentas and checks to make sure no fragments of placental tissue are left in the uterus. You are given Pitocin intravenously to make the uterus contract and halt the bleeding. The uterus and skin are then sutured closed. The entire operation takes about an hour, with the babies usually being born during the first 10 minutes.

MAXIMIZING THE JOY IN A CESAREAN DELIVERY

Some women don't mind having a cesarean delivery. "I confess that I'd been worried about labor because I'm a bit of a wimp. I even had to leave my husband alone in our childbirth class one time because I broke out in a cold, dizzy sweat when the teacher showed us the tool used to rupture the bag of waters. So when the doctor said I'd need a cesarean since both my girls were breech, I was actually kind of relieved," says Michelle Brow.

Other women, though, are disappointed to wind up with a cesarean birth. "When I had an emergency cesarean with my firstborn, I felt cheated out of an important maternal experience because I wasn't able to feel the actual moment of birth," Judy Levy explains. "With the twins, I was determined to feel more actively involved. So I talked ahead of time to another mother of multiples who'd had a C-section and asked her what she wished she had done differently. She gave me some great insights."

Here's what experienced moms of multiples recommend. Discuss these and any other preferences you might have with your obstetrician well before your delivery date. If all goes well, your doctor will probably be happy to take your wishes into consideration.

- Request that your obstetrician narrate the surgery as he goes along. Judy Levy says, "Hearing the doctor say, 'We're at the uterus now. Everything looks good. I can see both babies. Now I'm reaching in for this first child,' and so on, helped me to feel that I was aware of and participating in all that was going on."
- Ask to have the drape lowered for a moment after each baby is lifted from the uterus. "I wanted to get a good look at each little daughter the very moment she arrived in the world," says Judy Levy. "It was a thrill to think, 'This is my precious baby and she was *just born*.'"
- Though you probably won't be able to hold your multiples until after the surgery is over, it can be extremely satisfying to see your husband snuggling them. Stacy Moore says, "Right after the twins were born, the nurse showed them to me and then handed them to Tim. I cried with joy as I watched my husband hold our sweet babies at last."
- Get permission for your partner to take pictures during the surgery. "My obstetrician told me, 'You have full media rights. Make a video if you want to.' So instead of sitting near my head, my partner was down at the other end of the

operating table, with a camera," Judy explains. "These photos are such a treasure for me, because they let me connect to the actual moment of my twins' birth."

- Take pleasure and pride in your unique maternal experience. "When my older daughter was born, I worried that having a C-section somehow made me less of a mother," says Judy. "But with the twins, I didn't feel that way. I told myself, 'I am having *two* babies at once! What more could I possibly need in order to feel like a mother?' After all, I had done something not many mothers get to do—and it was truly miraculous."

Recovering from Children-Birth

Just as a multiple pregnancy is more challenging than a singleton pregnancy, the recovery period for postpartum mothers of multiples involves increased risk for complications. Although most new mothers of twins, triplets, or quads do not experience problems, you and your health care providers need to be on the lookout for warning signs and should take appropriate steps to minimize risk:

- A new mother of multiples may bleed more heavily after delivery because the uterus has been overstretched and because a greater portion of its surface area was covered by placental tissue. Alert the hospital staff if you are rapidly soaking your sanitary napkins or passing large blood clots. The obstetrician may have to check for retained placental tissue, treat you for uterine exhaustion (also called uterine atony), or suture a missed tear.
- Heavier postpartum bleeding, coupled with the extra demands a multiple pregnancy placed on your iron reserves, can increase the likelihood of postpartum anemia. Symptoms include dizziness, weakness, pallor, constant dull headache, and shortness of breath. "The first day after the twins were born, just sitting on the side of the bed made me so dizzy that my ears were ringing. There was no way I could have stood up without passing out. By the following day, though, I felt much better," says Heather Nicholas. Do not attempt to get out of bed unassisted until your doctor gives you the go-ahead. To combat anemia, continue to eat an iron-rich diet as you did during pregnancy.
- Uterine cramps are common after delivery because the uterus is still contracting as it descends back into the pelvis. Your extra-large uterus must contract all the more to get back to its former size, so you may experience stronger cramping than

does the mother of a singleton. Over-the-counter analgesics such as ibuprofen can alleviate discomfort. (Don't be concerned if you notice that cramps are strongest while breast-feeding. It is normal for the babies' suckling to trigger the release of oxytocin, the hormone that stimulates uterine contractions.)

- More problematic than uterine cramping is when the postpartum uterus does *not* contract normally. A nurse or doctor periodically palpates your abdomen to see if the uterus is firm. If not, you are examined again for retained placental tissue or injury to the uterus and perhaps given additional oxytocin. You may also be encouraged to periodically massage your own abdomen and to breast-feed, both of which stimulate uterine contractions.

- Fever higher than 100.4°F is a warning sign of infection. Tell the nurse or doctor immediately if you suspect you may be running a temperature.

- Pain on urination can be a sign of bladder or kidney infection. In addition to taking whatever antibiotics your physician prescribes, you can hasten recovery by drinking plenty of water. Bladder or urethral irritation can also occur in the absence of infection if a urinary catheter was used during your cesarean. This can be treated with cranberry juice or the medication Pyridium.

- If you had developed preeclampsia, you may need to continue on a medication called magnesium sulfate, given intravenously to prevent seizures, and have your blood pressure closely monitored for about 24 hours after delivery. During that time, you must stay in bed. Do not eat or drink anything unless your doctor says it is all right.

- Swelling of the feet is very common following the delivery of multiples. During pregnancy you retained a lot of extra fluid; during labor and delivery you received a lot of IV fluids. However, the increased urination necessary to get rid of this extra fluid often doesn't begin until three to five days after delivery. As a consequence, the swelling often gets worse before it gets better. It is generally not something to be concerned about. However, if swelling is accompanied by shortness of breath, it could be a sign of a rare but serious condition called postpartum cardiomyopathy, which warrants an immediate call to your doctor.

- Do not be surprised if your belly looks as big right after delivery as it was before. Sometimes with twins and frequently with triplets or quads, the greatly enlarged uterus stretches out the abdominal wall so much that a woman temporarily loses muscle tone and skin elasticity. After delivery and especially after a cesarean, distension of the bowels with gas makes the belly stick out. This will improve as your normal bowel activity returns and as you regain abdominal muscle tone.

Mothers of multiples who deliver by cesarean should also take note of the following points:

- During the first days after delivery, the incision usually does hurt, but no more so than if you had given birth to a singleton. Pain medication is provided and should be adequate to keep discomfort easily within tolerable levels—at or below a score of 3 on a pain rating scale of 0 to 10. Tell your doctor if you think you need more pain medication—or less. "After my first child was born by emergency C-section, I was given a morphine drip for the pain. But that made me feel so out of it that I couldn't help take care of my newborn," says Judy Levy. "That's why, in recovering from the planned C-section with the twins, I took only Tylenol and Motrin. To me, being slightly uncomfortable was a price worth paying in order to be alert and involved with my babies."
- About 12 hours after delivery, your obstetrician may encourage you to get out of bed and move around. To minimize discomfort, brace the incision site with your hands or a pillow, and try to maintain good posture. Do not attempt to leave your bed unaided before getting your doctor's approval.
- Sometimes staples are used to close the skin. These are typically removed three to five days postoperatively for a low transverse incision, or within five to seven days for a vertical incision. In the meantime, your incision site must be examined regularly for signs of infection, such as redness, increased tenderness, or discharge. Notify the medical staff if you notice any such symptoms. Be particularly vigilant about this if you're significantly overweight; obese women are three times more likely to develop an infection after a cesarean delivery.

Being discharged from the hospital does not mean that the postpartum recovery period is over. Once you're home, you must be careful not to overdo it—particularly if you had a cesarean delivery. That's no easy assignment when you've got twins, triplets, or quads to take care of, so line up plenty of help in advance (see Chapter 13 for tips), and be sure to follow these suggestions:

- Get as much rest as possible. This is a critical element of the recovery process, particularly in the first two weeks after delivery. Though uninterrupted slumber may be hard to come by, do make a point of sitting down and putting your feet up at every opportunity. Catch a nap whenever you can—and turn off the phone first so you won't be interrupted by well-meant but ill-timed calls of congratulations.
- Resume physical activity gradually. Check with your physician for recommended

limitations on lifting, stair-climbing, and housecleaning. Refrain from driving a car for a week to 10 days after delivery, if so instructed. And don't plan on rushing back to work too soon. "After the birth of my older daughter, I tried to do way too much, way too fast—taking care of chores around the house, handling much of the baby care on my own, and going back to law school after only one week. I was constantly exhausted, and it seemed like forever until my body felt good again," says Judy Levy. "I didn't want to make the same mistakes after the twins were born. This time, I did a minimum of housework, lined up lots of child-care helpers, and took a longer maternity leave. All that made quite a difference in how I felt, physically as well as emotionally."

Now that you know better what to expect during labor and delivery, try to relax in these last weeks of your pregnancy. Heather Nicholas shares her healthy philosophy: "There's so much unwarranted fear and negativity about labor. Sure, the pain can be bad, but childbirth is a beautiful experience, too. Remember that it's such a short event compared to the many months of pregnancy. And it's a blink of the eye in comparison to the wonderful years to follow, as you watch your babies grow—from tiny newborns, to adorable toddlers, to active school-agers, and all the way up to adulthood." Rather than dwelling on whatever worries you may have about giving birth, focus on the excitement of the present and on all the joys the future will bring.

Chapter Ten

Your Babies' Hospital Experience: The Nursery and the NICU

From conception, your multiples have been physically linked to you. You have shared with them your every breath, heartbeat, meal, and movement. But at the moment of birth, your babies begin an independent existence. For each, the first experiences in the outside world depend on his or her own state of health.

At the moment of delivery, each of your babies comes under the care of an individual health care team, which includes a neonatologist or pediatrician, a labor and delivery nurse, a neonatal nurse practitioner, and/or others. The team's first action is to clear the infant's airway. The baby is then placed on a radiant warmer, a small open crib with an overhead heat source, which provides the warmth a newborn needs while allowing the doctors and nurses full visual and physical access. Once under the warmer, the baby is completely dried to reduce heat loss.

Doctors use a rating scale called the Apgar score to assess how well a newborn is adapting to life outside the womb. This scale helps to quantify a baby's condition at birth and the need for additional medical intervention. The rating is done at one minute, five minutes, and sometimes again at ten minutes after birth.

There are five components to the Apgar score: heart rate, respirations, muscle tone, reflex irritability, and color. Each component is given a value of 0, 1, or 2, depending on the condition of the baby. These figures are then added to give the total score, on a scale of 0 to 10. If the one-minute score is less than 7, it indicates that the baby needs medical assistance in transitioning to life outside the uterus. For instance, the doctor gives resuscitative assistance to any baby who is not breathing on his or her own or whose heart rate is less than 80 to 100 beats per minute. Table 10.1 shows what each score means.

Apgar Scores

Component	0	1	2
Heart rate	Absent	Slow; less than 100 beats/minute	More than 100 beats/minute
Respirations	Absent	Weak	Good, strong cry
Muscle tone	Limp	Some bending	Active motion
Reflex irritability	No response	Grimace	Cough or sneeze
Color	Blue or pale	Body pink, extremities blue	Completely pink

Table 10.1

In between the one-minute and five-minute Apgar scores, or shortly thereafter, the health care teams perform routine newborn care for each baby. This includes the following:

- Weighing the baby.
- Measuring head circumference and overall length.
- Taking footprints.
- Placing identifying wristbands on the infants.
- Administering erythromycin ointment or silver nitrate eye drops to prevent eye infections.
- Giving an injection of vitamin K to prevent bleeding in the first hours and days of life. Vitamin K, which is necessary for the synthesis of blood-clotting factors, is produced by the intestinal flora. Because the intestinal tract is sterile at birth, a newborn lacks this vitamin. The injection provides an adequate supply until the baby can begin to produce his or her own.
- Taking a small sample of blood via a heel stick, or pinprick in the heel. The blood is sent to a laboratory to be checked for a variety of rare but serious diseases, including phenylketonuria and hypothyroidism. You and your pediatrician are notified if there are any problems. The blood may be taken soon after birth or at some later point, but it is required by law prior to discharge from the hospital. If

the test is done before your babies are 24 hours old, it must be repeated in two or three days, either in the hospital or, if your babies have been discharged, at your pediatrician's office.

The Well-Baby Experience

DR. LUKE: If all your babies are fine, they are soon handed over to you and your partner for some first snuggles—and first feedings. The issue of feeding is so important that we've devoted a full chapter to it. Please take time to read Chapter 11 *before* your multiples are born, so you can make an informed and careful decision about whether to feed by breast, bottle, or both.

If you have any problems during those first feedings, ask a nurse or the hospital's lactation consultant for help. They should be able to answer all your questions and offer suggestions and support. They can also assist you in finding feeding positions that don't place pressure on your incision, if you had a cesarean delivery.

ROOMING-IN WITH MULTIPLES

Rooming-in refers to the practice of keeping a mother and her baby—or babies, in your case—together during their hospital stay. Because an important goal of obstetrics today is to make all aspects of childbirth as natural as possible, rooming-in is now the norm at most hospitals around the country. The practice has a number of advantages. Studies have shown that mothers who share a hospital room with their newborns are more successful at breast-feeding and more sensitive to their infants' needs. Rooming-in also gives you confidence in your caretaking abilities as you learn routine baby-care skills like bathing and diapering through hands-on experience and under the supervision of nurses. You benefit physically, too, since recovery is hastened when a mother gets up and moves around soon after delivery.

Typically the babies sleep in small, separate cribs in the mother's room, but you may have other ideas.[1] "The nurses were going to put Benjamin and Madeleine into separate bassinets, but my husband said, 'No, they've been snuggled up to each other until now. They'd probably be happier sleeping together.' So the twins shared a bassinet while they roomed in with me," says Heather Nicholas, mother of boy/girl twins.

---

1. Tomashek KM, Wallman C; Committee on Fetus and Newborn. Cobedding twins and higher-order multiples in a hospital setting. Pediatrics 2007; 120:1359–66.

There may even be space in your hospital room for your husband. "Tim was able to sleep in my room, along with the babies and me, the whole time I was in the hospital," says Stacy Moore, mother of fraternal twin boys. "It was a wonderful experience for us all to be together as a family right from the beginning."

A potential disadvantage of rooming-in is lack of sleep for Mom. Remember that you always have the option of sending one or all of your babies to the nursery for a while. "After my singleton daughter was born, I wouldn't let the nurses take her away from me even for a few minutes. With the twins, though, I let up a bit. They were born at ten o'clock in the morning, and by three o'clock the following morning, I really needed to rest, so I asked the nurses to take care of the babies for a few hours," says Judy Levy, mother of fraternal twin girls. "Later I realized that this had set a healthy precedent, because it let me feel that it was okay to accept assistance. Once I was home, then, it was easier to say yes to friends who offered to help."

Many twins, if born healthy and mature, go home just a few days after delivery with their mothers. While the exact timing of discharge depends on your medical condition, laws mandate that health insurance companies pay for a minimum hospital stay of 48 hours after a vaginal delivery and 96 hours after a cesarean. Says Amy Maly, mother of identical twin girls, "We were extremely grateful that both our babies were able to be discharged from the hospital with me two days after they were born. We had been working toward that goal throughout the pregnancy and felt so fortunate that all had gone well. It was a wonderful homecoming."

If you too are taking your multiples home shortly after their birth, you can skip the rest of this chapter. But if one or more of your babies need special care, you'll want to read on to learn how to navigate through the neonatal intensive care unit (NICU) or special-care nursery. This truly will help you meet future challenges. As one mother explains, "Learning ahead of time about what happens in the NICU prepared me to handle the interventions that were necessary, gave me enough knowledge to ask the right questions, and helped me to accept without shock and fear the special needs of my newborns. If I hadn't done this, I would have been a basket case!"

What's What and Who's Who in the NICU

Even when born with a good birthweight and at a favorable gestational age, triplets and quads generally do stay in the NICU or the Level II (step-down) nursery for several days. Allison MacDonald's triplets, for example, were born at 36 weeks and had excellent birthweights for triplets, ranging from 4 lb., 11 oz. to 5 lb., 8 oz. Still, the biggest baby spent six days in the NICU, while the other two were in the NICU for eight days.

If you're expecting triplets or quadruplets, it is therefore prudent to prepare yourself psychologically for this eventuality. "The books I read while pregnant seemed to assume that multiple-birth babies would have to spend time in the NICU, yet I was in total denial about that. I planned to bring all my babies home from the hospital with me—but that's not how it ended up," says Ginny Seyler, mother of triplets. "In retrospect, I think the best approach is to maintain a positive and hopeful attitude during your pregnancy, but to keep your mind open to the possibility that some NICU time may be required. That way, if it happens, you'll feel more prepared emotionally."

If your multiples are born prematurely or have other medical problems, they are stabilized in the delivery room and then transferred via a portable incubator to the NICU, where medical care continues. Within the first few hours after birth, each baby receives a full physical examination. Samples of urine and stool are collected for analysis. Blood samples are drawn to determine each infant's blood type and Rh group, and to obtain data on levels of oxygen, carbon dioxide, glucose, and other essential factors. All of this information is used to evaluate the condition of your babies, and to plan for their care.

DR. LUKE: Some preemies need to stay in the NICU for just a few days, others for a few weeks, and some much longer. Regardless of whether they are singletons, twins, triplets, or quads, premature babies are just that—premature—which means they may not be ready to face the challenges of life outside the womb. In order to do so, they must receive a lot of intensive and specialized care.

This can leave parents feeling powerless, alone, and afraid. You may even feel reluctant to continue reading this chapter. Please understand, we are not sharing this information in order to frighten you. On the contrary, knowing the basics about the NICU will help you have a more confident and capable voice in your babies' care. To start, familiarize yourself with the following descriptions of the NICU equipment and personnel, and how each contributes to the care of your babies.

DR. NEWMAN: We absolutely understand how scary the NICU must seem to parents who are not familiar with such a setting. It must also be very disappointing to have imagined your multiples swaddled in a bassinet, but instead to see them in plastic isolettes, attached to wires, tubes, flashing lights, buzzers, and bells.

While this is initially overwhelming, it's important to remember what your babies need. Most of the equipment, and all of the staff, are there to immediately detect any problems before they become more serious or life-threatening. In that regard, a better name for the NICU would be the neonatal intensive *surveillance* unit. If your babies are premature or have complications, you want them to be under constant, close surveillance by the NICU staff along with the specialized equipment. Some of the anxiety you feel when you first observe the constant activity of the NICU is a direct result of the intense commitment that has been made to taking care of your babies. In a good NICU, each staff member recognizes that nothing is unimportant and nothing should be allowed to slide.

You also may feel intimidated because of how large the NICU is—but you do not have to worry about your babies getting lost in the crowd. That won't happen. In fact, it has been repeatedly demonstrated that the best NICUs are the largest NICUs. Such high-volume facilities allow staff to accumulate the experience and confidence they need to recognize and treat the many various complications newborns may have, and to provide your babies with truly superior care.

COMMON NICU EQUIPMENT

Body Temperature Equipment

A premature infant cannot regulate her body temperature very well, so in the NICU she is placed under an open radiant warmer that provides the heat she needs while also allowing doctors and nurses easy access should she require immediate assistance. Once stabilized, a preemie may be placed inside an *incubator* or *isolette,* which can be opened from the front or accessed via portholes. A temperature probe taped to the baby's skin provides feedback to the thermostat, which in turn controls heat output to provide a constant level of warmth.

Most isolettes are designed to accommodate one infant. However, some NICUs now have double isolettes designed especially for twins, with enough room and temperature monitors for two babies. Studies indicate that twins who are placed in the same isolette may gain weight faster and head home sooner.

Oxygen, Breathing, and Heart Rate Monitors

An infant at risk for *apnea* (cessation of breathing for 15 seconds or more) is placed on a cardiorespiratory machine that monitors heart rate and breathing rate. In addition, the baby may be put on a pulse oximeter, which measures the amount of oxygen in the blood via a sensor attached to a hand or foot. These machines have built-in alarms that sound when the heart rate, breathing rate, or level of oxygen falls below a specified level. The alarms are designed to buzz when these levels are still well within the safe range, so that the baby can be stabilized before a serious situation develops.

A transcutaneous monitor is another method of measuring the amount of oxygen and carbon dioxide in the bloodstream. It is placed on the baby's skin, and oxygen diffuses from the capillaries to the probe, resulting in a numerical value that is electronically calculated and displayed. This monitor allows the health care team to adjust respirator settings and oxygen levels without needing to draw blood as frequently.

Blood Pressure Monitor

Just as your blood pressure is taken by inflating a cuff around your arm, an infant's blood pressure can be measured the same way. The monitor automatically inflates at preset intervals and displays the blood pressure reading. Blood pressure can also be read via an umbilical arterial line.

Umbilical Lines

Each baby's umbilical cord contains two arteries and one vein. Normally the doctor ties off these blood vessels at birth. But when an infant is born prematurely, the doctor may instead thread the arteries with an umbilical arterial catheter. This can then be used to draw blood samples, give fluids and medications, and measure blood pressure.

Respiratory Equipment

Preemies often need oxygen in higher concentrations than the 21 percent level available in room air. Supplemental oxygen can be given in several ways. For a baby who has no difficulty breathing, oxygen may be given inside an *oxyhood* (a plastic box or hood placed over the baby's head) or a clear tent. Oxygen can also be delivered directly into the incubator or isolette, or via small nasal tubing.

When additional assistance is needed, oxygen may be delivered via continuous positive airway pressure, or CPAP (pronounced *see-pap*). A machine provides a steady supply of air and oxygen under pressure, thereby keeping the lungs partially inflated during exhalation and reducing the amount of physical effort required to draw a new breath. CPAP can be delivered via a mask that fits over the nose. If a baby has been intubated—meaning a tube has been threaded down the trachea (windpipe) and into the lungs—CPAP can be used to deliver supplemental oxygen directly into the lungs. For a preemie unable to breathe on her own, a ventilator or respirator is used to deliver a controlled mixture of air and oxygen, under pressure, at a regulated number of breaths per minute.

Feeding Methods

Many babies born before 34 weeks' gestation cannot suck effectively. These preemies are fed by *gavage*, a method in which a thin flexible tube called a nasogastric tube is inserted through the nose or mouth and threaded into the stomach. A vial of formula or breast milk is attached to the end of the tube, and gravity causes the milk to flow down into the baby's stomach. Babies fed this way are carefully monitored for distension of the abdomen, spitting up, and the amount of milk remaining in the stomach (called residuals) before the next feeding is given.

If your preemies cannot yet begin gavage feedings, they may be fed intravenously with a special formula containing all the essential nutrients. This is known as *parenteral nutrition* or *hyperalimentation*. A baby may receive some of his feedings by gavage and others by parenteral nutrition.

The decision on when to start nipple feedings or *nippling*—whether at the breast or the bottle—is based on the baby's developmental maturity and health status. Factors that are considered include the ability to coordinate breathing and swallowing, breathing rate, and growth pattern.

THE MEDICAL STAFF

Neonatologist

A neonatologist is a physician who specializes in the development, care, and diseases of newborns. A neonatologist has completed medical school, three years of pediatric residency training, and three more years of specialized training in the care of high-risk newborns.

At a Level III or Level IV hospital (facilities equipped to handle the sickest and smallest babies, as described in Chapter 2), the neonatologists take primary responsibility for the care of your premature multiples. They are usually present at the birth and lead the health care teams that resuscitate babies in the delivery room, if necessary. Once infants are transferred to the NICU, the neonatologists direct the treatment of any medical problems, adjust feedings, and coordinate on a daily basis the contributions of all other health care professionals involved in your babies' care.

Pediatrician

The pediatrician specializes in the development, care, and diseases of children. After graduating from medical school, these doctors complete at least a three-year residency training program in pediatrics. If a pregnancy lasts a minimum of 35 weeks, and if a baby weighs at least 5 lb., 8 oz. at birth, it is generally a pediatrician who handles his care, regardless of the level of the hospital. However, when a baby is premature or low birthweight (less than 5 lb., 8 oz.) or has unexpected complications, the pediatrician plays a secondary role during the NICU stay. The neonatologists should keep your pediatrician informed of any developments so that once your babies come home from the hospital, your pediatrician is prepared to take charge of their care.

Pediatric Neurologist

Also a pediatrician, this doctor has advanced training and experience in the diagnosis and treatment of conditions of the nervous system as they pertain to infants and children. He or she may be called in as a consultant when a baby has a sleeping or feeding problem, a metabolic disorder, poor muscle tone, partial paralysis, seizures, a breathing disorder, or a brain hemorrhage. The neurologist assesses the infant's motor strength, body and extremity movement, reflexes, and coordination of sucking and swallowing, and advises on the appropriate treatment.

Pediatric Ophthalmologist

An eye specialist, this physician has undergone advanced training in the diagnosis and treatment of vision disorders in infants and children. Your babies may have several eye exams by a pediatric ophthalmologist while in the NICU, particularly if they are hospitalized for an extended period of time. Because as many as one-third of preemies (particularly those with a birthweight of less than 2 pounds) develop a vision problem called *retinopathy of prematurity,* these eye examinations are extremely important for diagnosing this disorder. In addition, your babies are likely to have follow-up visits with this specialist after they are discharged from the hospital.

Radiologist

The radiologist administers and interprets the radiographic (X-ray) and ultrasonographic tests used to diagnose various medical conditions. Some of these procedures are performed routinely to detect any problems so that treatment can begin as early as possible. For example, an ultrasound of the brain is typically performed on all babies born before 34 weeks' gestation to check for brain hemorrhages. An ultrasonogram is also one of the first tests ordered if a physical problem is suspected, since it is noninvasive and does not involve the use of radiation. More sophisticated imaging techniques, such as computed tomography (CT) scans and magnetic resonance imaging (MRI), are also performed and interpreted by radiologists, some of whom are trained specifically in scanning children and newborns.

Interns, Residents, and Fellows

Medical school graduates who are enrolled in a residency program are called residents, except during the first year of their program, when they are called interns. The requirements, duration, and responsibilities of each type of residency program vary, depending on the specialty. The majority of residents working in the NICU are doing a pediatric residency, but you may also encounter residents from obstetrics, family practice, surgery, or internal medicine. Since they perform many of the routine procedures in the NICU, these are the doctors you are likely to see most often. Fellows are physicians who have finished their pediatric residency training and are now completing three extra years of training to become neonatologists. These neonatology fellows are also highly involved in the day-to-day management of babies in the NICU.

THE NURSING STAFF

Neonatal Nurses

Most neonatal nurses are registered nurses (RNs) with intensive care experience and special training in the care of preemies and other newborns with medical problems. Typically one nurse per shift is assigned as the primary care provider for a particular infant until discharge, handling about 90 percent of the care for that baby. The neonatal nurses are the health professionals with whom NICU parents interact most often and from whom you can learn the special parenting skills you need to care for your babies with confidence.

Certified Registered Nurses

RNs who have passed national specialty examinations in NICU nursing, critical care nursing, or mother-baby nursing are known as certified registered nurses. This level of training is required in some NICUs; in other cases, nurses opt to take these challenging exams from a personal sense of commitment to their specialty.

Nurse Practitioners

Nurse practitioners are registered nurses who have completed advanced education and training. Their ranks include neonatal nurse practitioners (NNPs), pediatric nurse practitioners (PNPs), and advanced registered nurse practitioners (ARNPs). Nurse practitioners work under the direction of a neonatologist and can provide some of the more advanced aspects of your babies' care.

Clinical Nurse Specialist

An RN with a master's degree, the clinical nurse specialist is a resource person for the nursing staff. He or she provides staff education, conducts nursing research, develops programs, and directs patient care.

Case Manager

Typically a case manager is a nurse who works with the NICU health care team to coordinate care, ensuring that everything necessary is completed to prepare for discharge.

ADDITIONAL HEALTH CARE TEAM MEMBERS

Physical Therapist/Occupational Therapist
The PT or OT works with premature babies who need help with their neuromuscular development, performing special exercises and other therapies. Depending on your babies' long-term health status, a PT or OT may be very involved in their follow-up developmental care.

Developmental Specialist
This is usually a nurse, physical therapist, or occupational therapist with advanced training and expertise in infant development. The developmental specialist evaluates some or all of the infants in the NICU, and can offer specific suggestions to parents, such as how to improve feedings and how to pick up on the babies' behavioral cues.

Audiologist
This medical professional is trained to detect, diagnose, and treat patients with impaired hearing. An audiologist may be called in as a consultant if any of your babies develop certain complications that could affect their hearing. Your infants are also likely to see an audiologist as part of their follow-up examinations after they are discharged from the NICU.

Neonatal Dietitian
A dietitian with special training in the nutritional needs of newborns, this person helps to formulate diets tailored to the changing needs of your babies, based on each one's medical condition, laboratory test results, and rate of growth.

Respiratory Therapist
Trained to assemble, calibrate, and monitor the respiratory equipment used in the NICU, this health professional sets up the equipment, changes the tubing daily, and monitors the air and oxygen flow-through. Respiratory therapists often attend early preterm births as part of the neonatal resuscitation team in case newborns need to be intubated.

Pharmacist
The hospital pharmacist works closely with the neonatologist and other members of the health care team to provide whatever medications each of your babies may need, in the appropriate form and dosage.

Technicians

These health care team members perform tests such as X-rays, ultrasounds, and blood and urine analyses to diagnose and monitor problems. Technicians provide important data to guide doctors' decisions about patient care.

PARENT SUPPORT STAFF

Social Worker

The social worker's role is to provide information, counseling, and emotional support to NICU parents and families. She or he helps you deal with any personal, medical, or financial problems related to your pregnancy and your babies' birth and acts as a liaison between you and the health care team.

Lactation Consultant

Typically a nurse with expertise in breast-feeding, including additional education and certification, the lactation consultant can arrange for you to rent or buy a breast pump and instruct you in its use and in how to safely store and transport your expressed milk to provide nourishment for your hospitalized babies. She also helps you solve any nursing problems that may arise and offers encouragement over the course of your multiples' hospital stay. Many NICUs have dedicated private rooms for breast pumping, as well as the ability to bank breast milk. The lactation consultant can familiarize you with these services.

Medical Complications of Prematurity

In general, the shorter a pregnancy, the more severe the newborn babies' health problems are likely to be. Gestational age at birth doesn't tell the whole story, however. In fact, it is not uncommon among multiples for one baby's health status to be significantly more problematic than that of his womb mates.

Triplet mom Ginny Seyler explains, "Heather and Brian had no serious problems at all. They were 'feeders and growers,' which meant they were basically fine but needed to get bigger and stronger. But Dillon didn't do as well as the other two babies, primarily because his lungs were underdeveloped. He was on a respirator for a day and needed several transfusions. He was just a very fragile little being for a long time."

Following is a brief discussion of the medical problems that are most common among premature and/or low-birthweight babies:

JAUNDICE

Jaundice is caused by the buildup of bilirubin, a greenish-yellow pigment formed during the normal breakdown of red blood cells. The liver removes bilirubin from the bloodstream, and, during pregnancy, the placenta and the mother's liver remove bilirubin from the baby. During the transition period immediately after birth, however, until the baby's own liver takes over, bilirubin may build up in the blood. This causes the skin to take on a yellowish tinge.

About half of all full-term newborns and about 80 percent of premature infants develop some degree of jaundice. Bilirubin levels usually peak within the first week, then fall to minimal levels in the second week. With appropriate feedings, ample water, and exposure to sunshine, mild jaundice usually does not require any special treatment.

An infant with bilirubin levels that are higher than normal, or whose levels are rising faster than normal, has a condition known as *hyperbilirubinemia,* which can be toxic to the baby's developing nervous system. In severe cases, an exchange blood transfusion may be required to cleanse the bilirubin from the newborn's blood. Usually, however, hyperbilirubinemia can be successfully treated with phototherapy: the use of light waves to break down bilirubin into components that the baby can eliminate in the urine. A baby receiving phototherapy is undressed to expose as much skin surface as possible, then placed for a set period of time under a bank of fluorescent lights known as bili-lights, or wrapped in what is called a bili-blanket. During this time, the baby's eyes are covered with protective pads or soft goggles. Because babies who receive phototherapy often have more frequent and looser bowel movements, additional fluids are given.

BODY TEMPERATURE PROBLEMS

Body heat is generated primarily by shivering, something newborns cannot do. Instead, babies have a special type of heat-generating body fat called brown fat, which is located around the shoulders and base of the neck and over the heart and kidneys. The inadequate stores of brown fat in premature infants, particularly those born before 30 weeks' gestation, are quickly used up. At that point, preemies must produce heat metabolically. This siphons off their supplies of oxygen and glucose, which in turn leads to weight loss, low blood sugar, and breathing difficulties.

Maintaining body temperature is a vital component of newborn care from the moment of birth and throughout the hospital stay. That's why temperature monitors are used along with radiant warmers and temperature-controlled incubators or isolettes. Whenever a premature baby is taken out of the isolette, he is wrapped in blankets and wears a stocking cap to prevent heat loss from his or her head.

HEART PROBLEMS

Before birth, a baby's blood flows through the ductus arteriosus, a short vessel connecting the pulmonary artery to the aorta. At the time of delivery, when the umbilical cord is cut, blood begins to flow through the baby's lungs to receive oxygen. This causes a pressure change in the pulmonary artery as the lungs expand and the ductus arteriosus closes to prevent the mixing of oxygenated and nonoxygenated blood.

When an infant is born prematurely, however, the fetal connection between the aorta and the pulmonary artery may not close properly. This condition, called *patent ductus arteriosus* (PDA), is the most common heart problem associated with prematurity. A neonatologist, often in conjunction with a pediatric cardiologist, makes the diagnosis of PDA. Treatment may include increasing the amount of supplemental oxygen, administering medications that can close the ductus, or surgically ligating the ductus.

PDA is also a factor in the breathing problems of prematurity.

BREATHING PROBLEMS

Throughout pregnancy, an unborn baby receives oxygen through the placenta as blood bypasses the fetal lungs and flows through the ductus arteriosus. During labor, uterine contractions squeeze a baby's chest, clearing fluid from the lungs as he passes through the birth canal. At the moment of birth, physical and chemical signals trigger the intake of the baby's first breath, filling his lungs with air. With each additional breath, some air remains in the lungs to keep them partially open. The lungs of a healthy full-term infant contain a fatty substance called *surfactant* that keeps the lungs' moist air sacs from collapsing. With the lungs thus partially expanded, breathing becomes easier with each subsequent breath.

A premature newborn, though, lacks sufficient surfactant to keep the lungs open. Increasing pulmonary pressure then forces blood back through the ductus arteriosus, maintaining the fetal circulation. When this occurs, nonoxygenated blood circulates throughout the body, and the baby can become oxygen-deprived. Without adequate surfactant, each breath is as difficult as the first, because with each inhalation the baby must completely inflate his collapsed lungs. Breathing becomes rapid and labored, the chest retracts (sucks in deeply), and the baby grunts as he tries to close off the back of his throat to prevent air from leaving the lungs. With each breath, additional lung tissue collapses, less oxygen enters the bloodstream, and breathing becomes progressively more difficult.

This is known as *respiratory distress syndrome* (RDS), and it is one of the most common complications of prematurity. As the baby's condition worsens, breathing becomes irregular and there may be periods of *apnea,* when breathing stops completely. Inadequate oxygen supply to the lungs further aggravates the situation, slowing down the production of new surfactant and hastening damage to the lung tissue.

To combat this problem, an artificial surfactant is placed directly into the lungs of a premature infant immediately after delivery, via an endotracheal tube. The artificial surfactant drains into the baby's alveoli (breathing sacs), where carbon dioxide and oxygen from the blood is exchanged, coating them and keeping them from collapsing. Artificial surfactant decreases the severity of RDS and can sometimes prevent it if administered early enough.

Over time, the baby's lungs begin to produce surfactant naturally. Until that occurs, the premature baby needs respiratory support. For this, various levels of oxygen and air can be delivered through an oxyhood, face mask, nasal tubing, or endotracheal tube inserted through the mouth and into the trachea.

Although respiratory therapy can get a premature baby past the critical early period of RDS, it can also cause some damage to the delicate lung tissue, a complication called *bronchopulmonary dysplasia* (BPD) or *chronic lung disease* (CLD). The damaged tissue forms scars that further impair air exchange. Until the lungs can heal and grow sufficiently, the baby remains dependent on respiratory therapy.

Infants who have had BPD are also more susceptible to colds, pneumonia, and other respiratory illnesses. The good news is that most children born prematurely outgrow their respiratory problems by school age.

NEUROLOGIC PROBLEMS

A baby's brain continues to grow and develop after birth, and consequently it is extremely sensitive to potential injury. Changes in pressure during a vaginal delivery, fluctuations in blood sugar levels and oxygen levels, hyperbilirubinemia, and the presence of infection can all cause some degree of brain injury.

A premature baby is particularly at risk because the fragile blood vessels in his brain may rupture and bleed. This event, known as *intraventricular hemorrhage* (IVH), happens most commonly within the first week after birth. IVH is relatively rare in babies born after 34 weeks' gestation, when an area of vascular growth called the *germinal matrix* becomes less vulnerable—but the smaller and more premature a baby is, the greater his chances of a hemorrhage. At highest risk are those born weighing 3 lb., 4 oz. or less.

IVH is categorized by four grades of severity:

- *Grade I:* The mildest hemorrhage, this involves a small amount of blood in the lining of the ventricle (one of the four cerebrospinal fluid-filled spaces in the brain). The origin of this bleeding is almost always the germinal matrix.
- *Grade II:* A small amount of blood enters the ventricles but does not cause them to enlarge.
- *Grade III:* A greater amount of blood enters the brain ventricles, causing them to enlarge temporarily. The resulting blood clot and tissue damage cause a blockage of the flow of spinal fluid into and out of the ventricles, resulting in hydrocephalus (swelling of the ventricles).
- *Grade IV:* The most severe type of hemorrhage, this involves bleeding that ruptures from the ventricles and extends into the brain tissue itself.

Symptoms of IVH include seizures, a bulging *fontanelle* (the soft spot on the top of the head), an enlarged head, breathing problems, vomiting, irritability, and an abnormal neurological exam. Ultrasound is typically used to diagnose IVH. A lumbar puncture (spinal tap), which detects blood in the spinal fluid, may also be necessary.

Once diagnosed, a hemorrhage is closely monitored. Treatment may include medication to decrease the size of the enlarged ventricle and to inhibit production of cerebrospinal fluid, thereby decreasing pressure on the brain. In severe cases, surgery is required to shunt the accumulating cerebrospinal fluid in the ventricles into the abdominal cavity via a plastic tube, thus relieving the pressure on the brain.

IVH can lead to developmental disabilities or delays, seizure disorders, and vision or hearing loss. The long-term consequences depend on a variety of factors, including the severity of the hemorrhage. But most babies, especially those with the more common Grade I or Grade II, do not experience major disabilities.

VISION PROBLEMS

The most common eye problem associated with preterm birth is called *retinopathy of prematurity* (ROP), sometimes also known as *retrolental fibroplasia*. It occurs when the blood vessels of the retina grow abnormally, triggering bleeding into the eye structure and causing scar tissue to form. This scar tissue may then block the lens of the eye, causing vision loss. It also may shrink, thereby tearing or detaching the retina.

Doctors are not sure exactly what causes ROP. The condition occurs most often among very small premature babies who are born weighing less than 1,000 grams (about 2 lb., 3 oz.), and among those born prior to 28 weeks' gestation. ROP is classified by stages, with Stage 1 being the mildest and Stage 5 being the most severe.

Fortunately, most cases of ROP are relatively mild and clear up without treatment. However, parents should be aware that premature babies, especially those who had ROP, are at a greater risk for developing *strabismus* (crossed eyes) and *amblyopia* (lazy eye) during early childhood. For this reason, annual eye exams are very important.

For more severe cases of ROP, treatment options include cryotherapy to freeze the abnormal blood vessels, which then shrink to allow new blood vessels to grow normally. Some cases may require surgery to reattach the retina. To minimize the risk of permanent, extensive loss of vision, early treatment is best.

HEARING PROBLEMS

Various medical conditions can contribute to hearing loss among newborns. These include intraventricular hemorrhage, severe jaundice, bacterial meningitis, and cranial or facial abnormalities. If hearing loss is detected, intervention should begin in infancy in order to minimize impairment of speech and language development. Significant progress has been made with the development of auditory cochlear implants that often can restore hearing in children with severe impediments.

INFECTIONS

Because preemies have immature immune systems, they are more prone to developing infections. These include *sepsis* (bacteria in the bloodstream), *pneumonia* (infection in the lungs), and *meningitis* (infection of the spinal cord and layers around the brain).

Some infections are contracted at birth as the baby passes through the birth canal. One such newborn infection is Group B streptococcus (GBS). This type of bacteria is a normal part of the flora of the gastrointestinal and genital tract, appearing in up to 40 percent of women and doing them no harm. However, if during the course of a vaginal delivery, GBS infects a baby, it can be potentially life-threatening. Fortunately, neonatal GBS infection can be quite effectively prevented by performing a GBS culture in the third trimester of pregnancy, then treating any expectant mother who tests positive with antibiotics such as penicillin.

A type of infection called *chorioamnionitis* (infection of the placental membranes) can be the result of premature rupture of the membranes prior to delivery. The mother may develop a fever and tenderness of the uterus, and usually labor also begins. In such cases, prior to delivery, a mother is given antibiotics that pass through the placenta to her baby or babies. After birth, these babies are immediately treated with antibiotics, even before laboratory results confirm the diagnosis.

An infection acquired from the hospital environment is termed a *nosocomial* infection. Even though hospital personnel and visitors scrub their hands and put on hospital gowns and masks before touching a patient, no one is germ-free. And even though hospital equipment is sterilized, it is not possible to eliminate all bacteria in the environment. Infectious agents can enter a preemie's body through a variety of sites, including a surgical incision, an intravenous line, a catheter, or a respirator. The smaller and more premature the baby, and the more medical and surgical intervention she requires, the greater the risk of infection.

FEEDING PROBLEMS

Like the other organ systems of the premature baby, the digestive system is not yet developed enough to handle its role of digesting food. Circulation to the digestive tract may be lower than normal because the baby's body is diverting blood to the more essential organs (the brain, lungs, heart, and kidneys). If anything were to be given by mouth to a very premature or very sick infant, it would be poorly digested and would trigger additional problems. For instance, oral feedings could increase the risk of *necrotizing enterocolitis* (NEC), in which poor circulation and infection contribute to the death of parts of the digestive tract, necessitating surgical removal of the affected sections of bowel.

Preemies also may be unable to suck effectively because this reflex generally does not develop until around the 34th week of pregnancy. The effort involved in sucking can, for a preemie, use up more calories than the feeding provides.

To prevent these problems, many premature babies are initially nourished intravenously. The very first feedings consist of sterile sugar water, given for calories and fluids. The amount given is carefully calculated based on how much the baby is urinating and on the concentration of the urine. Gradually other nutrients are added to the intravenous formula—sodium, potassium, calcium, protein, fat, vitamins—each of which has a vital role in growth and development. In fact, a premature infant's need for various nutrients exceeds that of his full-term nursery mates because of his lower nutrient stores, more rapid growth, and the stress of any complications he may be experiencing. To achieve just the right combination of nutrients, feedings are adjusted daily or even more frequently, based on the baby's clinical symptoms, blood levels, and growth.

As the premature baby develops, he makes a transition from intravenous to gavage feedings—receiving nourishment via a small, flexible tube inserted through the nose or mouth and into the stomach. First gavage feedings consist of sugar water, then progress to more enriched formulas.

Breast milk can be given by gavage, and in some NICUs, as many as 95 percent of babies are fed breast milk. Breast milk may be fortified with additional calcium or other nutrients through a process called *lacto-engineering*. The purpose is to promote maximum growth for the baby.

Before a premature infant can be breast-fed or bottle-fed, he must be able to suck, swallow, and breathe—all in the right sequence—without choking or turning blue or experiencing a resulting drop in heart rate. He must also be gaining weight and be medically stable. The transition from gavage feeding to nipple feeding may be done gradually, with the number of nipple feedings increasing each day until gavage is no longer needed. If all goes well, this may be achieved around the time the preemie reaches what would have been about the 35th week of pregnancy.

Parenting Your Hospitalized Babies

TAMARA: "Push!" my doctor commanded. But I didn't want to push. I didn't want my twins to be born, not yet. "It's way too soon, they're too little," I cried to my husband, Bill.

There was no stopping the labor, however. Nine weeks premature, my 3-pound son announced his arrival in the world with the faintest of cries. The nurse placed him on my abdomen, but I was so shocked by his minuscule size that I could barely react. Three minutes later, my 2-pound daughter was born. She wasn't breathing. "Intubate!" I heard someone order.

As soon as my twins were stabilized, they were rushed by ambulance from our little community hospital to a major NICU 35 miles away. I was not able to see them again for two days, until I was discharged.

Instead of delight at being a mother, what I felt most during those 48 hours was fear. If my preemies wound up being physically or mentally impaired, would I have what it takes to raise two disabled children? If one or both of my babies didn't survive, would my broken heart ever recover from the loss? I was terribly lonely, too. The Twin Tigers, as Bill and I had called the babies when they were safe and snug inside of me, were gone. In their place, I had only a jumbled memory of two tiny infants I had scarcely seen and never been allowed to hold.

Discharged at last, I was in a near panic of impatience as Bill drove me straight to the other hospital to visit my babies. Stepping into the NICU, I was overwhelmed by the sounds and sights: the buzzing alarms, the busy nurses, the bright lights, and in every isolette, an unbelievably tiny baby.

Bill guided me toward one particular incubator and lifted the lid. "Samantha, Mommy's here," I whispered. My miniature daughter turned her head, opened her eyes—and captured my heart. In an instant I knew, no matter how challenging or how fleeting our future together might be, I would treasure this child and her twin brother forever.

But the ordeal was far from over. Samantha came off the respirator, relapsed, and went back on. James had a small brain hemorrhage. Samantha's jaundice worsened. James's eyesight was threatened by retinopathy of prematurity. My babies' hold on life and health seemed perilously precarious.

Precarious too was my sense of myself as a mother. Surely I was less important to my children than were the doctors and nurses who guarded their lives. I couldn't breast-feed them, since they were too weak to suck. I couldn't hold them for long, since their body temperature was unstable outside the isolettes. Through the portholes, I tentatively stroked their bodies, fearful of dislodging the many tubes and wires. It was not what I had ever imagined motherhood to be.

Yet I adapted to this peculiar form of parenting. I learned to swaddle a baby without disturbing the cardiorespiratory monitor or temperature probe. I learned to hold the vial of the gavage tube high so that no air bubbles formed. In the NICU all day, every day, I rocked James for hours, then put him back in his isolette and walked to the next room to sing to Samantha. But each night in bed, fear for my babies would overwhelm me again.

The NICU staff knew not to promise parents a happy ending. But after two weeks, they were cautiously optimistic. Samantha was breathing well; James's hemorrhage had cleared on its own, and his eyes seemed better; both babies had escaped the most serious complications of prematurity. With encouragement from the nurses, I bought several preemie-size terrycloth suits. Seeing my twins dressed for the first time in something other than hospital-issue undershirts, the fear in my heart was at last outweighed by joyous hope.

A few weeks later, Bill and I brought our precious babies home.

DR. LUKE: Nothing can quite prepare a person for the emotional upheaval of being an NICU mom or dad, but it helps to know that you are not alone. It's also encouraging to realize that there is much you can do to take an active role in your babies' care during their hospital stay.

To start, vow that every time you visit the NICU, you will safeguard your infants by following all recommended procedures for preventing infection. Before entering the unit, scrub your hands and forearms thoroughly for several minutes and put a sterile gown over your street clothes. Also, don't try to bend the rules about visitors. Many NICUs grant access only to parents and perhaps grandparents. Visits by the babies' older siblings may be permitted provided that the children wear surgical masks and gowns, though policies vary greatly. Most important, remember that no one who has been exposed to or is experiencing an infectious disease should ever enter the NICU—not even the parents—until given a clean bill of health.

There's much more you can do as well. Some of our Multiples Clinic patients and other mothers and fathers of twins, triplets, and quads have described their NICU experiences. Their suggestions and insights can help you *feel* better—and can even help your babies *get* better.

How you may feel: *"I'm so lonely. I haven't been able to see my babies since they were born, and I miss them terribly."*

It's no wonder you are lonely! Your babies have been with you every moment for many months, and now suddenly you are apart. If you are in the same hospital as your multiples, ask politely but firmly to see them as soon as possible. Amid all the activity of a busy labor and delivery unit, the staff may have forgotten to arrange this. "I didn't get to see my twins for 11 hours after delivery because they had been whisked away to the NICU. I knew that I had given birth, but it almost seemed as if I hadn't, since there was no tangible evidence of my babies' existence," says Marcy Bugajski, mother of fraternal twin boys. "Finally, long after midnight, a nurse came into my room and asked if I had held my babies yet. When I told her I didn't even have a picture of them, she was appalled. Immediately she helped me into a wheelchair and wheeled me down to the NICU."

If your infants require major interventions such as a respirator, you may feel nervous about seeing them for the first time. Try not to delay. The longer you wait, the more time you have to imagine your worst fears coming true. Seeing your babies, on the other hand, gives you a chance to note all their positive features—this one's strength and alertness, that one's cowlick just like Grandpa's. Marcy adds, "I cried when I first saw my babies. They seemed so small, and they had these big tubes running down their throats from the ventilators. Yet at the same time, I was happy because they were alive. I couldn't believe that Dave and I had actually produced such beautiful little beings."

Your babies may have to be transported to another hospital if the one where you gave birth has no NICU, or if the NICU is filled to capacity or has an outbreak of infection. Should this occur, ask to be transferred to the same hospital where they are going, so you can finish your postpartum recovery in close proximity to your babies.

If a transfer is not possible, stay in touch by phoning the NICU often for updates. Don't worry about bothering the staff—they welcome calls from parents. Send your partner to the NICU to visit the babies, and have him call you on his cell phone (if the NICU permits this) or text-message you to deliver a detailed, moment-by-moment description of what's going on with each baby. Make sure he gets plenty of photos and some footprints to bring back to you.

How you may feel: *"I can't bear the thought of going home from the hospital without my babies."*

Admittedly, this can be a very painful experience. "Other couples were walking out of the hospital carrying carefully swaddled bundles, but I had to leave with empty arms. I felt like I was leaving a part of myself behind," says Marcy Bugajski.

There is a thin silver lining: Unlike most parents of newborns, you can get some uninterrupted sleep at night. Don't deny yourself this small advantage. Helen Armer, mother of triplets, explains, "My babies needed to stay in the hospital to be treated for jaundice. The nurses told me it was a blessing in disguise, and it turns out they were right. I was worn down physically from the pregnancy, and I really needed that week to recover while the babies were hospitalized. Emotionally it wasn't too bad because I knew they were not very sick."

Visit the NICU often. You'll naturally want to be with your babies as much as possible—and they'll benefit from your presence. In fact, studies show that premature infants who are touched or talked to daily experience more rapid weight gain and better brain development. "While my triplets were in the NICU, there wasn't any question about where I would be and what I would be doing. Every morning, I got up, went to the hospital, and stayed all day. I felt an urgent need to be there, helping to take care of them and following each baby's every little step forward or backward," Ginny Seyler says.

Of course, it's important to spend some time away from the NICU, too. A nonstop bedside vigil is exhausting. Realize that if your babies were at home, you wouldn't be sitting next to their cribs day and night. You need to take a breather sometimes, so go out to dinner or see a movie. Keep your cell phone with you so you'll know that the NICU staff can reach you if necessary.

How you may feel: *"I don't feel like a 'real' parent because I'm not the one taking care of my babies."*

Though your initial emotion may be one of powerlessness, you need to trust your ability to begin parenting. Learn to perform as many basic baby-care tasks as possible. Sure, those preemie diapers seem awfully small, but you can change them exactly as you would any diaper. The nurses are happy to have you help at bath time, too.

Even before your babies are ready for nipple feeding at the breast or bottle, you can participate in gavage feedings. Cradle one of your infants in one arm, and use the other hand to raise the vial of formula above the level of the baby's nose. "It was a sweet feeling to hold a baby who was getting formula through a nasogastric tube and to know that he was 'eating,'" says quad mom Anne Seifert.

Karen Danke, mother of fraternal twin boys, adds, "When your babies are in the NICU, it's important to be very involved with their care. Not only does this make you feel more like a parent, it is good training for when the babies are discharged and you have to manage on your own. They're so tiny—Jacob weighed only 3 lb., 14 oz. when he came home, for example—that it's intimidating to take care of them unless you've been practicing under the watchful eye of the hospital staff."

Some NICUs place multiple-birth siblings in separate rooms to minimize the risk that a feeding or treatment intended for Baby A Jones will inadvertently be given to Baby B Jones. Ask the nurse to arrange a few minutes of togetherness time for you, your husband, and all your babies. This simple pleasure can go a long way toward making you feel like real parents of multiples.

How you may feel: *"The doctors and nurses are much more important to my babies' well-being than I am."*

Karen Danke admits, "I was afraid the babies would think the doctors and nurses were their parents, instead of Chris and me. But that didn't happen. Right from day one, they definitely recognized our voices because they had been able to hear us during those last months of the pregnancy." Karen is right: Studies confirm that newborns recognize their mother's voice, and often their father's as well.

Recognize, too, that there are special things you can do for your babies. Most important is to hold them. "At first, I was afraid to touch my twins for fear of hurting them. But the doctor assured me that a parent's loving touch was very therapeutic in a way no technology could provide," says Lydia Greenwood, mother of boy/girl twins. With the help of a nurse to manage the tubes and wires, sit back and try to relax. Make sure to keep your baby well swaddled, and do not remove her stocking cap for more than a moment or two. If an alarm sounds, don't lose your cool. "It was frightening at first when an alarm would go off while I was holding one of the quads," says Anne Seifert. "But pretty soon I got to know which button was which, and then I didn't panic anymore. I knew the nurse would come right over and reattach the loose electrode or fix whatever problem there was."

You may also be encouraged to practice a therapeutic-touch technique called kangaroo care, which involves holding a baby skin-to-skin against your chest. Studies show that this practice often helps premature infants to regulate their breathing, heart rate, and body temperature.[2] It also improves babies' sleep quality, reduces crying, encourages weight gain and brain development, and contributes to earlier hospital discharge.[3] For parents, kangaroo care provides a greater sense of control and confidence, promotes bonding, and increases a mother's supply of breast milk.

Here's how it's done: Your baby, dressed only in a diaper and stocking cap, is snuggled between your bare breasts (or against Dad's bare chest), and covered with a blanket or your shirt. Your body heat keeps the baby warm as you stroke his skin and whisper to him.

Anne Seifert explains, "By the end of the second week, I was able to begin kangaroo care. The staff put a little drape around the isolette so no one could see, and I opened my loose top and slipped the baby in against my chest. All of my quads really responded to that, opening their little eyes and nuzzling close. I loved it, too."

In some NICUs, the policy is to wait until a baby is medically stable before beginning kangaroo care. In others, the practice is used from birth onward, if possible, even if the baby is connected to various monitors or machines. Ask your health care team if kangaroo care is an option for you and your babies.

Another way in which you and only you can contribute to your babies' well-being is by providing them with the best possible source of nourishment—your breast milk. Preemies in particular can benefit from the protection against infection and the greater digestibility that mother's milk provides. Ginny Seyler says, "While my triplets were in the NICU, I pumped my

2. Bosque EP, Brady JP, Affonso DD, Wahlberg V. Continuous physiological measurements of kangaroo versus incubator care in a tertiary level nursery. Pediatric Research 1988; 23:402A.
3. Charpak N, Ruiz-Peláez JG, Figueroa de C Z, Charpak Y. Kangaroo mother versus traditional care for newborn infants ≤2000 grams: A randomized, controlled trial. Pediatrics 1997; 100:682–8.

breasts every four hours and gave it to the nurses, who fed it to the babies through nasogastric tubes. It was very gratifying for me to be able to make this important contribution to their care." (For full information on breast-feeding, see Chapter 11.)

How you may feel: *"I don't know what's going on with my babies because I can't understand what the doctors say."*

"Physicians sometimes tend to talk above the average person's level of understanding. This can be intimidating, so you just nod and go along with whatever they are saying, even if you don't have a clue what it means," says Benita Moreno, mother of fraternal twin boys. "I learned that it's important not to be afraid to interrupt the doctor and say, 'I don't understand what you mean. Please explain it again in simpler terms.'"

Of course, while it's fine to ask questions, you do need to accept that answers may not always be immediately forthcoming. Test results take time, diagnoses are not always clear-cut, no one can predict the future—and sometimes there simply are no answers. Your best bet is to write down your questions, identify each of your babies' health care teams, and then direct your queries to them. Refrain from interrogating every doctor who walks by, even those who are not involved in your babies' care, in the hope of getting more encouraging answers.

Develop a mutually respectful relationship with each of your multiples' primary care nurses. They can keep you up to date about feedings, sleep patterns, and response to treatments. Nurses are also skilled at translating the stream of technical terms you may be hearing from the neonatologists and other health care team members. Remember, the neonatal nurses are taking care of your children 24 hours a day. If you wake up in the middle of the night and want a status report, you can phone the NICU and talk to the nurse in charge of each of your babies. These women and men are extraordinarily devoted and skilled caretakers, accustomed to handling not only the needs of physically fragile newborns, but also the needs of emotionally fragile parents.

DR. NEWMAN: The information in this chapter, and the insights and advice from other parents who have experienced NICU care for their multiples, can help you manage what may be the most challenging time you will ever experience in your life. As an obstetrician and maternal-fetal medicine specialist, I have the highest respect for what neonatologists and NICU staffs must do, and how well they do it.

I do know, however, that physicians, at times, get so deeply involved in the medical care issues that we forget about equally important factors such as emotional support and the family needs. There are always the pressures of the next patient to see and the next problem to address. However, we don't ever mind being reminded about the human element—so I can promise you that your neonatal care providers will never be put off by your suggestions for how they can better help to foster the bonds between you, your partner, and your babies in the NICU.

It also helps to familiarize yourself with the common NICU terminology presented in this chapter. You'll feel more confident speaking with your babies' doctors once words such as gavage, supplemental oxygen, hyperbilirubinemia, and phototherapy become an established part of your vocabulary. And because the NICU staff refer to their little patients' weight and size in grams and centimeters, you may want to keep at hand the conversion charts shown in Tables 10.2, 10.3, 10.4, and 10.5. With practice, you will soon be adept at thinking in metric terms rather than in pounds, ounces, and inches.

Conversion of Centimeters to Inches

Centimeters	Inches	Centimeters	Inches
1	0.39	45	17.72
2	0.79	50	19.69
3	1.18	55	21.65
4	1.57	60	23.62
5	1.97	65	25.59
10	3.94	70	27.56
15	5.91	75	29.53
20	7.87	80	31.50
25	9.84	85	33.46
30	11.81	90	35.43
35	13.78	95	37.40
40	15.75	100	39.37

Table 10.2

Conversion of Inches to Centimeters

Inches	Centimeters	Inches	Centimeters
10	25.4	20.5	52.1
10.5	26.7	21	53.3
11	27.9	21.5	54.6
11.5	29.2	22	55.9
12	30.5	22.5	57.2
12.5	31.8	23	58.4
13	33.0	23.5	59.7
13.5	34.3	24	61.0
14	35.6	24.5	62.2
14.5	36.8	25	63.5
15	38.1	25.5	64.8
15.5	39.4	26	66.1
16	40.6	26.5	67.4
16.5	41.9	27	68.7
17	43.2	27.5	69.9
17.5	44.4	28	71.2
18	45.7	28.5	72.5
18.5	47.0	29	73.8
19	48.3	29.5	75.1
19.5	49.5	30	76.4
20	50.8	30.5	77.6

Table 10.3

Conversion of Grams to Pounds and Ounces

	0 g	100 g	200 g	300 g	400 g	500 g	600 g	700 g	800 g	900 g
0 kg	0	3.5 oz.	7.0 oz.	10.6 oz.	14.1 oz.	1 lb., 1.6 oz.	1 lb., 5.2 oz.	1 lb., 8 oz.	1 lb., 12 oz.	2 lb.
1 kg	2 lb., 3.3 oz.	2 lb., 6.8 oz.	2 lb., 10.3 oz.	2 lb., 13.9 oz.	3 lb., 1.4 oz.	3 lb., 5 oz.	3 lb., 8.4 oz.	3 lb., 12 oz.	3 lb., 15.5 oz.	4 lb., 3 oz.
2 kg	4 lb., 6.5 oz.	4 lb., 10 oz.	4 lb., 13.6 oz.	5 lb., 1.1 oz.	5 lb., 4.7 oz.	5 lb., 8.2 oz.	5 lb., 11.7 oz.	5 lb., 15.2 oz.	6 lb., 2.8 oz.	6 lb., 6.3 oz.
3 kg	6 lb., 9.8 oz.	6 lb., 13.3 oz.	7 lb., 0.9 oz.	7 lb., 4.4 oz.	7 lb., 8 oz.	7 lb., 11.4 oz.	7 lb., 15 oz.	8 lb., 2.5 oz.	8 lb., 6 oz.	8 lb., 9.6 oz.
4 kg	8 lb., 13 oz.	9 lb., 0.6 oz.	9 lb., 4.2 oz.	9 lb., 7.7 oz.	9 lb., 11.2 oz.	9 lb., 15 oz.	10 lb., 2.3 oz.	10 lb., 5.8 oz.	10 lb., 9.3 oz.	10 lb., 12.8 oz.

Table 10.4

Conversion of Pounds and Ounces to Grams

Lb.	Oz. 0	1	2	3	4	5	6	7	8	9	10	11	12	13	14	15
1	454	482	510	538	568	596	624	653	681	709	737	765	795	823	851	880
2	908	936	966	994	1,022	1,050	1,078	1,107	1,135	1,163	1,191	1,219	1,249	1,277	1,305	1,334
3	1,362	1,390	1,418	1,446	1,476	1,504	1,533	1,561	1,589	1,617	1,645	1,673	1,703	1,731	1,759	1,786
4	1,814	1,843	1,871	1,900	1,928	1,956	1,984	2,013	2,041	2,070	2,098	2,126	2,155	2,183	2,211	2,240
5	2,268	2,296	2,325	2,353	2,381	2,410	2,438	2,466	2,495	2,523	2,551	2,580	2,608	2,637	2,665	2,693
6	2,722	2,750	2,778	2,807	2,835	2,863	2,892	2,920	2,948	2,977	3,005	3,033	3,062	3,090	3,118	3,147
7	3,175	3,203	3,232	3,260	3,289	3,317	3,345	3,374	3,402	3,430	3,459	3,487	3,515	3,544	3,572	3,600
8	3,629	3,657	3,685	3,714	3,742	3,770	3,799	3,827	3,856	3,884	3,912	3,941	3,969	3,997	4,026	4,054
9	4,082	4,111	4,139	4,167	4,196	4,224	4,252	4,281	4,309	4,337	4,366	4,394	4,423	4,451	4,479	4,508
10	4,536	4,564	4,593	4,621	4,649	4,678	4,706	4,734	4,763	4,791	4,819	4,848	4,876	4,904	4,933	4,961

Table 10.5

How you may feel: *"The NICU is so institutional. I'm heartbroken that my babies must spend their first weeks there instead of in the lovely nursery at home."*

Even though your babies are not yet ready for that beautiful nursery you've prepared at home, you can make their current environment cozier. Ask the nurse for guidelines on what's okay to bring into the NICU. Most hospitals allow parents to decorate the outside of the isolettes with family photos or simple black-and-white drawings, for instance, provided there is sufficient open space to observe the baby. A small mobile hanging above the incubator is also a nice touch. If you want to place a toy inside the isolette, choose one that can be sterilized, such as a soft plastic plaything. Skip any furry or stuffed toys that may harbor bacteria.

To help your babies look less like patients and more like the adorable little people they are, bring in some cute preemie clothing. Wardrobe items for the tiniest babies are available at many major department stores and some children's clothing stores. Or shop online at a number of websites, such as the Preemie Store and More: 1682 Roxanna Lane, New Brighton, MN 55112; Telephone 800-676-8469; website www.preemiestore.com.

How you may feel: *"I feel guilty about the outcome of my pregnancy. I must have done something wrong, and now my poor babies are paying the price."*

Please stop beating yourself up. Chances are that you did everything in your power to give your babies the healthiest start in life, and it's not your fault if things didn't turn out ideally. It does your babies no good (and does you much harm) to mull over the entire pregnancy and berate yourself for every steak left unfinished and every extra stairway climbed.

"I felt terribly guilty after the boys were born at 34 weeks, because I blamed myself for their prematurity. I kept thinking, 'I should have listened to my doctor and quit work when she told me to. This is all my fault.' That feeling lasted for a long time," admits Benita Moreno. "But finally I realized that I had to let go of the guilt and move on. I had done the best I could, and some things were simply beyond my control."

How you may feel: *"My friends don't know whether to offer congratulations or condolences. I feel so alone, like no one understands what I'm going through."*

It's natural to feel isolated from family and friends who have never experienced the NICU firsthand. They don't mean to be unkind, but they simply may not know what the right thing is to say. Particularly tough to take right now is the company of friends who have recently had healthy babies, because they are fretting about diaper rash and spit-up, while you are worrying about brain hemorrhages and collapsed lungs. "My advice is to ignore any insensitive comments," says Ginny Seyler. "People don't understand how much it hurts to hear remarks like 'Gosh, they are so tiny!'"

You want your own parents to visit the NICU with you, but you're afraid of how they'll react? You need to trust your instincts—but don't sell your folks short, either. "My in-laws are elderly, so I wasn't sure whether or not to encourage them when they asked if they were allowed in the NICU. It could be quite a shock for them to see a room full of tiny, sick babies," says Lydia Greenwood. "But when I voiced my concerns, my mother-in-law drew herself up and said, 'Of course we want to see our new grandchildren.' And they handled it beautifully, holding the twins without seeming bothered by the many tubes and monitors. After their visit, I felt cheered."

The best moral support, though, probably comes from other mothers and fathers whose babies have graduated from the NICU. Many hospitals offer support groups where you can connect with such parents. You can also find online chat rooms by entering the phrase *parents of preemies* into a search engine. Or contact the Mothers of Multiples Club, which may be able to help connect current NICU moms with those who've had similar experiences. If, despite these measures, you continue to feel extremely isolated or depressed, it would be wise to consult a mental health professional who is experienced at dealing with these types of family issues.

How you may feel: *"I'm overwhelmed at the thought of having to care for disabled children."*

There is a common saying in the NICU—"Babies often take two steps forward and one step back"—so try not to get discouraged. Ginny Seyler suggests, "It's important to understand that hospitalized infants have their good days and their bad days. To stay sane, you have to take it one day at a time and try to focus on their overall progress."

You may want to keep a daily log of each baby's weight, feedings, sleep patterns, and health status. When you feel dispirited, leaf back through its pages. You will probably see how far your babies have come since the first day they entered the NICU.

DR. NEWMAN: The NICU experience is a roller coaster. Premature babies are delicate and have many adaptations they must make to life outside the womb. Most preemies, especially the very low birthweight babies (less than 3 lb., 5 oz.), tend to progress in fits and starts. They have some improvement, then regress, then recover quickly—and lots of times these changes in condition happen from morning to afternoon, only to take another turn in the evening.

It is the job of the NICU staff to keep on constant alert for these subtle changes in how a baby is doing, to recognize what these changes may mean, and to be prepared to intervene if needed. But for parents, the constantly changing updates mean that one moment there is worry, the next relief, and then worry again. It's emotionally exhausting! And, of course, for parents with multiples in the NICU, this roller-coaster experience is magnified by the fact that each twin, triplet, or quad is taking his or her own course toward wellness.

My advice is to try to judge your babies' progress on a weekly basis rather than on a daily or hourly basis. That way, rather than being overwhelmed by the frequent fluctuations in your multiples' condition, you will be better able to maintain your emotional equanimity.

And if any of your babies do develop problems that potentially have long-term consequences, remember that help is available. You will be referred to specialists who can provide appropriate treatment or assistance. The outlook for today's preemies is brighter than ever before.

How you may feel: *"I live with a constant sense of terror that one or more of my babies won't survive."*

Try to cultivate an attitude of cautious optimism. Your babies may surprise you. "Despite my fears, my 3½-pounder did much better than I expected, considering that he weighed 2 pounds less than his brother," says Marcy Bugajski. "The doctor said it was due to the fact that little Ben was used to fighting for everything in utero, because big Alex had always gotten the lion's share of the nourishment."

Hospital support groups and social workers can help you handle your fears, particularly if they connect you to NICU graduates and their parents. To see a robust toddler who once lay where your babies are now can provide a powerful surge of confidence.

How you may feel: *"But what if the worst does happen? How will we cope?"*

The loss of a baby is a terrible tragedy; the loss of two or more is undeniably harder to bear. However, outsiders do not always understand the terribly complex mix of conflicting emotions faced by parents who must grieve the loss of one baby while celebrating the birth of the other (or others). Too often, sadness is compounded when family and friends offer misguided advice like "There's no reason to feel sad—you still have one baby to love." A professional grief counselor experienced in working with parents of multiples may be able to provide more understanding.

It can also be very helpful to connect with other parents who've experienced the loss of one or more of their multiples. Many NICUs provide lists of local parents who can help with this grieving process. Another option is to contact the Center for Loss in Multiple Birth (CLIMB), P.O. Box 91377, Anchorage, AK 99509; telephone 907-222-5321; email climb@climb-support .org; website www.climb-support.org. CLIMB provides support by and for parents and bereaved families, a quarterly newsletter, and samples of birth and memorial announcements.

Parents who've experienced the loss of an infant say that it is comforting to have photographs, a lock of hair, and footprints or handprints of the baby who died. Such mementos will also be important to the surviving child or children later in life, as they offer a means of connecting with their sibling.

It may help to find a meaningful way to honor a baby who had died. Many hospitals arrange memorial services or candle-lighting ceremonies. Some parents hold a private gathering for close family and friends, and devise a personal tribute to the lost twin. Other parents prefer to plant a tree in memory of the baby, or to wear a ring engraved with the child's name. Some parents make a memorial video. Writing about your feelings can help, too.

For some parents, the greatest comfort comes from cherishing their own personal memories of their child, no matter how brief the life may have been. Karen Danke, who lost a set of boy/girl twins the year before giving birth to her fraternal twin boys, shares her experience: "In my first pregnancy, I went for an ultrasound at 20 weeks, and the doctor realized that one of the babies had died already. The following week, I went into labor and delivered the twins. My little girl, the doctors estimated, had died about a month earlier. Though my son was born alive, there was no way to save him. The hospital staff encouraged us to hold our son and take his picture. At first, we didn't want to, but later we were glad we did. We counted his tiny little fingers and toes, and we named him—Kenneth Peter. Later, the nurses gave us both babies' receiving blankets and preemie outfits. We will always cherish those little treasures."

DR. LUKE: The death of a child touches us like nothing else, and the memory of that brief life stays in our hearts forever. When we grieve over the loss of a baby, we are also grieving for all the hopes and dreams that were never realized, and all the experiences and achievements that can never be.

Yet children always teach us lessons about ourselves, and the lessons learned from the children who have been in our lives for the shortest of times can be uniquely poignant. We need to honor those children by keeping our hearts open and free from bitterness, so that their memory can remind us every day of just how precious life is.

When Can Your Babies Go Home?

Discharge day is what most NICU parents dream of, pray for, and work toward hardest. Yet it's not always easy to predict just when that day will come. Barring serious complications, parents are often told to expect that their preemies will be ready to face the world outside the hospital around the time they should have been facing the world outside the womb—in other words, close to their original due date. Many preemies, though, are ready to leave even sooner. In general, here's what each baby must achieve in order to be discharged:

- All medical problems have been resolved or are under control.
- The baby practices demand feeding—deciding for herself when and how much to eat, and doing so about every two to three hours.
- The infant has shown steady, progressive weight gain over a period of several days to a week.
- A minimum weight (typically about 4 pounds) has been reached.
- The baby can maintain his body temperature in an open crib when covered only with a diaper, T-shirt, and blanket.
- There is good respiratory control, with no episodes of apnea.

"At our NICU, in order to be discharged, a baby had to do eight full feedings in a row, within 24 hours, in less than 20 minutes per feeding. At first our triplets couldn't do this because they would fall asleep in the middle of a feeding and have to finish by gavage," says Arlene McAndrew. "Little Kevin, who at 4 lb., 9 oz. was the smallest at birth, actually reached his feeding goal first and came home on day 10. The other two came home the following day."

In some cases, babies take a half-step toward home by being transferred out of the NICU and into a Level II or special-care nursery or what's called a low-maintenance room. This facility, while not equipped to handle the most serious neonatal needs, can provide a level of care more sophisticated than that of the typical nursery on a labor and delivery unit. Anne Seifert explains, "All four of our babies were in the NICU at the University of Michigan, which is a 90-minute drive from our house. After two weeks, though, they were strong enough to be transferred to the special-care nursery in a smaller hospital closer to home. That was much more convenient."

One increasingly common practice is to send home a baby who has a particular special need, but is otherwise ready for discharge, with equipment such as a respiratory support system or an apnea monitor. A visiting nurse or other health care professional closely supervises the infant, and parents are carefully instructed in the use of the equipment. Karen Danke says, "After 17 days in the NICU, Zachary came home from the hospital on supplemental oxygen, which he used during feedings. Without it, he didn't have the energy to eat enough, although other than that, he was fine."

Frequently one infant may be discharged before his siblings, particularly if the babies had different birthweights or health problems. "Heather came home after six weeks in the NICU, and Brian came home after seven weeks, but little Dillon was in the hospital for three months," Ginny Seyler recalls.

Work out the logistics so that you can continue to visit any babies who remain in the hospital. "Ed and I were concerned that we wouldn't be able to spend as much time visiting Holly after Alexander came home from the NICU," says Lydia Greenwood. "But soon we developed a system. Ed stopped to see her on his way to work each morning, while I stayed home all day with Alexander. Then Ed took care of Alexander in the evening, while I went to the hospital to be with Holly. That lasted for 11 days, until finally Holly came home, too."

Though you may feel conflicted about leaving one or more babies behind, try to look on the bright side: You have the chance to get used to taking care of just one infant at a time before facing the challenge of caring for them all at once. And sooner or later the day will come when you have all your multiples gathered around you—home at last.

Chapter Eleven

Feeding the Masses— Including the Breast-Feeding Mom

Certain baby-care skills can be acquired on an as-needed basis. You can muddle through the early days, learning as you go along and improving over time. After all, your babies are no worse off if your first attempts at diapering or dressing are amateurish. But when it comes to feeding your multiples, it's essential to get off to a good start. That's why you should look over this chapter *before* your babies are born. You have an important decision to make—breast, bottle, or both?—and you need to consider these options calmly and carefully. If you wait until delivery day, with all its hustle and bustle, you may get shunted toward a hasty decision that you will later find disappointing.

No matter how you choose to nourish your babies, though, understand that feedings are bound to be a bit crazy at first. It is for every new mother. And as with so many other aspects of parenting multiples, the more babies you have, the more hectic mealtimes may be.

Anne Seifert, mother of quadruplets, knows this from personal experience. "Mason came home from the NICU first, at eight weeks. My husband or I fed him every three hours, and that seemed pretty easy. When Sarah came home two days later, things got a little more complicated. But still, between Mark and me, we managed," says Anne. "Then Lindsey was discharged from the hospital. Was she colicky! It was nerve-wracking to try to feed and care for three 5-pound babies while one was screaming nonstop. Thank goodness, switching her formula eased her stomach distress. Finally little Andrew came home at nine and a half weeks. Because he was still tiny, he had to eat every two hours. Each feeding took 45 minutes, and still he got more milk on him than in him. The only way to handle it was to have Mark devote himself full-time to feeding and taking care of Andrew, while I took care of the other three babies."

To ensure that those early feedings go as smoothly as possible, gather your information and make your decision ahead of time. Then prepare whatever supplies you will need—whether nursing bras, breast pads and a breast pump, or bottles and formula, or all of the above. Also find an experienced mother of multiples who supports your decision and can troubleshoot with you should any difficulties arise.

Yes, You Can Nurse All Those Babies

TAMARA: Shortly after my premature twins were transported from the community hospital where they were born to a major medical center 30 miles away, my obstetrician came into my hospital room. Patting my hand, he said that he had called the NICU and been told that my babies were doing relatively well. Then he checked me over and assured me that my own physical recovery seemed to be on track.

As he headed for the door, he remarked, "Oh, I almost forgot to mention that I ordered the medication to dry up your breast milk. I imagine you aren't planning on nursing, are you? Breast-feeding twins can be tough, especially since no one knows how long your babies will be in the hospital, and . . ."

The doctor's voice trailed off as he noticed the look of horror on my face. "You didn't give me that medicine already, did you?" I cried.

"No, no," he quickly answered. "And of course I won't, if you don't want it."

"I *don't* want it. What I want is a breast pump. I am going to nurse my babies someday, so I'd better start building up my milk supply now."

And pump I did, for weeks. No, it wasn't the intimate bonding experience I had expected to have with my babies. In fact, sometimes I felt as physically attached to that pump as I was emotionally attached to my twins! Yet I knew that my breast milk was a lifeline that I—and *only* I—could throw to my babies, via nasogastric tubes, during their time in the NICU. Considering how much of their care I had to entrust to others, providing this unique form of nourishment helped me feel more like a real mother.

By the time my twins came home from the hospital, they had become champion nursers. And to me, breast-feeding had come to feel so natural that I continued until the twins were 14 months old. I weaned them on their due date—what would have been their first birthday if they'd gone full term. When we went to the hospital's Premature Baby Follow-up Clinic later that month, the pediatrician congratulated me on being "the mother of preemie twins who had nursed the longest." Her praise gave me a sweet sense of satisfaction.

DR. LUKE: One major difficulty for women who want to breast-feed is finding help and support—a role model who can offer practical advice on how to get started and how to resolve any problems. When it comes to child care, we automatically turn to our own mothers, and in most instances, they can provide sensible guidance based on personal experience. But back when your own mom was a new mother, the myriad benefits of breast milk were not as commonly recognized as they are today. If your mother was not encouraged to breast-feed back then, she may not be able to help you get started now.

Lack of an experienced role model is a problem that's magnified with a multiple pregnancy. New mothers of multiples tell me how often they hear discouraging comments like "With twins to take care of, you won't have time to breast-feed," or "Mothers of triplets or quads can't possibly make enough milk to nourish their babies properly." Even some health care professionals don't always encourage mothers of multiples to breast-feed, particularly in cases where the babies will be staying in the hospital for a while. This attitude is most unfortunate, especially since it is based on incorrect information—because the fact is that most mothers of multiples *can* breast-feed quite successfully, as many women have proven.

Strangely enough, discouragement also occasionally comes from people who supposedly support breast-feeding yet strongly discourage any plans to supplement nursing with formula. But for many mothers of twins and especially triplets and quads, supplementing is a reasonable option because it gives the babies the advantages of breast milk while affording the parents additional flexibility.

To overcome any discouragement or frustration, one of the best steps you can take is to seek the help and support of a lactation consultant. She is an essential member of your health care team, as discussed back in Chapter 2. Ideally you should meet with the lactation consultant early in your pregnancy and again when you are nearing delivery. This way, you will have established a relationship and can call upon her during the postpartum period when you actually begin breast-feeding.

Even if you do wait until after the babies are born, a lactation consultant can be immensely helpful. "The lactation consultants at the hospital where I delivered really empowered me mentally, emotionally, and physically," says Megan Ryerson, mother of boy/girl twins. "For instance, they taught me how to tandem-feed when my twins were just 20 hours old, which turned out to be a huge timesaver. They also told me that almost all babies lose a little weight in the first week, and that as long as the weight loss wasn't excessive and they started gaining soon, it did *not* mean the mother wasn't making enough milk. I ended up nursing my twins for 16 months, without ever using formula, and I think that the practical advice and encouragement I got from the lactation consultants were essential to my success."

DR. NEWMAN: In my early years as a physician, obstetricians often paid little attention to a mother's choice for or against breast-feeding. The issues of convenience and maternal discomfort were discussed as much as, if not more than, the health benefits of mother's milk.

Over the past several decades, however, there have been dramatic changes in attitude among obstetricians and pediatricians, as well as hospital nursery and NICU staff. On obstetrical services units, rooming-in and lactation consultants have become the standard of care. A medication called bromocriptine (Parlodel), which previously had been frequently used to suppress lactation, lost its FDA indication. The formerly ubiquitous free samples of infant formula have disappeared from hospital nurseries. Breast pumps are parked around every corner, and private rooms for breast-feeding or pumping are now part of the basic architectural footprint for any mother-baby unit.

Yet despite this sea change in our recognition of the benefits of breast-feeding, there are still barriers to be overcome—particularly when it comes to multiples and to newborns who require a stay in the NICU or special-care nursery. Even among some of my otherwise enlightened peers, I still sense concern and skepticism over the ability of mothers to successfully breast-feed twins, much less triplets or quads.

So let me emphasize this fact: With proper maternal nutrition after delivery, milk production increases in proportion to demand—even when a mother is breast-feeding two, three, or more infants.

Programs such as the UNICEF/World Health Organization Baby-Friendly Hospital Initiative support the evolution in evidence-based practice that favors breast-feeding.

Recognition as a Baby-Friendly hospital or birthing center requires that the facility provide education and counseling regarding the benefits of breast-feeding, and eliminate any institutional barriers to breast-feeding. That's why Chapter 2 included a recommendation to deliver your babies at a hospital that has achieved the Baby-Friendly designation. A list of such hospitals is available online at www.babyfriendlyusa.org.

Here are the 10 steps required to become a Baby-Friendly Hospital:

1. Have a written breast-feeding policy that is routinely communicated to all health care staff.

2. Train all health care staff in the skills necessary to implement this policy.
3. Inform all pregnant women about the benefits of breast-feeding.
4. Help mothers initiate breast-feeding within one hour of birth.
5. Show mothers how to initiate and maintain lactation, even if separated from their infants.
6. Give infants no food or drink other than breast milk, unless medically indicated.
7. Practice rooming-in—allow mothers and infants to remain together 24 hours a day.
8. Encourage breast-feeding on demand.
9. Give no pacifiers or artificial nipples to breast-feeding infants.
10. Foster the establishment of breast-feeding support groups and refer mothers to these groups upon discharge from the hospital or birthing center.

WHY BREAST IS BEST

Whether you choose to breast-feed exclusively or to supplement your nursing with formula, your babies stand to benefit greatly by receiving your breast milk. Medical professionals agree on this—including the American College of Obstetricians and Gynecologists, the American Academy of Pediatrics, and the Academy of Nutrition and Dietetics.[1,2,3]

For example, according to the American Academy of Pediatrics (AAP), the breast-fed infant is the reference against which all other feeding methods are measured regarding growth, health, development, and all other short- and long-term outcomes, and the premature infant benefits the most from this type of feeding. AAP recommends exclusive breast-feeding for about six months, followed by continued breast-feeding as complementary foods are introduced for one year or longer, as mutually desired by a mother and her infant (or infants). Similarly, the Academy of Nutrition and Dietetics states, "Exclusive breast-feeding provides optimal nutrition and health protection for the first six months of life, and breast-feeding with complementary foods from six months until at least 12 months is the ideal feeding pattern for infants."

Here are some of the many reasons why breast is best for babies:

• Breast milk is the ideal food for infants. It contains all the needed nutrients in exactly the right proportions.

1. American College of Obstetricians and Gynecologists. Committee opinion. Breastfeeding: Maternal and infant aspects. Obstetrics & Gynecology 2007; 109:479–80.
2. American Academy of Pediatrics. Policy statement. Breastfeeding and the use of human milk. Pediatrics 2012; 129:e827.
3. Academy of Nutrition and Dietetics. Position paper. Promoting and supporting breastfeeding. Journal of the Academy of Nutrition and Dietetics 2015; 115:444–9.

- Breast milk contains unique antibodies that protect babies against infection. These antibodies can't be manufactured any other way. Studies show that infants who are breast-fed are 50 to 75 percent less likely to develop gastrointestinal infections, respiratory infections, pneumonia, meningitis, middle-ear infections, and food allergies.
- The risk of sudden infant death syndrome (SIDS) is as much as 73 percent lower for breast-fed infants.
- Benefits of breast-feeding last way beyond weaning. For instance, people who were breast-fed as babies are as much as 30 percent less likely later in life to be obese or to develop intestinal disease or cancer.
- Breast milk may increase intelligence. Research reveals that premature infants who were tube-fed with breast milk scored an average of eight points higher on IQ tests given at age eight than did formula-fed preemies. Because all the children were fed through nasogastric tubes, scientists conclude that the results are the effect of the milk alone, and not the nurturing bond that nursing fosters.

DR. NEWMAN: One of my partners who just recently served as the president of the Society for Maternal-Fetal Medicine always referred to breast milk as *liquid gold*. I encourage all mothers of multiples to think of it that way, too.

Do be aware, though, that even if you are careful to get enough vitamin D yourself, very little vitamin D crosses to your babies through breast milk. That's why the American Academy of Pediatrics recommends that all breast-fed infants receive a vitamin D supplement of 400 IU per day, beginning within a few days of birth.[4] This supplementation should continue until such time as a baby is consuming 1,000 milliliters (about four cups) of either vitamin D–fortified infant formula or milk per day.

Breast-feeding has health advantages not only for babies, but also for nursing mothers. Consider this:

- Nursing helps you regain your figure faster by stimulating the uterus to contract—a real plus after your abdomen has been stretched by two, three, or four babies.[5]

---

4. Wagner CL, Greer FR. Prevention of rickets and vitamin D deficiency in infants, children and adolescents. Pediatrics 2008; 111:908.
5. Baker JL, Gamborg M, Heitmann BL, Lissner L, Sorensen TIA, Rasmussen KM. Breastfeeding reduces postpartum weight retention. American Journal of Clinical Nutrition 2008; 88:1543–51.

- Breast-feeding allows you to lose pregnancy pounds quicker. Producing milk for just a single baby requires as much as 500 calories a day, so if you're nursing multiples, your milk production could require up to an additional 1,000 to 2,000 calories a day beyond your own needs.
- Women who have breast-fed are at lower risk for developing rheumatoid arthritis, hypertension, cardiovascular disease, and diabetes, as well as breast and ovarian cancer.[6, 7, 8, 9]
- There is evidence that breast-feeding resets a woman's metabolism after pregnancy, significantly reducing her future risk for a multitude of chronic diseases—even decades later.[10]

Diet Tips for Nursing Moms of Multiples

Months before you find yourself in the delivery room looking into your newborns' eyes for the first time, Mother Nature starts preparing your body to feed your babies. Nutrient reserves are built up in anticipation of the day your babies will begin their lives outside the womb and take their first meal at your breast.

During pregnancy, you gained a certain amount of fat (as discussed in Chapter 3), particularly around your shoulder blades, thighs, and upper arms. The purpose of this fat is twofold. First, it's a ready reserve of concentrated calories for the last months of pregnancy, when you may not be able to eat enough to meet the nutritional demands of your growing babies. Second, this fat acts as a caloric warehouse, ready to be mobilized when required for milk production.

Fat reserves alone, however, can't handle the long-term demands placed on your body

6. Collaborative Group on Hormonal Factors in Breast Cancer. Breast cancer and breastfeeding: Collaborative reanalysis of individual data from 47 epidemiological studies in 30 countries, including 50,302 women with breast cancer and 96,973 women without the disease. Lancet 2002; 360:187–95.
7. Schwarz EB, Brown JS, Creasman JM, et al. Lactation and maternal risk of type 2 diabetes: A population-based study. American Journal of Medicine 2010; 123:863.e1–e6.
8. Karlson EW, Mandl LA, Hankinson SE, Grodstein F. Do breast-feeding and other reproductive factors influence future risk of rheumatoid arthritis? Results from the Nurses' Health Study. Arthritis & Rheumatology 2004; 50:3458–67.
9. Schwarz EB, Ray RM, Stuebe AM, et al. Duration of lactation and risk factors for maternal cardiovascular disease. Obstetrics & Gynecology 2009; 113:974–82.
10. Stuebe AM, Rich-Edwards JW. The reset hypothesis: Lactation and maternal metabolism. American Journal of Perinatology 2009; 26:81–8.

when you are nursing. For that, you need to eat right. Dietary guidelines for breast-feeding women are set with two goals in mind:

- *To allow healthy, full-term babies to double their birthweight within four to six months.* This requires that the mother produce a sufficient amount of milk. Generally that's not a problem because the driving force behind breast milk production is supply and demand. In other words, the more you nurse your babies, the more milk you will produce.
- *To keep nursing mothers in good health.* Meeting this goal can be more of a challenge. The nutrient content of breast milk is amazingly constant, whether the mother is underweight or overweight, anemic or well nourished—which means that if your diet is inadequate, your *own* health will suffer.

The Food and Nutrition Board of the National Academy of Sciences has established dietary reference intakes (DRIs) for women who are breast-feeding a single baby. These recommendations indicate that a nursing mother's calorie requirements increase about 500 calories per day, or 23 percent above nonpregnant levels. In addition, the need for certain nutrients (folic acid, riboflavin, thiamin; vitamins A, C, and D; and the minerals calcium, phosphorus, and zinc) increases by 50 percent or more. Other nutrient requirements (such as for niacin; vitamins B_6, B_{12}, and E; and the minerals iodine, iron, magnesium, and selenium) also increase, but by a lesser percentage.

DR. LUKE: Just as there are no current national dietary guidelines for women pregnant with multiples, there are as yet no official dietary guidelines for women breast-feeding multiples. Extrapolating from the DRIs for nursing mothers of singletons, however, I have made some educated estimates about the nutritional needs of women who are exclusively nursing twins, triplets, or quadruplets. These are shown in the top half of Table 11.1. To make your menu planning easier, I've also translated the data from grams per day into the more familiar terms of servings per day.

Nutrient needs vary depending on how much milk you produce—and that, of course, is determined by how many babies you have and whether you are supplementing with formula. The guidelines given in Table 11.1 are based on your estimated nutrient needs if you are exclusively breast-feeding your multiples. If you are supplementing with formula, these calorie counts should be adjusted downward, depending on how much supplementation your babies receive each day. For instance, if your quadruplets get half their feedings at the breast and the other half from formula, you can follow the guidelines for nursing twins.

Estimated Dietary Requirements: Nonpregnant Woman Versus a Woman Breast-Feeding Twins, Triplets, or Quads

		Active Nonpregnant Woman	Breast-Feeding Mother			
			Singleton	Twins	Triplets	Quads
Calories per day		2,200	2,700	3,200	3,700	4,200
Protein (grams)	20–25% of calories	110–138	135–169	160–200	185–231	210–263
Carbohydrate (grams)	45–50% of calories	248–275	304–338	360–400	416–463	473–525
Fat (grams)	30% of calories	73	90	107	123	140
Food groups	Serving size	Servings	Servings	Servings	Servings	Servings
Dairy (nonfat or low fat)	8 oz. milk or yogurt or 1 oz. cheese	6	8	10	12	14
Lean meat, poultry, fish, eggs	1 oz. or 1 medium egg	8	9	10	11	12
Vegetables	½ cup cooked or 1 cup fresh	4	4	5	6	7
Fruits	1 medium whole or ½ cup sliced	4	4	5	6	7
Grains, starchy vegetables*	1 slice bread or ½ cup	8	9	10	11	12
Fats, oils, nuts	1 tbsp. oil or butter, or 12 nuts	8	12	15	18	20

*Starchy vegetables include corn, potatoes, chickpeas, beans, and peas.

Table 11.1

If it's confusing to keep track of all these numbers, simplify matters by thinking of your nutritional needs in a familiar way—by calorie count. Compared to a prepregnancy diet, here are the higher calorie counts that nursing women need if their babies are exclusively breast-fed. (Again, remember that calorie counts go down when breast-feeding is supplemented with formula.)

- To nurse a singleton: an extra 500 to 600 calories a day.
- To nurse twins: an extra 1,000 to 1,200 calories a day.
- To nurse triplets: an extra 1,500 to 1,800 calories a day.
- To nurse quadruplets: an extra 2,000 to 2,400 calories a day.

If you've always been a weight-conscious calorie counter, these numbers may seem shockingly high. But in order to breast-feed successfully, you do need to eat—a lot! Remember, the extra calories you consume on a daily basis are being used in the production of breast milk; they are *not* being converted into unwanted and unnecessary fat stores.

If you do not consume enough calories, problems are likely to arise. Some moms learn this the hard way. "After my girls were born, I just wasn't as hungry as I had been during the pregnancy. I felt less motivated to eat, too—and I had less time for it, busy as I was taking care of the babies," says Amy Maly, mother of identical twin girls. "In hindsight, though, I realize that by not eating enough, I sabotaged my efforts at breast-feeding. Not only was I worried about producing too little milk, but I also felt drained and exhausted."

Are you concerned that the extra calories you need to take in when nursing will interfere with your ability to lose the pregnancy weight? Don't worry—that's not likely to happen. "My twins were breast-fed exclusively, and that helped me tremendously with losing the pregnancy weight. I think it's a big reason why, by the time of my six-week postpartum checkup, I weighed a little less than I did before I got pregnant," says Hannah Steele, mother of identical twin girls.

Arlene McAndrew, who breast-fed her triplets for seven months, agrees. "The whole time I was nursing, I felt super-hungry and I ate constantly, but still I had absolutely no problem losing the pregnancy weight. Clearly, breast-feeding three babies uses up a lot of calories," she says.

As a nursing mother of multiples, you need to eat the same foods as any other woman who is breast-feeding, but you should eat more often and have larger portions. In fact, you need almost as many calories to breast-feed as you did when you were pregnant. Yet, while the calorie counts are close, their food sources should be somewhat different when you are breast-feeding. Back in Chapter 4, which discussed what to eat while pregnant, the emphasis was on getting adequate calories, protein, and iron, with a focus on meats and a well-balanced diet overall.

Although your daily caloric needs have changed by only about 300 calories, the focus now is on getting enough calories and calcium, with *more dairy* and *less meat,* while still maintaining a balanced diet. Table 11.2 provides a sample menu comparing dietary needs during pregnancy with those appropriate while breast-feeding.

Sample Menu for Mothers of Multiples: Pregnancy Versus Breast-Feeding

Meal	Menu Suggestion	Twins Pregnancy/Nursing	Triplets Pregnancy/Nursing	Quads Pregnancy/Nursing
Breakfast	Scrambled eggs	2 eggs / 2 eggs	2 eggs / 2 eggs	2 eggs / 2 eggs
	Canadian bacon	1 oz. / 1 oz.	1 oz. / 1 oz.	1 oz. / 1 oz.
	Whole-wheat toast	2 slices / 2 slices	3 slices / 3 slices	3 slices / 3 slices
	Cheddar cheese	1 oz. / 1½ oz.	1½ oz. / 2 oz.	2 oz. / 2½ oz.
	Sliced bananas	1 banana / 1 banana	1 banana / 1 banana	1 banana / 1 banana
	Decaffeinated coffee	optional / optional	optional / optional	optional / optional
Midmorning	Whole-wheat toast	2 slices / 2 slices	2 slices / 2 slices	2 slices / 2 slices
	Peanut butter	2 tbsp. / —	2 tbsp. / —	2 tbsp. / 2 tbsp.
	Cheese	— / 1 oz.	1 oz. / 1½ oz.	2 oz. / 2½ oz.
	Apple slices	1 apple / 1 apple	1 apple / 1 apple	1 apple / 1 apple
	Milk	1 cup / 1½ cups	1½ cups / 2 cups	2 cups / 2 cups
Lunch	Tuna	2 oz / 2 oz.	2 oz. / 2 oz.	3 oz. / 3 oz.
	Swiss cheese	— / —	½ oz. / 1 oz.	1 oz. / 1 oz.
	Toasted rye	2 slices / 2 slices	2 slices / 2 slices	2 slices / 2 slices
	Lettuce/tomato salad	1 small / 1 small	1 small / 1 small	1 medium / 1 medium
	Potato salad	½ cup / ½ cup	½ cup / ½ cup	½ cup / ½ cup
	Ice cream	1 cup / 1 cup	1 cup / 1 cup	1 cup / 1½ cups
	Milk	1 cup / 1½ cups	1½ cups / 1½ cups	2 cups / 2 cups
	Orange sections	— / —	1 orange / —	1 orange / —

Meal	Menu Suggestion	Twins Pregnancy/Nursing	Triplets Pregnancy/Nursing	Quads Pregnancy/Nursing
Mid-afternoon	Whole-grain crackers	4 crackers / 4 crackers	8 crackers / 8 crackers	8 crackers / 8 crackers
	Liver pâté	1 oz. / —	1½ oz. / —	2 oz. / —
	Cottage cheese	— / ½ cup	— / ½ cup	— / 1 cup
	Fresh grapes	½ cup / ½ cup	½ cup / ½ cup	½ cup / ½ cup
Dinner	Broiled steak	5 oz. / 4 oz.	5 oz. / 4 oz.	6 oz. / 4 oz.
	Baked potato	1 small / 1 small	1 small / 1 small	1 medium / 1 medium
	Low-fat sour cream	1 tbsp. / 1 tbsp.	2 tbsp. / 2 tbsp.	3 tbsp. / 2 tbsp.
	Caesar salad	1 small / 1 small	1 medium / 1 medium	1 medium / 1 medium
	Dinner roll	1 roll / 1 roll	1 roll / 1 roll	1 roll / 1 roll
	Milk	1 cup / 1 cup	1 cup / 1 cup	1 cup / 1½ cups
	Tapioca pudding	1 cup / 1 cup	1 cup / 1 cup	1 cup / 1 cup
	Sliced strawberries	½ cup / —	½ cup / —	½ cup / ½ cup
After dinner	Ice cream	1 cup / 1 cup	1 cup / 1 cup	1 cup / 1 cup
Bedtime	Cereal	¾ cup / ¾ cup	¾ cup / ¾ cup	¾ cup / ¾ cup
	Milk	1 cup / 1 cup	1 cup / 1 cup	1 cup / 1 cup
	Fruit	½ cup / ½ cup	½ cup / ½ cup	½ cup / ½ cup

Table 11.2

FOURTH TRIMESTER: EMPHASIS ON CALCIUM, OMEGA-3S, ZINC, AND IODINE

Chapter 4 includes a discussion on the three trimesters of pregnancy, and the nutrients that are most vital during each time period. The postpartum period is sometimes referred to as the *fourth trimester,* and it too involves unique nutritional needs:

- Calcium requirements increase by 50 percent or more when you are nursing—and the more babies you're feeding, the more calcium you need. If your diet doesn't supply enough, this mineral will be drawn from your own bones, making them weaker, as well as potentially releasing lead into your bloodstream and breast milk. Good sources of calcium include dairy foods such as milk, cheese, and yogurt; sardines and salmon with bones; eggs; tofu; peanuts; spinach, beans, and potatoes. (And remember, for your body to appropriately mobilize and utilize calcium, you also need to ensure adequate postpartum intake of vitamin D—ideally, maintaining a blood level of 25-hydroxy vitamin D between 40 and 60 ng/ml, as discussed in Chapter 5.)

- Omega-3 fatty acids are important now because, while the quantity of fat in your breast milk remains fairly constant no matter what you eat, the type of fat in your milk depends on your diet. In order for your breast milk to be rich in the omega-3 fatty acids your babies need for proper visual and neurologic development, your diet also must be rich in these fatty acids. This is especially important if your babies were born prematurely. For instance, a study in the *Journal of the American Medical Association* found that when breast-feeding mothers' diets were high in the omega-3 docosahexaenoic acid, their preterm infants were at significantly less risk for developmental delays.[11] Even with full-term infants, the brain continues to add new cells and develop after birth and through the first year of life, and omega-3s are essential for that process. In fact, adequate maternal intake of omega-3s during both pregnancy and lactation has been strongly linked to optimal vision, behavior, and intelligence in offspring,[12] while low maternal intake has been associated with suboptimal fine motor coordination, communication, and social development.[13] So be sure your diet includes ample amounts of fish (the richest source of omega-3s), plus oils such as canola, safflower, flaxseed, and olive. Omega-3–enriched eggs are another good choice.

- Zinc is a critical component of many enzymes throughout the body. It also benefits your babies by promoting their neurologic development. In order for your breast milk to provide the zinc your multiples need, your diet should include beef, pork, lamb, poultry, seafood, and eggs. Zinc is also provided by plant sources such

---

11. Makrides, M., Gibson RA, McPhee AJ, et al. Neurodevelopmental outcomes of preterm infants fed high-dose docosahexaenoic acid: A randomized controlled trial. Journal of the American Medical Association 2009; 301:175–82.

12. Morse NL. Benefits of docosahexaenoic acid, folic acid, vitamin D and iodine on foetal and infant brain development and function following maternal supplementation during pregnancy and lactation. Nutrients 2012; 4:799–840.

13. Hibbeln JR, Davis JM, Steer C, et al. Maternal seafood consumption in pregnancy and neurodevelopmental outcomes in childhood (ALSPAC Study): An observational cohort study. Lancet, 2007; 369:578–85.

as whole-grain breads and cereals, beans, and nuts; however, the fiber in these foods results in less absorption.

- Iodine is essential for the production of thyroxine by the thyroid gland. This hormone regulates the rate of oxidation within cells and, in so doing, influences many aspects of your babies' health: body temperature control, metabolism of all nutrients, functioning of the nervous system and muscle tissue, and physical and mental development. Your breast milk will be rich in iodine if your diet includes fish and seafood, milk, enriched breads, and iodized salt.

With two or more babies to take care of, you have precious little time for meal planning. To make the task easier, refer to the following menu suggestions. (An asterisk indicates that the recipe appears at the back of this book.)

Menu Suggestions for the Fourth Trimester When Breast-Feeding

BREAKFAST
*Autumn Pancakes
French Toast with Applesauce
Grilled Ham and Cheese Sandwich
Oatmeal with Dried Cherries
*Pumpkin Waffles
Quiche Lorraine

LUNCH OR DINNER
Baked Manicotti
Cheeseburgers
Cheese Lasagna
Chicken Pot Pie
*Citrus Salmon
Gefilte Fish
Grilled Ham and Cheese Sandwich
London Broil
*Mini Meat Loaves

New England Clam Chowder
Pepper Steak
Pork Roast
Pot Roast
*Salmon Burgers
Spaghetti and Meatballs
Tuna Casserole
*Vegetarian Lasagna
*Vietnamese Steak Salad
Whitefish Salad

SNACKS
Apple Slices and Peanut Butter
*Basic Fruit Smoothie
*Basic Vegetable Smoothie
Deviled Eggs with Toast
Fruit Salad with Cheese and Crackers
Oatmeal-Walnut Cookies with Yogurt

DR. LUKE: In addition to the appropriate foods, you also need extra fluids. Nursing moms are typically very thirsty, even more so than during pregnancy. Drinking plenty of water and milk throughout the day helps to maintain your breast milk supply.

Within three to six months after delivery, you should be at your prepregnancy weight. If you're not and you want to continue to lose, decrease the amount of fat in your diet and reduce portion sizes for all the various foods *except dairy*. Chapter 12, "A Better Body after Babies," also details how to regain your figure through diet and lifestyle changes. For additional information on postpartum nutrition, consult another of our books, *Program Your Baby's Health: The Pregnancy Diet for Your Child's Lifelong Well-being*. Also, I invite you to get personalized nutrition counseling through my website, www.drbarbaraluke.com.

ARE YOUR BABIES GETTING ENOUGH TO EAT?

Back in the days when wet nurses were common, one woman would sometimes breast-feed as many as six children at once! Clearly, the female body is capable of nourishing more than one baby at a time. But because there are cases in which an infant does not get enough milk from nursing, you will want to be certain that your breast-fed babies are receiving the nourishment they need to thrive.

The quantity of breast milk or formula your multiples need for proper growth and development depends on their state of health, activity level, and metabolism. Most babies require 120 to 150 calories per kilogram of body weight, or about 55 to 68 calories per pound of body weight, in a 24-hour period. Both breast milk and infant formula contain about 20 calories per ounce. That means a 5-pound baby generally needs about 14 to 17 ounces per day, a 7-pound baby needs about 20 to 24 ounces per day, and a 10-pound baby needs about 28 to 34 ounces per day.

There's no way to measure in ounces the amount of breast milk your babies are taking in, unless you're pumping your breasts and feeding it to them with a bottle. But you can feel confident that your babies' intake is adequate if these other signs are present:

- Each baby soaks at least six diapers a day.
- Each baby has at least one bowel movement in a 24-hour period.
- Each baby gains ½ to 1 ounce per day, on average, during the first two to three months after he or she comes home from the hospital.

If any of your babies does *not* meet these criteria, be sure to alert your pediatrician without delay. There are a variety of factors that can undermine your milk production, and it's important that these be identified and remedied promptly:

- Fatigue, illness, stress, anger, or depression can sap the energy your body needs to produce an adequate supply of milk. These factors can also interfere with the *let-down reflex,* the normal hormonal mechanism by which milk is released from the milk-producing glands and moved into the milk ducts. If let-down is inhibited, your babies won't be able to draw the milk from your breasts, no matter how plentiful the supply. To resolve these problems, try lining up some help at home (see Chapter 13 for suggestions) and spending a day or two in bed, devoting yourself entirely to resting and nursing.

- Dieting seriously curtails milk production. If you've been skimping on meals, review Table 11.1 on recommended calorie counts and servings per day for nursing mothers of multiples.

- Excessive alcohol intake interferes with the let-down reflex, making it hard for your babies to get the milk out of your breasts. An occasional alcoholic beverage is okay, but you would be wise to limit your intake to no more than a drink or two per week.

- Inadequate stimulation of the breasts can impede milk production, so be sure to empty at least one breast at each feeding. If your babies are not strong sucklers, you may need to use a breast pump after feedings to completely empty your breasts. This sends your body a message to boost milk production.

- Resumption of estrogen-containing birth control pills has also been reported to reduce breast milk production. Once breast-feeding is well established, this reduction is probably minimal for mothers of singletons—but it may be more of an issue when you are trying to nourish twins, triplets, or quads. Contraceptive options that do not appear to reduce milk production include progesterone-only birth control pills, implants, IUDs, and barrier methods such as diaphragms and condoms.

The Mechanics of Breast-Feeding Multiples

With twins, the simplest way to divide your milk is to offer each baby one breast per feeding. For triplets or quads, devise a rotation system that allows each baby equal time at the breast.

Do be sure to alternate which side each baby suckles from. If you assign the same breast to the same infant every time, it limits that child's visual stimulation. It can also lead to lopsided breasts and a diminished milk supply on one side if one baby has a smaller appetite. "I noticed early on that my son was a much stronger sucker than my daughter, so I was careful to switch which breast he got from one feeding to the next. This helped me establish a good milk supply on both sides," says Megan Ryerson.

Another reason to switch sides at each feeding is that, if you don't, a baby may grow accustomed to a particular breast and refuse to nurse on the other. That can be a painful problem if you develop a clogged duct on one side and need the help of two or more babies to release the milk, or if one infant is unable to nurse for a few days, or if one child weans himself or herself earlier.

Full-term newborns usually nurse 10 to 12 times in 24 hours. Preemies may need to eat more often until they reach full-term size; your pediatrician can advise you on this. In any event, don't plan on feedings occurring like clockwork. Your babies will let you know when they're hungry—and this won't always happen at strictly regular intervals.

How long will each feeding last? That, too, may vary from baby to baby, from day to day, even from feeding to feeding. Typically a baby will suck eagerly, swallowing quickly, for the first 8 to 10 minutes of a feeding. Initially the baby receives the *foremilk,* or the milk that has collected in the breast since the last time you nursed. Foremilk is relatively thin and lower in fat.

Then, as milk flow slows and the baby's tummy starts to fill, she may start to doze off or appear to lose interest. Take that as a sign that it's time to burp her, then put the baby back on the breast for some additional, more leisurely sucking. Now the baby is receiving the richer *hindmilk,* which is higher in fat. Because hindmilk more effectively promotes the baby's weight gain, it's important that feedings last long enough to fully satisfy her hunger. Again, follow each baby's lead in determining how long a given feeding should last.

Does it sound like you'll be nursing around the clock? You're not alone in feeling that way. "At first, it seemed I spent every waking hour feeding babies—and almost all my hours were waking ones," says Lisa McDonough, a mother of boy/girl twins and two older children. No wonder: One study reports that it takes 10 to 15 hours daily to feed newborn twins if you feed the babies one at a time. With triplets or quads, of course, the time demands of nursing are even more challenging.

You can cut down significantly on the hours

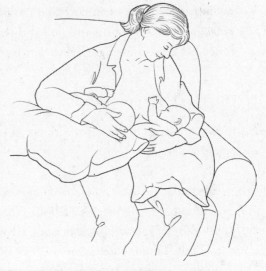

Simultaneous breast-feeding of multiples using the combination hold

spent feeding if you learn to nurse two babies simultaneously. First, get your shirt and bra out of the way, and have pillows strategically placed to support your arms and back. Then choose one of three positions:

- Both babies in the traditional cradle hold, bodies crisscrossed in front of you.
- Both in the football hold, legs tucked behind you.
- The combination hold, with one baby cradled and one held football-style.

Arrange pillows to support your arms and the babies' bodies. Or buy a special cushion designed for tandem nursing, such as the EZ-2-Nurse Twins nursing pillow from Double Blessings (telephone 800-584-8946; website www.doubleblessings.com).

TAMARA: My twins were so little that they didn't have much muscle tone those first months. Try to pick up a floppy baby with one arm while your other arm is busy holding another infant to your breast, and you'll see why I considered this business of moving the second baby into position to be the trickiest part of simultaneous nursing. It was no big deal, of course, if someone else was on hand to help me. But it took a lot of trial and error before I finally figured out how to manage it on my own.

Here's my method, using the combination hold. I sat on the sofa with James cradled in my left arm, my left elbow supported by the armrest. Samantha lay lengthwise on a pillow next to my right thigh, her head near my knee and her feet pointing toward my hips. Once James had latched on to my left breast, I encircled Samantha *and her pillow* with my right arm and pulled them onto my lap. Then with my right hand, I raised her head to my right breast, letting the pillow support her body.

IF YOU NEED HELP

If you have questions or problems with breast-feeding, help is readily available from the following organizations:

- International Lactation Consultant Association: 2501 Aerial Center Parkway, Suite 103, Morrisville, NC 27560. Telephone 888-ILCA-IS-U (888-452-2478) or 919-861-5577; email info@ilca.org; website www.ilca.org.
- La Leche League International: 35 E. Wacker Drive, Suite 850, Chicago, IL 60601. Telephone 800-LA-LECHE (800-525-3243); website www.llli.org. La Leche also publishes books, including *The Womanly Art of Breastfeeding*.

- Lactation Education Resources: 3621 Lido Place, Fairfax, VA 22031. Telephone 703-691-2069; email LERonline@yahoo.com; website www.LERon-line.com.
- U.S. Breastfeeding Committee: 4044 N. Lincoln Ave., #288, Chicago, IL 60618. Telephone 773-359-1549; email office@usbreastfeeding.org; website www.usbreastfeeding.org.

GETTING PRIMED TO PUMP

"Toward the end of my pregnancy, my brother, who is a family physician, offered to lend me the top-of-the-line electric breast pump he keeps on hand in case one of his patients should need it. Though at first I couldn't imagine ever using such a device, I took it just to be polite," says Lydia Greenwood, mother of boy/girl twins. "But it turned out to be a real boon to my breast-feeding efforts, particularly after I went back to work. Pumping during the day allowed me to keep up my milk supply, so I was able to nurse my babies a lot longer than I had ever thought would be possible."

There are a number of situations in which a breast pump can come in handy. One such circumstance is when babies are in the hospital. For premature newborns in the NICU, the effort involved in sucking from the breast or bottle can use up more calories than a feeding provides. That's why preemies are often fed through a nasogastric tube that runs from the nose directly down into the stomach. If you pump, your breast milk rather than formula can be given to your babies through this tube. Ginny Seyler says, "While my triplets were in the NICU, I pumped my breasts every four hours and gave it to the nurses, who fed it to the babies through nasogastric tubes. I wanted to be sure my babies got the benefits of breast milk, even though they were too little to suck."

Later, as your babies gain strength, they will begin to *nipple,* or drink from a tiny bottle with a special soft rubber nipple. Again, if you pump, breast milk rather than formula can be used for these feedings. (Don't be upset if the NICU staff suggests fortifying your milk. Although mother's milk is inarguably superior to formula, certain babies do best when breast milk is enhanced by specific extra nutrients.)

It's true that pumping lacks the emotional satisfaction nursing brings. But bear in mind that your milk is a precious gift *you alone* can provide for your hospitalized babies. For many women with babies in the NICU, this is a gratifying confirmation of motherhood. Plus, putting up with the hassle of pumping now will enable you to enjoy all the closeness and naturalness of nursing later, when your babies are stronger.

Usually the hospital staff is very supportive of a mother's pumping—but sometimes encouragement is not forthcoming. "I was determined to breast-feed, but there was little support for that at the NICU. The staff seemed surprised that I even wanted to try. They brought me a pump, but no one showed me how to use it. I watched a video on nursing, but still couldn't figure out how to get the boys to latch on properly. I pumped for six weeks and gave the breast milk to the boys in bottles. But it was so disappointing not to be able to really nurse that I eventually switched to formula," says Benita Moreno, mother of fraternal twin boys. "In hindsight, I wish I had called La Leche. I think a lactation consultant could have helped me work through the problems."

Pumping is also a convenient way to meet your babies' nutritional needs when you cannot be with them around the clock. Suppose you're ready to return to work but want to continue nursing. You can pump during the workday, refrigerate your milk, and have your caregiver feed it to your babies the following day, from bottles. Or suppose you want to get out of the house for the evening and have a much-deserved date with your partner. Again, the milk you pumped earlier can be fed to your babies in your absence. (Even if you don't plan to reserve your milk for your babies to drink later, you may at times need to pump or express your milk by hand. Three to four hours after your last nursing session, your breasts will grow uncomfortably full unless you relieve the engorgement by pumping or expressing milk.)

Frequent pumping also helps you establish and maintain a plentiful milk supply. Megan Ryerson says, "I pumped a *lot*—after each feeding, and whenever the babies napped for three hours at a stretch, and at nighttime even after they were sleeping through. At work, too, I stayed committed to my pumping schedule. This way I could be sure that I'd have plenty of milk, both in my breasts and in my freezer."

There may also be times when you are temporarily unable to breast-feed but want to maintain your milk supply in anticipation of resuming nursing as soon as possible. For instance, if you are sick and require medication that your doctor feels could pass through to your milk, you can pump and then discard that milk until you've completed your course of medication.

You may occasionally develop a plugged duct that refuses to be dislodged despite all your babies' best sucking efforts. In that case, the stronger suction of the pump can bring speedy relief. (Unplugging an obstructed milk duct can also be aided by taking a hot shower. While the hot water sprays on the affected breast, vigorously massage the affected area, stroking from the area of swelling and tenderness toward the nipple. If the area is extraordinarily tender and red and you have a fever, it could be an infection called mastitis or a breast abscess, which warrants an immediate call to your doctor.) "I developed mastitis when I was cutting back on breast-feeding in anticipation of weaning my twins after their first birthday. I took antibiotics for the infection, but it also helped to pump the affected breast a lot to keep it as empty as possible," says Hannah Steele.

Quickest, easiest, and most efficient are the electric breast pumps. They are expensive to buy (several hundred dollars or more), but they can be rented at reasonable rates from hospitals, pharmacies, or La Leche groups. Manually operated pumps are much cheaper, but are generally more difficult to use and less effective at emptying the breast. Under the Affordable Care Act, comprehensive breast-feeding support and counseling by a trained provider during pregnancy and/or in the postpartum period and the costs for renting breast-feeding equipment are covered—without having to pay a copayment, coinsurance, or a deductible.[14] Your doctor, lactation consultation, or a breast-feeding support group can recommend the best pump and instruct you in its use.

Two other items can make pumping easier and more efficient. The first is a vehicle lighter adapter that plugs into the cigarette lighter in your car, so that you can charge or use your electric breast pump while on the road. The second is a hands-free pumping bra that allows you to pump both breasts at once, without needing to hold onto anything—so you have both hands available to work at a computer, send texts, blow-dry your hair, cook, or do other tasks while sitting or standing near your electric pump. "These two products gave me back my freedom. They were key to my ability to nurse my twins for 13 months without ever using formula—so now I tell all my patients about them, too," says Hannah Steele, who is an obstetrician.

STORING BREAST MILK SAFELY

Before you begin to pump, wash your hands. Follow the pump manufacturer's instructions for cleaning the breast shield and tubing, and for sterilizing the container used to collect the milk.

Have on hand the special plastic bags designed for storing breast milk; these bags, which are available at pharmacies, do not interfere with the infection-fighting properties of your milk. Do not use regular plastic bags or other containers that haven't been sterilized. Label each bag with the date and time you filled it so you can use the oldest milk first. Limit the amount of milk in a bag to about 4 ounces.

Refrigerate breast milk as soon as possible after pumping. Breast milk can be safely stored in the refrigerator for 48 hours, in a refrigerator freezer for two weeks, or in a separate-door freezer for several months. Thaw milk by placing the container in a bowl of room-temperature water. Don't heat it on the stove or in the microwave; high temperatures reduce breast milk's nutritional content and present a risk of scalding. Once thawed, milk can be stored in the refrigerator for up to eight hours; it should never be refrozen.

If you're transporting breast milk to the NICU, pack it in ice for the journey. Be sure

---

14. http://hrsa.gov/womensguidelines/.

each bag is labeled with your babies' names and hospital identification numbers. You may also want to pump your breasts at the hospital each day so your babies will get some fresh milk, which is somewhat higher in nutrients and infection-fighting antibodies than milk that has been frozen.

Are you concerned about finding the time and a place to pump while at work? When the Patient Protection and Affordable Care Act was signed into law in 2010, the Break Time for Nursing Mothers law was created. This federal law applies to nursing mothers who are paid by the hour (rather than salaried), giving them the right to break time from work and a clean, private space that is not a bathroom in which to express milk during their child's first year of life.[15] At present, the federal law does not cover executive and administrative professionals, teachers, salaried employees, or those who have been on the job less than one year. However, some states do have laws related to breast-feeding, many of which provide additional support. Check with your human resources department to see what accommodations your employer makes for nursing mothers.

Supplementing: The Best of Both Worlds?

Some people argue that combining breast-feeding and bottle-feeding involves all the hassles of both methods and only half the benefits of either. But many nursing mothers of multiples find that supplementing their nursing with formula eases their load. Lydia Greenwood says, "Much as I enjoyed nursing, it was a relief to be able to have someone else feed the twins so I could sleep an extra hour or get out of the house occasionally. Supplementing was also a boon in public places. I could nurse one twin discreetly (for me, there was nothing discreet about simultaneous breast-feeding) while my husband gave a bottle to the other."

Particularly in families with older children, supplementing often makes sense. "I felt disappointed about how little I was able to mother my two-year-old while I was pregnant with the twins. Because I wasn't supposed to overexert myself physically, I couldn't pick her up or play actively. Then, after the twins were born, nursing exclusively proved to be so time-consuming that there wasn't much time left for their big sister," says one mother of twins. "So I started to supplement my breast-feeding with one bottle in the evening. This way, someone else could feed the babies while I read to my toddler or gave her a bath."

For most nursing mothers of triplets or quadruplets, supplementing with formula has great

---

15. US Department of Labor. Fact sheet #73: Break time for nursing mothers under the FLSA. Washington, DC; 2013. http://www.dol.gov/whd/regs/compliance/whdfs73.htm.

appeal. For one thing, it affords the babies the benefits of breast milk while alleviating any doubts as to whether or not everyone is receiving enough nourishment. What's more, it allows the mother to share the feeding workload with the babies' father or another helper—a very welcome option, considering how time-consuming it can be to feed triplets or quads. "Each of my triplets got about two-thirds breast milk and one-third formula. This worked so well that I was able to continue breast-feeding for seven months," says Arlene McAndrew.

Working mothers, too, often opt to supplement. "For the first three months, Benjamin and Madeleine were breast-fed exclusively. But then it was time for me to return to my job as an occupational therapist," says Heather Nicholas. "I started nursing in the mornings and evenings only, and they got formula during the day. This was a lot less hassle than it would have been to pump my milk at work. It was a good balance—so good that I nursed until the twins were eight months old."

A word to the wise: If you think you'll want to supplement eventually, it's best to introduce one daily bottle by age three to four weeks, if not sooner. If you wait too long, one or more of your babies may refuse the rubber nipple completely. For the first bottle-feedings, you might pump or express some breast milk and mix that with formula, to allow your babies to adjust gradually to the difference in taste and smell. Also, ask your partner or a helper to hold the babies during those initial offerings of the bottle. Otherwise, knowing that Mommy's breasts are nearby, your babies may reject their bottles and hold out for the real thing.

Bottle-Feeding Basics

Have you decided to supplement your nursing with an occasional bottle, or to forgo breast-feeding altogether in favor of formula? Then you'll need to know the basics of bottle-feeding. Any good manual on infant care can provide detailed instructions. But there are some additional points you should be aware of as a parent of multiples.

While no infant formula can claim to convey all the advantages of breast milk, the brands available today are nutritious and easy to prepare, and you needn't doubt that your babies can thrive on them. Most formulas are derived from cow's milk. If one of your babies has allergies or a sensitive stomach, however, that baby may do better on a soy-based or protein-hydrolysate formula. If this is the case, ask your pediatrician if it's all right to simplify your life by putting all your babies on that type of formula.

Most infant formulas come in three ways. Ready-to-pour is the most convenient but also the most expensive. Liquid formula concentrate is cheaper but must be mixed with sterilized water, and any unused portion has to be promptly refrigerated. Least expensive is powdered formula. The opened can of powder does not require refrigeration, but it, too, must be combined with sterilized water—and mixed well to prevent clumps.

Formula should be gently warmed before being given to your babies. Never heat bottles in the microwave oven; too many babies have had their mouths scalded this way. Instead, warm the bottles by placing them in a bowl of hot tap water for a few minutes. Before using, test the temperature on the inside of your wrist to make sure it is warm enough but not hot. If possible, it is preferable to feed your babies from glass bottles. If you must use plastic baby bottles, make sure the plastic does not contain bisphenol-A (BPA). This plasticizing agent, considered to be an endocrine-disrupting chemical, has been banned from baby bottles in some states in the United States and in many foreign countries. For the same reason, once your babies start eating other foods, it also is wise to use glass rather than plastic containers to store and heat their food. It is best never to microwave food in plastic containers because microwaving increases the leaching of these chemicals out of the plastic.

One other note of caution: Never put your babies to bed with bottles. If milk is allowed to pool in their mouths as they sleep, serious tooth decay can result once their baby teeth come in. There is also the danger of choking, should a baby bite through the rubber nipple while you are not there to immediately handle the emergency.

TIME-SAVING TIPS ABOUT BOTTLES

With two or more babies to feed, you'll want to make mealtimes as easy as possible. Take a tip from Kelly Kassab, an experienced mother of multiples: "Each evening, I cleaned the bottles and nipples, sterilized the water, mixed the formula, and poured it into enough bottles to get us through the next 24 hours. Then whenever the girls were hungry, all I had to do was warm up two bottles."

Another time-saving tactic is to feed your multiples simultaneously. This is simple if other people are on hand to give bottles to the other babies. But what if you're alone? Propping bottles is not recommended. Along with the nourishment a feeding provides, babies also need the emotional and physical closeness that comes from being held or touched as they eat. (If you feel you must prop bottles on occasion, be sure not to leave the babies unsupervised. A baby who begins to choke must be attended to at once.)

Here are several positions that allow you to feed two babies at the same time:

• Sit on the floor with your back against the wall. Open your legs in a V and place the babies between your knees, their heads supported by a pillow and their feet pointing toward you. Use your thighs as armrests while you hold the bottles in either hand, stroking the babies' cheeks with a free finger and gazing into their eyes.

- Sit in a comfortable armchair so you can prop your left elbow on the armrest. Support the babies' weight in your lap while supporting both their heads with your left arm and hand. Lean one baby's bottle against your chest or in the crook of your right arm, and hold the other bottle in your right hand.
- Cradle one baby, curling your left arm around her to support her head while your left hand holds her bottle. Lay the other baby with his head in your lap, and hold his bottle with your right hand.
- Lean back in an armchair and put both babies in a semiseated position on your lap, their backs and heads supported by your chest and arms. Hold one bottle in each hand.

What if several babies are screaming with hunger, yet you can't manage to feed simultaneously? Give the fussiest baby half a feeding to calm him, then feed the others, and then finish up with the first. To keep track of how much each child eats and avoid inadvertent bottle swaps between babies, use color-coded bottles.

ALL ABOUT BURPING

Whether your babies get breast milk or formula, you won't want to neglect an essential element of every feeding: the burp. An infant whose tummy is uncomfortably full of gas won't be able to take in the milk she needs to thrive. So be sure to burp your babies once or twice during each feeding, not just at the end.

If the traditional over-the-shoulder hold doesn't elicit the desired release of gas, try a different position. "Holly always belched whenever I patted her back, no matter how I held her. But her twin brother, Alexander, was trickier," says Lydia Greenwood. "Finally I found two positions that usually worked. I could lay him tummy side down across my lap and very gently move my knees up and down against his stomach. Or I could sit him in my lap, with one hand supporting his chest and head, and the other rubbing his back. One or the other technique usually brought up a very satisfying burp."

And satisfaction—for you and for all your babies—is what successful feeding is all about.

Chapter Twelve

A Better Body After Babies

Now that your journey through pregnancy and delivery is over, you're ready to reclaim your body! It's time to turn your attention not only to reshaping your figure, but also to making your body as strong and healthy as possible. This chapter is a practical guide to helping you become as fit and healthy as you have ever been—perhaps even more so than before this pregnancy.

This may not be nearly as challenging as you fear. "I gained 55 pounds during my twin pregnancy, and I had worried that I'd be stuck with lots of unwanted weight. But the pounds just dropped off of me! Within two weeks of delivery, I lost 45 of those 55 pounds. And the rest came off once I was able to get back to exercising regularly," says Megan Ryerson.

It is true that many women cite pregnancy as a sentinel event that began their lifelong struggle with weight. That experience has been confirmed by large, long-term studies like the CARDIA Study (Coronary Artery Risk Development in Young Adults)[1, 2] and the SPAWN Study (Stockholm Pregnancy and Women's Nutrition).[3, 4] This doesn't have to be the case, how-

1. Smith DE, Lewis CE, Caveny JL, Perkins LL, Burke GL, Bild DE. Longitudinal changes in adiposity associated with pregnancy: The CARDIA Study. Journal of the American Medical Association 1994; 271:1747–51.
2. Gunderson EP, Murtaugh MA, Lewis CE, Quesenberry CP, West DS, Sidney S. Excess gains in weight and waist circumference associated with childbearing: The Coronary Artery Risk Development in Young Adults Study (CARDIA). International Journal of Obesity 2004; 28:525–35.
3. Linne Y, Rossner S. Interrelationships between weight development and weight retention in subsequent pregnancies: The SPAWN Study. Acta Obstetricia et Gynecologica Scandinavica 2003; 82:318–25.
4. Linne Y, Dye L, Barkeling B, Rossner S. Weight development over time in parous women—The SPAWN Study—15 years follow-up. International Journal of Obesity 2003; 27:1516–22.

ever. The sooner you begin to take off the weight you put on during your multiple pregnancy—and the healthier the strategies you use in working toward this goal—the more successful you are likely to be.

During pregnancy, it is normal for a certain amount of body fat to be accumulated. This fat, which is used to meet the energy requirements of the mother and babies before birth and during lactation, is stored primarily in three areas—the triceps (upper arm), subscapular area (below the shoulder blades), and thighs.

If you followed the weight-gain guidelines for your prepregnancy body mass index (BMI), a significant amount of that fat was mobilized during the last trimester of your pregnancy, and you have been left with less postpartum weight to lose. But even if you gained more weight than you had expected or if your shape has changed in ways you hadn't planned, there's no need to feel discouraged.

The most important thing you can do is to prioritize your weight-loss and health-boosting goals. True, now that you are the mother of two or more children, your time and energy are at a premium, so it's all too easy to put your own needs last. That is a mistake. In order to take good care of your family, you must also take good care of yourself.

Studies show that a mother's body weight at one year postpartum is predictive of her subsequent risk for obesity, so the weight-loss efforts you make now are a wise investment in your future health. A word of caution, however: Do not try to lose weight *too* quickly, or your health will suffer—for instance, you may become run-down, more prone to infections, and less able to heal and recover. You will also adversely affect your ability to breast-feed effectively. So give yourself three to six months to regain your shape.

This may wind up being much easier than you think. One mother of twins reports, "I gained 63 pounds during my pregnancy. My twins made it the full 40 weeks and weighed 7 lb., 4 oz. each at birth. It wasn't hard to lose the pregnancy weight because chasing multiples around after they're born is quite a workout. Within six months, I was back to my prepregnancy weight—without having to do any extra exercise or calorie-cutting."

Even if you had triplets or quads, you can take off most if not all of the weight within three to six months. A mother of triplets says, "I closely followed the diet this book laid out for a healthy triplet pregnancy, and I managed to go a full 36 weeks. At birth, my triplets weighed in at 6 lb., 8 oz., 5 lb., 12 oz., and 5 lb., 7 oz. They had no health issues—no NICU time, no tubes, nothing—and came home from the hospital with me after just four days. I had gained a total of 81 pounds while pregnant, and now at five months postpartum, I have just seven left to lose."

The key to that kind of success is to develop the right habits. Bad habits (like overspending on credit cards) can get anyone into trouble. But habits can also be very positive—like regularly contributing to your retirement account or your children's college fund. In the same way, good habits will help you regain your figure. There are three essential good habits that are key to achieving long-lasting weight loss:

- A healthy diet.
- Regular exercise.
- Adequate sleep.

To be effective, these good habits must become part of your daily, long-term routine. Although it is human nature to want a quick fix for those extra pounds or that too-round tummy, there are no such speedy solutions. Instead, you need to commit to making good decisions about food, physical activity, and rest—day in and day out.

The National Weight Control Registry,[5] a nationwide study of more than 5,000 adults who have maintained a weight loss of at least 30 pounds for a year or more, demonstrates the power of healthy habits. Registry members report using the following strategies to lose weight and keep it off:

- 98% modified their food intake.
- 94% increased their physical activity, with walking being the form of exercise reported most often.
- 90% exercise for an average of one hour per day.
- 78% eat breakfast every day.
- 75% weigh themselves at least once a week.
- 62% watch less than 10 hours of television per week.

DR. LUKE: As a postpartum woman, you have a distinct advantage over other women—because you are in a metabolic state that favors weight loss. This is part of a natural process of healing and transformation that is already happening to you, so you just need to help it along to get the long-term results that you're hoping for.

As with any new diet and exercise program, get your doctor's approval before starting the regimen that follows.

---

5. The National Weight Control Registry can be accessed at www.nwcr.ws.

Postpartum Diet Principles

The same healthful dietary principles you followed during your pregnancy (as outlined in Chapters 4 and 5) still apply now—with a few modifications. Basically, you should continue to adhere to a diabetic diet. By stabilizing your blood sugar levels, this diet maximizes your energy while minimizing hunger pangs that could sabotage your weight-loss efforts.

The prescription for a postpartum diabetic diet includes getting 20 to 25 percent of your daily calories from protein, 30 percent from fats, and 45 to 50 percent from carbohydrates. Here are simple ways to apply the diabetic principles for stable blood sugar levels now that you have delivered:

- Eat often—at least three meals plus one to two snacks per day.
- Eat lean proteins, especially those rich in iron (such as lean red meats), as well as fish, poultry, dairy, eggs, and nuts.
- Eat healthy fats, such as mono- and polyunsaturated fats (found in olive oil, canola oil, nuts, and seeds), and omega-3 fatty acids (found in fish, enriched eggs, and flaxseed). Limit saturated fats and high-fat dairy. Avoid all sources of trans fats (such as hydrogenated vegetable shortening and some margarines).
- Eat carbohydrate-rich foods that are unrefined or minimally processed whenever possible. Focus on fresh fruits and vegetables, legumes, and whole grains; avoid refined carbohydrates (cookies, pastries, white bread) and starchy foods.
- Eat protein and carbohydrates together in every snack and every meal.
- Eat a bedtime snack that includes dairy.

In Table 12.1, these principles are applied to four healthy postpartum diets, ranging from 1,200 to 1,800 calories per day. Each of these diet prescriptions also is translated into the recommended number of daily servings of each major food group. (Note that these caloric intakes apply to *non-nursing* mothers. If you are breast-feeding, the caloric demands of nursing should put you at your prepregnancy weight within three to six months after delivery. If that does not happen and you want to continue to lose weight, decrease the amount of fat in your diet and reduce portion sizes for all the various foods *except dairy*, as discussed in Chapter 11.)

Estimated Nutrient Requirements and Recommended Servings per Day for Non-Nursing Postpartum Mothers of Multiples

	Percent of calories	For a 1,200-calorie diet	For a 1,400-calorie diet	For a 1,600-calorie diet	For a 1,800-calorie diet
Protein (grams)	20–25%	60–75	70–88	80–100	90–112
Carbohydrate (grams)	45–50%	135–150	158–175	180–200	202–225
Fat (grams)	30%	40	47	54	60
Food groups	**Serving size**	**Servings**	**Servings**	**Servings**	**Servings**
Dairy (nonfat or low fat)	8 oz. milk or yogurt, or 1 oz. cheese	3	4	4	4
Lean meat, poultry, fish, eggs	1 oz., or 1 medium egg	4	5	6	6
Vegetables	½ cup cooked, or 1 cup raw	6	7	8	8
Fruits	1 medium fruit, or ½ cup sliced	3	4	5	6
Grains, starchy vegetables*	1 slice bread, or ½ cup	2	2	2	3
Fats, oils, nuts	1 tbsp. oil or butter, or 12 nuts	5	6	6	7

*Starchy vegetables include corn, potatoes, chickpeas, beans, and peas.

Table 12.1

Following are three important strategies that will help you adhere to the guidelines:

- **Eat often enough.** To stabilize your blood sugar levels, minimize hunger, and promote weight loss, you need to eat at least four or five times a day, preferably every three to four hours throughout the day. Eat smaller meals plus larger, nutritionally balanced snacks.

- **Consume *enough* calories.** Although this advice might sound counterintuitive, eating fewer calories than your body's minimum daily requirement can actually cause you to *store* fat rather than lose it. To keep your metabolism humming and promote steady weight loss, aim for 1,200 to 1,400 calories a day if you delivered twins. If you are a new mother of triplets or quads, use the 1,600-calorie to 1,800-calorie guidelines—you will still lose weight, because your energy expenditures and caloric requirements will be much greater. (If you are nursing, add 500 calories per baby to these daily calorie counts.)

- **But do not eat *too many* calories.** Portion distortion seems to be the rule these days, as more and more people become overweight. A primary reason is that most people don't realize how many calories are on their plate. An excellent way to avoid overeating is to fill up on the less calorically dense foods first—for instance, by having a salad before eating pizza. When you do eat higher-calorie foods, reduce portion sizes. To do this without feeling deprived, it helps to include some low-calorie add-ons—for instance, extra veggies as the pizza topping. If you are going to have ice cream for dessert or a snack, fill a small bowl half full, and add fresh fruit. If you just can't resist the temptation of cookies, chips, or chocolate, limit the portions by buying prepackaged 100-calorie servings.

DR. NEWMAN: The preceding recommendations are particularly important if you were diagnosed with gestational diabetes during your multiple pregnancy. Even if postpartum testing reveals that your gestational diabetes has resolved after the birth of your babies, you are still at increased risk for long-term consequences. That's because a diagnosis of gestational diabetes is strongly associated with the subsequent development of adult-onset diabetes later in life. Between 20 and 50 percent of women diagnosed with gestational diabetes go on to develop impaired glucose tolerance (prediabetes) or full-blown diabetes within 10 to 20 years. Establishing appropriate habits regarding diet, exercise, and healthy behaviors, such as those presented in this chapter, is the only known way to reduce the long-term risk of developing type 2 diabetes.

Here's a bonus: These same healthy nutritional and exercise habits can also help prevent or reduce the severity of hypertensive disorders and other chronic health conditions down the road if you integrate them into your daily lifestyle now. There is no better time than right after the delivery of your babies to make such changes—because your babies are already bringing so many new changes to your lifestyle.

Making the Right Food Choices

What you eat is as important as how much and how often you eat in determining your weight-loss success. But since free time is practically nonexistent when you have two or more babies to take care of, you probably won't have much opportunity to plan menus or hunt for tasty, nutritious, slimming recipes. To simplify these tasks, refer to the following menu suggestions. An asterisk indicates that the recipe appears at the back of this book.

Menu Suggestions for the Fourth Trimester

BREAKFAST
*Asparagus Quiche
*Autumn Pancakes
Blueberry Muffins
Egg Burritos
French Toast with Applesauce
*French Toast with Ham and Cheese
Grilled Cheese and Tomato Sandwich
Grilled Ham and Cheese Sandwich
*Harvest Muffins
Oatmeal with Dried Cherries
*Oatmeal-Almond Pancakes
*Powerhouse Granola
*Pumpkin-Fruit Muffins
*Pumpkin Loaf
*Pumpkin Waffles
Quiche Lorraine
Scrambled Eggs and Raisin Toast
*Weekend Hash Browns
Whole-wheat Pancakes
Whole-Wheat Toast with Peanut Butter
*Wild Rice Omelet

LUNCH OR DINNER
*Arugula and Pear Salad
*Asian-Style Meatballs

*Asparagus Quiche
*Avocado Salad with Orange and Grapefruit
Baked Ham
Baked Manicotti
Beef and Barley Soup
*Beef and Bean Chili
Beef Brisket
*Beef Stew
*Beef Stroganoff
Beef Tacos
Beef Teriyaki
*Beet Salad with Goat Cheese
*Caesar Salad with Shrimp
*Caprese Salad
*Cashew Chicken Cheeseburgers
Cheese Lasagna
*Chicken and Dumplings
*Chicken and Sweet Potatoes
*Chicken and Wild Rice Casserole
*Chicken-Barley Soup
*Chicken-Citrus Salad
Chicken Pot Pie
*Chinese Chicken Salad
*Citrus Salmon
*Cobb Salad
Corned Beef and Cabbage

Gefilte Fish
Grilled Chicken
Grilled Pork Chops
Grilled Salmon
*Ginger Stir-Fry
*Golden Chicken Salad
*Greek Lemon Chicken
*Greek Salad
*Greek Spinach and Cheese Pie
*Ham and Pumpkin Quiche
*Honey Chicken Salad with Cherries
*Lamb and Lentil Stew
*Lamb Salad
*Lentil and Ham Salad with Walnuts
*Lentil Soup
*Linguine with Clams and Dried Tomatoes
London Broil
Manhattan Clam Chowder
Marinated Pork Tenderloin
*Maple Pork and Spinach Salad
*Mediterranean Sauté
*Mini-Meat Loaves
New England Clam Chowder
*Pasta with Chicken and Peanut Sauce
*Pasta with Green Sauce
*Pasta with Peas and Ham
*Pork and Cashew Bok Choy
*Pork with Apple Stuffing
Pepper Steak
Pork Roast
Pot Roast
*Salad Niçoise
*Salmon and Asparagus Salad
*Salmon Burgers
*Salsa Frittata
*Seasoned Baked Chicken
*Shrimp and Scallop Grill

*Spicy Beef
*Spicy Pork with Peanut Sauce
*Spicy Shrimp Salad
*Spinach and Pumpkin Casserole
*Steak and Arugula Salad
Shrimp Egg Foo Yung
Spaghetti and Meatballs
Sweet and Sour Pork
*Tomato Apricot Salad
Tuna Casserole
*Tuna Salad with White Beans
*Vegetarian Lasagna
*Vegetarian Stroganoff
*Vietnamese Steak Salad
*Waldorf Chicken Salad
Whitefish Salad

SNACKS
Apple Slices and Peanut Butter
Apple, Walnut, and Cheese Salad
Baked Apples with Cheddar Cheese
*Basic Fruit Smoothie
*Basic Vegetable Smoothie
*Chickpea Salad
Cottage Cheese and Fruit
Deviled Eggs with Toast
Fruit Salad with Cheese and Crackers
*Ginger Smoothie
*Golden Chicken Salad
Oatmeal-Walnut Cookies with Yogurt
*Pumpkin Custard
*Ratatouille
*Sunrise Bread Pudding
*Tabbouleh
Vanilla Yogurt with Walnuts and Wheat
  Germ
*Yogurt Guacamole

DR. LUKE: Among the 75 original recipes at the back of this book are a number of hearty salads. You also can design your own nutritious main-dish salads. One of my favorite ways to do this is to use the grid in Table 12.2. Start with a bowl of chopped leafy greens, add lots of vegetables, one or two protein foods, some nuts, and a fruit. For dressing, try a two-to-one mixture of balsamic vinegar (either white or regular) and olive oil.

Best Ways to Build a Salad

	Protein Foods	Nuts	Fruits	Vegetables	Leafy Greens
Portion Size	3 ½ oz.	½ oz.	½–1 cup fresh	½–1 cup	2 cups
Calories	About 200	About 100	About 50	About 25	About 25
	Beans	Almonds	Apples	Asparagus	Arugula
	Beef	Cashews	Apricots	Bamboo shoots	Basil
	Chicken	Hazelnuts	Avocado	Bean sprouts	Beet greens
	Cottage cheese	Peanuts	Banana	Beets	Boston lettuce
	Eggs	Pecans	Blackberries	Bell peppers	Butterhead lettuce
	Lamb	Pine nuts	Blueberries	Broccoli	Cilantro
	Pork	Pistachios	Cherries	Cabbage	Dandelion greens
	Salmon	Soybean nuts	Coconuts	Carrots	Endive
	Shellfish	Walnuts	Grapefruit	Celery	Escarole
	Tofu		Grapes	Chickpeas*	Mint
	Tuna		Lemons	Chives	Parsley
	Turkey		Limes	Corn**	Radicchio
			Mango	Cucumbers	Red leaf lettuce
			Melons	Fennel	Romaine lettuce
			Nectarines	Green beans	Spinach
			Oranges	Hearts of palm	Watercress

	Protein Foods	Fruits	Vegetables	Leafy Greens
Portion Size	2 oz.	½–1 cup fresh	½–1 cup	2 cups
Calories	About 200	About 50	About 25	
	Semi-soft and Hard Cheese:	Papaya	Mushrooms	
	Cheddar	Peaches	Olives	
	Edam	Pears	Onions	
	Feta	Pineapple	Pea pods	
	Goat	Plums	Peas**	
	Gouda	Pomegranates	Radishes	
	Monterey Jack	Raspberries	Tomatoes	
	Mozzarella	Strawberries	Water chestnuts	
	Muenster	Tomatoes		
	Parmesan			
	Swiss			

*Chickpeas have about 140 calories per ½ cup. **Corn and peas have about 60 calories per ½ cup.

Table 12.2

HOW FIBER HELPS

Another key to postpartum weight loss is to eat an adequate amount of fiber, which helps your body burn fat and stabilizes blood sugar and insulin levels. Adults should aim for *25 to 35 grams of fiber a day*—but most Americans get less than half that amount. Look for breads and grains that provide at least 3 grams of fiber per serving. Here are some examples:

- Oats contain 4 grams of fiber per ½ cup dry, or per 1 cup cooked.
- Seeds of Change microwaveable grains provide 4 to 5 grams of fiber per serving and come in a variety of flavors, such as Uyini Quinoa and Whole Grain Brown Rice, and Tigris—A Mixture of Seven Whole Grains.
- Feldkamp Famous German breads contain 6 grams of fiber per slice. Types include Whole Rye and Whole Rye with Muesli, Pumpernickel and Westphalian Pumpernickel, Fitness, Linseed, Sunflower Seed, and Three Grain.

- Thomas' English Muffins Double Fiber Honey Wheat provide 5 grams of fiber per muffin; the light version contains 8 grams of fiber and 125 calories.
- Brownberry Natural Health Nut Loaf has 3 grams of fiber per 100-calorie slice.
- Fruits with the highest amount of fiber per serving (5 to 6 grams) include prunes, raspberries, raisins, figs, and avocados. Fruits with 3 to 4 grams of fiber per serving include oranges, apples, pears, blueberries, and strawberries. Eat at least two to four servings of fruit daily.
- Vegetables with high fiber content include all varieties of beans (6 to 7 grams per serving), pumpkin (4 grams per serving), and chickpeas, squash, green peas, and fresh corn (3 grams per serving). Aim for at least two to four servings of vegetables every day.

The time of day at which you eat certain carbohydrate-rich foods also can affect how quickly you lose weight. The reason has to do with insulin sensitivity (the cells' ability to pick up and use insulin). The greater your insulin sensitivity is, the less pronounced are the fluctuations you experience in blood sugar and insulin levels. Insulin sensitivity is greatest early in the day. For this reason, starchy carbohydrates like bread and oatmeal—which are absorbed into the bloodstream more rapidly than other types of carbohydrates are—should be eaten earlier in the day, when the body is better able to keep blood sugar levels stable.

For an afternoon snack and at dinner, choose carbohydrates from fruits and vegetables, or from high-fiber grains like sweet potatoes, quinoa, millet, and wild rice. These will be absorbed more slowly than other carbohydrate-rich foods would, so they are appropriate for times of day when insulin sensitivity is reduced.

DESIGNING YOUR PLATE

DR. LUKE: One reason it's so easy to overindulge is that we tend to eat what we see, even if it fills us up way beyond the point needed to satisfy hunger. One simple way to reduce the urge to overeat is to design your plate—to fill it with predetermined proportions of particular types of foods. This concept is endorsed by various nutrition-oriented organizations. You can even buy special china plates and bowls with divisions for the types and quantities of foods recommended.

The idea is simple. First, reduce the size of your plate. Put away your regular dinner plates, or use them only as chargers beneath your luncheon plates and soup bowls. Second, fill your plate with specific amounts and types of food—one-third with low-fat protein and two-thirds with healthful carbohydrates (fruits, vegetables, and whole grains).

One of the diet experts I respect most is Dr. Brian Wansink, a consumer food behavior researcher and author of *Mindless Eating: Why We Eat More Than We Think.* He says, "The best diet is the one you don't know you're on." Along with the designed plate concept, Dr. Wansink recommends the following portion-control strategies.

- **Take 20 percent less—and 20 percent more.** Serve yourself a portion of food that is about 20 percent *less* than you usually eat—you probably won't even miss those extra bites. If the meal or snack looks too skimpy, dish out 20 percent *more* vegetables and fruits.

- **See everything you're going to eat.** Even if you're just having a snack, put everything on your plate before you begin eating—never eat directly out of the package or from the serving platter. As soon as you've served yourself, put away the food package or any leftovers. See what you're eating while you eat it, too. Don't clear away the chicken bones or empty bottles, for example. By serving as visual reminders of how much you have already eaten, they help keep you from overeating.

- **Downsize your food packages and reduce your food choices.** Food behavior research shows that the bigger the food package, the more a person typically eats. For instance, you're likely to eat 20 to 30 percent more cereal, pasta, crackers, or bread when the box or bag it comes in is large, compared to when the package is small. The same thing happens when there are lots of food selections—the more variety, the more likely you are to overeat.

- **Make overeating a hassle.** When you serve a meal, leave the serving platters in the kitchen or on a sideboard, not on the dining table—so second helpings of calorie-dense foods are beyond easy reach. For salads and vegetables, turn this strategy around—place the platters near you on the table, to encourage you to choose these foods if you want a second helping.

- **Don't eat while distracted.** Eat only at the table, even for snacks, so you can be mindful of what and how much you are consuming. Never eat in front of the television or while driving. When you're distracted, you're likely to eat far more than you intended without even realizing it.

- **Never eat the leftovers from anyone else's plate.** Many moms, not wanting food to go to waste, nibble on whatever their family members left uneaten on their plates. But you are better off saving or discarding those leftovers. Remember, it's better for other people's leftovers to go to waste than for them to go to *your* waist.

WHY YOU NEED WATER, WATER, WATER

There are several reasons why it is important to stay hydrated. First, drinking too little water throughout the day causes your metabolism to slow down, reducing your body's ability to burn fat. Second, when you think that you're hungry, you may in fact only be thirsty. If you drink a glass of water, you often will feel satisfied without having to reach for a snack. Third, if you are nursing, dehydration adversely affects your breast milk production.

How much water should a woman drink in a day? A simple guide is to take your current weight and divide by two—that's the number of ounces you should be getting every day. For example, if your current weight is 200 pounds, you should be drinking about 100 ounces of water (equal to 12½ cups, or a little more than 3 quarts, or about 3 liters). If your current weight is 160 pounds, you should be drinking about 80 ounces of water a day (equal to 10 cups, or about ½ gallon, or about 2.3 liters).

Fit-and-Firm Workout

Physical activity is another essential element for reclaiming your body—and it benefits more than just your figure. Here's what regular exercise can do for you:

- It helps you regain your strength. This is especially important if you were on bedrest during your multiple pregnancy, because muscles weaken when physical activity is limited for a prolonged period of time.
- Exercise boosts your metabolism, making it easier to lose weight.
- It increases your energy, so you feel less fatigued during the day—and it promotes better sleep, so you feel more rested (despite those frequent nighttime feedings).
- Aerobic activity benefits your cardiovascular system. Also, by improving circulation, it increases the delivery of nutrients and oxygen to all the cells of your body and helps prevent blood clots in the legs (which you are at increased risk for during the first month or two postpartum).
- Being active promotes optimal function of your immune system, helping to keep you healthy.
- Exercise promotes psychological well-being by triggering the release of mood-boosting endorphins.

The simplest way to ease back into exercise after childbirth is to walk. Put your newborns in their stroller and take them out for a walk every day. When the weather doesn't cooperate, take your walk inside a mall. An added advantage to walking while pushing a stroller is that you also get an upper-body workout. Don't get discouraged if you can manage only 10 minutes or so at first. Just keep at it and your endurance will soon increase. Gradually build up until you are walking for 45 to 60 minutes daily.

In addition to walking, you'll want to do specific exercises that help you tone, strengthen, and stretch. This is particularly important for your abdominal muscles, which were very stretched out during your multiple pregnancy. Several of the exercises that follow are Pilates techniques, which utilize balance and resistance to build strong core muscles in your abdomen and back.

The following regimen includes six different exercises. For exercises that alternate sides of the body, one repetition (or rep) equals doing the move once to each side. For each exercise (unless otherwise indicated), start with five to eight reps and gradually build up until you can do 15 reps. When you can complete one set of 15 reps, try for two sets of eight reps, again gradually increasing until you can do two sets of 15 reps for each exercise. Always move slowly, in a controlled fashion, and never force a stretch. Don't forget to breathe! For the floor exercises, place a mat or towel on the floor. Try to do the whole series of exercises every day or at least every other day.

1. Windmill Stretch

Stand tall, arms at your sides, feet about hip-width apart. Bend forward at the waist, keeping your knees straight. Reach your right hand down to touch (or try to touch) your left foot, while reaching your left arm straight over your head. Hold for a count of three. Return to standing position. Repeat with the left hand touching the right foot.

2. Progressive Push-ups

Here are four options, labeled A through D, which get progressively more challenging. Move to the next level once you can do two sets of 15 reps at the easier level.

A. Wall Push-up: Stand facing a wall, about an arm's length away. Place your palms flat against the wall at shoulder height, arms straight, fingers pointing up. Slowly bend your elbows, keeping your heels on the floor and your spine straight, and bringing your upper body to within a few inches of the wall. Hold for 1 to 2 seconds, then push back to the starting position.

B. Forearm Push-up: Get down on your hands and knees. To get into the starting position, carefully walk your hands forward until you can lower yourself onto your forearms, so your knees are on the floor and your hips, back, and head are aligned at a diagonal to the floor. Next, slowly lower your body until it is within a few inches of the floor, then push back to the starting position.

C. GIRL's PUSH-UP: Get down on your hands and knees. To get into the starting position, walk your hands forward until your hips, back, and head are aligned at a diagonal to the floor. (Your knees should still be on the floor.) Next, slowly lower your body until it is within a few inches of the floor, then push back to the starting position.

D. CLASSIC PUSH-UP: Get down on your hands and knees. To get into the starting position, straighten one leg and then the other so your toes and balls of the feet are on the floor. Your arms should be straight, hands directly beneath your shoulders, and your hips, back, and head should be aligned and nearly parallel to the floor. Trying to keep as straight as a plank, bend your elbows, lowering your body to within a few inches of the floor, then straighten your arms and push yourself back up to the starting position.

---

3. Spine Twist

Sit on the floor with your legs straight and spread as wide as you comfortably can. Extend your arms straight out to the sides at shoulder height, palms facing down. Next, twist at the waist to rotate your upper body as far as possible to the left without moving your hips or legs. Gently pulse three times, twisting a little farther each time. Return to the starting position, then repeat by twisting to the right.

---

4. Single Leg Stretch and Tummy Toner

Lie flat on your back, arms straight and stretched toward the ceiling above you, legs straight and together. Inhaling, use your abdominal muscles to lift your head and shoulder blades off the floor. At the same time, keeping your right leg straight and extended on the floor, bend your left leg to bring your left knee to your chest. Holding the left knee with both hands, exhale as you pulse three times, lifting your upper body a little farther off the floor and pulling your knee closer with each pulse. (The idea is to use your abdominal muscles and increase hip flexibility, not to yank on your knee.) Return to starting position, then repeat with the other leg.

---

5. Double Leg Stretch and Tummy Toner

Lie flat on your back, arms straight and stretched toward the ceiling, legs straight and together. Inhaling, use your abdominal muscles to lift your head and shoulder blades off the floor. At the same time, bend both legs and bring both knees toward your chest, placing your hands on your shins and tucking in your chin. Exhale and hold this position for the count of three, then return to starting position.

6. The Hundred

Lie flat on your back, arms straight at your sides. Beginners' version: Lift your legs off the ground and bend your knees at about a 90-degree angle, so your shins are nearly parallel to the floor. Using your abdominal muscles to lift your head and shoulder blades off the floor, bring your chin to your chest and raise your arms so that they are straight out in front of you, a few inches above the floor. Keep your pelvis stable and focus on using your abdominal muscles, not your lower back muscles. It helps to perform Kegel exercises at the same time (see Chapter 6). Inhale to a count of five, then exhale to a count of five, pumping your arms up and down about 6 to 8 inches on each count. Do 10 to 20 pumps, then relax. Work up to 100 pumps (hence the name of the exercise). Intermediate version: Do the exercise as described, but keep your legs straight and stretched toward the ceiling, so they are at a 90-degree angle to the floor. Advanced version: Do the exercise as described, but keep your legs straight and stretched out on a diagonal, so they are at a 45-degree angle to the floor.

Plot Your Progress

It is very motivating to monitor how your body is changing as you lose weight and build muscle. Weigh yourself regularly—at least once a week.

In addition, you'll want to take certain measurements. As discussed earlier, during pregnancy body fat is stored at the triceps (upper arms), subscapular area (below the shoulder blades), and thighs. Each week, record your weight and the following circumference measurements (as taken with a nonstretch tape measure):

- Upper bust: at your underarms.
- Mid bust: at fullest part of your bust, wearing a bra.
- Lower bust: just under your breasts.
- Upper arm: midway between shoulder and elbow.
- Waist: at the smallest point.
- Hips: at the widest point.
- Upper thigh: three-fourths of the way up the thigh, between knee and hip.
- Mid thigh: halfway between knee and hip.
- Knee: just above the kneecap.
- Calf: halfway between ankle and knee.

Use Table 12.3 to track your progress over a six-month period.

Postpartum Progress Report

Date	Week	Weight	BMI	Bust Upper	Bust Mid	Bust Lower	Mid-Upper Arm	Waist	Hips	Waist-to-Hip Ratio	Thigh Upper	Thigh Mid	Knee	Calf
	1													
	2													
	3													
	4													
	5													
	6													
	7													
	8													
	9													
	10													
	11													
	12													
	13													
	14													
	15													

Date	Week	Weight	BMI	Bust			Mid-Upper Arm	Waist	Hips	Waist-to-Hip Ratio	Thigh		Knee	Calf
				Upper	Mid	Lower					Upper	Mid		
	16													
	17													
	18													
	19													
	20													
	21													
	22													
	23													
	24													
	25													
	26													

Table 12.3

As gratifying as it is to see the number on the bathroom scale move steadily downward, good health requires that you keep track of several other important numbers, too. One of these is your body mass index (BMI), a calculation based on weight and height. An ideal BMI is between 18.5 and 24.9. For an online BMI calculator, go to http://www.nhlbi.nhi.gov/health/educational/lose_wt/BMI/bmicalc.htm. Table 12.3 includes a column for recording your BMI week to week.

Another number to consider is your percentage of body fat. Ideally, women should have about 22 to 26 percent body fat—but the average woman in the United States has about 32 percent or more. To put this in perspective, elite gymnasts average about 14 percent, aerobic instructors about 17 percent, and swimmers about 20 percent.

Your waist-to-hip ratio (waist circumference divided by hip circumference) is also an indicator of health. An ideal ratio is less than 0.80.

Table 12.4 lists the ranges in body weight and hip measurements, by height, associated with 22 to 26 percent body fat and normal-weight BMI.

Target Weight and Hip Measurements by Height

Height	Weight (pounds)	Hip Measurement (inches)
4'10"	108–120	30–32.5
4'11"	110–123	31–33.5
5'	112–126	31.5–34
5'1"	115–129	32–34.5
5'2"	118–132	32.5–35
5'3"	121–135	33.5–36
5'4"	124–138	34–36.5
5'5"	127–141	34.5–37
5'6"	130–144	35.5–38
5'7"	133–147	36–38.5
5'8"	136–150	36.5–39.5
5'9"	139–153	37.5–40
5'10"	142–156	38–40.5
5'11"	145–159	38.5–41
6'	148–162	39.5–42

Table 12.4

When the Weight Goes but the Belly Stays

Some postpartum women, especially those who have given birth to multiples, find that even after they lose the pregnancy weight, their bellies continue to bulge. Here's why: During pregnancy, the growing uterus stretches the muscles in the abdomen as well as the overlying skin. This can cause the two large parallel bands of muscles (the *rectus abdominus* muscles) that meet in the middle of the abdomen to separate. This condition, called *diastasis recti* or *diastasis recti abdominis,* typically develops in late pregnancy but becomes most noticeable after delivery.

When the abdominal muscles separate this way, the uterus, bowels, and other organs have just a thin band of connective tissue holding them in place. In mild cases, there may be a ridge in the middle of the abdomen that is noticeable only when the ab muscles are tense (such as during coughing or straining), and the condition may resolve itself as the muscles naturally regain their tone and strength. In more severe cases, however, the belly bulge is pronounced enough that a woman may feel as though she still looks pregnant many months after delivery. The weakened abdominal muscles can lead to lower back pain. Hernias also may develop, and these can be painful as well.

You are at increased risk for diastasis recti if you:

- Are age 35 or older.
- Have a BMI of 30 or greater.
- Had excess amniotic fluid (polyhydramnios) during your pregnancy.
- Delivered babies with a high combined birthweight.
- Gave birth to triplets or quads.

If you have symptoms that suggest diastasis recti, talk to your doctor. Certain exercises may help you regain abdominal strength and reduce the separation between the muscles, especially if the condition is not too severe. Arlene McAndrew, mother of triplets, says, "I didn't have any pain or hernias from my diastasis recti, but the separation in the muscles was as wide as five fingers. I went to a physical therapist, who showed me specific exercises to do. They really helped—the separation decreased to just one and a half fingers wide, and has continued to improve."

In severe cases, particularly if the diastasis recti is interfering with your daily activities or if you develop a painful hernia, surgery may be recommended to repair the muscle separation. "Even though I had no trouble dropping the pregnancy weight, my belly stayed big because of the diastasis recti. A year after delivery, I still felt like I looked six months pregnant. I also was in a lot of discomfort and I wasn't digesting food properly. Ab exercises didn't help—in fact, they were painful. It turned out that I didn't just have a 'pooch.' I had several hernias, one of which was among the biggest my doctor had ever seen. He said I needed surgical repair for the hernias, plus abdominoplasty to tighten the abdominal muscles," says Megan Ryerson. "There's a stigma associated with getting a tummy tuck, and my insurance didn't cover the whole cost of the operation because they claimed it was partially cosmetic. But I'm so glad I did it! The surgery gave me my life back. I can run fine again, food doesn't bother me anymore, and my body looks pretty much like it did before I had children."

DR. LUKE: We have been able to get insurance to cover postpartum tummy tucks for many of our Multiples Clinic moms because diastasis recti is so common among mothers of twins, triplets, and quads. Particularly when a woman develops back pain or other symptoms, a strong case can be made that the surgery is therapeutic and not simply cosmetic.

The Importance of Sleep

The third essential element in reshaping your postpregnancy body is rest. Sleep deprivation has metabolic effects that predispose a person to weight gain—and also to depression. Research has shown that brain functions that affect energy levels, eating behaviors, and metabolism are strongly linked to circadian rhythms and sleep. Disruption of this circadian clock can have adverse metabolic effects—including a drop in satiety-promoting hormones and a rise in appetite-promoting hormones.

As a mother of newborns, your circadian rhythm is already disrupted. To minimize the effects of this, you should use every opportunity to rest, and try to sleep whenever possible. Creating those opportunities is a primary focus of the next chapter. The more you can incorporate the suggestions from Chapter 13 into your life, the more well-rested and less stressed you're likely to be. These strategies, along with the diet and exercise tips presented here, will help to give you a healthier, slimmer, fitter body than ever before.

Chapter Thirteen

The Crazy First Months at Home

Ruth Markowitz looked around the nursery and broke into a cold sweat. There was the changing table, but she scarcely knew how to fasten a diaper. There was the infant bathtub, but she panicked at the thought of holding a wet, wiggling baby. There was the crib, where newborn Nicola was screaming with hunger. And there was the other crib, where Evan was mingling his cries with those of his twin. "I was petrified," confesses Ruth. "How would I manage to feed, carry, clean, and soothe two babies at once? I was afraid to touch them." There's a word for what Ruth was feeling: *twinshock*. If you've just brought home two babies, you probably feel it, too.

Of course, the impact increases exponentially for parents in the throes of *tripletshock* and *quadshock*. Anne Seifert, the mother of quadruplets, says, "During the pregnancy, I hadn't let myself worry about how I'd manage to take care of four babies at once, because I didn't want the stress to trigger contractions. Once the quads were born, though, reality hit. I had several panic attacks just thinking about the hurdles that lay ahead."

To get past the anxiety and take pleasure in your babies, you need more than a pep talk. You need specific strategies for coping during those challenging first months.

How to Recruit Help

DR. LUKE: After talking with hundreds of mothers of multiples, I'm convinced of one basic truth: You will need help, especially during those first hectic weeks after the babies come home. And the more babies you've got, the more assistance you'll require.

One Australian study, for instance, showed that it takes 197 hours per week to care for infant triplets and do household chores—yet there are only 168 hours in a week!

Help is particularly vital if you've had little previous experience in taking care of an infant. For instance, Stacy Moore said to me, "Before my twins were born, I had changed maybe two diapers in my entire life. The first time I saw a newborn's bowel movement, I looked at that sticky black meconium in horror and thought, 'Is this what baby poop always looks like?' It was intimidating to have to learn everything from scratch."

There's nothing self-indulgent about seeking help; it's truly in your babies' best interests. If you try to do everything yourself, you'll quickly sink into such extreme exhaustion that you won't be able to take good care of your babies. Even if you are a superwoman, you'll simply run out of time. It is also wise to not forget that other people—including your spouse and older children—may suffer if you attempt to meet 100 percent of your babies' all-consuming demands on your own. So consider the following alternatives, and select the ones best suited to your situation.

Hire a professional.

If you can afford it, a baby nurse is an excellent option—particularly one who specializes in multiples. (Despite the title, this person is usually an experienced caregiver, not a registered nurse.) While details of the arrangement vary, you can probably count on certain basics. The typical baby nurse lives in your home for as long as you request, whether a couple of weeks or many months. Some work 12-hour shifts; others work around the clock except for a few hours off during the day. If you're breast-feeding, she gets up at night to help. Otherwise, she manages night feedings herself so you can sleep. She takes care of the babies, their laundry, and their room, but does not shop or clean house.

One mother of boy/girl twins hired a nurse who stayed three months. Says she, "The baby nurse taught me to breast-feed, give baths, even recognize thrush. And she took care of me as I recovered from my C-section."

Even experienced moms often regard professional help as a necessity when they're trying to meet the needs of their older children as well as newborn multiples. "For the first six weeks after the triplets were born, I had some help during the day, but I was on my own every night. My husband couldn't get any time off work, and I also had to take care of our three-year-old daughter. On average, I was getting two hours of sleep a night. It was really tough," admits Helen Armer. "Then I hired an overnight nanny for eight weeks. Each weekday evening, she came at 11 P.M. and stayed till 7 A.M., handling all the triplets' needs during that time. I couldn't sleep the entire eight hours, of course. I stayed up till midnight paying bills or doing laundry, then woke up at 6 A.M. to get my daughter ready for nursery school. But at least I was able to rest for six hours, five nights a week."

Such help isn't cheap, unfortunately. The more babies you have, the more you pay. "The baby nurse cost me a lot of money," says Helen, "but it was worth it. I'm not sure how I would have survived without her!"

Locate a qualified baby nurse through word of mouth, do an Internet search for "Baby Nurse" plus your state name, or find a baby-nurse placement agency in the yellow pages under Child Care. Several months before your due date, meet with the agency director to discuss duties, hours, and payment—and don't be shy about confirming that all of the agency's baby nurses have undergone criminal background checks.

If live-in or overnight help isn't financially feasible, hire a daytime babysitter to come for much of the day, or arrange her schedule to overlap your babies' fussiest time. Through your local Mothers of Multiples Club, you may find a levelheaded teenager or twenty-something sitter who has twin or triplet siblings herself and is experienced at handling more than one baby at a time. Even more economical is a mother's helper—typically a preteen who, though not mature enough to be left alone with the babies, can help you feed and change your newborns and entertain them while you take a shower or relax with a cup of tea.

But do beware of falling into the trap where the babysitter plays while the mom cleans. Says Lydia Greenwood, the mother of boy/girl twins, "I found myself scrubbing floors one afternoon, while my hired help played peek-a-boo with Alexander and Holly. *That* didn't seem quite fair! So I negotiated a change in the sitter's duties to include kitchen cleanup, vacuuming, and clutter control—giving me more free time to enjoy my twins." If such an arrangement doesn't sit well with your sitter, have a cleaning service or housekeeper take up the slack.

And don't let yourself feel guilty about it. "Since I don't work outside the home, at first I felt sheepish about spending my husband's hard-earned paycheck on a housekeeper," says one mother of twins and an older child. "But I stopped feeling guilty when my husband pointed out that my 'job responsibilities' had virtually tripled overnight, and it was okay to outsource some of my duties."

Invite relatives to stay for a week, a month, or longer.

You may prefer that your mother and/or mother-in-law stay with you those first weeks, as Ruth Markowitz did. "At first, I left the child care in their experienced hands, but once they showed me what to do, I realized it wasn't that hard," she recalls.

The more babies you have, the more help you'll need. "My mother-in-law stayed with us for the last several months of my triplet pregnancy, taking care of my toddler and me. Then once the babies came home from the NICU, my father and mother and mother's cousin came for three months. They just dropped their own lives so that they could help us," says Arlene McAndrew. "At that point, most of my time was spent pumping breast milk, so my relatives handled almost everything else. I knew that I could trust them, so I didn't obsess about exactly how and when things had to be done."

TAMARA: Afraid it's an imposition to take so much of someone's time? Instead of asking a favor, offer a job.

My twins came home in late spring, which turned out to be great timing. My college-age sister needed a summer job, and I needed around-the-clock assistance. She became the nanny, living with us all summer and helping take care of the babies, and I paid her as much as she would have made at any other job. I was so sorry to see her go in the fall—not only because she had made life immeasurably easier, but also because we had grown much closer emotionally.

Although my little sister has many nieces and nephews now, I know that my kids—the only people in the world who call her Aunt Nanny—hold a special place in her heart.

Let friends lend a helping hand.
When a friend offers to help, give her a specific assignment or let her choose from a list you've prepared. For example, she can:

- Feed one baby a bottle or amuse her while she waits her turn at the breast.
- Dress one infant while you bathe another.
- Take the babies for a walk while you nap.
- Accompany you to the pediatrician.
- Fold laundry or wash dishes while you chat.
- Bring a bag of groceries or replenish your stock of diapers and wipes.
- Take your older child to the playground or preschool so you can concentrate on the babies.
- Drop off a frozen meal or covered dish, or prepare dinner in your own kitchen. Best are the one-handed meals—hamburgers, salads, casseroles, things that don't require a knife—so parents can each hold a fussy baby while still managing to get some food into their own mouths.

Hang on to your sense of humor when asking for help. For instance, Ginny and David Seyler's answering machine bears this message: "Hi. We can't come to the phone right now. But if you'd like to come over and diaper a baby or two or three, feel free! Otherwise, leave a message."

If you feel shy about asking again and again for assistance, just ask once, as Judy Levy did when her twin daughters were born. "I told a friend that even though many people had offered to help, I was embarrassed to follow through. She made a list of the names and phone numbers of everyone who had volunteered, and established a schedule whereby a different person dropped off a meal each Wednesday and Sunday. With the leftovers, we only had to cook once or twice a week. That was the greatest!"

You have three or four babies? You'll need more than dinner delivery. Again, try to find someone who's willing to take charge of coordinating the volunteers. "My friend Janice would work everything out for the week, then call me and say, 'Get your calendar and write all this down. Sue is coming Monday to help with laundry, Mary will be there Tuesday to clean the house, Jane will bring groceries on Wednesday,' and so on," explains quad mom Anne Seifert. "It was hard to open my house to all these people, but I am so thankful for them. I simply could not have managed everything myself."

Seek out other unpaid volunteers.

Call your local college and ask if any student might be interested in a hands-on research project on multiples, or whether an entire sorority might want to adopt your family to fulfill its community service requirement. Find out if the high school would allow a student who assists you to earn extra credit for a child-care or cooking class. A Girl Scout troop or local youth group could be approached about helping with errands, shopping, or other household chores, while an elderly neighbor could play surrogate grandparent.

Make sure your partner participates fully in the babies' care.

"Tim took two weeks off work after the twins were born, and that was the most helpful thing for me," says Stacy Moore. "We learned together how to take care of the babies, encouraging each other and saying, 'Yeah, that looks right!' whenever we mastered a new skill."

Urge Dad to take as much time off from work as possible in those first challenging weeks after the babies come home—you might be surprised at how accommodating employers can be when a family is dealing with new multiples. Your partner can assist with feedings and baths, change diapers, clean up spit-up, empty the diaper pail, and soothe a crying baby or two. If he doesn't know how to do basic baby-care tasks, teach him. Chances are he's already used to doing the vacuuming, cooking, and food shopping, since you were cautioned against overexerting yourself during the pregnancy—so let him continue with these jobs now.

Nocturnal duties can also be shared. If you're bottle-feeding, take turns on the night shift, assigning one parent to handle all infant care while the other sleeps through, and then switching roles the next night. "At first, Mark and I would both get up to take care of the quads, but that meant neither of us got any decent sleep at all," says Anne Seifert. "Then we started switching off, letting one person sleep for six hours while the other handled all the babies' needs. It was far more manageable."

Another option is to split the night shift. "I quickly exhausted myself handling all the twins' nighttime needs alone," says Lydia Greenwood. "My husband, Ed, came up with a great system. In the evenings, we shared baby-care duties until we went to bed at 10 P.M. It was my job to wake up and handle anything that needed to be done between bedtime and 4 A.M. Any cries that came after that, Ed answered until he left for work in the morning. Typically this meant that I nursed the twins at 2 A.M., Ed gave them bottles at 6 A.M., and then I nursed again at 9 A.M. Once we hit upon this schedule, my fatigue eased dramatically."

Even if you're exclusively breast-feeding, your partner can still share the load. Let him be the one to get up when a hungry baby howls. He can bring the child to your bed, so you can continue to doze as she nurses. When she's done, he can burp her, change her if necessary, and settle her back to sleep—then repeat the process when the next baby needs to be fed. Just be sure you both agree on Dad's responsibilities before going to bed, because 2 A.M. is not the best time to negotiate.

Sanity-Saving Schedules

If your babies were hospitalized after birth, they may already be used to a schedule. Ask the staff to outline it for you before the babies are discharged. "The NICU had our triplets on a good schedule, so once the babies came home, we just kept them on that same schedule," says Kevin McAndrew.

But for most parents, life with newborn multiples at first seems to have no rhythm—no pattern to when the babies sleep or eat, and no way to predict the course of the day. This can be frustrating. You think that you finally have five minutes to jump into the shower, but then one baby suddenly wakes up from his nap. You struggle to get everyone bundled up and into the stroller, only to be forced to cut the walk short when someone starts screaming with hunger before you've gone a block.

The solution is to ease your babies toward similar schedules. During the day, when one baby is hungry, feed the others, too. Do the same at night, even if it means waking a sleeping baby or two in order to feed them at the same time or in close order.

But what about the common recommendation to feed on demand rather than on a schedule? While it's true that feeding on demand is generally recommended, it's simply not always realistic with multiples, particularly for nighttime feedings. For instance, if you allow twins total control over the schedule, you may find yourself feeding the first one at 1 A.M. and the second at 2:30 A.M.—which means that by 4 A.M., the first one will be hungry again. You'll never get more than an hour of uninterrupted sleep. And if you have triplets or quads, you'll be dragging yourself out of bed every half hour.

Once your babies reach the age of three months, however, one, if not all, may be ready to sleep five or six hours at a stretch. At that point, experiment for a few nights to see what happens if you don't wake the other baby or babies along with the first. If another baby screams to be fed 20 minutes after you've returned her brother or sister to bed, go back to feeding them together for a few more weeks. But if you're lucky, one or more babies will sleep through the night—and you'll be that much closer to a full night's sleep yourself.

You'll also want to coax your babies toward similar sleep schedules during the day as well as at night. When one is ready to nap, try to settle the whole crew in their cribs. The reward: You gain a few free hours to yourself.

Do the same in the evening by getting your babies ready for bed at the same time. A pleasant bedtime ritual encourages babies to settle down more easily. "To help get our infant twins on the same schedule, we established a nightly routine of bath-bottle-bed. The girls were down by 8 P.M. every evening, giving my husband and me some adult time," notes Kelly Kassab, mother of twin girls and another child.

If you have trouble synchronizing your multiples, try keeping a daily log. It helps you spot the regularities and similarities in your babies' schedules, so you can build on these emerging patterns. Record the time and the number of minutes each child nurses or the ounces of formula consumed, when each nap starts and ends, how many wet and dirty diapers each baby has, when each baby is bathed, and when vitamins or other medications are given. Also leave space to jot down your babies' milestones, as well as any questions you may have for the pediatrician.

TAMARA: As I studied my twins' daily logs, I realized that both babies typically napped for two hours in the morning, but James fell asleep around 11 and Samantha closer to noon. I postponed his nap by actively entertaining him for half an hour, and moved hers up to 11:30 by cutting short the midmorning games and rocking her instead. Within a week, they were accustomed to falling asleep at about the same time—most mornings anyway.

It was such a luxury to have that hour to myself when both babies were napping. Usually I'd nap, too. But if I was feeling relatively energetic, I could check in at the office, call a friend, clean the house, or just relax with a magazine.

For easier comparison, I used a side-by-side format for my twins' log, a sample of which appears here. You can adjust it as needed for the number of babies in your family.

A Day in the Life: Keeping a Log

Establishing a routine is half the task when it comes to parenting twins, triplets, or quads. To record your children's daily habits, first devise a master sheet covering a 24-hour period. Start and end the page at whatever time you consider the start of the day. Some parents set up an Excel spreadsheet. If you prefer a paper log, use paper large enough to accommodate all your babies' information side by side for easy comparison, and post it in a convenient place, such as on the refrigerator or the door to the nursery. Table 13.1 shows a partial-day sample that you can adapt to suit your own situation.

Date: June 8

Time	James					Samantha			
	Feed	Diaper	Sleep	Bath		Feed	Diaper	Sleep	Bath
5 A.M.	Formula, 7 oz.	Wet	Up 5:10 Down 5:45	—		Formula, 6 oz.	BM	Up 5:10	—
6 A.M.	—	—	—	—		—	—	Down 6:15	—
7 A.M.	—	—	—	—		—	—	—	—
8 A.M.	Nurse, 15 mins.	BM	Up 8:10	—		Nurse, 25 mins.	Wet	Up 8:10	—
9 A.M.	—	—	—	Tub		—	—	—	Sponge
10 A.M.	Nurse, 20 mins.	—	Down 10:50	—		Formula, 8 oz.	—	—	—
11 A.M.	—	—	—	—		—	BM	—	—
Noon	—	—	—	—		—	—	Down 12:05	—
Notes:	Ask doctor about spitting up					Diaper rash improving			
Meds:	Vitamins					Vitamins, diaper ointment			
News:	James found his fingers!					Samantha's first smile (or was it gas?)			

Table 13.1

Sleep Strategies

If you're going to get your babies on the same general schedule, it makes sense to work toward a routine that's as convenient as possible for you. That means a schedule in which the babies are most eager to play during the day and most inclined to sleep at night.

This will make an enormous difference in your own sense of well-being. "At first, when the twins were up at all hours of the night, I was so sleep-deprived that I felt weepy much of the time. That was weird, because normally I'm a happy person," admits Amy Maly, mother of identical twin girls. "This lasted about five or six weeks, until the twins were sleeping better at night—which of course meant I was sleeping better, too. Getting a decent amount of rest made me feel human and happy again."

Unfortunately, infants are not born with an instinctive sense of day versus night. Instead of automatically coordinating their body rhythms to those of the sun and moon, your multiples may often reverse those cycles—snoozing most of the day away and then feeling alert and hungry half the night.

Such an out-of-sync schedule is a pain. It's frustrating to hang around the house all day while one or more babies indulge in interminable naps. Worse, their nighttime antics leave you exhausted, since midnight demands for attention interfere with your own rest.

Fortunately, you can solve this problem. By helping your babies differentiate between day and night, you give them a good start toward sleeping through the night (a milestone typically reached around age three to four months). The key: Within a week of birth, most infants begin to have one long stretch of sleep that lasts from three to five hours—and your challenge is to make sure that, for all your babies, this long rest period occurs at night.

Show that daytime is playtime.
To consolidate their sleep into nighttime, your babies must also consolidate their wakefulness into daytime. So keep your multiples active when the sun's up. Establish a rise-and-shine routine for morning. As you lift your babies from their cribs, greet them with a big smile and a cheerful, "Good morning!" With excitement in your voice, tell your babies of your plans for the day. Make a show of raising the window shades and turning on their music box.

Make daytime feedings fun. Beginning with breakfast and continuing with each feeding throughout the day, your multiples' meals should be social occasions. Sing or talk to them as they nurse. Gaze into their eyes and tell them how happy you are to hold them.

After a feeding, don't just plunk them in their cribs. Entertain them instead with a game of This Little Piggy, a waltz around the room, or a guided tour of their new home. Need to shower? Line up the bouncy seats in the bathroom and let your multiples absorb the sight of each other and the sound of the running water. When the weather allows, a trip to the yard or around the block in their stroller will help the babies stay alert as they take in the feel of the sun's warmth on their faces, hear the sounds of the neighborhood, and see all that the world has to offer.

Make naps distinct from nighttime slumber.

You don't want to go overboard in your efforts to keep your multiples awake during the day, of course. They do need to nap. Your job is simply to teach them that daytime sleep is different from—and briefer than—nighttime slumber.

To start, keep the nursery well-lit at naptime. Light is the major clue that tells us when we're supposed to be awake. With the window shades up and curtains open, the sun reminds your babies that siestas shouldn't last all afternoon.

Don't be too insistent about hushing household noises. By imposing a ban on noise, you encourage infants to sleep for hours on end during the day—the opposite of your true goal. What's more, you force everyone else in the house to tiptoe. Babies learn to sleep under whatever conditions they are introduced to from the beginning. Go ahead and turn on the CD player, run the vacuum, allow the phone to ring, and let siblings play in the next room. Don't use a white-noise machine or other sound-canceling device during daytime slumber.

Cut naps short if they last too long. For weary parents of multiples desperate for a few hours of peace, the idea that their infants might nap too long seems ludicrous. But it isn't—not when prolonged napping interferes with the babies' ability to sleep well at night. A good rule of thumb is to limit daytime naps to no more than three hours at a stretch. This helps your children learn to save their longest sleep period for nighttime. So try not to groan when one baby, waking from her nap, startles her sister or brother into wakefulness, too.

If one of your babies continues to nap past that three-hour mark, try picking him up, patting his back, changing his diaper, stripping off his clothes, rubbing under his chin, or tickling his toes. If you simply cannot rouse him no matter what you do, he's probably in a deep-sleep stage. Wait 15 minutes to give him time to cycle into a lighter sleep stage, then try again to wake him.

Let evening be transition time.

Your babies can learn that the evening routine is prelude to an extended rest. Be careful not to begin bedtime preparations too soon, however. The earlier in the evening you tuck them in, the earlier they're likely to awaken.

A vital step is to establish a soothing bedtime ritual. Human circadian rhythms operate on a 25-hour day. To click back to a 24-hour schedule, adults watch the clock. But your babies can't tell time. For them, a nightly ritual signals that it's time to wind down. Change each one into pajamas, as a sign that the day is done. Help them grow sleepy by rocking, reading aloud, and singing a soothing song.

Ready the nursery for nighttime, too. Let your infants watch as you pull down the window shades and draw the curtains. Turn off all lights except for a night-light; remember, darkness is a cue for sleep. Now is the time to keep the house fairly quiet. Set the CD player or television volume on low, and save noisy chores such as vacuuming for morning.

Before the final tucking in, make sure each baby is comfortable. During the day, it doesn't matter much if some slight discomfort wakes a baby—and his wails then wake the others— since naps shouldn't be overlong anyway. But before laying your multiples down at night, try to ensure that they're cozy enough to sleep a good while.

Change any diaper that is wet or soiled. If you use cloth diapers, make sure there's no Velcro closure scratching a tiny waist. For disposables, be certain the tabs aren't stuck to anyone's skin, that the corners of the tabs aren't poking a tummy, and that the edges aren't digging into a delicate thigh.

Next do climate control. Check each baby's hands. If they feel cold, switch to warmer pajamas. Is the back of anyone's neck damp? That baby is too warm and needs lighter-weight pajamas.

A sudden belch can startle a baby out of slumber, so be sure to burp everyone after feeding. And be on the lookout for other discomforts that could interfere with sleep. Might a hand or foot get stuck between the mattress and crib slats? Cushioned crib bumpers can prevent this. Has the neck or crotch of the biggest baby's pajamas grown too tight? It's time for a larger size.

Keep nighttime calm and quiet.

When your multiples are newborns, their stomachs hold only enough to satisfy them for three to four hours (or even less if they were low birthweight or premature). They need to be fed at least once each night for several months. You should not attempt to prevent those normal hunger-induced awakenings. But you can help your babies understand that a nighttime feeding is not an invitation to party.

Feed the babies in their bedroom. Infants learn to associate the nursery with sleep. If you take them to the living room to nurse, they may be so excited by this new environment that they won't be able to drop off again when the meal is over.

Don't turn on the lights. You don't need 100-watt illumination in order to offer a breast or bottle. The soft glow of a night-light or filtered rays from the hallway will suffice. This semi-darkness cues the babies that it will soon be time to sleep again.

Keep things quiet. If you turn on the TV or CD player for entertainment while you nurse, your babies will be entertained, too—and they won't want to settle back to bed once their tummies are full. Think twice about serenading your little one with lullabies; instead, save your songs for daytime. And take a tip from Lydia Greenwood: "I don't even talk to my twins much during nighttime feedings. I figure we have plenty of time to chat during the day."

Skip the fun and games, too—2 A.M. is not the time to indulge in a round of Pop Goes the Weasel. If a nighttime feeding takes more than 20 minutes per baby, handling or burping is excessive. If a diaper is wet or soiled, change it, but without any fanfare. You're not being cold or cruel; you're simply letting your babies know that at this time of night grown-ups are very boring. Don't feel guilty. You'll more than make up for any missed fun the next morning.

If your multiples share a bedroom, there is one exception to the rule about keeping nighttime quiet. Hannah Steele, an obstetrician and mother of identical twin girls, says, "One of my patients who also has twins clued me in to the fact that it's best to let the babies get used to each other's nighttime crying. Your impulse might be to grab the wailing baby and whisk her out of the bedroom so she doesn't wake up her sibling—but if you do, the babies don't learn how to keep right on sleeping when the other one cries."

TAMARA: Premature babies often have unique sleep patterns and problems, as I found out in the weeks after my twins came home from the hospital. Like every parent, I had looked forward to saying, "The baby slept through the night!" But preemies usually take longer to achieve this magical milestone, in part due to the corrected age phenomenon. While most full-term babies are developmentally capable of sleeping through the night by about three to four months of age, preemies are unlikely to be ready until they are five, six, or even seven months old—in other words, about three to four months after their original due date.

Another way in which prematurity affects sleep has to do with nutritional needs. Premature infants need to eat more often. When my twins were discharged from the NICU, they weighed just over 4 pounds. No way could their tiny tummies hold enough milk to carry them through for four hours, so I was given strict instructions to feed them every two hours. Not until your babies' weight has climbed to about 9 pounds will your pediatrician give you the go-ahead to stretch feedings to every three to four hours. Until that happens, expect catnaps to be the order of business.

Preemies are particularly prone to mixing up their days and nights. This stems from the fact that in the hospital, certain routine procedures such as bathing are often performed on the late-night shift. By the time your babies come home, they may be used to snoozing the day away and splashing around at midnight. You'll have to work harder to reverse this pattern.

You also may have to put some extra effort into helping your premature babies adjust to a quiet, dimly lit nursery. The first evening my son was home from the hospital, after all the well-wishers had departed, I sat with him in the nursery and quietly rocked him as I watched the sunlight gradually fade. It dawned on me then that little James had never before experienced darkness or silence. The neonatal intensive care unit had been a brightly lit ward filled with beeping vital-signs monitors, ringing phones, and constant conversation between parents and staff.

If your preemies seem fretful in the unfamiliar quiet of home, try leaving a light on in the nursery. Near the cribs, place a radio, ticking clock, or white-noise machine. Then over the next week or so, gradually dim the light and turn down the sound, until your babies adapt to a more tranquil way of life.

Do Multiples Need Mountains of Equipment?

Twins, triplets, or quads will need more equipment and supplies than a singleton, of course—but not necessarily two, three, or four times as much stuff. Here are tips on what to buy and how to save:

EACH BABY NEEDS HIS OWN . . .

- **Car seat:** Choose seats narrow enough to fit side by side in your car. Many parents prefer infant car seats (where the base stays belted inside the car and the seat lifts out) because this makes it possible to carry twins together for short distances, putting the seats on the ground in order to open doors. The babies can snooze undisturbed as you move them around, and stairs aren't the problem they would be for a stroller. If you have preemies coming home from the NICU or nursery, don't forget about the need for car seats. More than a few anxious parents have been disappointed on discharge day when they realize they've forgotten to buy car seats.
- **Crib:** Two babies may be able to share a single crib for the first three months or so, but then it gets overcrowded. Be sure your cribs meet current federal safety standards.
- **Stroller seat:** Before you buy, assess what kind of use you expect the stroller to get. Each style has its own advantages and disadvantages. A tandem-style twin stroller has two forward-facing seats and fits easily through doorways, but it

can be heavy. A face-to-face stroller lets twins share toys on a center tray, but it may not collapse for easy storage. Side-by-side strollers often are lightweight and collapsible, but may not fit through doorways and aisles. Umbrella side-by-side models are narrower and lightweight, but they may not provide the back support and full recline that newborns need. If possible, select a style with individually reclining seats. Another option to consider is an all-terrain or jogging stroller—so you can get a brisk workout for yourself while the babies enjoy an outing. For triplets or quads, choices are more limited, so go with whatever seems sturdiest.

- **Infant seat:** Separate seats are easier to carry and move around than double or triple styles. Bouncers provide extra fun.
- **High chair:** A one-handed tray release mechanism is essential, since you may have more babies than hands. Extra-large trays make handy play tables when multiples are being kept conveniently immobilized. But before you buy, make sure the big trays won't crowd your kitchen.

DUPLICATES ARE NICE BUT NOT ESSENTIAL

- **Swing:** Motorized styles are quieter than manual cranks, and they generally stay in motion longer, too. Gliders take up less space, but some babies seem to prefer the motion of the swing. Choose a model that has several position options for the back of the seat, including a reclining position for newborns and an upright position for older babies.
- **Front pack or sling:** Having one baby in a front pack and the other in a single stroller makes it easier to maneuver twins through a crowd. Two packs let each parent carry a load while keeping hands free. A double front pack may seem smart, but the twins' combined weight could prove too cumbersome.

ONE WILL DO

- **Playpen or play yard:** Choose an extra-large model.
- **Rocking chair:** Make sure it's wide enough for you to cuddle at least two babies at a time.
- **Diaper bag:** Go for jumbo, with a shoulder strap. Or try a diaper backpack; it holds lots and leaves your hands free.
- **Infant bathtub:** You can bathe only one baby at a time.

Find Deals, Save Dollars

You can borrow furniture, clothes, and equipment, or buy it gently used at tag sales, consignment shops, Goodwill stores, or online exchanges like eBay or Craigslist. The best deals (along with helpful advice) may come from other mothers of multiples whose twins or triplets have outgrown their specialized equipment. These moms will be sympathetic to your needs and anxious to declutter their own homes by getting rid of equipment they no longer need. You can meet these people at local or regional Mothers of Twins clubs or online.

Here are more money-saving suggestions:

- When buying new, ask the store for a discount on items purchased in duplicate.
- To cut down on your initial expenditure, delay purchases of equipment that won't be needed immediately, such as the high chairs and playpen. Even that second crib can wait a few months if necessary.
- Comparison shop. Store-brand disposable diapers can save you money; powdered formula is cheaper than ready-to-feed. Find out if a local price club sells baby food in bulk. It may be a good time to get a membership to a warehouse store such as Costco or Sam's Club.
- Check magazines for blow-in cards from manufacturers, inviting you to join their mailing lists to receive coupons and special offers. Or call the companies direct and request extra discount coupons. Online, do a search for baby product coupons.
- If you're using cloth diapers, find a diaper service that charges a flat fee for delivery, with only a modest increase for additional diapers.
- Each baby will need her own snowsuit, jacket, shoes, and sun hat. But everyone can share a wardrobe of play clothes and pajamas.
- Most in-home caregivers charge only slightly more (not twice as much) for twins. Many day-care centers offer a sibling discount.
- Your pediatrician may give you a two-for-one break on fees. It never hurts to ask.

Stretch Your Living Space

Even a small nursery can accommodate multiples. To create a play area in the center of the room, arrange twins' cribs in an L in the corner. If you have triplets, arrange cribs in a U shape along three walls.

- To increase closet capacity, install a second rod 2 feet below the first, and hang a shoe bag inside the door to store booties, bonnets, and pacifiers.
- Sling saddlebags over the changing table to hold diapers, wipes, and ointment, leaving drawers free for clothes and blankets.
- Use shelves rather than toy boxes to keep playthings organized without sacrificing floor space.
- Raise the rod in your coat closet, and use the space beneath to store the stroller.
- If having two or more high chairs in the kitchen leaves no room for anyone else to eat, install a wall-mounted table that flips up and out of the way when not in use.

Stress-Busters for Busy Parents

TAMARA: What kept me from stressing out completely was learning to catnap whenever and wherever opportunity presented itself. If I'd driven the twins to the pediatrician or the park, for instance, they were both sure to fall asleep on the way home. I knew from experience that if I tried to move them into the house, one or both would wake up, and I'd lose any chance of catching a nap myself.

Instead, I'd park in my driveway, turn off the engine, crank back the driver's seat, and snooze right there until one baby or the other woke up. My neighbors thought it was funny, but I didn't care. I logged a lot of shut-eye this way, and felt better for it.

I shared this tip at one Mother of Twins Club meeting, and soon everyone was offering stress-reducing suggestions of their own. Following are some smart ones to try:

Save steps.

The less you have to run around the house, the more energy you'll have for playing with your babies. Spread the baby equipment throughout the house—infant seats in the family room, swings in the dining room, playpen in the den—so your multiples are readily accommodated no matter what room you're in. Store some diapers, wipes, and clean clothes downstairs. That way, you don't have to run up to the nursery every time a baby needs changing. "I keep spit-up cloths in every room, handy for emergencies. My home isn't going to be featured in the pages of *House Beautiful,* but I have what I need where I need it," says Lisa McDonough, mother of boy/girl twins and two older children.

To spare yourself those 2 A.M. treks to the kitchen, put several bottles of sterilized water and a can of powdered formula in the nursery before you go to bed. If you use ready-to-serve formula, which must be kept refrigerated once it's opened, invest in several bottle warmers—you'll still have to go to the fridge, but you won't have to wait long for the bottles to warm up when the babies are ready to eat.

Home delivery can be a boon. Shop for baby clothes, toys, and child-proofing supplies by catalog or online. Find a pharmacy that delivers formula, diapers, and other supplies.

Avoid interruptions.

For your voicemail message, record your newborns' vital statistics or progress reports as they grow. Program your phone to go straight to voicemail when you're resting or feeding or bathing the babies. Use a nursery monitor during the babies' naps so you can work undisturbed anywhere in the house, without constant hikes to the nursery to check on the children.

Eliminate unnecessary tasks.

You don't need to give each baby a full tub bath daily. You can alternate days as long as the diaper area, hands, and face are wiped clean. Once the babies can handle the big bathtub, bathe one right after the other; don't bother to change the water unless it's really dirty. When your babies can sit with complete steadiness, bathe them all together.

Don't let germ patrol drive you to distraction.

To avoid illness, wash your hands often, wash toys, and ask friends with sick tots to stay away. But unless your babies have compromised immune systems, don't make yourself crazy. Lisa McDonough reports, "At first, I used separate spoons and bowls for each twin, but meals took forever, dirty dishes were everywhere, and I'd mix up the spoons anyway. Then my pediatrician pointed out that the babies were bound to catch each other's colds. So when the twins seemed healthy and I was crunched for time, I made do with a single spoon and bowl. Mealtimes were a lot simpler."

Get out of the house.

"For the first five weeks after my twin girls were born, I didn't get out of the house with the babies for anything other than doctor appointments," Judy Levy says. She's not exaggerating: One study from England showed that mothers of young twins leave the house far less often than do mothers of singletons. This isolation compounds the emotional strains of parenting multiples. Make a point of getting out for fresh air and a change of scenery as often as possible.

True, it's not easy to get two or more babies fed, changed, dressed, and alert enough to enjoy the wide world simultaneously. Yet once outings become part of the pattern of the day, the effort involved eases significantly. It needn't be an elaborate adventure. A walk in the park, a visit with a neighbor, or a stroll through the mall can lift spirits. "After being stuck in the house for days, a trip to the dry cleaner's seems exotic," says Lydia Greenwood.

Key to cutting down on prep time is a well-stocked diaper bag. Prepare a checklist: two diapers per baby, plus wipes, ointment, and changing pad; a clean outfit, bib, and blanket for each baby; spit-up cloths (and baby bottles if you're not nursing); pacifiers, teethers, and small toys; your wallet, cell phone, and keys; and whatever else you need. Lydia adds, "I restock my bag each evening. It still takes hours to get out the door the next morning, but at least the packing is done."

Figure out what time of day works best for an excursion, given your babies' schedules. "At first, I made myself frantic trying to get errands done in the morning—an impossibility, considering my twins' eating and napping routines," says Lydia Greenwood. "Once I started scheduling their doctor's appointments and play dates for afternoons only, outings with the babies got much easier."

A note of caution: You never want to leave one baby alone in the stroller or car while you go back inside to finish dressing another. Get everyone completely ready to roll, then quickly settle them into their stroller or car seats.

Stay connected to the world.

Finding time for friends may seem like a pipe dream when you barely have time to go to the bathroom. But maintaining your social connections, to whatever extent is possible, truly will help reduce your stress levels. "I had heard many new moms of singletons complain about their lack of a social life. With triplets, I figured the problem would be three times worse unless I took steps to prevent it," says Arlene McAndrew. "So I told all my friends, 'Please keep calling and inviting me along to whatever you're doing. Most of the time, I may have to say no—but sometimes I can say yes.' And they did keep calling. Their friendship allowed me to have a life outside of the babies."

Safeguarding Your Babies' Health

DR. NEWMAN: After all you went through to ensure that your babies would arrive in this world as healthy as possible, you certainly don't want to risk any accidents now that they're here. While the task of keeping two or more babies safe and sound may seem daunting at first, with some forethought and basic training, you'll rise to the challenge.

Be sure to program the phone number for your pediatrician and the local poison control center into your cell phone. I also urge you to take a class in infant first aid and cardiopulmonary resuscitation (CPR), or at least order the Infant CPR Anytime Personal Learning Program—which includes a how-to DVD and practice mannequin—from the American Heart Association (877-AHA-4CPR, www.shopcpranytime.org). I hope you never need to use these skills, but it's wise to be prepared for an emergency.

SKILLS YOU NEED TO LEARN

Any good manual on baby care describes these essential skills in detail. Whether you're taking care of one baby or four, the basics remain the same. You do have an advantage, however, over all those singleton families—as a parent of multiples, you'll more quickly gain the practice you need to perform all these tasks expertly. Check out the instructions on how to:

- Feed your babies.
- Bathe your babies.
- Diaper your babies.
- Recognize and treat diaper rash.
- Recognize and treat cradle cap.
- Use a bulb syringe to clear a baby's stuffy nose.
- Take a baby's temperature.
- Give a baby medicine, orally or rectally.

THE WELL-STOCKED MEDICINE CABINET

When a baby (or two or three) spikes a fever, it's a bad feeling to discover that your medicine cabinet is bare. Use this checklist to shop ahead, so you're ready whenever supplies are needed:

- Infant ear or forehead thermometer. (If rectal thermometers are used, have one per baby, labeled with each child's name.)
- Calibrated medicine dropper or syringe for measuring dosage. (Do *not* use kitchen spoons; they vary greatly in size and may result in giving too much or too little medicine.)
- Bulb syringes for suctioning mucus from tiny stuffed-up noses.
- Tweezers for removing splinters.
- Sterile bandages in various sizes and shapes.
- Gauze pads and adhesive tape.

- Infant acetaminophen (Tylenol) or other liquid aspirin substitute. (Never give baby aspirin or any other type of aspirin to a child—it can lead to Reye's syndrome, a potentially fatal neurological disease.)
- Pedialyte or other rehydration liquid, to avoid dehydration from diarrhea.
- Liquefied charcoal and syrup of ipecac, to induce vomiting. (Use it only if recommended by your pediatrician or local poison control center.)
- Diaper ointment or cream for diaper rash.
- Antiseptic spray or ointment (such as Neosporin) for minor cuts or scrapes.
- Calamine lotion or 0.5 percent hydrocortisone cream for insect bites and itchy rashes.
- Sunscreen. (Sunscreen is recommended for babies over six months old. Prior to that, be especially careful to avoid excessive sun exposure, using a minimal amount of sunscreen on the infant's face and backs of the hands only when adequate protective clothing and shade are not available.)

Before You Call the Pediatrician

Of course, you should call the doctor anytime a baby seems to have a medical problem. But in order for the pediatrician to advise you, she'll need certain information. Before you pick up the phone, jot down the following information regarding the baby about whom you are concerned:

- The symptoms and when they began.
- The baby's temperature, when it was taken, and what type of thermometer you used.
- When, what, and how much the baby ate last.
- The time of the baby's last wet or dirty diaper.
- Whether and when that baby—or any of your babies—might have been exposed to a sick person.

Baby-Proofing Basics Times Two (or More)

"As soon as my twins became mobile, I realized how quickly one could crawl toward danger while I was busy chasing, changing, or feeding the other," says Lydia Greenwood. "Basic baby-proofing clearly wasn't enough in our household. We needed that extra measure of thoroughness I call twin-proofing." To make your home safe for your multiples, follow these guidelines:

Throughout Your Home

On all electrical outlets, install covers that automatically snap closed to conceal the outlet opening whenever the plug is removed, or use box-shaped covers that fit over outlet plates to prevent your children from removing the plug from the outlet. Tack down cords to all lamps, air conditioners, and other appliances; chewing on cords can lead to disfiguring or even life-threatening burns. Put breakables up high or out of sight. Store out of reach any small items that might present a choking hazard—chess pieces, small knickknacks, coin collections. Shorten window cords from blinds or draperies by tying them with secure knots or using wrap-around cord shorteners. Place a gate at the *top and bottom* of stairs. Don't place a toy box—or anything else—beneath a window where it could be used as a stepladder to climb out. Install window guards on all windows above the first floor.

Living Room

Replace glass coffee tabletops with Plexiglas, or add cushioning. Add baby bumpers to the sharp corners of any low table or desktop. Bolt cabinets and bookshelves to the wall so they don't topple over if a child tries to climb them. Install a latch to keep swinging doors open so they don't pinch tiny fingers.

Dining Room

Use place mats rather than a tablecloth; with their combined strength, your tots could easily yank on the corner of a tablecloth and pull a hot casserole down onto themselves. When setting the table, lay out knives for the adults only after all the babies are safely strapped into their high chairs. Put locks on china cabinets to keep little ones away from breakables like goblets and candlesticks. Never leave a half-finished glass of an alcoholic beverage where your children can reach it. Just a few swallows can be harmful.

Kitchen

Store all toxic products—polishes, drain cleaner, scouring powder—in the highest cupboards. Install baby-proof latches on any cabinet that holds breakable items. Keep electric appliances (mixer, blender, food processor, carving knife, waffle iron, toaster, microwave oven) out of reach. Never leave knives in the dishwasher where curious crawlers could easily reach them. Always put pots on back burners. Install stove knob covers to keep kids from turning on burners. Store unused plastic trash bin liners out of reach. Before discarding any plastic bag, fold it lengthwise and tie tight knots in the center. Keep the garbage can inside a latched cabinet, place the trash bin on a high counter, or use a garbage pail with a locking mechanism similar to that on a diaper pail. Otherwise, your tots may paw through the garbage, encountering sharp cans or choking hazards like chicken bones.

Nursery

Once your babies can stand, move their crib mattresses to the lowest position to thwart attempts to climb out. Remove pictures from walls that are within reach of the cribs; you don't want the children to cut themselves on the glass or sharp corners. Be sure the toy chest has holes for ventilation, in case the kids climb inside, and hinges that hold the cover securely in any position to prevent the lid from slamming on a small hand or head.

Bathroom

Empty the tub immediately when bath time is over. *Never* leave any of the children alone in a bathtub, even for an instant. Turn the thermostat on the hot water heater down to 120 degrees so your babies won't scald themselves if they turn on the faucet. Pad the sharp spout of the tub with a soft spout cover. Put a nonskid mat on the bottom of the tub. Keep all electrical appliances such as hair dryers and curling irons (and their cords) out of reach. Install a latch on the toilet lid. Keep all medications in a locked box. Lock up all toxic products, including perfumes, mouthwash, aftershave, cosmetics, cleansers, and disinfectants.

TAMARA: If you're still feeling overwhelmed by all the time and energy required to take care of your multiples, don't despair. You're not alone. In that first chaotic year after my twins were born, a triumphant day was one in which I accomplished *anything* beyond the all-consuming baby-care essentials. Often, even a single load of laundry was more than I could manage.

Trust me—things do get easier with time as you and your babies settle into a manageable routine. In the meanwhile, don't worry about those days when nothing gets done. If you've made time to cherish your babies and give them good care, you've done all you really need to do.

DR. NEWMAN: I see and hear from my patients often enough after they deliver to know that the first year with twins, triplets, or quads can be a challenging, exhausting, even an overwhelming experience for some parents. Try to keep in mind that you will get some payback down the road for the overtime you're putting in now. For instance, with at least one playmate already in place, your multiples will require somewhat less of your time as they get older—because they'll be able to entertain each other. And if at some point you end up having another child, taking care of a singleton infant will seem like a piece of cake to you. Best of all, raising multiples is an accomplishment of which you will always be very proud. It truly is one of the most deeply moving and life-affirming experiences a parent can ever have.

Chapter Fourteen

Becoming One Big Happy Family

Every pregnant woman imagines that magical moment: Seconds after birth, her baby (or babies!) will be placed in her arms, and she'll be immediately overwhelmed by love. This ideal has been promoted for more than four decades, since early research on parent-infant bonding sparked a revolution that gave fathers access to the maternity ward and mothers more control over labor.

Sounds wonderful to fall instantly, effortlessly, in love with your newborns? Sure. The problem is that parents of singletons and multiples alike have come to *expect* that enchanted moment—yet studies show that only about 25 percent actually experience it.

The reasons are myriad. Some mothers are simply too exhausted to feel anything more profound than a sense of relief that the ordeal of labor is over. For others, disappointment may cloud that first encounter. Perhaps you and your husband had always longed for a daughter but wound up with a trio of boys. Maybe you hoped to experience natural childbirth but, like 50 percent of mothers of twins and nearly all mothers of triplets and quads, ended up having a cesarean delivery. Or possibly the opportunity to immediately bond with your newborns was interrupted by the babies' need for special medical care in the NICU.

"I expected the textbook bonding experience—go to the hospital, have the babies, breast-feed the twins right on the delivery table, and bond with both at that very instant," says Amy Maly, mother of identical twin girls. "But that just didn't happen. I wanted to deliver vaginally, but I wound up with a cesarean. Because I wasn't able to see the twins as they were delivered, I had this weird sense of alienation—'Gosh, did those babies really come out of *me*?' Afterward I was too groggy from the anesthesia to be able to nurse well. Then I was afraid that I had missed the golden opportunity and that we'd never really bond quite right."

Bonding with All Those Babies

DR. LUKE: In the days following delivery, many of our patients at the Multiples Clinic have expressed concerns similar to Amy's. Fortunately, such worries are usually dispelled fairly quickly as the parents' love for their babies blossoms.

Research has shown that parent-infant bonding is an ongoing process that evolves over time. It is not a bolt-from-the-blue moment that must occur at the moment of birth in order for the relationship to thrive. It is more like falling in love—that first rush is like a crush, but true intimacy develops over the months as you get to know each other.

It's important to accept this fact because with multiples, the bonding issue can be extra complicated. Who expects to fall in love with two, three, or four people at the same time? Yet this is precisely the challenge that parents of multiples must confront. No wonder that bonding with twins, triplets, or quadruplets may take longer than with a singleton. Here's why:

Time limitations interfere with enjoyment.
A study from Israel showed that mothers of twins spend 35 to 39 percent of their time on infant-related tasks, whereas mothers of one baby spend only 22 to 29 percent. This means that parents of multiples have less time for playing, snuggling, talking, and especially the one-on-one interacting so essential to the bonding process.

"I didn't bond with my triplets nearly as quickly as I did with my first child," admits Helen Armer. "It was mainly the fatigue. In the beginning, I had enough to do just taking care of their basic needs. I sometimes joked, 'All I can do is feed, burp, and change each baby, then plunk it back in the crib'—but it wasn't really funny. There was no time to play." For Helen, the situation eased and affection grew once she and her triplets were getting more sleep at night, leaving everyone with more energy for daytime fun.

To maximize your pleasure in parenthood, tune in to your babies' quiet alert periods, when infants are at their most engaging. Take note of how your babies respond to you by following your movements with their eyes, molding their body to yours, and exploring your skin with their hands. Stick out your tongue or open your mouth, then wait patiently; within a minute, one or more of your babies may imitate you. Talk to your little ones, too, using a soft high-pitched tone. Infants won't understand the words, but they'll recognize a loving tone.

One-on-one time is difficult to come by.

Ginny Seyler, another mother of triplets, says, "I worried about how I would be able to make my babies understand that I loved each and every one of them. How do you look into the eyes of three babies at a time? How do you hold them all when they all need cuddling at once?"

The answer to that dilemma is to seize every opportunity to give each child your undivided attention. Diaper changes and baths are, of necessity, performed on one baby at a time—so make the most of those chances to talk and play one on one. Even during simultaneous feedings, you can have a one-on-one moment with one infant simply by making eye contact and smiling. Perhaps exempt one or two daily feedings from the simultaneous system, setting aside the extra time needed to gaze into just one little face for the full feeding. Use a front pack or sling around the house (not just on excursions out), and alternate which baby you carry in it. This allows you to stay physically close and helps you learn to read each baby's unique signals. As you become more adept at interpreting and responding to their needs, your babies will cry less—leaving more opportunities for pleasant interaction with each one.

It may be comforting to remember that your babies expect a crowd and are used to sharing you. Although they may not always get quite as much individual parental attention as singletons do, multiples enjoy a unique benefit—the warm relationship they have with their wombmates. Anne Seifert says, "I can't always give my quadruplets as many hugs and kisses as I'd like to. I can hold two at a time, but I can't hold all four. Yet it's comforting to see how much affection they get from one another. They love to laugh together, play together, and snuggle up close together. They're the best of friends now, and I hope they always will be."

Mothers and fathers may get caught up in *unit bonding*.

Parents may feel attached to their multiples as a matched set rather than as separate individuals. One warning sign of unit bonding is when parents insist on always dressing their babies identically. While there's no harm in coordinating the babies' outfits on occasion, do beware of overdoing it. If you find yourself changing all the kids' clothes every time one soils her suit, you're probably overinvested in the idea of presenting your babies to the world as a matched set.

What to do with all those matching outfits your babies received as gifts? "At our baby shower, it was fun to open two of this, two of that. But there's no law saying we have to dress the boys in those identical outfits on the same day," says Stacy Moore, mother of fraternal twin boys. "If Brandon wears his bunny overalls on Monday, I'll wait till Thursday to have Steven wear his. Those matching gifts get used and are very much appreciated—they just don't get used at the same time."

Studies suggest that unit bonding is more problematic with identicals than with fraternals, since parents may have trouble telling the babies apart. Don't feel guilty if you're not sure on sight which baby is which—this is a very common problem—but do devise some way to prevent identity mix-ups. You might leave on the babies' hospital bracelets for the first week or two, or keep a dab of red nail polish on one baby's toenail for a month or so, until you identify some distinguishing features. Does this child have a longer face? Does that one have a small birthmark or a distinctive hair swirl? "It was impossible to tell my babies apart until I noticed that their eyes were a slightly different color," says one mother of identical twin boys. Once you've figured out how to tell the babies apart, clue in friends and relatives.

Consider also whether it's in your babies' best interests to have matching names. Though one U.S. study found that 40 percent of parents choose alliterative or rhyming names for their multiples, it may be easier for everyone to regard your children as individuals if their names are quite distinct. Too late now because the babies are already born and named? Stay open to the possibility that in the future it may prove expedient to begin referring to Camille and Lucille as Cammy and Lucy, or to stretch Donny and Danny to Donald and Daniel. Whatever monikers are chosen, consciously call your babies by name rather than referring to them as *the twins* or *the quads*.

Bonding with your infants as individuals is also enhanced when you make the effort to appreciate each baby's unique qualities. Notice each child's preferences for certain activities, sounds, or textures. Try to determine which baby is most energetic, which loves to be tickled on the toes, and which one can yell the loudest. But don't feel guilty if such recognition takes time. "At first I felt overwhelmed by the challenge of bonding with two babies at once, and disappointed that I wasn't able to point out lots of distinctions between my twins," says Judy Levy, mother of fraternal twin girls and an older daughter. "But then I realized that all I really needed to do in the beginning was to give them love and tenderness. Their personalities would emerge over time."

Favoritism may come into play.
Most parents expect to love their children equally, so you may be shocked to find yourself drawn more to a particular baby. Perhaps one of your multiples has a temperament that fits more easily with yours. Maybe she's prettier, or easier to soothe, or developmentally more advanced. With boy/girl twins, you might prefer the child of the sex you'd hoped for. If one twin is hospitalized longer, you might feel closer to the baby who's already at home—or to the little

one who's still in the NICU. One mother of twins even confessed that because she had wanted just one child, it took months to overcome her resentment of the second-born twin.

Whatever triggers favoritism, take steps to overcome it as soon as you can. If one child has a difficult temperament, focus on his or her positive traits. Accept that developmentally multiples are not clones; one may be crawling while the others are still learning to sit. Even if you don't love all the babies equally at first, if you treat them fairly and lovingly, genuine affection for each will follow.

Infertility treatments can complicate bonding.

Because parents of multiples are often infertility patients, they may experience unique emotional concerns about bonding, especially if the babies were conceived using donor sperm or donor eggs. "For more than a decade, I tried various infertility treatments, including Pergonal and in vitro fertilization, but never managed to carry a pregnancy past seven weeks. Finally, when I was 42, my fertility specialist suggested using donor eggs from a younger woman, which could be fertilized with my husband's sperm. That's when I conceived quadruplets," says Sarah Turner.

Given that the quads were not genetically related to Sarah, her doctor suggested that she talk to a counselor about any conflicting emotions she might have. "That would be good advice for anyone concerned about bonding," says Sarah, "but honestly, I haven't had the slightest bit of trouble falling in love with these babies. With all I went through to bring them into this world, I feel like a full-fledged, bona fide mother."

Developmental delays may lead to disappointment.

Another common hindrance to bonding stems from the fact that many multiples are born prematurely. Parents who expect their children to keep pace developmentally with their peers may feel cheated when their babies fail to smile, sit, or walk on schedule.

To get past this disappointment, understand that it's normal during pregnancy for expectant parents to develop a mental picture of their babies. One early task of parenting is to resolve the discrepancy between this idealized image and the real infants. When newborns have medical problems, this task is harder. Parents must mourn the loss of the dreamed-of infants—a process that may take weeks—before they can bond with the children they actually have.

For this reason, it is essential that you think of your preemies in terms of their corrected age, or the age they would be now if they had been born at full term. Sure, your girlfriend's six-week-old singleton is already bestowing those heart-melting first smiles on Mommy. You'll see first smiles, too—but probably not for about six weeks after your babies' original due date.

It's also very important to have a daily visit with any baby who remains hospitalized, even if this means leaving at-home infants with a sitter. This way, you can witness and rejoice in each step of your hospitalized baby's progress.

TAMARA: The deepest shock I ever felt was at first sight of my premature twins. My son's head was no larger than a lemon; red, wrinkled flesh draped his bony 3-pound frame. My daughter lay still, blue, not even breathing. My heart, overwhelmed with fear, had little room to register love.

Separation intensified my anxiety and pain. My twins were rushed to a major medical center miles away, while I stayed behind for two days at the hospital where I'd given birth. I felt desperately lonely. The Twin Tigers, as I had called them when they were snug inside me, were gone. Yet the James and Samantha who had replaced them—babies I'd scarcely seen and never held—seemed far less real.

That started to change when I was discharged. I spent endless hours each day in the NICU, scurrying between the twins' separate rooms—holding them, feeding them, singing to them, sitting by their isolettes hour after hour. But still, overshadowing everything was the constant fear that my babies wouldn't survive.

The turning point came two weeks later. I was holding my son when a nurse walked into his room unannounced and said, "Samantha wants to meet James." She placed my daughter—who had been momentarily freed from the many monitors that connected her to her isolette—into my empty arm. For the first time, I saw my twins together. Suddenly I felt confident that they would live. My dread turned to hope, my disappointment to joy, my loneliness to an overwhelming love. I felt like a real mother at last.

In the months that followed my twins' homecoming, my adoration for them grew ever deeper. Yet occasionally I'd wonder: "Is there some small part of a mother's heart that can be given only in those euphoric first moments after giving birth? Would I have loved my twins even more if I hadn't had to endure those days of separation and those weeks of anxious uncertainty?"

The answer came two years later, when I delivered my third child, a healthy 7½-pounder. Little Jack and I had a glorious first embrace just moments after he was born, and my passion for him is profound—yet no more profound than my passion for the twins. Though James and Samantha and I were denied a blissful experience at their birth, ours is a comradeship shared only by those who face disaster together and triumph. And I believe that, having known the fear of losing my twins, I can now offer *all* my children even more patience, compassion, and love than I might otherwise have found in my heart.

How to Help a Big Brother or Sister Adjust

For an older sibling, the arrival of twins, triplets, or quads can be traumatic. Not one baby but several have displaced him as the center of his parents' universe. Eager to admire the infants, visiting relatives and friends—to say nothing of strangers on the street—often ignore him. And just when he finally has Mommy to himself for a moment, some baby or another cries to be fed or changed.

When one baby is born, the father usually compensates the older sibling for the mother's lack of time and attention. But with multiples, Dad is needed to help with the newborns, so the older child may end up feeling abandoned. Helen and Tom Armer can relate to that. Says Helen, "Caroline had just turned three when the triplets were born, and she was pretty jealous at first. She wanted a lot more attention from Mom and Dad than we were able to give her, and that led to all kinds of tantrums."

Parents naturally wind up feeling guilty for causing an older child pain. Those guilt feelings may arrive at the same moment your multiples do. Judy Levy confesses, "When I delivered my twins, I was put in the same recovery bay on the maternity ward where I had been when my first child was born two years earlier. When they handed me the twins, I kept flashing back to Rianna's birth. I felt so guilty and I wondered, 'How can I love these little newborns and still keep loving my first baby?'"

For other parents, guilt grows along with their awareness of the demands of caring for multiples. One mother of twins recalls, "About three weeks after the babies were born, I was nursing them as my 18-month-old daughter stood next to me. She started to sob, and soon her tears were soaking the edge of my nursing pillow. I promised her I would play soon, but she couldn't understand why Mommy wouldn't play *now*. It broke my heart to think she was being cheated."

To minimize such problems, take steps to ease a sibling's adjustment to her expanded family. Some ideas to try:

- The first time your older child meets the multiples, present him or her with a small gift and say that it is from the babies. Thereafter, let the older child open any gifts that well-wishers may bring for the newborns. Says Judy, "Two-year-old Rianna didn't care what was in the box. She just liked the thrill of the unwrapping."
- Spend time alone with your firstborn every day—reading, playing, talking together, or whatever your child enjoys most. Build this ritual into your routine. Helen explains, "Now that the triplets are here, my three-year-old daughter and I cherish our private morning time together, eating breakfast, packing her lunchbox, and then driving to her preschool."

- If a big brother or sister enjoys fetching diapers or holding bottles for the babies, express your thanks enthusiastically. But don't make it seem as though he or she must accept this responsibility in order to stay in your good graces.
- Read storybooks about sibling rivalry to your older child to encourage him or her to express any resentment. Share your own frustration—"Boy, these babies cry a lot, don't they?"—to show that you understand how the older child is feeling.
- Explain that you are so busy because two or more babies take extra time, not because multiples are special. Ask friends not to tell the older child that he is special because he has twin or triplet siblings—he needs to be appreciated for his own unique qualities.
- Let your older child share play sessions or outings with just one of the multiples at a time, so she can form her own one-on-one relationship with each new sibling.
- Remind visitors to talk to the older child. "We have a rule that anyone who comes to the house has to play with Rianna before they even are allowed to see the babies," Judy Levy reports.
- On outings, attach a sign to the stroller that says, "The babies won't mind if you greet their older brother first." Or let your toddler and one twin sit in the stroller, while the other twin rides in a front pack or sling. This makes the babies' twinship less obvious.
- If a passerby remarks on the babies' big blue eyes, for example, you can say, "Yes, they have beautiful eyes just like their big sister."
- Make sure your firstborn has an exciting, enjoyable life outside the home. Says Helen, "Caroline felt less neglected once she started nursery school. It gave her friends and activities of her own—a world apart from the triplets."

If You're Feeling Blue

"After my babies were born, my emotions were all mixed up. I was thrilled to be a mother, but I often felt weepy, too. I'd start to cry if anyone even looked at me cross-eyed," says Meredith Alcott, mother of identical twin girls. "Thank goodness, within a few weeks I started to feel like myself again."

Meredith is far from alone. Postpartum mood disorders affect as many as 50 to 80 percent of mothers in the United States. The mildest form is known as the new-baby blues—

or among mothers of multiples, the new-babies blues. That let-down, quick-to-cry feeling usually begins within a few days of delivery, and typically abates within 10 to 14 days. No treatment is required for the postpartum blues other than reassurance that it will disappear soon.

Most new moms can feel better fast by doing one simple thing—spending a few minutes each day mothering *themselves*. Yes, it's hard to find a free moment, but you need nurturing, too. Set aside time every day to read a novel, phone a friend, play an instrument, chat online, or indulge in some other relaxing activity. To ease that chained-to-the-nursery feeling, hire a babysitter every week or two, and treat yourself to a professional manicure or massage, a lunch date with a friend, or a movie matinee. The sooner such activities are worked into your regular routine, the sooner you'll start feeling more like yourself.

Another excellent option is to exercise, because the hormones released during a workout provide a boost to your mood. If you can't find time to hit the gym, bundle the babies in their stroller and take a brisk walk. Do some simple stretches and sit-ups while the babies nap. Or put the babies in their bouncy seats in the TV room, and let them watch while you work out to an aerobics DVD. (For more ideas, see Chapter 12.)

Is It Postpartum Depression?

In some cases, postpartum mood disorders are more severe than simple new-baby blues. From 10 to 20 percent of new mothers suffer from postpartum depression (PPD), symptoms of which are similar to those of clinical depression. If you experience several of the following symptoms for more than two weeks, you may have PPD:

- Uncontrollable weeping.
- Despondency or hopelessness.
- Feelings of inadequacy.
- Loss of interest in activities that used to be enjoyable.
- Inability to concentrate.
- Memory problems.
- Food cravings or loss of appetite.
- Loss of interest in normal activities, such as personal grooming or speaking with friends.
- Having trouble sleeping even when given the chance (insomnia) or sleeping too much (hypersomnia).

There is no clear-cut answer as to why some postpartum women get depressed, but the most likely explanation involves a mix of physiological, genetic, and lifestyle factors. Scientific evidence suggests the following:

- Hormone levels, particularly of estrogen and progesterone, shift dramatically after childbirth. These hormones are known to affect mood. There are also postpartum changes in corticosteroid hormone secretion that can affect mood.
- Genetics play a part. A family history of mood disorders increases a woman's odds of developing PPD.
- Personal history is also a risk factor. If you had PPD following an earlier pregnancy, you have a 30 to 50 percent chance of experiencing it again after the birth of your multiples.
- Mothers who have complicated pregnancies, require a cesarean delivery, or give birth to babies who are premature and/or require special medical care are also at greater risk for PPD.
- Women who lack social support are more likely to develop PPD.
- Marital conflict and financial problems contribute to depression.
- Diabetes is another risk factor. A study from Harvard Medical School found that having diabetes during pregnancy nearly doubled a woman's chances of experiencing PPD.[1]
- Diet has a role. A study from the National Institutes of Health suggests that women who consume fewer omega-3 fatty acids are at higher risk for PPD.[2] Omega-3s are crucial ingredients in the biochemical processes that produce brain neurotransmitters such as serotonin and dopamine, which affect mood. Fish is high in omega-3s, so eat fish at least three times a week. Also consider taking daily fish oil supplements that provide at least 1,000 mg of combined eicosapentaenoic acid and docosahexaenoic acid (EPA/DHA).
- Thyroid hormone levels also drop significantly in the postpartum period. Low thyroid levels are associated with symptoms of depression. If your depression is accompanied by other signs of low thyroid (such as increased sensitivity to cold,

1. Kozhimannil KB, Pereira MA, Harlow BL. Association between diabetes and perinatal depression among low-income mothers. Journal of the American Medical Association 2009; 301(8):842–7.
2. Freeman MP, Hibbeln JR, Wisner KL, Brumbach BH, Watchman M, Gelenberg AJ. Randomized dose-ranging pilot trial of omega-3 fatty acids for postpartum depression. Acta Obstetricia et Gynecologica Scandinavica 2006; 113:31–5.

constipation, pale dry skin, thinning or loss of hair, failure to lose weight after delivery, or muscle and joint pain), ask your doctor about blood tests to check your thyroid levels.

New mothers of multiples may be more susceptible to postpartum mood disorders. A study from Johns Hopkins University found that, nine months after delivery, 16 percent of mothers of singletons and 19 percent of mothers of multiples had moderate to severe depressive symptoms.[3] There are several possible explanations for this increased risk. The hormonal shifts that follow a multiple pregnancy may be more dramatic than for mothers of singletons. One Swedish study found that the more complications a woman experienced during pregnancy, the more likely she was to develop PPD—and mothers of multiples are more prone to pregnancy complications, including gestational diabetes.[4] Likewise, some research suggests an association between cesarean deliveries and a higher incidence of PPD—and again, many mothers of twins and almost all mothers of triplets or quads have had cesarean deliveries. All these factors may be compounded by the more challenging physical, emotional, and financial demands involved in taking care of two or more newborns.

Unfortunately, too many moms suffer in silence. The Johns Hopkins study found that, among mothers of both singletons and multiples, only 27 percent of those who had symptoms of PPD reported talking about the problem with their physician or a mental health specialist.

One mother of twins says, "I had expected motherhood to be the most fulfilling experience of my life. But less than a week after the twins were born, I found myself feeling either sad or mad most of the time. I was so ashamed that I couldn't bring myself to talk to anyone about it." Even when a woman does broach the subject with family or friends, she may be told, "Snap out of it. You're a mother now, and you're responsible for these babies."

Yet if you are suffering from PPD, it is very important to get help. If you're reluctant to seek help for yourself, do it for your babies' sake: Studies show that maternal depression early in an infant's life can have significant negative effects on the child's psychological, social, and intellectual development.

The most serious form of postpartum mood disorder is called postpartum psychosis. Here, the distinguishing symptom is a break with reality—the woman loses the ability to distinguish what is real from what is not. As a result of the psychotic state, she may become a threat to

---

3. Choi Y, Bishai D, Minkovitz CS. Multiple births are a risk factor for postpartum maternal depressive symptoms. Pediatrics 2009; 123:1147–54.
4. Vadlimarsdottir U, Hultman CM, Harlow B, Cnattingius S, Sparen P. Psychotic illness in first-time mothers with no previous psychiatric hospitalizations: A population-based study. PLOS Medicine 2009; 6:194–201.

herself and her babies. Immediate treatment is necessary, usually involving hospitalization and antipsychotic medications. Fortunately, this condition is rare, occurring in less than 1 in 1,000 postpartum women, and the risk decreases after the first month following delivery.

The vast majority of women with PPD can be helped far more easily. Treatment typically includes short-term cognitive behavioral therapy (CBT) and/or antidepressant medication, such as selective serotonin reuptake inhibitors (SSRIs). These two approaches appear to be equally effective; some women benefit most from a combination of both. Help is also available from the following groups:

- Center for Postpartum Health: 13743 Riverside Drive, Sherman Oaks, CA 91423. Telephone 818-887-1312; website www.postpartumhealth.com.
- Postpartum Health Alliance: P.O. Box 927231, San Diego, CA 92192-7231. Telephone 619-254-0023; email info@postpartumhealthalliance.org; website www.postpartumhealthalliance.org.
- Postpartum Support International: 6706 SW 54th Ave., Portland OR 97219. Telephone 800-944-4773; email PSIOffice@postpartum.net; website www .postpartum.net.

DR. NEWMAN: Many women suffering from PPD wait too long to seek treatment. This is a mistake, because unaddressed depressive disorders often worsen over time. In addition, with both CBT and antidepressant SSRI medications, improvement may not be noticeable for several weeks after treatment begins.

The rule of thumb is that if your baby blues haven't eased within three weeks of delivery, it's time to speak to your doctor. After all, you've been through a lot in order to bring these babies into the world—and you deserve to enjoy them to the fullest.

Married . . . with Multiples

TAMARA: One evening a few months after the twins came home, I was having dinner with my husband and my sister. As I chattered on and on about the babies—how much they had grown, how adorable they were, how intensely in love I was with both of them—Bill was uncharacteristically quiet. Suddenly he excused himself from the table, said he wanted to take a walk, and left the house.

I looked at my sister in surprise. "What's with him?" I asked. My sister said simply, "I think he misses his wife."

For a marriage to stay strong after two, three, or four new members suddenly join the family, the partners have to devote some time to nurturing and nourishing their relationship. That's not to say you need to escape for a two-week cruise together. With newborn multiples to take care of, a getaway is probably not an option—but neither is it necessary, psychologists believe. Studies show that one big romantic blitz does less to reduce marital stress than do small loving moments together, repeated day after day. So carve out a few minutes to reconnect.

Encourage your partner to take paternity leave.

The more time he can take off work, the more involved he'll feel with the babies, and the more he'll enjoy them. The bonus: He'll also have more in common with you. But be sure not to hover over him with instructions on how to handle the babies. Treat him like a competent equal.

Make contact during the day.

When you're apart, try to phone, text message, or email each other at least once daily. Don't just say, "Please pick up some diapers on the way home from work." Give each message some affectionate content, like "I'm so glad I am married to you." When your husband walks into the house, give him a hug *before* you thrust a crying baby or two into his arms. He wants to feel like a partner in love, not just a partner in parenthood.

Share a meal.

Sit down to one intimate meal together each day, even if it's just a bowl of cereal before the babies wake up. Spend at least part of that time talking about something other than your multiples.

Hang onto your sense of humor.

Finding ways to laugh together can help transform the difficulties you are facing into sources of, if not joy, then at least mutual amusement. Just be sure to laugh *with* each other, not *at* each other. Keep a good attitude about your new parenting skills. You will both make plenty of small mistakes that are funny in retrospect.

DR. NEWMAN: One of my triplet moms happened to be a writer. In a candid discussion of some of her marital challenges in the months after the babies arrived, she joked that she was planning a new book. She wasn't sure how it was going to end, but she already had the title: *Triplets: The Meltdown of the Nuclear Family.* She and her husband had a lot of fun talking about how to turn marital misadventures into fodder for the book. I'm glad to say that they got through that tricky first year and are still happily married.

Compliment each other.

"Lydia and I are facing a lot of challenges right now. Not only do we have the kids to take care of, but she's trying to start up a home-based business, and I've just taken a new job," says Ed Greenwood, father of boy/girl twins. "Whenever I feel stressed out, she reminds me of all we've accomplished already, and I do the same for her. When we confirm our confidence in each other, the demands of our lives seem less daunting."

Reconnect as lovers.

First, ask your doctor when it's okay to resume having sex. In general, physicians recommend that women wait four to six weeks after delivery, so the cervix can close and vaginal tissues can heal. If you had a cesarean, your physical recovery may take a little longer.

For many women, though, the bigger issue is emotional readiness. You're tired and stressed out; you're worried that lovemaking may hurt; and you're getting as much skin-to-skin contact as you can handle just from rocking, soothing, and feeding all those babies. Your husband, on the other hand, is probably eager to resume an active sex life.

Try to be open to feelings of romance. Instead of fretting about colic while you wash your hair, let your mind linger on the memory of the last time your husband and you shared a long, slow kiss. A fantasy that provides a 60-second sabbatical from the demands of parenting can refresh your romantic spirit and rekindle your desire.

TAMARA: My husband, Bill, and I have always had a really good relationship. But I'll admit that the first year after the twins' birth was a challenging time in our marriage. I wondered, "What's wrong here? Do other couples handle this better than we do?"

Then I went to a meeting of the Mothers of Twins Club, and I was shocked to learn how many of the members' marriages had split up in the first few years after their multiples were born. But at the same time, it was encouraging to hear from numerous other moms that the task of parenting multiples gets much easier over time, if you can stick together through the initial adjustment.

When I got home that night, I sat down at the dining room table with Bill, and we talked for hours and hours. We agreed to remind ourselves and each other daily that we were in love, that we adored our children, and that *together* we could get through the toughest of times. And we have.

DR. LUKE: Some years ago, I was involved in a field study on the childhood growth of twins at the annual Twins Days Festival in Twinsburg, Ohio. Over the course of the study, which lasted several years, we weighed and measured nearly 1,000 twin children. We also interviewed their parents regarding the pregnancy as well as each child's birthweight and health during infancy. The results of our research showed that children are amazingly resilient. Most multiples grew to be within the normal range for weight and height, even if they had been born prematurely and/or at a low birthweight.

But what was even more striking was the resilience and strength of the mothers. They were the most organized, calm, unflappable women I had ever met. Because the festival takes place the first full weekend in August, it's typically hot and muggy—the perfect recipe for irritable kids and aggravated parents. Yet despite the hassles of helping kids take off their shoes to be weighed and measured, and answering our many questions—all while soothing whining children who were overheated, overstimulated, and overtired—never once did a mother lose her temper. Nor did anyone forget the details of her children's arrival in this world, down to the exact minute of birth, birthweight, and birth length.

The fathers, likewise, were the most knowledgeable and easygoing dads I had ever seen. Never once did a man turn to his wife and insist, "*You* help the kids with their shoes," or bark at a child who was being uncooperative. Often they remembered, in almost as much detail as the moms, the specifics of their children's birth. It was obvious how proud these couples were of their kids, and how confident and relaxed they were in their roles as parents.

Of course, there were single-parent families present. During the interviews, some of them confided that the stress—of infertility treatments, or of months-long vigils in the NICU, or of having a houseful of colicky newborns—had torn their marriages apart. Yet in some ways these single parents seemed to have an even closer bond with their children.

Although I had never met any of these mothers or fathers before the interviews, my heart went out to each of them as they told me their unique stories. I was particularly touched by those who had had complicated pregnancies and coped courageously with weeks of bedrest, difficult deliveries, or months of visiting their multiples in the NICU. These parents seemed to know their children better than most parents do, because they had endured so much to get to this stage. They remembered every little victory and loved their children all the more for being survivors.

Because my work with the University Consortium on Multiple Births is primarily in the field of obstetrics, I rarely get to see this metamorphosis—this transformation from anxious parents-to-be coping with a challenging pregnancy to confident, well-adjusted, loving mothers and fathers. The experience was both heartening and humbling.

Parenthood is one of life's most profound and rewarding adventures, and as parents of multiples, you will experience it even more intensely. Couples open to this opportunity for personal growth will find their marriages immeasurably enriched.

Given how rapidly your family has expanded, it may take some time to see yourselves as one big happy family. But when you do, the feeling will be like nothing you've experienced before. For as often as you are overwhelmed by the demands of having multiples, you and your partner will be more often overwhelmed with joy—with wonderment at your babies' beauty, with pride as you watch them grow, and with profound gratitude at having been multiply blessed.

Best Recipes for Moms-to-Be of Multiples

One of the most common questions asked by expectant mothers of multiples is "What should I eat to make sure I'm getting all the calories and nutrients my unborn babies need?" To answer that question as thoroughly as possible, this fourth edition of *When You're Expecting Twins, Triplets, and Quads* includes 75 recipes. Each has been developed by Dr. Barbara Luke to provide excellent nutrition, delicious flavor, and easy preparation. To help you meet your daily calorie intake goal, all recipes include a per-serving calorie count. Also listed are the amounts of protein, carbohydrate, fat, and fiber per serving.

You'll notice that many of the recipes include egg whites rather than whole eggs, and low-fat or nonfat versions of dairy products like milk, cheese, yogurt, and mayonnaise. The point is not to cut calories. Rather, such ingredients allow for a higher proportion of protein for the calories provided, while reducing saturated fats and cholesterol, and utilizing healthier monounsaturated and polyunsaturated fats.

In addition, for easy reference, each recipe receives two ratings. First is the Blue-Ribbon Rating, which shows the number of specific nutrients each serving provides at 20 percent or more of the recommended dietary allowance (RDA) for pregnancy. You can also refer to the chart "Summary of Nutrient Content of Recipes" to find out which recipes provide the specific nutrients you may be looking for (again, at 20 percent or more of the RDA) to round out the day's diet. For instance, if you know you need more calcium today, check the chart to find out which specific recipes—27 of them, in this case—can provide you with a healthy calcium boost. Likewise for iron—there are 21 delicious recipes that provide 20 percent or more of the RDA for iron per serving.

The second rating for each recipe is the All-Star Rating. This shows the number of Top 25 Food All-Stars (as described in Chapter 4) that are included in the recipe. Many of the common Food All-Stars—eggs, milk, vegetables, meat—can be readily found in most cookbook recipes. Other All-Stars—pumpkin, legumes, oats, nuts, and tofu—appear less frequently in typical cookbooks. That's why so many of the original recipes included in this section contain these often-overlooked nutritional powerhouses.

Bon appétit!

Index to Recipes

Index to Recipes

Summary of Nutrient Content of Recipes

(✓ indicates recipe provides 20% or more of the RDA for that nutrient per serving)

	Protein	Vitamins A, C, or E	B-Vitamins	Calcium	Iron	Other Minerals	Fiber
Beef and Lamb Entrées							
Asian-Style Meatballs	✓	✓	✓		✓	✓	
Beef and Bean Chili	✓	✓	✓		✓	✓	✓
Beef Stew	✓	✓	✓			✓	✓
Beef Stroganoff	✓		✓	✓	✓	✓	
Lamb and Lentil Stew	✓		✓			✓	✓
Lamb Salad	✓	✓	✓	✓	✓	✓	✓
Mini Meat Loaves	✓	✓	✓			✓	
Spicy Beef	✓	✓	✓			✓	✓
Steak and Arugula Salad	✓	✓	✓	✓	✓	✓	✓
Vietnamese Steak Salad	✓	✓	✓		✓	✓	✓
Pork Entrées							
French Toast with Ham and Cheese		✓	✓	✓		✓	✓
Ham and Pumpkin Quiche	✓	✓	✓	✓		✓	
Lentil and Ham Salad with Walnuts	✓	✓	✓		✓	✓	✓
Maple Pork and Spinach Salad	✓	✓	✓	✓	✓	✓	✓
Pasta with Peas and Ham	✓	✓	✓			✓	
Pork and Cashew Bok Choy		✓	✓			✓	
Pork with Apple Stuffing	✓		✓			✓	✓
Spicy Pork with Peanut Sauce	✓		✓			✓	

	Protein	Vitamins A, C, or E	B-Vitamins	Calcium	Iron	Other Minerals	Fiber
Poultry Entrées							
Cashew Chicken	✓	✓	✓			✓	
Chicken and Dumplings	✓		✓	✓		✓	
Chicken and Sweet Potatoes	✓	✓	✓			✓	✓
Chicken and Wild Rice Casserole	✓		✓	✓		✓	
Chicken-Barley Soup	✓	✓	✓			✓	✓
Chicken-Citrus Salad		✓	✓			✓	✓
Chinese Chicken Salad	✓	✓	✓	✓	✓	✓	✓
Cobb Salad	✓	✓	✓		✓	✓	✓
Golden Chicken Salad	✓	✓					
Greek Lemon Chicken	✓	✓	✓			✓	✓
Honey Chicken Salad with Cherries	✓	✓	✓	✓	✓	✓	✓
Pasta with Chicken and Peanut Sauce	✓	✓	✓			✓	
Seasoned Baked Chicken	✓	✓	✓			✓	✓
Waldorf Chicken Salad	✓	✓	✓		✓	✓	✓
Seafood Entrées							
Caesar Salad with Shrimp	✓	✓	✓	✓	✓	✓	✓
Citrus Salmon	✓		✓			✓	
Linguine with Clams and Dried Tomatoes		✓				✓	
Salad Niçoise	✓	✓	✓		✓	✓	✓
Salmon and Asparagus Salad	✓	✓	✓			✓	✓

	Protein	Vitamins A, C, or E	B-Vitamins	Calcium	Iron	Other Minerals	Fiber
Salmon Burgers	✓	✓	✓	✓		✓	
Shrimp and Scallop Grill	✓	✓	✓		✓	✓	
Spicy Shrimp Salad	✓	✓	✓		✓	✓	✓
Tuna Salad with White Beans	✓	✓	✓		✓	✓	✓
Dairy and Vegetarian Entrées							
Arugula and Pear Salad	✓	✓	✓	✓		✓	✓
Asparagus Quiche	✓	✓	✓	✓		✓	
Autumn Pancakes		✓	✓	✓		✓	
Avocado Salad with Orange and Grapefruit		✓				✓	✓
Beet Salad with Goat Cheese		✓		✓		✓	✓
Caprese Salad	✓	✓	✓	✓		✓	✓
Ginger Stir-Fry	✓	✓	✓			✓	
Greek Salad	✓	✓	✓	✓		✓	✓
Greek Spinach and Cheese Pie	✓	✓	✓	✓	✓	✓	✓
Lentil Soup		✓	✓		✓	✓	✓
Mediterranean Sauté	✓		✓			✓	✓
Oatmeal-Almond Pancakes	✓	✓	✓	✓		✓	
Pasta with Green Sauce	✓	✓			✓	✓	✓
Pumpkin Waffles		✓	✓				✓
Ratatouille		✓	✓			✓	✓
Salsa Frittata	✓	✓	✓	✓		✓	
Spinach and Pumpkin Casserole	✓	✓	✓	✓		✓	✓

	Protein	Vitamins A, C, or E	B-Vitamins	Calcium	Iron	Other Minerals	Fiber
Tomato Apricot Salad		✓	✓			✓	✓
Vegetarian Lasagna	✓	✓	✓			✓	
Vegetarian Stroganoff	✓	✓	✓			✓	✓
Wild Rice Omelet	✓	✓	✓		✓	✓	✓

Side Dishes and Snacks

	Protein	Vitamins A, C, or E	B-Vitamins	Calcium	Iron	Other Minerals	Fiber
Chickpea Salad		✓	✓			✓	✓
Harvest Muffins		✓				✓	
Powerhouse Granola		✓	✓			✓	✓
Pumpkin Custard	✓	✓	✓	✓		✓	✓
Pumpkin-Fruit Muffins		✓					
Pumpkin Loaf		✓	✓			✓	✓
Sunrise Bread Pudding		✓	✓			✓	✓
Tabbouleh		✓	✓			✓	✓
Weekend Hash Browns	✓	✓	✓	✓		✓	
Yogurt Guacamole			✓			✓	✓

Smoothies

	Protein	Vitamins A, C, or E	B-Vitamins	Calcium	Iron	Other Minerals	Fiber
Basic Fruit Smoothie	✓	✓	✓	✓		✓	
Basic Vegetable Smoothie	✓	✓	✓	✓		✓	
Ginger Smoothie		✓					

Beef and Lamb Entrées

Asian-Style Meatballs

MAKES 4 SERVINGS

3 tablespoons low-sodium soy sauce

¾ cup orange juice

1 tablespoon hoisin sauce

1 tablespoon honey

1 clove garlic, minced

1 pound lean ground beef

½ cup rolled oats

8 ounces canned water chestnuts, drained, sliced, and chopped

2 egg whites

½ teaspoon salt

In a large saucepan combine soy sauce, orange juice, hoisin sauce, honey, and garlic. In a separate bowl, mix ground beef, oats, water chestnuts, egg whites, and salt. Using an ice cream scoop, form meat mixture into 1-inch to 2-inch balls, and add to the sauce. Cook over medium heat until done, about 15 to 20 minutes.

All-Star Rating: 4 Stars ★		Nutrient Content per Serving	
Beef		Calories	390 kcal
Egg		Protein	39 g
Oats		Carbohydrate	38 g
Orange		Fat	8 g
		Fiber	1 g

Blue-Ribbon Rating: 11 Ribbons 🎗			
Iron	Selenium		
Manganese	Vitamin B$_6$		
Niacin	Vitamin B$_{12}$		
Phosphorus	Vitamin C		
Protein	Zinc		
Riboflavin			

Beef and Bean Chili

MAKES 4 SERVINGS

1 pound lean ground beef
2 medium onions, chopped
1 green pepper, chopped
2 8-ounce cans diced tomatoes
1 tablespoon chili powder
¼ teaspoon cayenne pepper

¼ teaspoon paprika
¾ cup canned pinto beans, drained
¾ cup canned red kidney beans, drained
¾ cup canned Great Northern beans, drained
Salt and pepper to taste

In a large skillet, cook the ground beef, onions, and green pepper until the meat is browned and the onions are tender; drain off the fat. Stir in the tomatoes, chili powder, cayenne, paprika, and beans; cover and simmer for 15 to 20 minutes. Add salt and pepper to taste.

All-Star Rating: 3 Stars ★		*Nutrient Content per Serving*	
Beans		Calories	375 kcal
Beef		Protein	44 g
Tomatoes		Carbohydrate	31 g
		Fat	8 g
Blue-Ribbon Rating: 15 Ribbons 🎗		Fiber	9 g
Fiber	Selenium		
Iron	Thiamin		
Magnesium	Vitamin A		
Manganese	Vitamin B$_6$		
Niacin	Vitamin B$_{12}$		
Phosphorus	Vitamin C		
Potassium	Zinc		
Protein			

Beef Stew

MAKES 6 SERVINGS

3 tablespoons olive oil

1½ pounds lean stew beef, trimmed and
cut into bite-size pieces

1 medium onion, cut into 1-inch pieces

2 tablespoons all-purpose flour

1 garlic clove, chopped

¼ teaspoon dried thyme

½ teaspoon paprika

½ teaspoon ground black pepper

3 cups beef broth

2 medium carrots, cut into 1-inch pieces

2 cups celery, cut into 1-inch pieces

8 ounces potatoes, peeled and cut into
1-inch cubes

1½ cups green peas

In a large Dutch oven, heat the oil; add the beef and cook for 2 to 4 minutes, stirring, until the meat is browned. Stir in the onion, flour, garlic, and seasonings. Add the broth and bring to a boil. Reduce the heat, cover, and cook for about 1½ hours, or until the meat is tender. Add the carrots, celery, potatoes, and peas. Cook until the vegetables are tender, about 15 minutes.

All-Star Rating: 2 Stars ★		*Nutrient Content per Serving*	
Beef		Calories	329 kcal
Peas		Protein	28 g
		Carbohydrate	19 g
Blue-Ribbon Rating: 12 Ribbons		Fat	15 g
Fiber	Selenium	Fiber	4.1 g
Thiamin	Vitamin A	Calcium	75 mg
Niacin	Vitamin B$_6$	Iron	4 mg
Phosphorus	Vitamin B$_{12}$		
Protein	Vitamin C		
Riboflavin	Vitamin K		

Beef Stroganoff

MAKES 4 SERVINGS

1 tablespoon olive oil

½ pound sliced mushrooms

1 medium onion, minced

1 clove garlic, minced

1 pound beef tenderloin or flank steak,
    ½-inch thick, thinly sliced

1 package dry onion soup mix

1 cup nonfat plain Greek yogurt

2 cups cooked long-grain and wild rice

In a large skillet heat the oil; add the mushrooms, onion, and garlic. Cook until the onion is tender, and then remove from the skillet. In the same pan, cook the beef until done; remove from the skillet. In the same pan, stir in 1¼ cups water and soup mix. Bring to a boil; reduce heat and cook for 5 minutes. Stir in mushroom mixture and beef. Remove from heat; stir in yogurt. Serve over rice.

All-Star Rating: 2 Stars ★		Nutrient Content per Serving	
Beef		Calories	400 kcal
Yogurt		Protein	39 g
		Carbohydrate	34 g
Blue-Ribbon Rating: 9 Ribbons		Fat	12 g
Calcium	Selenium	Fiber	2 g
Iron	Vitamin B$_6$		
Niacin	Vitamin B$_{12}$		
Phosphorus	Zinc		
Protein			

Lamb and Lentil Stew

MAKES 8 SERVINGS

1 pound lean lamb, cut into 1-inch cubes	2 teaspoons balsamic vinegar
1 clove garlic, minced	1 teaspoon salt
2 medium tomatoes, peeled, seeded, and diced	2 cups beef broth
1 cup dried green lentils	2 cups water
1 teaspoon chopped fresh rosemary leaves	½ cup chopped fresh cilantro

In a slow cooker, combine all ingredients except cilantro. Cover and cook on low heat for 7 to 8 hours or until the lentils are tender. Sprinkle with cilantro.

All-Star Rating: 3 Stars ★		*Nutrient Content per Serving*	
Lamb		Calories	360 kcal
Lentils		Protein	39 g
Tomatoes		Carbohydrate	32 g
		Fat	8 g
Blue-Ribbon Rating: 9 Ribbons 🎗		Fiber	15 g
Fiber	Selenium		
Manganese	Thiamin		
Niacin	Vitamin B$_{12}$		
Phosphorus	Zinc		
Protein			

Lamb Salad

MAKES 2 SERVINGS

¼ red onion, chopped

1 clove garlic, minced

1 cup nonfat Greek yogurt

5 ounces boneless lamb meat, cut into
bite-sized pieces

4 cups romaine lettuce, torn into
bite-sized pieces

12 cherry tomatoes

1 ounce nonfat feta cheese, crumbled

1 tablespoon olive oil

½ lemon, juiced

1 tablespoon chopped mint

In a medium bowl, combine the red onions, garlic, and yogurt. Add the lamb, stir, cover, and marinate 4 to 6 hours or overnight. Arrange the lamb in a shallow pan and place under the broiler for 8 to 12 minutes, or until done. Remove from heat and cool. Toss the lamb, lettuce, tomatoes, and cheese in a medium salad bowl. In a small bowl, mix the oil, lemon juice, and mint; pour over the salad.

All-Star Rating: 4 Stars ★		Nutrient Content per Serving	
Cheese		Calories	400 kcal
Lamb		Protein	35 g
Tomatoes		Carbohydrate	35 g
Yogurt		Fat	14 g
		Fiber	12 g

Blue-Ribbon Rating: 14 Ribbons 🎗	
Calcium	Potassium
Fiber	Riboflavin
Iron	Thiamin
Magnesium	Vitamin A
Manganese	Vitamin B$_6$
Niacin	Vitamin B$_{12}$
Phosphorus	Vitamin C

Mini Meat Loaves

MAKES 2 MINI LOAVES, OR 8 SERVINGS

2 pounds extra-lean ground beef

¾ cups spaghetti sauce

1 cup seasoned bread crumbs

½ cup chopped fresh parsley

½ cup chopped celery

4 large egg whites, beaten

1 envelope dried onion soup mix

12 ounces nonfat evaporated milk

Preheat the oven to 375°F. In a large bowl, combine all the ingredients. Divide the mixture into two small loaf pans. Bake, uncovered, for 45 to 60 minutes, or until a meat thermometer inserted into the center of a loaf reaches 180°F. Pour off the grease; let stand for 10 minutes before serving.

All-Star Rating: 4 Stars ★		*Nutrient Content per Serving*	
Beef		Calories	390 kcal
Egg whites		Protein	30 g
Milk		Carbohydrate	21 g
Tomato (sauce)		Fat	20 g
		Fiber	1.7 g
Blue-Ribbon Rating: 8 Ribbons 🏅		Calcium	180 mg
Magnesium	Protein	Iron	3.3 mg
Selenium	Vitamin B$_6$		
Niacin	Vitamin K		
Phosphorus	Zinc		

Spicy Beef

12 ounces boneless beef sirloin steak

¼ cup hot bean sauce or hot bean paste

¼ cup dry white wine

2 tablespoons soy sauce

½ teaspoon ground black pepper

½ teaspoon cornstarch

1 teaspoon chili oil

1 tablespoon canola oil

2 medium carrots, bias sliced

1 garlic clove, minced

1½ cups snow peas

6 ounces fresh mushrooms, thinly sliced

2 cups hot cooked rice

2 green onions, cut into slivers

Trim the fat from the beef. Thinly slice across the grain into bite-size strips. (For easier slicing, partially freeze the beef first.) Set aside. For the sauce, in a small bowl, stir together the bean sauce or paste, wine, soy sauce, black pepper, cornstarch, and chili oil. Set aside. Pour the canola oil into a wok or large skillet. (Add more oil as necessary during cooking.) Preheat over medium-high heat. In the hot oil, stir-fry the carrots and garlic for 2 minutes. Add the snow peas; stir-fry for 2 minutes. Add the mushrooms; stir-fry for 1 to 2 minutes, or until the vegetables are crisp-tender. Remove the vegetables from the wok. Add the beef to the wok. Stir-fry for 2 to 3 minutes or to the desired doneness. Push the beef from the center of the wok. Stir the sauce. Add the sauce to the center of the wok. Cook and stir until thickened and bubbly. Return the cooked vegetables to the wok. Stir all the ingredients together to coat with the sauce. Cook and stir for 1 minute more, or until heated through. Serve immediately with the rice. Garnish with the green onions.

All-Star Rating: 2 Stars ★		Nutrient Content per Serving	
Beef		Calories	468 kcal
Snow peas		Protein	26 g
Blue-Ribbon Rating: 15 Ribbons 🏅		Carbohydrate	49 g
Fiber	Thiamin	Fat	18 g
Folate	Vitamin A	Fiber	4.1 g
Magnesium	Vitamin B₆	Calcium	59 mg
Niacin	Vitamin B₁₂	Iron	4.5 mg
Phosphorus	Vitamin C		
Protein	Vitamin K		
Riboflavin	Zinc		
Selenium			

Steak and Arugula Salad

MAKES 4 SERVINGS

½ head romaine lettuce

1 large Belgian endive

3 cups fresh baby arugula

½ red onion, thinly sliced

12 cherry tomatoes

1 12-ounce jar marinated artichoke hearts, drained and sliced

½ cup sliced fresh mushrooms

1 ounce chopped walnuts

2 tablespoons olive oil

1 tablespoon red wine vinegar

1 clove garlic, minced

1 tablespoon lemon juice

Salt and pepper to taste

½ pound steak, broiled and sliced

¼ cup shredded Parmesan cheese

In a large salad bowl, combine the romaine lettuce, endive, arugula, onion, tomatoes, artichoke hearts, mushrooms, and walnuts. In a small bowl, mix the oil, vinegar, garlic, and lemon juice; add salt and pepper to taste. Pour dressing over the salad. Arrange the steak slices over the salad; sprinkle with the cheese.

All-Star Rating: 4 Stars ★	Nutrient Content per Serving	
Cheese	Calories	350 kcal
Steak	Protein	30 g
Tomatoes	Carbohydrate	23 g
Walnuts	Fat	16 g
	Fiber	12 g

Blue-Ribbon Rating: 13 Ribbons 🎗	
Calcium	Riboflavin
Fiber	Thiamin
Iron	Vitamin A
Magnesium	Vitamin B_6
Manganese	Vitamin B_{12}
Phosphorus	Vitamin C
Potassium	

Vietnamese Steak Salad

2 green onions, cut into 2-inch pieces

1 pound lean steak, cooked and cut into
  1-inch by ½-inch strips

½ teaspoon minced fresh ginger

½ teaspoon salt

½ teaspoon pepper

2 tablespoons olive oil

1 tablespoon rice wine vinegar

2 tablespoons lemon juice

3 cups finely shredded cabbage

In a large salad bowl, mix all ingredients.

All-Star Rating: 2 Stars ★	
Beef	
Cabbage	

Blue-Ribbon Rating: 14 Ribbons	
Fiber	Protein
Iron	Selenium
Magnesium	Thiamin
Manganese	Vitamin B$_6$
Niacin	Vitamin B$_{12}$
Phosphorus	Vitamin C
Potassium	Zinc

Nutrient Content per Serving	
Calories	335 kcal
Protein	34 g
Carbohydrate	10 g
Fat	17 g
Fiber	5 g

Pork Entrées

French Toast with Ham and Cheese

MAKES 2 SERVINGS

2 large egg whites	2 slices lean boiled ham
¼ cup skim milk	2 slices Muenster cheese
½ teaspoon ground cinnamon	1 teaspoon butter
4 slices cinnamon-raisin bread	1 cup chunky applesauce

In a small bowl, whisk together the egg whites, milk, and cinnamon. Make two sandwiches with the bread, ham, and cheese. Add the sandwiches to the egg mixture, turning to soak thoroughly. In a small skillet, melt the butter. Add the soaked sandwiches, cooking until the undersides are browned and the cheese is melted, 5 to 7 minutes. Turn the sandwiches and cook for 5 to 7 minutes on the other side, or until browned. Serve topped with the applesauce.

All-Star Rating: 5 Stars ★		*Nutrient Content per Serving*	
Apples		Calories	580 kcal
Cheese		Protein	26 g
Eggs		Carbohydrate	100 g
Ham		Fat	11 g
Milk		Fiber	10.8 g
		Calcium	252 mg
Blue-Ribbon Rating: 11 Ribbons		Iron	5.5 mg
Calcium	Riboflavin		
Fiber	Selenium		
Folate	Thiamin		
Magnesium	Vitamin B$_{12}$		
Niacin	Zinc		
Phosphorus			

Ham and Pumpkin Quiche

15 ounces canned pumpkin

4 ounces extra-lean ham (5 percent fat), chopped

½ cup finely chopped onion

1 cup sliced fresh mushrooms

4 large egg whites

12 ounces nonfat evaporated milk

½ cup grated Parmesan cheese

2 tablespoons all-purpose flour

1 unbaked 10-inch pie shell

Preheat the oven to 375°F. In a medium bowl, combine the pumpkin, ham, onion, mushrooms, and egg whites; mix well. Gradually add the milk, stirring until well blended. Toss the cheese with the flour; fold into the pumpkin mixture. Pour into the pie shell; bake for 60 minutes, or until a knife inserted in the center comes out clean.

All-Star Rating: 4 Stars ★		*Nutrient Content per Serving*	
Cheese		Calories	303 kcal
Eggs		Protein	17 g
Ham		Carbohydrate	31 g
Pumpkin		Fat	12 g
		Fiber	3.6 g
Blue-Ribbon Rating: 10 Ribbons 🏅		Calcium	339 mg
Calcium	Selenium	Iron	2.6 mg
Magnesium	Thiamin		
Phosphorus	Vitamin A		
Protein	Vitamin B$_{12}$		
Riboflavin	Vitamin K		

Lentil and Ham Salad with Walnuts

MAKES 2 SERVINGS

¾ cup lentils, rinsed and sorted

½ carrot, chopped

½ yellow onion, chopped

1 stalk celery, chopped

2 ounces sliced ham, chopped

1 tablespoon lemon juice

2 tablespoons balsamic vinegar

1 tablespoon olive oil

1 tablespoon chopped fresh parsley

1 ounce chopped walnuts

Salt and pepper to taste

Place the lentils, carrot, and onion in a large saucepan; cover with two quarts of water and bring to a boil. Cover and reduce heat; simmer about 15 to 20 minutes or until lentils are tender, stirring occasionally. Drain lentils and vegetables; place in a medium salad bowl; stir in celery and ham. In a small bowl, mix lemon juice, vinegar, and oil; pour over the lentil mixture. Top with parsley and walnuts; salt and pepper to taste.

All-Star Rating: 3 Stars ★		*Nutrient Content per Serving*	
Ham		Calories	380 kcal
Lentils		Protein	21 g
Walnuts		Carbohydrate	36 g
		Fat	18 g
Blue-Ribbon Rating: 8 Ribbons 🎗		Fiber	17 g
Fiber	Selenium		
Iron	Thiamin		
Manganese	Zinc		
Phosphorus	Vitamin A		

Maple Pork and Spinach Salad

MAKES 2 SERVINGS

3 cups fresh baby spinach

8 ounces cooked pork tenderloin, sliced into bite-size pieces

2 tablespoons chopped pecans

1 ounce shredded Gouda cheese

1 tablespoon olive oil

1 tablespoon maple syrup

2 tablespoons cider vinegar

Place fresh spinach in a medium salad bowl. Top with pork, pecans, and cheese. In a small bowl, mix the oil, maple syrup, and vinegar; pour over the salad.

All-Star Rating: 4 Stars ★		*Nutrient Content per Serving*	
Cheese		Calories	360 kcal
Pecans		Protein	35 g
Pork		Carbohydrate	10 g
Spinach		Fat	20 g
		Fiber	6 g

Blue-Ribbon Rating: 12 Ribbons 🎗	
Fiber	Selenium
Iron	Thiamin
Manganese	Vitamin A
Niacin	Vitamin B$_6$
Phosphorus	Vitamin C
Riboflavin	Zinc

Pasta with Peas and Ham

MAKES 8 SERVINGS

1 tablespoon whipped butter
2 tablespoons all-purpose flour
2 teaspoons brown mustard
2½ cups skim milk
1 cup shredded Colby cheese
1 cup shredded Monterey Jack cheese

8 ounces uncooked enriched macaroni
8 ounces lean boiled ham, cut into
  bite-size pieces
1 pound canned sweet peas
½ cup seasoned bread crumbs

Preheat the oven to 375°F. In a large saucepan, melt the butter; add the flour and mustard, mixing well. Add the milk, and stir until the sauce is smooth and slightly thickened. In a small bowl, toss together the shredded cheeses. Set aside ½ cup of the cheese mixture. To the saucepan, add the remaining 1½ cups cheese and heat until melted, stirring occasionally. Cover and remove from the heat. Cook the macaroni according to the package directions; drain. In a 2-quart casserole, combine the sauce with the macaroni, ham, and peas. Sprinkle the remaining cheese and the bread crumbs on top. Bake, uncovered, for 20 to 25 minutes, or until browned and bubbly.

All-Star Rating: 4 Stars ★		Nutrient Content per Serving	
Cheese		Calories	355 kcal
Ham		Protein	22 g
Milk		Carbohydrate	35 g
Peas		Fat	14 g
		Fiber	2.9 g
Blue-Ribbon Rating: 10 Ribbons 🎗		Calcium	318 mg
Calcium	Riboflavin	Iron	2.9 mg
Folate	Selenium		
Niacin	Thiamin		
Phosphorus	Vitamin A		
Protein	Vitamin B$_{12}$		

Pork and Cashew Bok Choy

MAKES 6 SERVINGS

12 ounces lean boneless pork

4 tablespoons soy sauce

2 teaspoons peeled, grated fresh ginger

2 garlic cloves, minced

½ cup hoisin sauce

½ cup water

1 tablespoon cornstarch

1 teaspoon sugar

1 tablespoon canola oil

2 medium onions, cut into thin wedges

1 Chinese cabbage (bok choy), cut
    diagonally into 1-inch pieces

4 cups hot cooked rice

¼ cup dry-roasted cashews

Trim the fat from the pork. Thinly slice across the grain into bite-size strips. (For easier slicing, partially freeze the pork first.) In a medium bowl, stir together pork, 2 tablespoons of soy sauce, ginger, garlic. Cover and refrigerate for 1 to 2 hours. For the sauce, in a small bowl stir together hoisin sauce, water, remaining soy sauce, cornstarch, and sugar. Set aside. Pour canola oil into a wok or large skillet and preheat over medium-high heat. (Add more oil as necessary during cooking.) Stir-fry onions, cabbage in hot oil for 1 minute. Remove vegetables from wok. Add pork mixture to the hot wok. Stir-fry for 2 to 3 minutes, or until no pink remains. Push pork from the center of the wok. Stir the sauce and add it to the center of the wok. Cook and stir until the sauce is thickened and bubbly. Return cooked vegetables to the wok. Stir all ingredients together to coat with the sauce. Cover and cook for 1 minute more, or until heated through. Serve immediately with the rice. Sprinkle with the cashews.

All-Star Rating: 3 Stars ★		Nutrient Content per Serving	
Cabbage		Calories	554 kcal
Cashews		Protein	30 g
Pork		Carbohydrate	61 g
Blue-Ribbon Rating: 12 Ribbons 🎗		Fat	20 g
Folate	Thiamin	Fiber	3.6 g
Magnesium	Vitamin A	Calcium	113 mg
Niacin	Vitamin B$_6$	Iron	4.1 mg
Phosphorus	Vitamin B$_{12}$		
Riboflavin	Vitamin C		
Selenium	Zinc		

Pork with Apple Stuffing

MAKES 4 SERVINGS

4 boneless pork loin chops, 1 inch thick
(approximately 4 ounces each)

1 teaspoon salt

1 tablespoon butter

1 medium celery stalk, diced

1 large onion, diced

2 large Golden Delicious apples, peeled,
cored, and diced

4 slices firm white bread, cut into
½-inch pieces

½ cup apple juice

1 teaspoon poultry seasoning

1 large egg

¼ cup raisins

Preheat the oven to 325°F. Slice each pork chop nearly through to create a pocket in the center and sprinkle with the salt. Roast in a pan for 30 minutes. Meanwhile, in a large saucepan, melt butter over medium heat. Add celery and onion and cook until tender, about 10 minutes, stirring often. Add apples and cook for 6 to 8 minutes more, until softened. Remove from the heat; stir in the bread, apple juice, poultry seasoning, egg, and raisins. After the chops have cooked for 30 minutes, remove from the oven. Spoon stuffing into the center of each chop. Place remaining stuffing in a greased 1½-quart casserole. Return pork chops and stuffing to the oven. Cook for 30 minutes more, or until a meat thermometer inserted in the thickest part of a chop reaches 155°F. (If the stuffing browns too quickly, cover it loosely with foil.) Let the chops stand for 5 minutes; the internal temperature of the meat will rise to 160°F upon standing.

All-Star Rating: 3 Stars ★		*Nutrient Content per Serving*	
Apples		Calories	536 kcal
Egg		Protein	36 g
Pork		Carbohydrate	48 g
Blue-Ribbon Rating: 12 Ribbons 🎗		Fat	21 g
Fiber	Selenium	Fiber	5.6 g
Folate	Thiamin	Calcium	119 mg
Niacin	Vitamin B$_6$	Iron	3.5 mg
Phosphorus	Vitamin B$_{12}$		
Protein	Vitamin K		
Riboflavin	Zinc		

Spicy Pork with Peanut Sauce

MAKES 4 SERVINGS

8 ounces uncooked enriched linguine

4 boneless pork loin chops, 1 inch thick (approximately 4 ounces each)

¼ teaspoon ground black pepper

½ teaspoon salt

4 green onions, cut into 1-inch diagonal slices

1 tablespoon peeled, minced fresh ginger

3 garlic cloves, crushed with a garlic press

3 tablespoons creamy peanut butter

1 tablespoon soy sauce

½ teaspoon ground red pepper

¾ cups water

Cook the linguine according to the package directions. Drain, cover, and keep warm. Sprinkle the pork chops with the pepper and ¼ teaspoon of the salt. Heat a large skillet over medium-high heat until hot. Add the pork chops and cook for 4 minutes; turn the chops over and cook 4 minutes longer. Transfer the pork to a platter; cover with foil to keep warm. To the same skillet, add the green onions and the remaining ¼ teaspoon salt. Cook over medium heat for 4 minutes, stirring frequently. Stir in the ginger and garlic; cook for 1 minute. Return the pork to the skillet. In a small bowl, stir the peanut butter, soy sauce, ground red pepper, and water until blended. Pour the peanut-butter mixture into the same skillet; heat to boiling over medium-high heat. Reduce the heat to low; simmer for 1 minute. Serve with the peanut sauce poured over the chops.

All-Star Rating: 2 Stars ★		*Nutrient Content per Serving*	
Peanut butter		Calories	481 kcal
Pork		Protein	43 g
		Carbohydrate	47 g
Blue-Ribbon Rating: 12 Ribbons		Fat	12 g
Folate	Selenium	Fiber	2.7 g
Magnesium	Thiamin	Calcium	39 mg
Niacin	Vitamin B$_6$	Iron	4.5 mg
Phosphorus	Vitamin B$_{12}$		
Protein	Vitamin K		
Riboflavin	Zinc		

Poultry Entrées

Cashew Chicken

MAKES 6 SERVINGS

½ cup chicken broth

3 tablespoons oyster sauce (such as Kame)

1½ tablespoons cornstarch

1½ tablespoons honey

1 tablespoon soy sauce

2 teaspoons white wine vinegar

2 tablespoons oil

1 cup chopped green onions

1 small onion, cut into 8 wedges

½ cup diagonally sliced carrots

1 cup snow peas

1 pound boneless, skinless chicken breasts, cut into 1½-inch pieces

¼ cup canned pineapple chunks in juice, drained

¼ cup cashews

6 cups hot cooked rice

Combine the first 6 ingredients in a small bowl; set aside. Heat 1 tablespoon of the oil in a stir-fry pan or wok over medium-high heat. Add ½ cup of the green onions and the onion wedges; stir-fry for 1 minute. Add the carrots; stir-fry for 2 minutes. Add the snow peas; stir-fry for 2 minutes. Remove the vegetables from the pan; keep warm. Heat the remaining 1 tablespoon oil in the pan over medium-high heat. Add the chicken; stir-fry for 5 minutes. Add the broth mixture, cooked vegetables, the pineapple, and cashews; bring to a boil and cook for 1 minute, or until thick. Stir in the remaining ½ cup green onions. Serve with the rice.

All-Star Rating: 3 Stars ★		Nutrient Content per Serving	
Cashews		Calories	391 kcal
Chicken		Protein	22 g
Peas		Carbohydrate	52 g
		Fat	10 g
Blue-Ribbon Rating: 10 Ribbons		Fiber	10 g
Folate	Selenium	Calcium	47 mg
Magnesium	Vitamin A	Iron	2.6 mg
Niacin	Vitamin B$_6$		
Phosphorus	Vitamin C		
Protein	Vitamin K		

Chicken and Dumplings

MAKES 4 SERVINGS

1 tablespoon safflower or olive oil
1 pound cooked, diced chicken
1 cup chopped onions
1 cup chopped carrots
1 cup chopped celery
1 cup chicken broth

1½ cups reduced-fat all-purpose
  baking mix
½ cup cornmeal
¾ cup skim milk
¼ cup sliced green onions
½ cup shredded Parmesan cheese

In a large skillet or Dutch oven, heat the oil and sauté the cooked chicken pieces until golden. Add the onions, carrots, celery, and chicken broth. Bring to a boil; reduce the heat. Cover and simmer for 5 minutes, stirring occasionally. In a medium bowl, combine the baking mix, cornmeal, milk, and green onions. Mix until a soft dough forms; drop by rounded spoonfuls onto the chicken mixture. Cook, uncovered, for 10 minutes. Sprinkle with the cheese. Cover and cook for an additional few minutes, or until the cheese has melted.

All-Star Rating: 3 Stars ★		*Nutrient Content per Serving*	
Cheese		Calories	513 kcal
Chicken		Protein	38 g
Milk		Carbohydrate	47 g
		Fat	18 g
Blue-Ribbon Rating: 13 Ribbons ♟		Fiber	2.6 g
Calcium	Thiamin	Calcium	305 mg
Magnesium	Vitamin B₆	Iron	2.6 mg
Niacin	Vitamin B₁₂		
Phosphorus	Vitamin E		
Protein	Vitamin K		
Riboflavin	Zinc		
Selenium			

Chicken and Sweet Potatoes

MAKES 4 SERVINGS

4 boneless, skinless chicken breast halves
   (approximately 1 pound)
Garlic powder to taste
Salt and ground black pepper to taste
½ cup all-purpose flour
1 tablespoon olive or canola oil
1 cup peeled, cubed sweet potatoes

1 cup chopped onions
1 cup chopped green bell peppers
1 cup chopped celery
½ cup golden raisins
¾ cup chicken broth
¾ cup apple cider

Rinse and pat dry the chicken. Cut the chicken into ½-inch pieces. Sprinkle with garlic powder, salt, and pepper. Dip the chicken into the flour to coat well. In a large skillet or Dutch oven, heat the oil and brown the chicken on all sides until golden. Remove the chicken and set aside. Add the sweet potatoes, onions, bell peppers, celery, and raisins; sauté until the onions are tender. Stir in the chicken broth and apple cider. Add the browned chicken and bring to a boil. Reduce the heat, cover, and simmer for 25 to 30 minutes, or until the chicken is cooked and the potatoes are tender.

All-Star Rating: 2 Stars ★		*Nutrient Content per Serving*	
Chicken		Calories	535 kcal
Sweet potatoes		Protein	26 g
		Carbohydrate	56 g
Blue-Ribbon Rating: 13 Ribbons		Fat	21 g
Biotin	Riboflavin	Fiber	6.1 g
Fiber	Selenium	Calcium	118 mg
Folate	Thiamin	Iron	3.2 mg
Magnesium	Vitamin B$_6$		
Niacin	Vitamin C		
Phosphorus	Vitamin K		
Protein			

Chicken and Wild Rice Casserole

1 6.2-ounce package fast-cooking
   long-grain and wild rice mix
1 pound chicken breasts, roasted and
   cut into bite-size pieces
1 10.75-ounce can condensed cream of
   chicken soup

½ cup skim milk
1 cup sliced fresh mushrooms
1 cup frozen green peas
1 cup shredded Muenster cheese

Preheat the oven to 350°F. Prepare the rice according to package directions, omitting the butter. Add the chicken, soup, milk, mushrooms, and peas; mix well. Pour into a 2-quart casserole. Bake, covered, for 30 minutes. Uncover; sprinkle with the cheese. Bake, uncovered, for an additional 5 to 10 minutes, or until the cheese is melted.

All-Star Rating: 4 Stars ★
Cheese
Chicken
Milk
Peas

Blue-Ribbon Rating: 11 Ribbons	
Calcium	Selenium
Magnesium	Vitamin A
Niacin	Vitamin B_6
Phosphorus	Vitamin B_{12}
Protein	Zinc
Riboflavin	

Nutrient Content per Serving	
Calories	470 kcal
Protein	40 g
Carbohydrate	37 g
Fat	17 g
Fiber	3.2 g
Calcium	243 mg
Iron	2.7 mg

Chicken-Barley Soup

MAKES 6 SERVINGS

½ cup lentils

2 tablespoons salted margarine or butter

1 cup chopped onions

1 garlic clove, minced

6 cups chicken broth

¼ teaspoon crushed dried rosemary

¼ teaspoon ground black pepper

1½ cups cooked, diced chicken

½ cup finely chopped fresh parsley

½ cup green peas

1½ cups sliced carrots

½ cup uncooked quick-cooking barley

Rinse and drain the lentils; set aside. Melt the margarine or butter in a large saucepan or Dutch oven. Sauté the onions and garlic until tender but not brown. Stir in the chicken broth, rosemary, pepper, and lentils; bring to a boil. Reduce the heat and simmer, covered, for 20 minutes. Stir in the chicken, parsley, peas, carrots, and barley. Simmer, covered, for about 20 minutes more, or until the carrots are just tender.

All-Star Rating: 3 Stars ★		Nutrient Content per Serving	
Chicken		Calories	397 kcal
Lentils		Protein	35 g
Peas		Carbohydrate	41 g
		Fat	11 g
Blue-Ribbon Rating: 13 Ribbons 🎀		Fiber	12.5 g
Fiber	Thiamin	Calcium	80 mg
Magnesium	Vitamin A	Iron	4.9 mg
Niacin	Vitamin B$_6$		
Phosphorus	Vitamin B$_{12}$		
Protein	Vitamin C		
Riboflavin	Vitamin K		
Selenium			

Chicken-Citrus Salad

4 cups mixed baby greens

½ teaspoon finely chopped fresh ginger

½ teaspoon finely chopped fresh garlic

1 tablespoon orange marmalade

¼ cup orange juice

¼ cup grapefruit juice

1 tablespoon olive oil

6 ounces cooked chicken breasts, skinned and shredded

½ red onion, chopped

1 stalk of celery, chopped

1 orange, peeled and cut into segments

½ red grapefruit, peeled and cut into segments

2 tablespoons chopped peanuts

Place greens in a medium salad bowl. In a separate bowl, combine ginger, garlic, marmalade, orange juice, grapefruit juice, and olive oil. To the juice mixture, add the chicken, onion, celery, orange segments, and grapefruit segments; mix well. Spoon mixture on top of greens; sprinkle with chopped peanuts.

All-Star Rating: 4 Stars ★		*Nutrient Content per Serving*	
Chicken		Calories	400 kcal
Grapefruit		Protein	29 g
Orange		Carbohydrate	30 g
Peanuts		Fat	18 g
		Fiber	10 g

Blue-Ribbon Rating: 9 Ribbons 🏵	
Fiber	Thiamin
Niacin	Vitamin A
Phosphorus	Vitamin B$_6$
Potassium	Vitamin C
Selenium	

Chinese Chicken Salad

MAKES 2 SERVINGS

¼ head cabbage, shredded
¼ head iceberg lettuce, shredded
1 tablespoon chopped fresh cilantro
1 stalk chopped scallions
1 tablespoon olive oil
1 tablespoon rice wine vinegar
1 teaspoon soy sauce

1 tablespoon honey
8 ounces cooked chicken breasts,
   skinned and shredded
2 tablespoons honey-roasted peanuts,
   chopped
1 tablespoon toasted sesame seeds

Combine the cabbage, lettuce, cilantro, and scallions in a medium bowl. In a separate bowl, combine the oil, vinegar, soy sauce, and honey; add the chicken and mix well. Add the chicken mixture to the greens. Top with the peanuts and sesame seeds.

All-Star Rating: 3 Stars ★		*Nutrient Content per Serving*	
Cabbage		Calories	375 kcal
Chicken		Protein	36 g
Peanuts		Carbohydrate	12 g
		Fat	20 g
Blue-Ribbon Rating: 12 Ribbons 🎗		Fiber	10 g
Calcium	Phosphorus		
Fiber	Potassium		
Iron	Selenium		
Magnesium	Thiamin		
Manganese	Vitamin B$_6$		
Niacin	Vitamin C		

Cobb Salad

MAKES 2 SERVINGS

¼ head romaine lettuce

¼ head Boston lettuce

½ bunch watercress, coarse stems removed

2 slices crisp turkey bacon, chopped

4 ounces cooked skinless chicken or
  turkey breast, diced

2 tomatoes, cubed

½ ripe avocado, pitted, peeled, and sliced
  lengthwise

2 hard-boiled eggs, whites only, chopped

1 tablespoon chopped fresh chives

1 ounce grated Swiss cheese

1 tablespoon red wine vinegar

1 tablespoon olive oil

½ teaspoon Dijon mustard

Salt and pepper to taste

Combine the romaine, Boston, and watercress greens in a medium salad bowl. Over the greens arrange the bacon, chicken or turkey, tomato, and avocado; garnish with the chopped eggs and chives. In a small bowl, mix the cheese, vinegar, oil, and mustard together; add salt and pepper to taste. Pour over the salad.

All-Star Rating: 5 Stars ★		*Nutrient Content per Serving*	
Avocado		Calories	360 kcal
Cheese		Protein	30 g
Chicken		Carbohydrate	15 g
Egg		Fat	20 g
Tomato		Fiber	12 g
Blue-Ribbon Rating: 14 Ribbons 🎗			
Fiber	Riboflavin		
Iron	Selenium		
Magnesium	Thiamin		
Manganese	Vitamin A		
Niacin	Vitamin B$_6$		
Phosphorus	Vitamin B$_{12}$		
Potassium	Vitamin C		

Golden Chicken Salad

MAKES 4 SERVINGS

1 cup canned pumpkin

½ cup fat-free mayonnaise

1 teaspoon lemon juice

1 teaspoon salt

¼ teaspoon ground black pepper

3 cups cooked, chopped chicken

2 ounces chopped almonds

Combine the pumpkin, mayonnaise, lemon juice, salt, and pepper; mix well. Add the chicken and almonds; mix lightly; chill.

All-Star Rating: 3 Stars ★		Nutrient Content per Serving	
Almonds		Calories	288 kcal
Chicken		Protein	21 g
Pumpkin		Carbohydrate	10 g
		Fat	17 g
Blue-Ribbon Rating: 3 Ribbons 🎀		Fiber	3 g
Protein	Vitamin K	Calcium	69 mg
Vitamin A		Iron	2.7 mg

Greek Lemon Chicken

MAKES 6 SERVINGS

3 pounds bone-in chicken parts
½ cup Roditis wine (Greek white wine)
½ cup olive oil
¼ cup lemon juice
2 tablespoons dried oregano
1 teaspoon dried thyme

1 teaspoon dried basil
1 teaspoon salt
½ teaspoon ground black pepper
1 14-ounce can artichoke hearts, drained
1 lemon, sliced
3 cups hot cooked white rice

Rinse the chicken and pat dry with paper towels. In a large baking dish, combine the wine, olive oil, lemon juice, and seasonings. Add the chicken; cover and marinate for at least 3 hours, or overnight. Preheat the oven to 350°F. Add the artichoke hearts and lemon slices. Bake for 1 hour, basting occasionally. Serve over the rice.

All-Star Rating: 1 Star ★		Nutrient Content per Serving	
Chicken		Calories	426 kcal
		Protein	53 g
		Carbohydrate	31 g
Blue-Ribbon Rating: 14 Ribbons 🎗		Fat	10 g
Fiber	Selenium	Fiber	4.7 g
Folate	Thiamin	Calcium	100 mg
Magnesium	Vitamin B₆	Iron	4.9 mg
Niacin	Vitamin B₁₂		
Phosphorus	Vitamin C		
Protein	Vitamin E		
Riboflavin	Zinc		

Honey Chicken Salad with Cherries

MAKES 2 SERVINGS

3 cups romaine lettuce

6 ounces roasted chicken, skinned and
    sliced into bite-sized pieces

½ cucumber, peeled and sliced

¼ cup fresh cherries, pitted

1 tablespoon chopped pecans

1 ounce shredded Parmesan cheese

2 tablespoons cider vinegar

1 tablespoon olive oil

1 tablespoon honey

Place greens in a medium salad bowl. Top with chicken slices, cucumber, cherries, pecans, and cheese. In a small bowl, mix the vinegar, oil, and honey; pour over the salad.

All-Star Rating: 4 Stars ★		*Nutrient Content per Serving*	
Cheese		Calories	360 kcal
Cherries		Protein	34 g
Chicken		Carbohydrate	18 g
Pecans		Fat	17 g
		Fiber	10 g
Blue-Ribbon Rating: 8 Ribbons 🎗			
Calcium	Phosphorus		
Fiber	Selenium		
Manganese	Vitamin B$_6$		
Niacin	Vitamin C		

Pasta with Chicken and Peanut Sauce

MAKES 4 SERVINGS

8 ounces uncooked enriched pasta

2 cups chicken broth

2 tablespoons soy sauce

1 tablespoon cornstarch

¼ cup creamy peanut butter

1 tablespoon canola oil

½ cup thinly sliced onions

2 garlic cloves, minced

4 boneless, skinless chicken breast halves (approximately 1 pound), cut into 1-inch pieces

2 green onions, sliced

¼ cup chopped peanuts

Cook the pasta according to the package directions. Drain; keep warm; set aside. In a medium mixing bowl, stir together the chicken broth, soy sauce, and cornstarch. Stir in the peanut butter until smooth. Set the sauce aside. In a wok or large skillet, heat the canola oil over medium-high heat. Add the onions and garlic to the hot oil; stir-fry for 2 to 3 minutes. Remove the onion mixture from the skillet. Add the chicken to the wok. Stir-fry for about 3 minutes, or until the chicken is no longer pink. Push the chicken from the center of the wok. Stir the sauce; add to the center of the wok. Cook and stir for 4 minutes, or until thickened and bubbly. Return the onion mixture to the skillet; stir all the ingredients together. Arrange the pasta on individual plates or a large platter. Spoon the chicken mixture over the pasta. Sprinkle with the green onions and peanuts.

All-Star Rating: 3 Stars ★		*Nutrient Content per Serving*	
Chicken		Calories	561 kcal
Peanut butter		Protein	33 g
Peanuts		Carbohydrate	54 g
		Fat	24 g
Blue-Ribbon Rating: 13 Ribbons 🎗		Fiber	3.8 g
Folate	Thiamin	Calcium	50 mg
Magnesium	Vitamin B$_6$	Iron	4 mg
Niacin	Vitamin B$_{12}$		
Phosphorus	Vitamin E		
Protein	Vitamin K		
Riboflavin	Zinc		
Selenium			

Seasoned Baked Chicken

MAKES 4 SERVINGS

1 cup plain bread crumbs

1 envelope dried onion soup mix

½ teaspoon ground black pepper

½ teaspoon ground red pepper

4 boneless, skinless chicken breast halves
  (approximately 1 pound)

½ cup light mayonnaise

2 cups diced carrots

2 baking potatoes, peeled and quartered

Preheat the oven to 425°F. Combine the bread crumbs, onion soup mix, and seasonings. Coat the chicken breast halves with the mayonnaise, then coat in the bread crumb mixture. Place in a baking dish; add the carrots and potatoes. Bake for 20 to 30 minutes, or until the potatoes are tender and the chicken is cooked through.

All-Star Rating: 1 Star ★		*Nutrient Content per Serving*	
Chicken		Calories	563 kcal
		Protein	43 g
Blue-Ribbon Rating: 13 Ribbons		Carbohydrate	60 g
Fiber	Thiamin	Fat	16 g
Magnesium	Vitamin A	Fiber	6.4 g
Niacin	Vitamin B$_6$	Calcium	99 mg
Phosphorus	Vitamin B$_{12}$	Iron	4.5 mg
Protein	Vitamin C		
Riboflavin	Vitamin K		
Selenium			

Waldorf Chicken Salad

MAKES 2 SERVINGS

½ head Boston lettuce

6 ounces roasted chicken, skinned and
    chopped

1 stalk celery, chopped

2 Granny Smith apples, cored and cut into
    bite-size pieces

¼ cup dried cherries

1 ounce chopped walnuts

1 tablespoon plain yogurt

1 tablespoon light mayonnaise

1 tablespoon lemon juice

Salt and pepper to taste

Divide the lettuce onto two medium salad plates. In a large bowl combine the chicken, celery, apples, cherries, and walnuts. In a small bowl, mix the yogurt, mayonnaise, and lemon juice; pour over the chicken mixture. Add salt and pepper to taste. Serve over the greens.

All-Star Rating: 4 Stars ★		*Nutrient Content per Serving*	
Apples		Calories	360 kcal
Cherries		Protein	29 g
Chicken		Carbohydrate	25 g
Walnuts		Fat	17 g
		Fiber	8 g

Blue-Ribbon Rating: 12 Ribbons 🎗	
Fiber	Potassium
Iron	Selenium
Niacin	Thiamin
Magnesium	Vitamin A
Manganese	Vitamin B$_6$
Phosphorus	Vitamin C

Seafood Entrées

Caesar Salad with Shrimp

MAKES 2 SERVINGS

4 cups romaine lettuce

½ cup croutons

¼ cup shredded Parmesan cheese

8 ounces chilled cooked shrimp, peeled
and deveined

2 tablespoons olive oil

1 teaspoon Dijon mustard

½ lemon, juiced

1 clove garlic, minced

Dash of Worcestershire sauce

Salt and pepper to taste

Place lettuce in a medium salad bowl. Add croutons, cheese, and shrimp; toss well. In a small bowl, combine the oil, mustard, lemon juice, garlic, and Worcestershire sauce; add salt and pepper to taste. Pour over the salad.

All-Star Rating: 2 Stars ★		*Nutrient Content per Serving*	
Cheese		Calories	330 kcal
Shrimp		Protein	30 g
		Carbohydrate	9 g
Blue-Ribbon Rating: 9 Ribbons 🎗		Fat	19 g
Calcium	Selenium	Fiber	6 g
Fiber	Vitamin A		
Iron	Vitamin B$_{12}$		
Niacin	Zinc		
Phosphorus			

Citus Salmon

1 6.2-ounce package fast-cooking
   long-grain and wild rice mix

3 tablespoons orange marmalade

1 teaspoon ground cumin

1 teaspoon ground coriander

¾ teaspoon salt

¾ teaspoon grated fresh lemon peel

¼ teaspoon ground black pepper

1 teaspoon very hot water

4 salmon fillets, ¾ inch thick
   (approximately 6 ounces each),
   skin removed

Lemon wedges

Preheat the grill. Cook the rice according to the package directions. Cover and keep warm. In a small bowl, mix the marmalade, cumin, coriander, salt, lemon peel, pepper, and 1 teaspoon very hot water until blended. With tweezers, remove any bones from the salmon. Brush the marmalade mixture all over the salmon pieces. Place the salmon on the grill over medium heat and cook for 4 minutes. With a wide metal spatula, carefully turn the salmon over; cook for 4 to 5 minutes more, until the salmon turns opaque throughout and flakes easily when tested with a fork. Serve over the hot rice. Garnish with lemon wedges.

All-Star Rating: 1 Star ★		Nutrient Content per Serving	
Salmon		Calories	350 kcal
		Protein	32 g
Blue-Ribbon Rating: 8 Ribbons		Carbohydrate	43 g
Magnesium	Selenium	Fat	5g
Niacin	Thiamin	Fiber	1.2 g
Phosphorus	Vitamin B$_6$	Calcium	45 mg
Protein	Vitamin B$_{12}$	Iron	1.9 mg

Linguine with Clams and Dried Tomatoes

MAKES 4 SERVINGS

8 ounces uncooked linguine, fettuccine, or
    spaghetti
1 pound canned minced clams
2 tablespoons olive oil
2 garlic cloves, minced

½ cup dry white wine
½ cup oil-packed dried tomatoes,
    drained and cut into strips
½ cup grated Parmesan cheese

Cook the pasta according to the package directions. Drain; keep warm; set aside. For the sauce, drain the clams, reserving the liquid; set the clams aside. In a medium saucepan, heat the olive oil; stir in the garlic. Stir in the reserved clam liquid and the wine. Bring to a boil. Simmer for 10 minutes, or until the sauce is reduced to about 1 cup. Stir in the clams and tomatoes; heat through. Arrange the pasta on individual plates or a large platter. Spoon the sauce over the pasta. Sprinkle with the cheese.

All-Star Rating: 3 Stars ★		*Nutrient Content per Serving*	
Cheese		Calories	420 kcal
Clams		Protein	30 g
Tomatoes		Carbohydrate	49 g
		Fat	13 g
Blue-Ribbon Rating: 7 Ribbons 🍴		Fiber	2.2 g
Folate	Selenium	Calcium	194 mg
Niacin	Thiamin	Iron	4.3 mg
Phosphorus	Vitamin C		
Riboflavin			

Salad Niçoise

MAKES 2 SERVINGS

½ head Boston lettuce

½ pound green beans, cooked and drained

12 cherry tomatoes

¼ pound new potatoes, cooked and
    quartered

1 6-ounce can chunk light tuna, drained

1 hard-boiled egg, halved

¼ cup small black olives

2 flat anchovy filets (optional)

1 tablespoon capers

2 tablespoons olive oil

1 tablespoon lemon juice

1 tablespoon white balsamic vinegar

Place the lettuce leaves on two medium salad plates. Arrange the green beans, tomatoes, potatoes, tuna, egg, olives, and anchovies on top of the lettuce; garnish with capers. In a small bowl, mix the oil, lemon juice, and vinegar; pour over the salads.

All-Star Rating: 3 Stars ★		*Nutrient Content per Serving*	
Egg		Calories	400 kcal
Tomatoes		Protein	32 g
Tuna		Carbohydrate	48 g
		Fat	14 g
Blue-Ribbon Rating: 13 Ribbons		Fiber	12 g
Fiber	Selenium		
Iron	Thiamin		
Magnesium	Vitamin A		
Manganese	Vitamin B$_6$		
Niacin	Vitamin B$_{12}$		
Phosphorus	Vitamin C		
Riboflavin			

Salmon and Asparagus Salad

MAKES 2 SERVINGS

4 ounces cooked or canned salmon, flaked

½ pound cooked fresh asparagus, cut into 2-inch pieces

1 carrot, chopped

6 hard-boiled eggs, whites only, cut into wedges

1 scallion, chopped

2 tablespoons chopped pecans

1 tablespoon olive oil

1 tablespoon white wine vinegar

1 tablespoon lemon juice

½ teaspoon Dijon mustard

Salt and pepper to taste

In a large bowl, mix together the salmon, asparagus, carrot, egg, scallion, and pecans. In a small bowl, mix the oil, vinegar, lemon juice, and mustard; add salt and pepper to taste. Pour over salmon mixture.

All-Star Rating: 4 Stars ★		Nutrient Content per Serving	
Asparagus		Calories	320 kcal
Egg		Protein	27 g
Pecans		Carbohydrate	12 g
Salmon		Fat	18 g
		Fiber	8 g

Blue-Ribbon Rating: 12 Ribbons 🎀	
Fiber	Selenium
Magnesium	Thiamin
Manganese	Vitamin A
Niacin	Vitamin B$_{12}$
Phosphorus	Vitamin C
Riboflavin	Zinc

Salmon Burgers

MAKES 4 SERVINGS

1 pound canned red or pink salmon, drained and flaked

1 green onion, sliced

3 tablespoons prepared white horseradish

¼ cup seasoned bread crumbs

2 tablespoons chopped fresh parsley

1 tablespoon soy sauce

¼ teaspoon ground black pepper

1 tablespoon olive oil

8 ounces enriched orzo, cooked

In a medium bowl, with a fork, lightly mix all the ingredients except the olive oil and orzo. Shape the mixture into four 3-inch round patties. Heat the olive oil in a skillet over medium heat until hot. Add the salmon cakes, and cook for about 5 minutes per side, or until golden and hot. Serve over the warm orzo.

All-Star Rating: 1 Star ★		*Nutrient Content per Serving*	
Salmon		Calories	465 kcal
		Protein	28 g
Blue-Ribbon Rating: 12 Ribbons 🎗		Carbohydrate	49 g
Calcium	Selenium	Fat	17 g
Magnesium	Thiamin	Fiber	2.2 g
Niacin	Vitamin B$_{12}$	Calcium	287 mg
Phosphorus	Vitamin D	Iron	2.5 mg
Protein	Vitamin E		
Riboflavin	Vitamin K		

Shrimp and Scallop Grill

MAKES 6 SERVINGS

1 tablespoon brown sugar	8 ounces sea scallops
1 tablespoon soy sauce	2 large onions, each cut into 6 chunks
1 tablespoon vegetable oil	2 green bell peppers, each cut into 6 chunks
2 teaspoons Chinese five-spice powder	
¼ teaspoon ground black pepper	12 cherry tomatoes
1 pound large shrimp, shelled and deveined	4 cups hot cooked white rice

Preheat the grill. In a large bowl, mix the brown sugar, soy sauce, vegetable oil, Chinese five-spice powder, and pepper; add the shrimp and scallops, tossing to coat. Onto 6 long metal skewers, alternately thread the shrimp, onions, scallops, bell peppers, and cherry tomatoes. Place the skewers on the grill over medium heat. Grill for 10 to 12 minutes, until the shrimp and scallops turn opaque throughout, turning the skewers occasionally and brushing the shrimp and scallops with any remaining spice mixture halfway through cooking. Serve over the rice.

All-Star Rating: 3 Stars ★		*Nutrient Content per Serving*	
Scallops		Calories	419 kcal
Shrimp		Protein	37 g
Tomatoes		Carbohydrate	48 g
		Fat	8 g
Blue-Ribbon Rating: 13 Ribbons 🎗		Fiber	2.3 g
Folate	Vitamin A	Calcium	105 mg
Iron	Vitamin B$_{12}$	Iron	5.7 mg
Magnesium	Vitamin C		
Niacin	Vitamin D		
Phosphorus	Vitamin E		
Protein	Vitamin K		
Selenium			

Spicy Shrimp Salad

MAKES 2 SERVINGS

1 tablespoon olive oil

1 tablespoon minced fresh ginger

1 lime, juiced

1 tablespoon soy sauce

1 teaspoon honey

¼ teaspoon crushed red pepper flakes

¼ cup chopped fresh cilantro

8 ounces cooked medium shrimp, peeled and deveined

4 cups mixed baby greens

1 carrot, chopped

2 hard-boiled eggs, finely chopped

2 tablespoons cashews, chopped

In a large bowl combine the oil, ginger, lime juice, soy sauce, honey, red pepper flakes, and cilantro. Stir in the shrimp; cover and refrigerate for 2 to 3 hours. Divide the greens between two medium salad plates; top with shrimp mixture. Sprinkle with carrot, egg, and cashews.

All-Star Rating: 3 Stars ★		Nutrient Content per Serving	
Cashews		Calories	320 kcal
Egg		Protein	32 g
Shrimp		Carbohydrate	12 g
		Fat	16 g
Blue-Ribbon Rating: 9 Ribbons 🎗		Fiber	9 g
Fiber	Selenium		
Iron	Vitamin A		
Niacin	Vitamin B$_{12}$		
Phosphorus	Zinc		
Riboflavin			

Tuna Salad with White Beans

MAKES 2 SERVINGS

3 cups mixed baby greens

1 6-ounce can chunk light water-packed
tuna, drained and flaked

1 8-ounce can white beans, drained

2 tomatoes, cored and chopped

½ cup chopped sweet onion (Vidalia)

1 hard-boiled egg, chopped

2 tablespoons chopped fresh parsley

2 tablespoons olive oil

1 tablespoon white wine vinegar

1 tablespoon lemon juice

Salt and pepper to taste

Divide baby greens onto two medium salad plates. In a large bowl mix the tuna, white beans, tomatoes, onion, egg, and parsley. In a small bowl, mix the oil, vinegar, and lemon juice; pour over the tuna mixture. Add salt and pepper to taste. Serve over the greens.

All-Star Rating: 4 Stars ★		*Nutrient Content per Serving*	
Beans		Calories	390 kcal
Egg		Protein	34 g
Tomatoes		Carbohydrate	27 g
Tuna		Fat	16 g
		Fiber	10 g

Blue-Ribbon Rating: 14 Ribbons 🎀	
Fiber	Riboflavin
Iron	Selenium
Manganese	Thiamin
Magnesium	Vitamin A
Niacin	Vitamin B$_6$
Phosphorus	Vitamin B$_{12}$
Potassium	Vitamin C

Dairy and Vegetarian Entrées

Arugula and Pear Salad

MAKES 2 SERVINGS

4 cups fresh arugula greens

2 firm Bartlett or d'Anjou pears, sliced

1 ounce walnuts

6 ounces nonfat feta cheese

1 tablespoon white balsamic vinegar

1 tablespoon olive oil

¼ teaspoon Dijon mustard

Salt and pepper to taste

Place greens in a medium salad bowl. Top with pear slices, walnuts, and cheese. In a small bowl, combine the vinegar, oil, mustard, salt and pepper; pour over the salad.

All-Star Rating: 2 Stars ★		Nutrient Content per Serving	
Cheese		Calories	385 kcal
Walnuts		Protein	26 g
		Carbohydrate	38 g
Blue-Ribbon Rating: 12 Ribbons 🏅		Fat	15 g
Calcium	Riboflavin	Fiber	8 g
Fiber	Vitamin A		
Magnesium	Vitamin B$_6$		
Manganese	Vitamin B$_{12}$		
Phosphorus	Vitamin C		
Potassium	Zinc		

Asparagus Quiche

MAKES 6 SERVINGS

1 pound fresh asparagus, trimmed and
  cut into ¾-inch pieces
1 unbaked 10-inch pie shell
2 large eggs, or 4 large egg whites
2 cups skim milk

⅛ teaspoon ground black pepper
Pinch of ground nutmeg
1 cup coarsely shredded low-fat Swiss
  cheese

Preheat the oven to 425°F. In a 2-quart saucepan, boil 4 cups water. Add the asparagus and cook for 6 to 8 minutes, until tender. Drain the asparagus and rinse with cold running water. Drain again and set aside. Line the pie shell with foil and fill with pie weights or uncooked rice. Bake the pie shell for 10 minutes; remove the foil with the weights, and bake for 7 to 10 minutes more, until the crust is golden. Reduce the oven temperature to 350°F. Meanwhile, in a medium bowl, with a wire whisk or fork, mix the eggs, milk, pepper, and nutmeg until well blended. Sprinkle the asparagus and cheese into the pie shell. Pour the liquid mixture over the asparagus and cheese. Place a sheet of foil underneath the pie plate to catch any drips during baking. Bake the quiche for 40 to 45 minutes, until a knife inserted in the center comes out clean.

All-Star Rating: 4 Stars ★		*Nutrient Content per Serving*	
Asparagus		Calories	355 kcal
Cheese		Protein	24 g
Eggs		Carbohydrate	26 g
Milk		Fat	17 g
		Fiber	1.8 g
Blue-Ribbon Rating: 13 Ribbons 🎗		Calcium	455 mg
Calcium	Vitamin A	Iron	2.1 mg
Folate	Vitamin B$_{12}$		
Magnesium	Vitamin C		
Protein	Vitamin E		
Riboflavin	Vitamin K		
Selenium	Zinc		
Thiamin			

Autumn Pancakes

MAKES 15 PANCAKES, OR 5 SERVINGS

2 tablespoons canola oil
2 cups all-purpose flour
1 tablespoon baking powder
1 teaspoon salt
1½ cups low-fat (1%) milk
½ cup canned pumpkin-pie mix
2 large egg whites

Preheat a lightly oiled griddle to 375°F. In a large bowl, combine the flour, baking powder, and salt. In another bowl, combine the milk, pumpkin-pie mix, and egg whites; add to the dry ingredients, stirring until just moistened. For each pancake, pour ¼ cup batter onto the hot griddle. Spread the batter into a 4-inch circle before it sets. Cook until the surface bubbles and appears dry; turn and continue cooking for 2 to 3 minutes. Serve with butter and maple syrup.

All-Star Rating: 3 Stars ★		*Nutrient Content per Serving*	
Eggs		Calories	294 kcal
Milk		Protein	9 g
Pumpkin		Carbohydrate	49 g
		Fat	7 g
Blue-Ribbon Rating: 7 Ribbons 🎗		Fiber	3.6 g
Calcium	Selenium	Calcium	312 mg
Folate	Thiamin	Iron	2.7 mg
Niacin	Vitamin A		
Phosphorus			

Avocado Salad with Orange and Grapefruit

MAKES 2 SERVINGS

4 cups mesclun or mixed baby greens

½ tablespoon Dijon mustard

2 tablespoons lemon juice

1 tablespoon avocado or olive oil

2 tablespoons cider vinegar

½ ripe avocado, pitted, peeled, and sliced
    lengthwise

1 large red grapefruit, pith removed and
    sliced into segments

1 orange, pith removed and sliced into
    segments

Salt and pepper to taste

3 tablespoons chopped cashews

Place greens in a medium salad bowl. In a small bowl, mix the mustard, lemon juice, oil, and vinegar. Dip the avocado slices in the vinaigrette to keep them from turning brown. Arrange the avocado and grapefruit sections on the greens; top with the dressing and sprinkle with the cashews.

All-Star Rating: 4 Stars ★		*Nutrient Content per Serving*	
Avocados		Calories	310 kcal
Cashews		Protein	6 g
Grapefruit		Carbohydrate	27 g
Orange		Fat	20 g
		Fiber	10 g
Blue-Ribbon Rating: 5 Ribbons 🎗			
Fiber	Vitamin A		
Magnesium	Vitamin C		
Phosphorus			

Beet Salad with Goat Cheese

MAKES 2 SERVINGS

2 medium beets, scrubbed, trimmed, and
cut in half

2 medium Belgian endives

2 ounces reduced fat goat cheese, coarsely
crumbled

1 Granny Smith apple, cored and sliced
into bite-size pieces

¼ cup chopped walnuts

1 tablespoon honey

1 tablespoon lemon juice

2 tablespoons white balsamic vinegar

1 tablespoon olive oil

Place the beets in a saucepan, add enough water to cover, and boil for 20 to 30 minutes, or until tender. Drain and cool; cut into ¼-inch slices. Place the endive leaves in a medium salad bowl. Top with the goat cheese, sliced apples, and walnuts. In a small bowl, mix the honey, lemon juice, vinegar, and oil; pour over the salad.

All-Star Rating: 3 Stars ★		Nutrient Content per Serving	
Apple		Calories	335 kcal
Cheese		Protein	12 g
Walnuts		Carbohydrate	32 g
		Fat	20 g
Blue-Ribbon Rating: 6 Ribbons 🎗		Fiber	6 g
Calcium	Manganese		
Fiber	Potassium		
Magnesium	Vitamin C		

Caprese Salad

MAKES 2 SERVINGS

2 large tomatoes, sliced

4 ounces part-skim mozzarella cheese,
    drained and sliced

12 leaves fresh sweet basil, chopped

1 tablespoon pine nuts

1 tablespoon olive oil

Salt and pepper to taste

Alternate tomato and mozzarella slices around a salad plate. Sprinkle with chopped basil and nuts. Drizzle oil over salad; add salt and pepper to taste.

All-Star Rating: 3 Stars ★		Nutrient Content per Serving	
Cheese		Calories	300 kcal
Nuts		Protein	18 g
Tomato		Carbohydrate	10 g
		Fat	20 g
Blue-Ribbon Rating: 12 Ribbons		Fiber	5 g
Calcium	Phosphorus		
Fiber	Potassium		
Iron	Thiamin		
Magnesium	Vitamin A		
Manganese	Vitamin B$_6$		
Niacin	Vitamin C		

Ginger Stir-Fry

MAKES 4 SERVINGS

1 cup vegetable broth

¼ cup dry white wine

2 tablespoons soy sauce

2 tablespoons cornstarch

1 tablespoon canola oil

2 teaspoons peeled, grated fresh ginger

1½ cups sliced zucchini

1 pound fresh asparagus, cut into 1-inch pieces, or 1 10-ounce package frozen cut asparagus, thawed and well drained

2 green onions, sliced

1 10½-ounce package extra-firm tofu (fresh bean curd), cut into ½-inch cubes

1 ounce pine nuts or chopped almonds, toasted

2 cups hot cooked brown rice

For the sauce, in a small bowl, stir together the broth, wine, soy sauce, and cornstarch. Set aside. Pour the canola oil into a wok or large skillet; preheat over medium-high heat. Stir-fry the ginger in the hot oil for 15 seconds. Add the zucchini and fresh asparagus (if using); stir-fry for 3 minutes. Add the green onions and thawed asparagus (if using); stir-fry for 1½ minutes more, or until the asparagus is crisp-tender. Remove the vegetables from the wok. Add the tofu to the hot wok. Stir-fry for 2 to 3 minutes, or until lightly browned. Remove from the wok. Add the sauce to the hot wok. Cook and stir until thickened and bubbly. Return the vegetables and tofu to the wok. Stir all the ingredients together for 1 minute more, or until heated through. Stir in the nuts. Serve over the rice.

All-Star Rating: 3 Stars ★		Nutrient Content per Serving	
Asparagus		Calories	352 kcal
Nuts		Protein	16 g
Tofu		Carbohydrate	51 g
		Fat	9 g
Blue-Ribbon Rating: 11 Ribbons 🎗		Fiber	4.7 g
Folate	Selenium	Calcium	97 mg
Magnesium	Thiamin	Iron	3.5 mg
Niacin	Vitamin C		
Phosphorus	Vitamin E		
Protein	Vitamin K		
Riboflavin			

Greek Salad

MAKES 2 SERVINGS

2 tomatoes cut into wedges

1 small cucumber, cut into thick
   half-moons

8 kalamata olives

½ red onion, sliced into rings

½ green pepper, cut into bite-size pieces

4 ounces nonfat feta cheese, cut into
   small cubes

½ clove garlic, minced

2 tablespoons olive oil

1 tablespoon lemon juice

¼ teaspoon oregano

¼ teaspoon sea salt

¼ teaspoon black pepper

In a medium salad bowl combine the tomatoes, cucumber, olives, onion, green pepper, and feta cheese. In a small bowl, mix the garlic, oil, lemon juice, oregano, salt, and pepper; pour over the salad.

All-Star Rating: 2 Stars ★	
Cheese	
Tomatoes	

Blue-Ribbon Rating: 12 Ribbons 🎗	
Calcium	Phosphorus
Fiber	Potassium
Magnesium	Vitamin A
Manganese	Vitamin B$_6$
Niacin	Vitamin B$_{12}$
Riboflavin	Vitamin C

Nutrient Content per Serving	
Calories	350 kcal
Protein	31 g
Carbohydrate	20 g
Fat	16 g
Fiber	8 g

Greek Spinach and Cheese Pie

MAKES 6 SERVINGS

¼ cup olive oil

2 pounds fresh spinach (approximately 3 10-ounce bags)

1 large onion, finely chopped

4 large eggs

8 ounces feta cheese, crumbled

8 ounces part-skim-milk ricotta cheese

¼ cup chopped fresh parsley

17 sheets phyllo pastry (thawed, if frozen)

3 tablespoons butter, melted

In a skillet, heat the oil. Sauté the spinach and onion until the onion is clear and tender; remove from the heat. In a medium bowl, beat the eggs. Stir in the feta and ricotta cheeses, parsley, and onion-spinach mixture. Lightly grease a 13- × 9-inch baking pan. Lay 1 sheet of phyllo in the pan; brush with the butter. Layer 8 more sheets of phyllo, one at a time, brushing each with the melted butter. Cover evenly with the spinach mixture. Top with the 8 remaining sheets of phyllo, one at a time, brushing each with the melted butter. Refrigerate for 30 minutes. Preheat the oven to 350°F. Bake the pie for 35 to 40 minutes, or until golden brown. Cut into 12 pieces, each about 3 × 4 inches.

All-Star Rating: 4 Stars ★		Nutrient Content per Serving	
Eggs		Calories	303 kcal
Feta cheese		Protein	18 g
Ricotta cheese		Carbohydrate	6 g
Spinach		Fat	23 g
		Fiber	14 g
Blue-Ribbon Rating: 15 Ribbons 🎗		Calcium	430 mg
Calcium	Selenium	Iron	11.3 mg
Fiber	Vitamin A		
Iodine	Vitamin B$_6$		
Iron	Vitamin B$_{12}$		
Magnesium	Vitamin C		
Phosphorus	Vitamin E		
Protein	Zinc		
Riboflavin			

Lentil Soup

MAKES 6 SERVINGS

1 pound lentils
1 cup chopped celery
1 medium onion, chopped
2 garlic cloves, finely chopped
½ cup olive oil
1 6-ounce can tomato paste

1 tablespoon chopped fresh parsley
1 teaspoon salt
Ground black pepper to taste
1 bay leaf
2 tablespoons white vinegar

Rinse and soak the lentils in warm water for 2 hours; drain. To a large saucepan, add 8 cups water, the lentils, celery, onion, and garlic. Bring to a boil, cover, and simmer for 30 minutes. Add the olive oil, tomato paste, parsley, salt, pepper, and bay leaf. Simmer for 20 minutes, or until the lentils are tender. Remove the bay leaf and discard. Add the vinegar before serving.

All-Star Rating: 2 Stars ★	
Lentils	
Tomato paste	

Blue-Ribbon Rating: 12 Ribbons	
Fiber	Thiamin
Folate	Vitamin B$_6$
Iron	Vitamin C
Magnesium	Vitamin E
Phosphorus	Vitamin K
Protein	Zinc

Nutrient Content per Serving	
Calories	450 kcal
Protein	23 g
Carbohydrate	51 g
Fat	19 g
Fiber	25 g
Calcium	72 mg
Iron	7.7 mg

Mediterranean Sauté

1 tablespoon butter

1 tablespoon olive oil

1 garlic clove, finely chopped

1 cup chopped celery

¼ teaspoon fennel seed

6 green onions, chopped

½ cup golden raisins

1 cup uncooked quick-cooking barley

1 15-ounce can garbanzo beans, rinsed and drained

2 cups vegetable broth

1 cup chopped fresh parsley

½ cup chopped walnuts

Heat the butter and oil in a large skillet. Add the garlic and cook until golden brown. Add the celery, fennel seed, and green onions. Cover and cook over medium heat until the vegetables are tender. Add the remaining ingredients except the parsley and walnuts. Bring to a boil; cover and reduce the heat. Cook for 10 minutes, or until the barley is tender. Stir in the parsley and walnuts.

All-Star Rating: 3 Stars ★		Nutrient Content per Serving	
Barley		Calories	503 kcal
Garbanzo beans		Protein	14 g
Walnuts		Carbohydrate	77 g
		Fat	16 g
Blue-Ribbon Rating: 6 Ribbons 🎗		Fiber	15.1 g
Fiber	Protein	Calcium	106 mg
Folate	Selenium	Iron	3.5 mg
Magnesium	Vitamin K		

Oatmeal-Almond Pancakes

MAKES 12 PANCAKES, OR 4 SERVINGS

2½ cups skim milk

1 cup rolled oats

1 cup all-purpose flour

½ cup whole-wheat flour

¼ cup toasted wheat germ

2 ounces ground almonds

¼ cup firmly packed brown sugar

2 teaspoons baking powder

1 teaspoon baking soda

1 teaspoon ground cinnamon

½ teaspoon salt

4 large egg whites, beaten

2 teaspoons flaxseed oil

Applesauce

Combine the milk and oats in a small bowl. Let stand for 30 minutes to soften the oats. In a large bowl, stir together all remaining dry ingredients. To the dry mixture, add the oat mixture and eggs; stir gently until blended. Brush a large skillet with the oil; heat over medium heat. Using ¼ cup batter for each pancake, pour the batter onto the skillet; cook until the underside is browned; flip. Transfer to a platter and keep warm. Repeat with the remaining batter, brushing the skillet with more oil as necessary. Serve hot with applesauce.

All-Star Rating: 5 Stars ★		Nutrient Content per Serving	
Almonds		Calories	525 kcal
Eggs		Protein	22 g
Milk		Carbohydrate	72 g
Oats		Fat	16 g
Wheat germ		Fiber	6 g
		Calcium	422 mg
Blue-Ribbon Rating: 12 Ribbons ⚜		Iron	4.4 mg
Calcium	Riboflavin		
Fiber	Selenium		
Magnesium	Thiamin		
Niacin	Vitamin B$_{12}$		
Phosphorus	Vitamin E		
Protein	Zinc		

Pasta with Green Sauce

MAKES 4 SERVINGS

1 cup frozen chopped spinach	¼ cup grated Parmesan cheese
1 cup vegetable broth	1 garlic clove, chopped
½ cup part-skim-milk ricotta cheese	1 pound uncooked enriched linguine
¼ cup chopped fresh parsley	2 ounces pine nuts

Mix all the ingredients except the pasta and nuts together in a food processor or blender until well blended. Cook the pasta according to the package directions; drain well. Pour the sauce over the pasta; toss to coat. Garnish with pine nuts.

All-Star Rating: 4 Stars ★		*Nutrient Content per Serving*	
Parmesan cheese		Calories	530 kcal
Pine nuts		Protein	26 g
Ricotta cheese		Carbohydrate	70 g
Spinach		Fat	16 g
		Fiber	4.5 g
Blue-Ribbon Rating: 6 Ribbons 🎗		Calcium	254 mg
Calcium	Protein	Iron	6 mg
Fiber	Vitamin A		
Iron	Vitamin K		

Pumpkin Waffles

2 cups sifted cake flour	1½ cups low-fat (1%) milk
4 teaspoons baking powder	1 cup canned pumpkin-pie mix
1 teaspoon salt	½ cup finely chopped pecans
6 large egg whites	

Preheat a waffle iron. Into a large bowl, sift the flour, baking powder, and salt. In a medium bowl, beat the egg whites; add the milk, pumpkin-pie mix, and nuts; mix well. Pour the pumpkin mixture into the bowl with the flour mixture; stir gently until all the ingredients are blended. Lightly oil the waffle iron, or spray with nonstick cooking spray. Pour 1 cup batter onto the waffle iron. Cook for 3 to 5 minutes, or until the waffles are golden brown and steam no longer rises from the waffle iron. Repeat with the remaining batter.

All-Star Rating: 4 Stars ★		Nutrient Content per Serving	
Eggs		Calories	287 kcal
Milk		Protein	10 g
Pecans		Carbohydrate	46 g
Pumpkin		Fat	7 g
		Fiber	5.2 g
Blue-Ribbon Rating: 5 Ribbons 🎗		Calcium	152 mg
Folate	Thiamin	Iron	3.4 mg
Fiber	Vitamin A		
Riboflavin			

Ratatouille

MAKES 4 SERVINGS

4 tablespoons olive oil

1 medium eggplant (approximately
    1 pound), peeled and cut into
    1-inch cubes

1 zucchini (approximately 1 pound),
    cut into 1-inch cubes

1½ cups sliced onions

3 garlic cloves, chopped

2 red bell peppers, cut into bite-size pieces

1½ cups peeled, chopped tomatoes

3 sprigs fresh thyme

1 bay leaf

¼ cup chopped fresh basil

4 cups hot cooked saffron rice

Salt and ground black pepper to taste

In a large saucepan, heat 2 tablespoons of the oil. Add the eggplant and zucchini, and sauté over medium heat until tender. Remove the vegetables to a bowl; set aside. In the same saucepan, heat the remaining 2 tablespoons oil. Add the onions and sauté until tender. Add the garlic and bell peppers; cook until tender. Add the tomatoes, thyme, and bay leaf. Reduce the heat to low, cover, and cook for 5 minutes. Add the eggplant and zucchini; cook for 20 minutes more. Stir in the basil. Remove the bay leaf and discard. Season with salt and pepper. Serve over the saffron rice.

All-Star Rating: 1 Star ★		Nutrient Content per Serving	
Tomatoes		Calories	430 kcal
		Protein	9 g
Blue-Ribbon Rating: 10 Ribbons 🎗		Carbohydrate	68 g
Fiber	Selenium	Fat	15 g
Thiamin	Vitamin A	Fiber	8 g
Folate	Vitamin B$_6$	Calcium	103 mg
Magnesium	Vitamin C	Iron	3.8 mg
Niacin	Vitamin E		

Salsa Frittata

MAKES 4 SERVINGS

1 teaspoon olive oil

1 pound sweet potatoes or yams, peeled and cut into ½-inch cubes

3 large eggs or 6 large egg whites

1 jar medium-hot salsa (approximately 12 ounces)

½ teaspoon salt

¼ teaspoon ground black pepper

1 cup shredded sharp Cheddar cheese

1 medium tomato, diced

Preheat the oven to 425°F. In a large skillet with an oven-safe handle (or cover the handle with heavy-duty foil for baking in the oven later), heat the olive oil over medium-high heat. Add the sweet potatoes and cook, covered, until they are tender and golden brown, about 10 minutes, stirring occasionally. Meanwhile, in a medium bowl, with a wire whisk or fork, beat the eggs with ¼ cup of the salsa (chopped, if necessary), the salt, and the pepper. Stir in the cheese; set aside. Stir the diced tomato into the remaining salsa. Stir the egg mixture into the sweet potatoes in the skillet. Cover and cook over medium heat, without stirring, for 3 minutes, or until the egg mixture begins to set around the edges. Remove the cover and place the skillet in the oven. Bake for 4 to 6 minutes, until the frittata is set. To serve, invert the frittata onto a cutting board. Cut into wedges and top with the salsa mixture.

All-Star Rating: 4 Stars ★		Nutrient Content per Serving	
Cheese		Calories	415 kcal
Eggs		Protein	21 g
Sweet potatoes or yams		Carbohydrate	44 g
Tomato		Fat	17 g
Blue-Ribbon Rating: 9 Ribbons 🎗		Fiber	2.3 g
Calcium	Vitamin A	Calcium	246 mg
Phosphorus	Vitamin B$_{12}$	Iron	2.6 mg
Protein	Vitamin C		
Riboflavin	Vitamin E		
Selenium			

Spinach and Pumpkin Casserole

MAKES 4 SERVINGS

½ cup fat-free mayonnaise
½ cup all-purpose flour
1½ cups low-fat (1%) milk
8 large egg whites
1 cup canned pumpkin

1 10-ounce package frozen chopped
  spinach, cooked and drained
6 slices white or whole-wheat toast,
  cut into cubes
1½ cups shredded sharp Cheddar cheese

Preheat the oven to 350°F. In a medium saucepan, combine the mayonnaise and flour; mix well. Add the milk and egg whites; cook over low heat, stirring constantly, until thickened. Stir in the pumpkin and spinach. In the bottom of a 12- × 8-inch baking dish, layer the toast cubes. Top with half the cheese and half the pumpkin mixture; repeat. Bake for 45 to 50 minutes, or until thoroughly heated.

All-Star Rating: 5 Stars ★		Nutrient Content per Serving	
Cheese		Calories	455 kcal
Eggs		Protein	28 g
Milk		Carbohydrate	49 g
Pumpkin		Fat	16 g
Spinach		Fiber	5.2 g
		Calcium	586 mg
Blue-Ribbon Rating: 12 Ribbons 🎗		Iron	4.1 mg
Calcium	Selenium		
Fiber	Thiamin		
Folate	Vitamin A		
Magnesium	Vitamin B$_{12}$		
Protein	Vitamin E		
Riboflavin	Vitamin K		

Tomato Apricot Salad

MAKES 2 SERVINGS

4 cups fresh baby spinach

1 8½-ounce package microwaveable quinoa and whole grain brown rice

3 fresh apricots, pitted and chopped

3 fresh tomatoes, cored and chopped

¼ cup chopped red onion

2 tablespoons olive oil

2 tablespoons roasted pine nuts

Divide the spinach into two medium salad plates. Microwave the quinoa and rice according to package directions; pour mixture into a large bowl. To the quinoa mixture, add the apricots, tomatoes, onion, oil, and pine nuts; mix well. Serve over the spinach.

All-Star Rating: 3 Stars ★		*Nutrient Content per Serving*	
Pine nuts		Calories	350 kcal
Spinach		Protein	9 g
Tomatoes		Carbohydrate	34 g
		Fat	20 g
Blue-Ribbon Rating: 11 Ribbons		Fiber	8 g
Fiber	Thiamin		
Magnesium	Vitamin A		
Manganese	Vitamin B$_6$		
Niacin	Vitamin C		
Phosphorus	Zinc		
Potassium			

Vegetarian Lasagna

MAKES 8 SERVINGS

1 tablespoon olive oil

½ cup chopped onions

½ cup chopped green bell peppers

½ cup chopped celery

1 teaspoon crushed garlic

2 15-ounce cans tomato sauce

¼ cup chopped fresh cilantro

1 12-ounce package low-fat (1%) cottage cheese

1 8-ounce package reduced-fat cream cheese (or Neufchâtel), softened

½ cup nonfat sour cream

9 packaged enriched lasagna noodles, cooked and drained

Preheat the oven to 350°F. In a large skillet, heat the oil and sauté the onions, bell peppers, celery, and garlic; cook until tender. Add the tomato sauce and cilantro; heat well. In a medium bowl, combine the cottage cheese, cream cheese, and sour cream. Grease a 13- × 9-inch baking dish with butter or margarine. Arrange 3 lasagna noodles on the bottom of the dish. Top with one-third of the sauce and one-third of the cheese mixture. Repeat the layers twice, topping with the cheese mixture. Bake, uncovered, for 40 to 45 minutes. Let stand for 10 minutes before cutting.

All-Star Rating: 2 Stars ★		Nutrient Content per Serving	
Cheese		Calories	442 kcal
Tomato sauce		Protein	21 g
Blue-Ribbon Rating: 8 Ribbons 🎗		Carbohydrate	59 g
Niacin	Thiamin	Fat	13 g
Protein	Vitamin A	Fiber	3 g
Riboflavin	Vitamin B$_{12}$	Calcium	122 mg
Selenium	Vitamin C	Iron	3.8 mg

Vegetarian Stroganoff

MAKES 4 SERVINGS

10 ounces uncooked enriched spinach fettuccine

1 tablespoon butter

1 tablespoon olive oil

2 pounds fresh mushrooms, sliced

1 cup chopped onions

1 garlic clove, finely chopped

¼ cup all-purpose flour

2 cups vegetable broth

¼ cup tomato paste

1 cup nonfat sour cream

½ cup chopped walnuts

Cook the fettuccine according to the package directions; drain and keep warm. In a large saucepan, melt the butter and olive oil. Sauté the mushrooms, onions, and garlic until tender. Mix in the flour, vegetable broth, and tomato paste, stirring constantly until the mixture comes to a boil. Reduce the heat and stir in the sour cream and walnuts. Cook, without boiling, until thoroughly heated. Pour the sauce over the hot fettuccine.

All-Star Rating: 3 Stars ★		*Nutrient Content per Serving*	
Spinach (pasta)		Calories	500 kcal
Tomato paste		Protein	21 g
Walnuts		Carbohydrate	65 g
		Fat	20 g
Blue-Ribbon Rating: 10 Ribbons 🎗		Fiber	6.7 g
Fiber	Riboflavin	Calcium	127 mg
Folate	Thiamin	Iron	3.9 mg
Niacin	Vitamin A		
Phosphorus	Vitamin B$_6$		
Protein	Vitamin D		

Wild Rice Omelet

MAKES I SERVING

¾ cup All-Whites (pasteurized liquid
 egg whites)
1 green onion, sliced
1 ounce skim milk
Salt and ground black pepper to taste

1 teaspoon butter
½ cup cooked long-grain and wild rice
¼ cup shredded Muenster cheese
1 tomato, sliced
¼ cup chopped walnuts

Combine the egg whites, green onion, milk, salt, and pepper in a medium bowl. Melt the butter in a medium skillet. Pour in the egg mixture and cook over medium-low heat until the omelet is set. Lift the edges with a spatula to allow the uncooked egg mixture to flow underneath. Place the rice and cheese on half of the omelet and fold the other half over the filling. Continue cooking until the cheese has melted. Garnish with the tomato slices and chopped walnuts.

All-Star Rating: 5 Stars ★		Nutrient Content per Serving	
Cheese		Calories	450 kcal
Eggs		Protein	23 g
Milk		Carbohydrate	51 g
Tomato		Fat	19 g
Walnuts		Fiber	25 g
		Calcium	72 mg
Blue-Ribbon Rating: 12 Ribbons 🎗		Iron	7.7 mg
Fiber	Thiamin		
Folate	Vitamin B$_6$		
Iron	Vitamin C		
Magnesium	Vitamin E		
Phosphorus	Vitamin K		
Protein	Zinc		

Side Dishes and Snacks

Chickpea Salad

MAKES 4 SERVINGS

2 cups canned chickpeas, rinsed and drained

½ cup chopped onions

¼ cup chopped fresh parsley

3 tablespoons lemon juice

2 tablespoons olive oil

1 teaspoon Dijon mustard

1 medium carrot, chopped

4 cups shredded romaine lettuce

½ cup chopped almonds

Stir all the ingredients together except for the lettuce and almonds. Serve over the shredded lettuce. Garnish with the chopped almonds.

All-Star Rating: 2 Stars ★		*Nutrient Content per Serving*	
Chickpeas		Calories	282 kcal
Almonds		Protein	11 g
		Carbohydrate	27 g
Blue-Ribbon Rating: 7 Ribbons 🎗		Fat	15 g
Fiber	Vitamin C	Fiber	8.7 g
Folate	Vitamin E	Calcium	115 mg
Magnesium	Vitamin K	Iron	2.7 mg
Vitamin A			

Harvest Muffins

MAKES 1 DOZEN MUFFINS

1 cup canned pumpkin-pie mix

1 cup low-fat (1%) milk

¼ cup butter, melted

¼ cup honey

1 tablespoon vanilla extract

2 large egg whites

¾ cup firmly packed brown sugar

2 cups all-purpose flour

1 tablespoon baking powder

¼ teaspoon salt

1 cup chopped walnuts

½ cup raisins

Preheat the oven to 400°F. Line a muffin tin with 12 paper liners. In a medium bowl, combine the pumpkin-pie mix, milk, butter, honey, vanilla, egg whites, and brown sugar; mix well. Into a large bowl, sift together the flour, baking powder, and salt. Add the pumpkin mixture to the flour mixture, stirring gently until just blended. Stir in the nuts and raisins. Spoon the batter into the muffin tin, filling each cup about half full. Bake for 15 to 20 minutes, or until a toothpick inserted in the center comes out clean.

All-Star Rating: 2 Stars ★		Nutrient Content per Serving	
Eggs		Calories	278 kcal
Milk		Protein	5 g
Pumpkin		Carbohydrate	44 g
Walnuts		Fat	9 g
		Fiber	3 g
Blue-Ribbon Rating: 2 Ribbons 🎗		Calcium	144 mg
Phosphorus	Vitamin A	Iron	1.8 mg

Powerhouse Granola

MAKES 8 CUPS, OR 8 SERVINGS

3 cups rolled oats

½ cup wheat germ

½ cup chopped almonds

2 tablespoons ground flaxseed

1 12-ounce can apple juice concentrate, thawed

¼ cup firmly packed brown sugar

½ cup chopped dried apricots

½ cup chopped dried apples

1 cup dried cherries

Preheat the oven to 300°F. In a large bowl, combine the oats, wheat germ, almonds, and flaxseed. In a small bowl, combine the apple juice concentrate and brown sugar. Add the juice mixture to the oat mixture and mix thoroughly. Spread on a baking sheet and bake, stirring occasionally, for 40 to 50 minutes, or until golden brown. Stir in the apricots, apples, and cherries. Bake for 5 minutes more. Let cool; store in an airtight container.

All-Star Rating: 5 Stars ★		Nutrient Content per Serving	
Almonds		Calories	417 kcal
Apples		Protein	10 g
Cherries		Carbohydrate	72 g
Oats		Fat	11 g
Wheat germ		Fiber	7.1 g
		Calcium	72 mg
Blue-Ribbon Rating: 6 Ribbons 🎗		Iron	3.4 mg
Fiber	Thiamin		
Magnesium	Vitamin E		
Phosphorus	Zinc		

Pumpkin Custard

4 large egg whites, lightly beaten
1 pound canned pumpkin-pie mix
½ teaspoon salt
12 ounces nonfat evaporated milk
¼ cup chopped almonds

Preheat the oven to 350°F. In a large bowl, mix the egg whites, pumpkin-pie mix, salt, and evaporated milk. Pour into 8 greased 6-ounce custard cups. Set the custard cups in a shallow pan; fill the pan with hot water. Bake for 45 to 50 minutes, or until a knife inserted in the center of the custard comes out clean. Chill. Top with the chopped almonds.

All-Star Rating: 4 Stars ★		*Nutrient Content per Serving*	
Almonds		Calories	248 kcal
Eggs		Protein	13 g
Milk		Carbohydrate	42 g
Pumpkin		Fat	4 g
		Fiber	10 g
Blue-Ribbon Rating: 7 Ribbons 🍴		Calcium	337 mg
Calcium	Riboflavin	Iron	1.7 mg
Fiber	Vitamin A		
Phosphorus	Vitamin D		
Protein			

Pumpkin-Fruit Muffins

MAKES 12 MUFFINS

1 cup uncooked old-fashioned rolled oats

½ cup skim milk

2½ cups all-purpose flour

1 cup firmly packed brown sugar

1 tablespoon baking powder

½ teaspoon baking soda

½ teaspoon ground cinnamon

2 cups canned pumpkin

½ cup raisins

2 large eggs

¼ cup flaxseed oil

1 teaspoon vanilla extract

Preheat the oven to 350°F. Line a muffin tin with 12 paper liners. Combine the oats and milk; mix well. Set aside. In a large bowl, combine the flour, brown sugar, baking powder, baking soda, and cinnamon; mix well. Stir in the pumpkin, raisins, oat mixture, eggs, flaxseed oil, and vanilla; mix just until the dry ingredients are moistened. Pour into the muffin tin. Bake for 20 to 30 minutes, or until the muffins are golden and a toothpick inserted in the center comes out clean.

All-Star Rating: 4 Stars ★		*Nutrient Content per Serving*	
Eggs		Calories	310 kcal
Milk		Protein	6 g
Oatmeal		Carbohydrate	52 g
Pumpkin		Fat	7 g
		Fiber	1.6 g
Blue-Ribbon Rating: 2 Ribbons 🎗		Calcium	40 mg
Vitamin A	Vitamin E	Iron	1.7 mg

Pumpkin Loaf

MAKES 2 LOAVES, OR 12 SERVINGS

2 cups all-purpose flour

2 cups whole-wheat flour

4 teaspoons baking powder

1 teaspoon baking soda

2 teaspoons salt

2 cups canned pumpkin-pie mix

¼ cup firmly packed brown sugar

1 cup milk

8 large egg whites

½ cup canola oil

2 cups chopped walnuts or pecans

Preheat the oven to 350°F. Grease two 9- × 5-inch loaf pans. Into a large bowl, sift together the white flour, wheat flour, baking powder, baking soda, and salt. In another large bowl, combine the pumpkin-pie mix, brown sugar, milk, egg whites, and oil. Add the pumpkin mixture to the flour mixture; stir gently just until the dry ingredients are moistened. Stir in the nuts. Pour the batter into the loaf pans. Bake for 60 to 65 minutes, or until a toothpick inserted in the center comes out clean. Let cool for 10 minutes; remove from the pans.

All-Star Rating: 4 Stars ★		Nutrient Content per Serving	
Eggs		Calories	324 kcal
Milk		Protein	7 g
Nuts		Carbohydrate	38 g
Pumpkin		Fat	17 g
		Fiber	6.3 g
Blue-Ribbon Rating: 7 Ribbons 🎗		Calcium	120 mg
Fiber	Thiamin	Iron	2.1 mg
Magnesium	Vitamin A		
Phosphorus	Vitamin E		
Selenium			

Sunrise Bread Pudding

MAKES 4 SERVINGS

1½ cups canned pumpkin-pie mix
½ cup low-fat (1%) milk
4 large egg whites
8 slices raisin bread, cubed
1 teaspoon ground cinnamon
½ teaspoon ground nutmeg

Preheat the oven to 325°F. In a large bowl, combine the pumpkin-pie mix, milk, and egg whites; stir in the bread and spices. Spoon into a 1-quart casserole. Bake for 50 minutes, or until a knife inserted in the pumpkin mixture comes out clean.

All-Star Rating: 3 Stars ★		*Nutrient Content per Serving*	
Eggs		Calories	277 kcal
Milk		Protein	10 g
Pumpkin		Carbohydrate	56 g
		Fat	3 g
Blue-Ribbon Rating: 5 Ribbons 🎗		Fiber	10.6 g
Fiber	Selenium		
Folate	Vitamin A		
Riboflavin			

Tabbouleh

MAKES 4 LARGE SALADS

4 cups boiling water

1 cup uncooked fine bulgur

1 cup finely minced fresh parsley

½ cup finely minced fresh mint leaves

1 large tomato, chopped

¼ cup olive oil

¼ cup lemon juice

1 teaspoon salt

Ground black pepper to taste

1 head romaine lettuce

In a large pot, pour the boiling water over the bulgur and let stand for 2 hours. Drain and squeeze out the excess water; place in a large bowl. Stir in all the other ingredients except the lettuce; let stand for 1 hour before serving. Divide the lettuce among 4 plates; top with the tabbouleh.

All-Star Rating: 2 Stars ★		*Nutrient Content per Serving*	
Bulgur		Calories	275 kcal
Tomato		Protein	7 g
		Carbohydrate	34 g
Blue-Ribbon Rating: 7 Ribbons 🎗		Fat	14 g
Fiber	Vitamin C	Fiber	9.3 g
Folate	Vitamin E	Calcium	83 mg
Magnesium	Vitamin K	Iron	3.3 mg
Vitamin A			

Weekend Hash Browns

MAKES 4 SERVINGS

1 tablespoon safflower oil

2 cups frozen shredded hash brown
potatoes, thawed

¾ cup sliced green onions

4 slices white or whole-wheat toast, cut into
small cubes

2 large eggs plus 6 large egg whites,
beaten

1 cup shredded Muenster cheese

Salt and ground black pepper to taste

In a large skillet, heat the oil; add the hash browns and ½ cup of the green onions. Cook, stirring occasionally, until the potatoes are a deep golden brown. Add the toast cubes, eggs and egg whites, cheese, salt, and pepper. Cook until the eggs are set. Garnish with the remaining ¼ cup green onions.

All-Star Rating: 2 Stars ★		Nutrient Content per Serving	
Cheese		Calories	352 kcal
Eggs		Protein	20 g
		Carbohydrate	33 g
Blue-Ribbon Rating: 9 Ribbons		Fat	15 g
Calcium	Vitamin B₁₂	Fiber	3.3 g
Phosphorus	Vitamin C	Calcium	270 mg
Protein	Vitamin E	Iron	2.9 mg
Riboflavin	Vitamin K		
Selenium			

Yogurt Guacamole

MAKES 6 SERVINGS

3 ripe avocados (approximately 1½ pounds)

2 garlic cloves, finely chopped

2 tablespoons lemon juice

1½ cups plain low-fat yogurt

2 tablespoons medium-hot salsa

¼ teaspoon ground cumin

¼ cup chopped fresh cilantro

Salt and ground black pepper to taste

6 pita breads, split

In a large bowl, mash the avocados. Stir in the remaining ingredients except the pita breads. Serve on the pita breads.

All-Star Rating: 3 Stars ★		Nutrient Content per Serving	
Avocados		Calories	244 kcal
Tomatoes (salsa)		Protein	10 g
Yogurt		Carbohydrate	42 g
		Fat	6 g
Blue-Ribbon Rating: 5 Ribbons 🎗		Fiber	7.4 g
Fiber	Selenium	Calcium	131 mg
Magnesium	Thiamin	Iron	2.2 mg
Phosphorus			

Smoothies

Basic Fruit Smoothie

MAKES 1 LARGE SMOOTHIE

2 ounces Silken tofu, soft (approximately ½ cup)

1 cup plain or vanilla nonfat yogurt

½ cup cut-up fresh or frozen fruit

½ cup fruit juice

1 tablespoon lemon or lime juice

2 All-Whites (pasteurized liquid egg whites)

2 tablespoons nonfat dry milk solids

1 tablespoon flaxseed oil

4 ice cubes, crushed

Put all the ingredients in a blender. Process until smooth and blended.

All-Star Rating: 5 Stars ★		*Nutrient Content per Serving*	
Eggs		Calories	414 kcal
Fruit		Protein	26 g
Milk		Carbohydrate	44 g
Tofu		Fat	15 g
Yogurt		Fiber	2 g
		Calcium	582 mg
Blue-Ribbon Rating: 10 Ribbons 🎗		Iron	1.5 mg
Calcium	Selenium		
Magnesium	Vitamin B$_{12}$		
Phosphorus	Vitamin C		
Protein	Vitamin E		
Riboflavin	Zinc		

Note: With each Basic Fruit Smoothie, you can meet your daily requirement of:

1 serving of meat or meat equivalents—from the 2 ounces tofu + 2 egg whites.

2 servings of dairy—from the 1 cup yogurt + 2 tablespoons nonfat dry milk.

2 servings of fruit—from the ½ cup fresh or frozen + ½ cup juice.

1 serving of fat—from the 1 tablespoon flaxseed oil.

VARIATIONS ON THE BASIC FRUIT SMOOTHIE

Fruit
Apples
Applesauce
Apricots
Bananas
Blackberries
Blueberries
Cherries
Cranberries
Dates, rehydrated
Mangoes
Oranges
Papayas
Peaches
Pears
Pineapple
Prunes, rehydrated
Strawberries

Fruit Juice
Apple
Cranberry
Grape

Guava nectar
Orange
Pear nectar
Pineapple

Optional Nutrient Boosters
Brewer's yeast, 1 teaspoon
Old-fashioned rolled oats, 1 tablespoon
Wheat germ, 1 tablespoon

Optional Flavorings
Almond extract
Carob powder
Cinnamon
Cloves
Coffee or tea, brewed
Ginger, freshly grated
Honey
Mint or peppermint extract
Maple syrup
Nutmeg
Vanilla extract

Basic Vegetable Smoothie

MAKES 1 LARGE SMOOTHIE

2 ounces Silken tofu, soft (approximately ½ cup)

1 cup plain low-fat yogurt

½ cup cut-up vegetables

½ cup vegetable juice

1 tablespoon lemon or lime juice

2 All-Whites (pasteurized liquid egg whites)

2 tablespoons nonfat dry milk solids

1 tablespoon flaxseed oil

Seasoning (optional, add 1 or more): balsamic vinegar, celery salt, onion salt, Tabasco sauce

4 ice cubes, crushed

Put all the ingredients in a blender. Process until smooth and blended.

All-Star Rating: 5 Stars ★		Nutrient Content per Serving	
Eggs		Calories	416 kcal
Milk		Protein	28 g
Tofu		Carbohydrate	35 g
Vegetables		Fat	19 g
Yogurt		Fiber	2.3 g
Blue-Ribbon Rating: 14 Ribbons 🎗		Calcium	648 mg
Calcium	Thiamin	Iron	1.9 mg
Folate	Vitamin A		
Magnesium	Vitamin B_6		
Phosphorus	Vitamin B_{12}		
Protein	Vitamin C		
Riboflavin	Vitamin E		
Selenium	Zinc		

Note: With each Basic Vegetable Smoothie, you can meet your daily requirement of:

1 serving of meat or meat equivalents—from the 2 ounces tofu + 2 egg whites.

2 servings of dairy—from the ½ cup yogurt + 2 tablespoons nonfat dry milk.

2 servings of vegetables—from the ½ cup fresh + ½ cup juice.

1 serving of fat—from the 1 tablespoon flaxseed oil.

Ginger Smoothie

MAKES 1 LARGE SMOOTHIE

2 ounces Silken tofu, soft (approximately ½ cup)

½ cup lemon sorbet

½ cup ginger ale

1 teaspoon peeled, grated fresh ginger

1 tablespoon honey

1 tablespoon lemon juice

Put all the ingredients in a blender. Process until smooth and blended.

All-Star Rating: 1 Star ★		*Nutrient Content per Serving*	
Tofu		Calories	270 kcal
		Protein	4 g
Blue-Ribbon Rating: 1 Ribbons 🎗		Carbohydrate	61 g
Vitamin C		Fat	2 g
		Fiber	0.4 g
		Calcium	91 mg
		Iron	1.2 mg

Note: The Ginger Smoothie is excellent for easing nausea.

Birthweight References for Twins

	Week	Mean Weight (grams)	Standard Deviation	Percentile						
				5th	10th	25th	50th	75th	90th	95th
Both Genders	20	320	132	113	157	238	313	390	486	579
	22	491	142	275	318	397	482	567	670	761
	24	687	152	454	500	583	678	776	888	967
	26	909	173	641	691	791	897	1014	1133	1223
	28	1152	204	836	898	1015	1144	1280	1419	1520
	30	1424	238	1045	1130	1265	1412	1578	1732	1833
	32	1721	278	1264	1382	1540	1711	1906	2078	2182
	34	2037	323	1512	1650	1825	2030	2252	2444	2564
	36	2375	360	1791	1930	2132	2363	2613	2831	2984
	38	2659	398	2019	2154	2405	2657	2893	3160	3363
	40	2854	395	2319	2333	2550	2847	3114	3420	3470

	Week	Mean Weight (grams)	Standard Deviation	Percentile						
				5th	10th	25th	50th	75th	90th	95th
Females	20	312	127	114	155	234	304	382	472	546
	22	480	136	277	306	389	472	557	657	719
	24	673	150	452	489	570	664	762	860	949
	26	890	172	376	631	772	882	995	1116	1188
	28	1131	204	811	879	1001	1123	1257	1398	1484
	30	1397	237	1018	1093	1239	1387	1556	1707	1796
	32	1691	272	1253	1335	1504	1681	1868	2050	2149
	34	2001	317	1489	1593	1792	2001	2209	2408	2539
	36	2329	351	1755	1882	2088	2316	2557	2788	2890
	38	2621	392	1973	2079	2352	2616	2868	3101	3359
	40	2823	392	2319	2345	2531	2779	3128	3300	3390
Males	20	328	137	112	159	241	320	399	497	593
	22	502	146	275	325	404	494	577	696	776
	24	700	153	465	517	594	688	791	906	978
	26	927	173	656	714	811	911	1029	1167	1240
	28	1172	203	853	925	1041	1160	1296	1435	1555
	30	1448	236	1081	1165	1285	1433	1596	1758	1866
	32	1751	280	1308	1419	1562	1737	1925	2098	2225
	34	2071	325	1576	1680	1848	2053	2286	2481	2610
	36	2421	364	1884	1980	2163	2404	2656	2891	3011
	38	2702	400	2060	2224	2452	2700	2988	3207	3406
	40	2881	404	2322	2333	2631	2850	3002	3470	3470

Adapted from Min S-J, Luke B, Gillespie B, Min L, Newman RB, Mauldin JG, et al. Birthweight references for twins. American Journal of Obstetrics & Gynecology 2000; 182:1250–7.

Birthweight References for Triplets

	Week	Mean Weight (grams)	Standard Deviation	Percentile						
				5th	10th	25th	50th	75th	90th	95th
All	20	319	105	129	184	267	324	380	446	487
	22	474	118	266	319	408	474	549	622	663
	24	652	140	419	472	565	656	747	825	884
	26	853	169	584	657	747	857	971	1053	1148
	28	1080	203	766	848	947	1084	1213	1317	1405
	30	1330	242	929	1060	1186	1335	1484	1619	1726
	32	1619	292	1125	1287	1440	1626	1810	1959	2091
	34	1876	344	1278	1529	1710	1893	2091	2262	2368
Mono- and Dichorionic	20	316	107	129	173	258	329	380	429	484
	22	470	122	257	281	406	479	547	591	645
	24	647	143	402	425	568	662	726	812	862
	26	855	174	548	607	761	880	965	1060	1095

	Week	Mean Weight (grams)	Standard Deviation	Percentile						
				5th	10th	25th	50th	75th	90th	95th
Mono- and Dichorionic	28	1079	209	705	811	950	1097	1192	1317	1395
	30	1335	252	880	1051	1197	1336	1474	1622	1674
	32	1597	313	1024	1271	1405	1601	1760	1959	2088
	34	1822	384	1067	1249	1641	1869	2082	2217	2330
Trichorionic	20	330	91	186	237	282	326	396	446	466
	22	486	109	308	361	417	480	554	619	662
	24	664	134	455	504	574	670	752	822	894
	26	865	165	624	668	751	867	978	1051	1120
	28	1099	201	766	848	969	1105	1225	1350	1441
	30	1354	238	929	1054	1205	1372	1499	1646	1752
	32	1657	271	1180	1325	1475	1667	1847	1978	2149
	34	1954	298	1396	1592	1784	1964	2190	2299	2472
Females	20	302	100	122	170	257	307	357	422	487
	22	455	112	257	308	398	464	518	578	642
	24	631	133	406	465	550	630	716	777	862
	26	828	162	584	631	719	820	935	1014	1120
	28	1051	195	768	841	921	1035	1181	1279	1369
	30	1299	231	932	1051	1144	1272	1451	1570	1669
	32	1590	277	1151	1271	1429	1588	1748	1902	2044
	34	1851	304	1339	1529	1691	1845	2037	2223	2279

Males	20	336	107	136	200	277	345	402	464	489
	22	494	122	281	341	421	497	578	645	674
	24	674	143	447	488	586	679	769	842	902
	26	880	173	597	679	780	894	993	1086	1156
	28	1109	208	705	889	984	1120	1251	1370	1441
	30	1363	249	902	1100	1227	1376	1538	1661	1742
	32	1649	305	1119	1325	1490	1666	1865	1992	2091
	34	1901	379	1067	1536	1755	1939	2172	2330	2390

Adapted from Min S-J, Luke B, Min L, Misiunas R, Nugent C, Van de Ven C, et al. Birthweight references for triplets. American Journal of Obstetrics & Gynecology 2004; 191:809–14.

Resources for Parents of Multiples

Bedrest and High-Risk Pregnancy

Sidelines National High Risk Pregnancy Support Network: P.O. Box 1808, Laguna Beach, CA 92652. Telephone 888-447-4754; email sidelines@sidelines.org; website www.sidelines .org. *Support group for women with high-risk pregnancies.*

Breast-Feeding

Baby-Friendly Hospital Initiative: 125 Wolf Rd., Suite 402, Albany, NY 12205. Telephone 518-621-7982; email info@babyfriendlyusa.org; website www.babyfriendlyusa.org. *Referrals to medical facilities that provide education and counseling regarding the benefits of breast-feeding, and that eliminate any institutional barriers to breast-feeding.*

Gromada, Karen Kerkhoof. *Mothering Multiples: Breastfeeding & Caring for Twins or More.* 3rd edition. La Leche League International, 2007.

International Lactation Consultant Association: 2501 Aerial Center Parkway, Suite 103, Morrisville, NC 27560. Telephone 888-ILCA-IS-U (888-452-2478) or 919-861-5577; email info@ilca.org; website www.ilca.org. *Education resources and referrals to consultants in your area.*

La Leche League International: 35 E. Wacker Drive, Suite 850, Chicago, IL 60601. Telephone 877-4-LA-LECHE (877-452-5324); website www.llli.org. *Breast-feeding information for parents; referrals to local support groups. Books include The Womanly Art of Breastfeeding.*

Lactation Education Resources: 3621 Lido Place, Fairfax, VA 22031. Telephone 703-691-2069; email LERonline@yahoo.com; website www.LERon-line.com. *Educational materials.*

United States Breastfeeding Committee: 4044 N. Lincoln Ave., #288, Chicago, IL 60618. Telephone 773-359-1549; email office@usbreastfeeding.org; website www.usbreast feeding.org. *Educational materials.*

Childbirth Preparation

Bradley Method (aka American Academy of Husband-Coached Childbirth): P.O. Box 5524, Sherman Oaks, CA 91413-5224. Telephone 800-4-A-BIRTH (800-422-4784); website www .bradleybirth.com. *Information and referrals to classes in your area.*

Hypnobabies: Telephone 714-894-BABY (714-894-2229); email info@hypnobabies.com; website www.hypnobabies.com. *Information, self-study materials, and referrals to classes in your area.*

International Childbirth Education Association: 2501 Aerial Center Parkway, Suite 103, Morrisville, NC 27560. Telephone 800-624-4934; website www.icea.org. *Referrals to childbirth educators, doulas, and classes in your area.*

Lamaze International (aka American Society for Psychoprophylaxis in Obstetrics): 2025 M Street NW, Suite 800, Washington, DC 20036-3309. Telephone 800-368-4404; website www.lamaze.org. *Information and referrals to classes in your area.*

Diet and Pregnancy

Academy of Nutrition and Dietetics Hotline: 120 South Riverside Plaza, Suite 2000, Chicago, IL 60606-6995. Telephone 800-877-1600; website www.eatright.org. *Referrals to dietitians in your area.*

Erick, Miriam. *Managing Morning Sickness: A Survival Guide for Pregnant Women.* Bull Publishing, 2004.

Luke, Barbara, Sc.D., M.P.H., R.N., R.D.: website www.drbarbaraluke.com. *Personalized nutrition counseling.*

Luke, Barbara, Sc.D., M.P.H., R.D., and Tamara Eberlein. *Program Your Baby's Health: The Pregnancy Diet for Your Child's Lifelong Well-Being.* Ballantine Books, 2001.

Nutrition Source—Harvard School of Public Health: 677 Huntington Avenue, Boston, MA 02115. Telephone 617-495-1000; website www.hsph.harvard.edu/nutritionsource/. *Guidelines for healthful eating.*

Women, Infants, and Children (WIC) Special Supplemental Nutrition Program: website www.fns.usda.gov/wic. *Supplemental foods, health care referrals, and nutrition education for low-income pregnant and postpartum women.*

Fetal Therapy

North American Fetal Therapy Network; email information@NAFTNet.org; website www.naftnet.org. *An association of medical centers in the United States and Canada that perform advanced in utero fetal therapeutic procedures.*

Twin to Twin Transfusion Syndrome Foundation, 411 Longbeach Parkway, Bay Village, OH 44140; phone 800-815-9211; email info@tttsfoundation.org; website www.tttsfoundation.org. *Provides educational, emotional, and financial support to families, medical professionals, and other caregivers before, during, and after a diagnosis of TTTS. For a list of medical centers that perform laser surgery for TTTS, visit www.tttsfoundation.org/laser_centers.php.*

Food Products

Bob's Red Mill: www.bobsredmill.com. *Whole-grain, high-fiber foods and recipes.*

Eggland's Best: www.egglandsbest.com. *Omega-3-fortified eggs.*

Fage: www.fageusa.com. *Greek strained yogurt.*

Ginger People: www.gingerpeople.com. *Ginger products.*

Kashi: www.kashi.com. *Healthful snacks, including Kashi TLC (Tasty Little Chewies).*

Kind Bars: www.kindsnacks.com. *Convenient, nutritious snacks.*

Lactaid: www.lactaid.com. *Lactose-free dairy products and recipes.*

Lärabar: www.larabar.com. *Whole-grain snack bars.*

Seeds of Change: www.seedsofchangefoods.com. *Organic foods.*

Vita Foods: www.vitafoodproducts.com. *Herring and salmon products and recipes.*

Grief and Bereavement

Center for Loss in Multiple Birth (CLIMB): P.O. Box 91377, Anchorage, AK 99509. Telephone 907-222-5321; email climb@climb-support.org; website www.climb-support.org. *Support by and for parents and bereaved families; quarterly newsletter; relevant articles; samples of birth and memorial announcements.*

Health Information

American Board of Medical Specialties: 353 North Clark St., Suite 1400, Chicago, IL 60654. Telephone 866-ASK-ABMS (866-275-2267) or 312-436-2600; website www.abms .org. *Verification of an individual doctor's status as a board-certified specialist.*

American College of Obstetricians and Gynecologists: P.O. Box 70620, Washington, DC 20024-9998. Telephone 800-673-8444 or 202-638-5577; website www.acog.org. *Information on pregnancy, childbirth, and women's health.*

BMJ infographic, "Neurodevelopmental Consequences of Preterm Birth": website www .bmj.com/content/350/bmj.g6661/infographic. *Illustrates risk level for various neurodevelopmental consequences based on degree of prematurity.*

March of Dimes: 1275 Mamaroneck Avenue, White Plains, NY 10605. Telephone: 914-997-4488; website www.marchofdimes.com. *Information on preventing prematurity, birth defects, and infant mortality.*

National Healthy Mothers, Healthy Babies Coalition: Telephone 703-838-7552; email NationalHMHBCoalition@gmail.com; website www.hmhb.org. *Educational materials.*

National Institute of Child Health and Human Development; P.O. Box 3006, Rockville, MD 20847. Telephone 800-370-2943; email NICHDInformationResourceCenter@mail.nih .gov; website www.nichd.nih.gov. *Educational materials and research updates from the National Institutes of Health.*

Office on Women's Health, U.S. Dept. of Health and Human Services. Telephone 800-994-9662; website www.womenshealth.gov. *Educational materials from the federal government.*

Multiple Birth

Bowers, Nancy. *The Multiple Pregnancy Sourcebook*. Contemporary Books/McGraw-Hill, 2001.

International Society for Twin Studies: Queensland Institute of Medical Research, Post Office, Royal Brisbane Hospital, Brisbane 4029, Australia. Email ists@qimr.edu.au; website www.ists.qimr.edu.au. *Research information.*

Multiples of America (formerly National Organization of Mothers of Twins Clubs): 2000 Mallory Lane, Suite 130-600, Franklin, TN 37067-8231. Telephone 248-231-4480; email Info@MultiplesofAmerica.org; website multiplesofamerica.org. *Information, support, and referrals to local chapters.*

Raising Multiples (formerly Mothers of Supertwins): P.O. Box 306, East Islip, NY 11730. Telephone 631-859-1110; website www.raisingmultiples.org. *Information support and referrals to local chapters.*

Twin Services: P.O. Box 10066, Berkeley, CA 94709. Telephone 510-524-0863; email twinservices@juno.com; website www.twinservices.org. *Publications and counseling.*

Twins magazine: 30799 Pinetree Road, #256, Cleveland, OH 44124. Telephone 855-758-9467; website www.twinsmagazine.com.

Nutrition References and Cookbooks

America's Test Kitchen. *The Complete Vegetarian Cookbook*. America's Test Kitchen, 2015.

Bittman, Mark. *The Food Matters Cookbook*. New York: Simon & Schuster, 2010.

Bittman, Mark. *How to Cook Everything Vegetarian*. Houghton Mifflin, 2007.

Jamieson, Patsy. *The Essential EatingWell Cookbook: Good Carbs, Good Fats, Great Flavors*. Countryman, 2006.

Luke, Barbara, and Tamara Eberlein. *Program Your Baby's Health: The Pregnancy Diet for Your Child's Lifelong Well-Being*. Ballantine Books, 2001.

Nestle, Marion. *Food Politics*. University of California Press, 2013.

Nestle, Marion. *What to Eat*. North Point Press, 2007.

Ottolenghi, Yotam, and Jonathan Lovekin. *Plenty: Vibrant Vegetable Recipes from London's Ottolenghi*. Chronicle Books, 2011.

Ottolenghi, Yotam, and Sami Tamimi. *Jerusalem: A Cookbook*. Ten Speed Press, 2012.

Parker, Katie, and Kristen Smith. *The High Protein Vegetarian Cookbook*. Countryman Press, 2015.

Pollan, Michael. *Cooked: A Natural History of Transformation*. Penguin Press, 2014.

Pollan, Michael. *In Defense of Food: An Eater's Manifesto*. Penguin Press, 2008.

Pollan, Michael. *The Omnivore's Dilemma: A Natural History of Four Meals*. Penguin Press, 2007.

Price, Jessie. *EatingWell's Comfort Foods Made Healthy: The Classic Makeovers Cookbook*. Countryman Press, 2008.

Rolls, Barbara. *The Volumetrics Eating Plan: Techniques and Recipes for Feeling Full on Fewer Calories*. HarperCollins, 2005.

Rolls, Barbara, and Mindy Hermann. *The Ultimate Volumetrics Diet*. William Morrow, 2013.

Romanoff, Jim. *The EatingWell Healthy in a Hurry Cookbook: 150 Delicious Recipes for Simple, Everyday Suppers in 45 Minutes or Less*. Countryman Press, 2006.

Sears, Barry. *The Mediterranean Zone*. HarperCollins, 2014.

Sears, Barry. *The Omega Zone: The Miracle of the New High-Dose Fish Oil*. HarperCollins, 2002.

Wansink, Brian. *Mindless Eating: Why We Eat More Than We Think*. Bantam, 2007.

Waters, Alice. *The Art of Simple Food: Notes, Lessons, and Recipes from a Delicious Revolution*. Clarkson Potter, 2007.

Waters, Alice. *The Art of Simple Food II: Recipes, Flavor, and Inspiration from the New Kitchen Garden*. Clarkson Potter, 2013.

Willett, Walter C., and P.J. Skerrett. *Eat, Drink, and Be Healthy: The Harvard Medical School Guide to Healthy Eating*. Free Press, 2005.

Nutrition Websites

Academy of Nutrition and Dietetics: www.eatright.org

American Egg Board: www.aeb.org

Body mass index (BMI) calculator: http://www.nhibi.nih.gov/health/educational/lose_wt/BMI/bmicalc.htm

Environmental Defense Fund (including a guide for choosing seafood): www.edf.org

Food and Drug Administration: www.fda.gov

International Food Information Council Foundation: www.foodinsight.org

National Dairy Council: www.nationaldairycouncil.org

National Fisheries Institute: www.aboutseafood.com

National Weight Control Registry: www.nwcr.ws

Nutrition Source (information on healthy eating from the Harvard School of Public Health): www.hsph.harvard.edu/nutritionsource

Whole Grains Council: www.wholegrainscouncil.org

Nutritional Supplements and Supplement Drinks

Carlson Laboratories: 600 W. University Dr., Arlington Heights, IL 60004. Telephone 888-234-5656; website www.carlsonlabs.com. *Quality nutritional supplements.*

Carnation: Telephone 800-289-7313; website www.carnationbreakfastessentials.com. *Carnation Instant Breakfast brand.*

Nestlé HealthCare Nutrition: Consumer & Product Support, 445 State Street, Fremont MI 49412. Telephone 800-247-7893 or 888-240-2713; website www.boost.com or www.nestlenutritionstore.com. *Boost brand nutritional drinks.*

National Institutes of Health Office of Dietary Supplements; website https://ods.od.nih.gov. *Information on supplements.*

Ross/Abbott Nutrition: 625 Cleveland Avenue, Columbus, OH 43215-1724. Telephone 800-227-5767 or 800-986-8501; website www.abbottnutrition.com or www.ensure.com. *Ensure, Promote, and TwoCalHN brands.*

U.S. National Library of Medicine Dietary Supplement Label Database: http://www.dsid.nlm.nih.gov. *Information on supplements.*

Physical Therapy

American Physical Therapy Association: 1111 North Fairfax Street, Alexandria, VA 22314-1488. Telephone 800-999-2782 or 703-684-2782; website www.apta.org. *Referrals to physical therapists.*

Physician Referrals

American College of Obstetricians and Gynecologists: P.O. Box 70620, Washington, DC 20024-9998. Telephone 800-673-8444; website www.acog.org. *Referrals to maternal-fetal medicine specialists.*

Society for Maternal-Fetal Medicine: 409 12th Street, SW, Washington, DC 20024. Telephone 202-863-2476; email smfm@smfm.org; website www.smfm.org (click on "Find an MFM"). *Referrals to maternal-fetal medicine specialists.*

Postpartum Depression

Center for Postpartum Health: 13743 Riverside Drive, Sherman Oaks, CA 91423. Telephone 818-887-1312; website www.postpartumhealth.com. *Information and support.*

Postpartum Health Alliance: P.O. Box 927231, San Diego, CA 92192-7231. Telephone 619-254-0023; email info@postpartumhealthalliance.org; website www.postpartumhealth alliance.org. *Information and support.*

Postpartum Support International: 6706 SW 54th Ave., Portland, OR 97219. Telephone 800-944-4773; email PSIOffice@postpartum.net; website www.postpartum.net. *Information and support.*

Prenatal Multiples Programs

The following is a partial list of well-respected prenatal multiples programs in the United States. It is not meant to be all-inclusive—certainly there are many other health care providers and groups who have accumulated a great deal of experience in managing multiple pregnancies—but it does give you a place to start your search.

In addition, see the section on page 515 called Fetal Therapy. Members of the organizations cited there also have a lot of experience in the medical management of multiple gestations. Another option is to contact the Society for Maternal-Fetal Medicine, listed above in the section called Physician Referrals.

Associates in Advanced Maternal-Fetal Medicine LLC, 7765 SW 87th Ave, Suite 200, Miami, FL 33173; website www.advancedmfm.com.

Banner Good Samaritan Hospital, Dept. of Maternal-Fetal Medicine, 1111 E. McDowell Rd., Phoenix, AZ 85006.

California Pacific Medical Center, 3698 California St., San Francisco, CA 94118.

Eastside Maternal Fetal Medicine, 1110 112th Ave. NE, Suite 100, Bellevue, WA 98004.

Hackensack University Medical Center, Dept. of Childbirth Education, 30 Prospect Avenue, Hackensack, NJ 07601.

Indiana University Health, 11700 N. Meridian St., C453, Carmel, IN 46032.

Maine Medical Center, OB Parent Education Program/Expecting Multiples: Bundles of Joy, 22 Bramhall St., Portland, ME 04101.

Medical University of South Carolina, Dept. of Ob-Gyn/Prenatal Wellness Center, 135 Cannon St., Charleston, SC 29425.

Missouri Baptist Medical Center, Childbirth and Parenting Education Program/Multiples and More Class, 3015 North Ballas Rd., St. Louis, MO 63131.

Morristown Medical Center, Parent Education/Twins, Triplets and More, 100 Madison Ave., Morristown, NJ 07960.

Newton Medical Center, Parent Education/Twins, Triplets and More, 175 High St., Newton, NJ 07860.

New York University Langone Medical Center, Maternal-Fetal Medicine Associates PLLC, 70 E. 90th St., New York, NY 10128; website www.nyulangone.org.

Northwestern Medicine/Prentice Women's Hospital, Division of Maternal-Fetal Medicine, 250 E. Superior St., Chicago, IL 60611.

Obstetrix Medical Group of San Jose, 900 E. Hamilton Ave., Suite 220, Campbell, CA 95008.

Ochsner Health System, Multifetal Pregnancy Center, 1514 Jefferson Hwy., Clinic Tower 6th floor, New Orleans, LA 70121; website www.ochsner.org/services/multifetal-pregnancy-center.

Overlook Medical Center, Parent Education/Twins, Triplets and More, 99 Beauvoir Ave., Summit, NJ 07902.

Prentice Women's Hospital, Northwestern University, 250 East Superior St., Room 03-2201, Chicago, IL 66011.

Savannah Perinatology Associates, Memorial University Medical Center, Provident Building, Suite 302, 4750 Waters Ave., Savannah, GA 31404; website www.memorialhealth.com/savannah-perinatology-associates.aspx.

Sutter Medical Center, Dept. of Ob-Gyn/Sutter Moms of Multiples Center, 5151 F St., Sacramento, CA 95819.

Swedish Medical Center, Birth and Family Education/Preparation for Multiples, 747 Broadway, 5 East, Seattle, WA 98122.

University of Alabama at Birmingham, Women and Infants Center, 1700 6th Ave. South, Birmingham, AL 35249; website www.obgyn.uab.edu.

University of California, San Diego, Dept. of Ob-Gyn/Fetal Surgery Program, 200 West Arbor Drive, San Diego CA 92103-8433.

University of California, San Francisco Medical Center, Dept. of Ob-Gyn/Twins and More Program, 505 Parnassus Ave., San Francisco, CA 94122.

University of Michigan, Dept. of Ob-Gyn, 1500 East Medical Center Dr., Floor 1, Reception E, Ann Arbor, MI 48109-5384.

University of Washington, Prematurity Prevention Program, 1959 NE Pacific St., Seattle, WA 98195

Valley Perinatal Services, 9440 E. Ironwood Square Dr., Scottsdale, AZ 85258; website www.valleyperinatal.com.

Products

Affiliated Genetics: 2749 Parleys Way, Salt Lake City, UT 84109. Telephone 800-362-5559; email info@affiliatedgenetics.com; website www.affiliatedgenetics.com. *Provides cheek-swab, mail-order genetic test used to determine twin type ($150 plus $10 handling for twins; $75 more for each additional multiple).*

Double Blessings: 1425 30th St., Suite H, San Diego, CA 92154. Telephone 800-584-8946; email info@doubleblessings.com; website www.doubleblessings.com. *Mail-order products for multiples, including nursing pillows.*

Genex Diagnostics: #180–4616 25th Avenue NE, Seattle, WA 98105. Telephone 888-262-2263; email lab@genexdiagnostics.com; website www.genexdiagnostics.com. *Provides cheek-swab, mail-order genetic test used to determine twin type ($180 for testing twins; $275 for triplets).*

Infant CPR Anytime Personal Learning Program: From the American Heart Association. Telephone 800-233-1230; email AHAcustomerservice@workflowone.com; website www.shopcpranytime.org. *Instructional DVD and mannequin for learning cardiopulmonary resuscitation (CPR).*

Preemie Store and More: 1682 Roxanna Lane, New Brighton, MN 55112. Telephone 800-676-8469; website www.preemiestore.com. *Clothing and products for premature infants.*

Doctor to Doctor:
A Research Update

BY ROGER B. NEWMAN, M.D.

About the author of this appendix:

This Research Update was written by Roger B. Newman, M.D., Professor of Obstetrics and Gynecology and Maas Endowed Chair for Reproductive Sciences at the Medical University of South Carolina (MUSC). A nationally recognized expert in high-risk obstetrics and the care of women pregnant with multiples, Dr. Newman has directed the MUSC Prenatal Wellness Center Multiple Pregnancy Program since its inception in 1987. He has published nearly 150 scientific articles and 20 book chapters, primarily on the care of multiples, has held leadership positions in the American Congress of Obstetrics and Gynecology, and is a past president of the Society for Maternal-Fetal Medicine.

• • •

The information presented here, intended primarily for health care professionals, addresses some of the thornier management issues that arise when caring for women who are pregnant with multiples. All of these issues are touched on in the appropriate chapters of *When You're Expecting Twins, Triplets, or Quads*, in language geared toward a lay audience. However, many of these medical management issues are both complex and serious, and in some cases controversial. That's why I have added this appendix to the fourth edition of the book, to cover some of these topics in greater depth and explore the details of the scientific literature. My hope is that the reader who is pregnant with multiples will share this appendix with her obstetrician or maternal-fetal medicine specialist, so that doctor and patient can then discuss in detail any concerns pertinent to her individual situation.

Admittedly, this appendix is not all-inclusive of potential problems. My intention is to focus specifically on some of the complications of monochorionic or monoamniotic twins, strategies for prevention of preterm birth, and questions that often come up regarding delivery options.

For further information on current obstetrical opinion regarding these and other questions and complications beyond the scope of a relatively brief appendix, I would refer colleagues to a recent symposium that I edited, "Multiple Pregnancies," *Clinical Obstetrics and Gynecology*.[1] The chapters of this symposium address topics in depth, such as first-trimester ultrasound and screening for chromosomal abnormalities in multiples, multifetal pregnancy reduction, nutrition for multiples (by Dr. Barbara Luke), diagnosis and management of twin-twin transfusion syndrome and other monochorionic twin complications, issues unique to monoamniotic twins, spontaneous preterm birth prevention, issues unique to higher-order multiples, appropriate fetal surveillance, timing of delivery, and route of delivery. As editor, I am very proud of its content and believe that it can serve as a fabulous resource.

Complications Unique to Monozygotic Gestations

Multifetal gestations present numerous challenges for obstetricians and their patients—because virtually every possible fetal or maternal complication occurs with greater frequency in multiple as compared to singleton gestations.

In addition to an increased frequency of usual obstetric complications, multiple gestations also present a variety of unique pregnancy problems encountered only in monozygotic (identical) multiples. Some practitioners may have limited experience with monozygotic complications, so we begin our discussion here.

FETAL ANOMALIES

Fetal structural defects occur more frequently in multiple gestations than in singletons. In a large review of fetal malformations among twin pregnancies, four important observations

---

1. Newman RB. Multiple pregnancies. Clinical Obstetrics and Gynecology 2015; 58:556–702.

could be made.[2] First, the prevalence of congenital malformation is 1.2 to 2.0 times higher among twin fetuses compared to singletons. Second, the higher prevalence occurs primarily among like-sex twin sets or among known monozygotic twins when that information was provided. Third, in 80 to 90 percent of twin sets, the fetuses are discordant for any structural defect. This discordance persists even if the twins are identical, although the concordance rate for anomaly is slightly higher among monozygotic twins.[3] Fourth, the most common defects are cardiac malformations, neural tube defects, facial clefting, gastrointestinal anomalies, and anterior abdominal wall defects including cloacal and bladder exstrophy.

Of interest, however, is a recent analysis of congenital heart disease that took advantage of the Danish Twin Registry, which is one of the oldest twin registries in the world, containing information on twins born in Denmark for more than a century. The Danish Twin Registry has consistently used questionnaire data to assign zygosity and has proven superior to other large public health data sets that use like-sex twins as a proxy for zygosity. Unlike previous studies, the Danish Twin Registry did not demonstrate a higher risk of congenital heart disease among monozygotic twins compared to dizygotic twins.[4] This finding suggests that the intrauterine environment of a multiple gestation may predispose to the development of congenital heart disease rather than assuming it is only related to the monozygotic twinning process.

As has been discussed previously in this book, twin gestations represent a major maternal nutritional challenge. Nutrient and micronutrient intake during pregnancy has been linked to fetal congenital heart defects.[5] Early maternal nutritional depletion may affect not only fetal growth in multiple gestations but, potentially, fetal anomalies as well. It is also likely that nutritional deficiencies can make the fetus more susceptible to other environmental or prenatal exposures that may be teratogenic. This concern underscores the importance of preconception and early pregnancy vitamin supplementation, especially with the B vitamins. Preconception folic acid has been proven to prevent recurrent spina bifida, and many believe that it reduces the risk of congenital heart disease as well.

Birth defects among monozygotic twin gestations are frequently categorized as occurring by one of three mechanisms. The first mechanism is midline structural defects believed to be a consequence of the underlying stimulus to zygote splitting. Examples of such midline

2. Kohl SG, Casey G. Twin gestation. Mt. Sinai Journal of Medicine 1975; 42:5239.
3. Luke B, Keith LG. Monozygotic twinning as a congenital defect and congenital defects in monozygotic twins. Fetal Diagnosis and Therapy 1990; 5(2):61–9.
4. Herskind AM, Pedersen DA, Christensen K. Increased prevalence of congenital heart defects in monozygotic and dizygotic twins. Circulation 2013; 128:1182–8.
5. Shaw GM, Carmichael SL, Yang W, Lammer EJ. Periconceptional nutrient intakes and risks of conotruncal heart defects. Birth Defects Research Part A: Clinical and Molecular Teratology 2010; 88:144–51.

anomalies include conjoined twins, facial clefting, neural tube defects, sirenomelia, holopros-encephaly, and bladder exstrophy.

The second category includes defects that are a consequence of abnormal monochorionic placental development resulting in vascular interconnections. The classic example is the acar-diac twin, or twin reversed arterial perfusion (TRAP) sequence, as it is now known. Vascular exchanges are also involved in the genesis of malformations associated with the demise of one monochorionic twin. Demise of a monochorionic twin is believed to cause hypotension or vascular thrombosis in the surviving twin. Congenital abnormalities potentially caused by this ischemic injury include microcephaly, hydrocephalus, intestinal obstruction, renal dysplasia, aplasia cutis, and limb amputations.

The third category of defects includes those resulting from intrauterine crowding associ-ated with the presence of multiple fetuses. These include foot deformities, dislocation of the hip, and asymmetry of the skull.

Interventions to improve pregnancy outcome for fetal anomalies require that those anoma-lies be detected. Virtually all twin pregnancies undergo a fetal anatomic survey usually between 18 and 22 weeks of gestation. At our own institution we reviewed almost 250 consecutive twin gestations and successfully used ultrasound to identify 21 of 24 anomalous fetuses. There were no false-positive diagnoses, and both the specificity and positive predictive values were 100 percent.

Prenatal diagnosis of congenital malformation in a multiple pregnancy allows for interven-tions that may include increased antepartum fetal testing; a change in the timing, location, or mode of delivery; consultation with various neonatal and pediatric subspecialists; and, in some cases, interventions such as fetal therapy, selective multifetal reduction of the abnormal twin, or termination of the pregnancy. Selective multifetal reduction versus expectant management can become an extremely complex issue in multiple pregnancies discordant for a potentially lethal fetal structural abnormality.

Acardiac Twin (TRAP Sequence)

Twin reversed arterial perfusion (TRAP) sequence, also known as an acardiac twin, is an ex-tremely rare anomaly that, like conjoined twins, occurs only with a monochorionic placenta. An acardiac twin is believed to occur in approximately 1 in 100 monozygotic twin pregnancies, or about 1 in 35,000 pregnancies overall. Acardia results from an umbilical artery-to-artery anastomosis between monochorionic twin fetuses. The acardiac twin, which is only partially developed, relies on the normal twin (or pump twin) to provide circulation through a reversal of blood flow in the artery-to-artery anastomosis. The reversed flow in the umbilical artery can be identified using Doppler ultrasound.

The need to provide a blood supply to the acardiac co-twin puts tremendous strain on the normal twin. The prognosis for the normal twin is best predicted by the size of the acardiac twin. In one review, when the estimated weight of the acardiac twin was 70 percent or more of the normal pump twin, the risk of pregnancy loss of both fetuses was high. In those cases, 40 percent were complicated by polyhydramnios, 30 percent of pump twins developed congestive heart failure, and almost all delivered prematurely.[6] When the birthweight ratio was less than 70 percent, the preterm delivery rate was still very high (75 percent) and polyhydramnios still complicated 30 percent of the births, but congestive heart failure occurred in only 10 percent of the normal pump twins.

Management options include invasive procedures designed to interrupt the cardiovascular anastomosis between the two twins and expectant observation. In high-risk cases, fetoscopic cord occlusion has been achieved by means of both cord ligation and laser ablation of the vascular connection.[7, 8] Ultrasound guided techniques have also been used to occlude the vascular communication between the two fetuses. Successful techniques have included the injection of absolute alcohol or helical thrombogenic metal coils into the umbilical artery of the acardiac twin. These invasive techniques are recommended for those twin sets where the estimated acardiac twin weight is 70 percent or more of the estimated pump twin weight. Invasive techniques should also be considered when there is ultrasound evidence of polyhydramnios or congestive heart failure of the pump twin at a previable gestational age. The ideal group for expectant observation would be those twin sets where the acardiac twin is estimated to be less than 50 percent of the size of the normal twin, with almost 90 percent survival.[9]

Conjoined Twins

Conjoined twinning is another exceedingly rare complication uniquely associated with monozygotic twinning. It has a reported incidence of between 1 in 50,000 and 1 in 100,000 deliveries. Conjoined twins are reliably detected with ultrasonography as a result of failure to identify separation between the fetuses in a monoamniotic/monochorionic twin gestation. It

6. Moore TR, Gale S, Benirschke K. Perinatal outcomes of forty-nine pregnancies complicated acardiac twinning. American Journal of Obstetrics & Gynecology 1990; 163:907–12.
7. Pagani G, D'Antonio F, Khalil A, et al. Intrafetal laser treatment for twin reversed arterial perfusion sequence: Cohort study and meta-analysis. Ultrasound in Obstetrics & Gynecology 2013; 42:6–14.
8. Lee H, et al.; for the North American Fetal Therapy Network (NAFTNet). The North American Fetal Therapy Network registry data on outcomes of radiofrequency ablation for twin reversed arterial perfusion sequence. Fetal Diagnosis and Therapy 2013; 1:1–6.
9. Jelin E, Hirose S, Rand L, et al. Perinatal outcomes of conservative management versus fetal intervention for twin reversed arterial perfusion sequence with a small acardiac twin. Fetal Diagnosis and Therapy 2010; 27:138–41.

is important to carefully examine both of the fetuses because of the high frequency of associated anomalies not associated with the fusion. A fetal echocardiogram is particularly valuable because delineation of any congenital heart disease is important in evaluating the possibility of survival.

Conjoined twins are categorized based on the location and degree of fusion. The main types of conjoined twins are thoraco-omphalopagus (25 percent; joined at the chest and abdomen), thoracopagus (18 percent; joined at the chest), pygopagus (20 percent; joined at the rear end), omphalopagus (10 percent; joined at the umbilicus), craniopagus (6 percent; joined at the head), and ischiopagus (5 percent; joined at the hip).

The combination of ultrasonography and magnetic residence imaging (MRI) can be used to define the extent of organ involvement and assess the possibility of extrauterine separation. Approximately 40 percent of conjoined twins are stillborn and another 35 percent die within the first 48 hours of life. The prognosis for survival depends on the degree of shared organs, the vital nature of those organs, and their amenability to surgical separation. In thoracopagus twins, the degree of heart fusion determines the outcome. Congenital heart disease is found among 75 percent of thoracopagus twins, and a common ventricle is incompatible with survival of either fetus.

Omphalopagus twins usually have the best chance for surgical separation and survival unless other severe associated anomalies are found. An omphalocele is present in one-third of these twins, and congenital heart defects are present in about one-fourth. The liver is shared in approximately 80 percent of sets. The best situation is when there is only a skin or muscle bridge connecting the two fetuses and there are no shared organs.

Craniopagus twins have an unpredictable outcome because it's difficult to assess the degree of intracranial fusion and the vascular connections before delivery. Pygopagus twins have a fairly good outcome because sharing of vital organs does not occur. These twins are usually joined at the buttocks and lower spine, often sharing a common rectum, anus, and external genitalia. Ischiopagus twins present more complex problems because they often share abdominal and pelvic organs and are more technically difficult to separate. These twins often have a common pelvis and may have four legs (ischiopagus tetrapus) or three legs (ischiopagus tripus). Their lower gastrointestinal tracts join at the terminal small bowel and empty into a single large bowel. They commonly share a bladder and urethra and frequently have rectovaginal abnormalities.

If there is a possibility of postdelivery survival, conjoined twins should be delivered by elective cesarean. Even if the conjoined twins are not expected to survive, cesarean delivery is usually needed to avoid maternal trauma; however, before viability, induced vaginal delivery of conjoined twins may be possible because of the smaller combined fetal size. When the diagnosis of conjoined twins is made in the first or early second trimester, it is appropriate to consider the option of pregnancy termination.

It is recommended that conjoined twins be delivered at a tertiary center because of the complex and multidisciplinary postdelivery evaluation and care that these infants will require. Unless an emergency exists, attempts at separation should be delayed to allow the twins to become larger, other abnormalities to be detected, and the operation to be carefully planned.

Any planned attempt at separation can be anticipated to present extremely difficult decisions for the family in the postpartum period. These decisions should be supported not only by the patient's obstetrician and neonatologist, but also by other pediatric subspecialists, members of the hospital ethics committee, and/or a chaplain. Survivors of separation are likely to need long-term rehabilitation for orthopedic, neurologic, gastrointestinal, genitourinary, and gynecologic disabilities.

Conjoined twinning is believed to be a random event with negligible risk of recurrence. There has never been a reported case of a conjoined twin having conjoined offspring.

Monoamniotic Twins

Monoamniotic twins complicate less than 1 percent of monozygotic gestations, occurring in approximately 1 in every 25,000 to 30,000 pregnancies. The importance of monoamnionicity is found in the high fetal mortality rate associated with this type of placentation. Since both fetuses are in the same amniotic sac, cord entanglement is present in virtually all monoamniotic twin sets. Knotting of the cords can result in sudden, unexpected fetal demise.

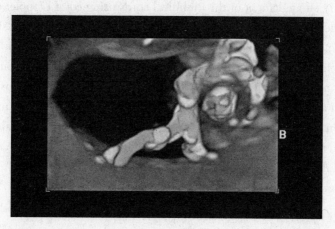

Second trimester monoamniotic, monochorionic twins with entangled umbilical cords because both twins are in the same amniotic sac. Although not shown, first trimester mo/mo twins would usually have only a single yolk sac.

Other causes of perinatal mortality in monoamniotic twins include birth defects and twin-twin transfusion syndrome (TTTS). Older studies (conducted before ultrasound allowed for the prenatal diagnosis of this condition) report a stillbirth rate of almost 50 percent associated with monoamniotic placentation. More recent studies have reported lower perinatal mortality rates between 10 and 20 percent.[10]

In early pregnancy it is easy to differentiate monochorionic from dichorionic twins with ultrasound. What is more difficult is differentiating diamniotic/monochorionic from mono-amniotic/monochorionic twins, as both of these conditions are associated with only a single placenta and fetuses of the same gender. If the splitting of the embryo occurs more than 7 days following conception, the result is a monoamniotic/monochorionic twin pregnancy. If the division occurs more than 12 days after conception, the monoamniotic, monochorionic (mo/mo) twins may be conjoined.

Key ultrasound findings to help diagnose monoamniocity are the presence of a single yolk sac and the absence of a thin amniotic membrane separating the two fetuses. While it has been classically taught that monoamniotic twins have only a single yolk sac, there is a very narrow window of time during which splitting of the embryo can result in a single amniotic sac but two yolk sacs. The dividing amniotic membrane can also be very hard to see in the first trimester. It is common to be unable to identify the dividing amniotic membrane until at least 12 to 13 weeks of gestation. The diagnosis of monoamniotic twins probably cannot be certain until at least 14 to 16 weeks. Even at that time, efforts should continue to identify the dividing amniotic membrane in all future ultrasound scans, given that diamniotic/monochorionic twins are 30 times more common than monoamniotic twins. By the second trimester it is also frequently possible to identify entanglement of the umbilical cords using color Doppler ultrasound.

A new diagnosis of monoamniotic twins after 16 weeks of gestation should be viewed skeptically and emergently evaluated. A mid-trimester diagnosis of monoamniotic twins could easily be a complication of a diamniotic/monochorionic twin set commonly referred to as *stuck twin* syndrome. A stuck twin can be a manifestation of twin-twin transfusion syndrome (TTTS), wherein nearly all of the amniotic fluid is missing from the sac of one twin, resulting in the amniotic membrane being closely applied to the fetus like plastic wrap. The other twin is freely mobile in its own amniotic sac with polyhydramnios, while the movement of the stuck twin is restricted. If the stuck twin syndrome is not identified, the opportunity for potentially effective treatment options for TTTS can be missed.

---

10. Rodis JF, McIlveen PF, Egan JFX, et al. Monoamniotic twins: Improved perinatal survival with accurate prenatal diagnosis and antenatal fetal surveillance. American Journal of Obstetrics & Gynecology 1997; 177:1046–9.

Four significant questions need to be answered regarding management of a monoamniotic gestation:

1. Should monoamniotic twins be monitored on an inpatient or an outpatient basis?

Because of the risk of dual fetal loss due to constriction of umbilical cord blood flow, increased fetal surveillance has been recommended for monoamniotic twins. Recent studies have supported the routine admission of monoamniotic twins to the hospital for daily fetal monitoring. Heybourne reported on 96 sets of monoamniotic twins, of which 87 still had two surviving fetuses at 24 weeks' gestation.[11] Forty-three of these twin sets were admitted electively for fetal monitoring multiple times each day. The other 44 monoamniotic twin sets were followed as outpatients with fetal monitoring two to three times per week; admission was reserved for the usual obstetrical indications. The monoamniotic twins electively admitted to the hospital experienced no stillbirths, compared to a 15 percent risk for those twins managed as outpatients. Inpatient admission was also associated with a greater gestational age at delivery and an increased birthweight. Other, smaller studies have also compared inpatient versus outpatient mortality and found similar results.[12] Combining these studies, the overall outpatient mortality was 15.3 percent versus 0 percent for those monoamniotic twins admitted to the hospital. Consequently, approximately one fetal death is prevented for every five women admitted to the hospital pregnant with monoamniotic twins.

If inpatient management is chosen, then a decision will be necessary as to when. Some physicians advise admission at the point of viability, approximately 24 weeks' gestation. At MUSC, we routinely recommend admission at approximately 26 weeks' gestation when survivability is higher—but ultimately that decision is up to the patient. This decision can be aided by reviewing the NIH morbidity and mortality calculator specific for these extremely early gestational weeks. This information can be accessed at the following NIH-sponsored website: http://www.nichd.nih.gov/about/org/der/branches/ppb/programs/epbo/pages/epbo_case.aspx.

Prior to hospital admission for inpatient monitoring, the patient should be

11. Heybourne KD, Porreco RP, Garite TJ, Phair K, Abril D; Obstetrix/Pediatrix Research Study Group. Improved perinatal survival of monoamniotic twins with intensive inpatient monitoring. American Journal of Obstetrics & Gynecology 2005; 192:96–101.
12. DeFalco LM, Sciscione AC, Megerian G, et al. Inpatient versus outpatient management of monoamniotic twins and outcomes. American Journal of Perinatology 2006; 23:205–11.

told that that the duration of hospitalization could be months. At the time of admission, we recommend enhancement of lung maturity with antenatal cortico-steroids because of the possibility of an unpredictable emergent delivery.

2. How should monoamniotic twins be monitored?

In the Heyborne study, those monoamniotic twins admitted to the hospital were monitored two to three times a day for an hour. One of the smaller studies also monitored patients three times per day, while another one attempted to do continuous monitoring.

We have not found it reasonable or possible to do continuous monitoring. Also, there are no data documenting that continuous fetal monitoring improves outcome. If monoamniotic twins are monitored as outpatients, the usual recommendation is for a nonstress test three times per week. Fetal nonstress testing can reveal evidence of umbilical cord constriction as well as evidence of fetal hypoxia. In one report of 13 sets of monoamniotic twins followed as outpatients, all had cord entanglement at birth, and for 8, the sole indication for delivery was nonreassuring results following fetal heart rate testing.[13] These findings included persistent moderate-to-severe variable decelerations (four cases), persistent fetal bradycardia (one case), and a persistently nonreactive nonstress test result with a nonreassuring fetal biophysical profile (two cases). Two other sets of twins were delivered because of premature labor, one associated with intrauterine growth restriction, and two were electively delivered after documentation of fetal lung maturity.

3. How should monoamniotic twins be delivered?

The recommended route of delivery has typically been cesarean for fear of intrapartum complications. This recommendation is based primarily on expert opinion, as there have been no published studies with adequate statistical power to answer this question. There have been small case series published that describe monoamniotic twins delivered vaginally. If vaginal delivery is desired, it would be optimal for both twins to be cephalic and well grown. If vaginal delivery is attempted, continuous fetal monitoring during labor is essential because acute fetal distress can develop rapidly, caused by constriction of a knotted umbilical

---

13. Rodis JF, McIlveen PF, Egan JFX, et al. Monoamniotic twins: Improved perinatal survival with accurate prenatal diagnosis and antenatal fetal surveillance. American Journal of Obstetrics & Gynecology 1997; 177:1046–9.

cord as the first baby descends through the pelvis. That said, our preference is to deliver monoamniotic twins by cesarean due to the almost universal presence of entangled umbilical cords.

4. When should monoamniotic twins be delivered?

As with any other high-risk pregnancy, delivery should be timed to minimize both maternal risk and fetal risk. Fetal interests are best served when the decision regarding the timing of delivery is guided by an understanding of the risk of neonatal death from prematurity, balanced against the risk of intrauterine death. With outpatient fetal monitoring, the risk of stillbirth between 32 and 34 weeks is approximately 5 percent. With inpatient monitoring, the risk of stillbirth is close to zero. Most experts recommend delivery of monoamniotic twins between 32 and 34 weeks of gestation.

VanMieghem and coworkers recently reviewed the obstetric and perinatal outcomes for 193 monoamniotic twin pregnancies.[14] Fetal and neonatal outcomes were compared between fetuses followed in an inpatient setting and those undergoing increased outpatient follow-up between 26 and 28 weeks of gestation until planned cesarean between 32 and 35 weeks of gestation. The risk of stillbirth was compared with the risk of serious neonatal complications. Of 144 ongoing pregnancies with two live fetuses at 26 weeks of gestation, 53 were managed primarily as outpatients and 71 were electively admitted for fetal monitoring. Five fetuses in the outpatient management group died, while two fetuses were lost in the inpatient management group. The loss in the inpatient management group was a double intrauterine fetal demise at 33 weeks and 6 days, one day before a scheduled cesarean. In this review, the prospective risk of nonrespiratory neonatal complication was lower than the prospective risk of stillbirth after 32 weeks and 4 days. VanMieghem and colleagues concluded that with close fetal surveillance the risk of stillbirth is minimized, as well as the risk of neonatal death or serious neonatal complication by delivery at 33 weeks of gestation. Heyborne and colleagues, based on the results of their review, felt that the optimal time for delivery was probably somewhere between 34 and 36 weeks of gestation.[15] Taken together,

14. VanMieghem T, DeHaus R, Lewi L, et al. Prenatal management of monoamniotic twin pregnancies. Obstetrics & Gynecology 2014; 124:498–506.
15. Heyborne KD, Porreco RP, Garite TJ, Phair K, Abril D; the Obstetrix/Pediatrix Research Study Group. Improved perinatal survival of monoamniotic twins with intensive inpatient monitoring. American Journal of Obstetrics & Gynecology 2005; 192:96–101.

these investigations suggest that the optimal time for delivery for intensively managed monoamniotic twins would be between 33 and 34 weeks of pregnancy.

In my view, the management of monoamniotic/monochorionic twins requires an accurate diagnosis and thorough consultation with the patient regarding the risks and possible interventions to reduce them. Ultrasonography to rule out fetal anomalies, and particularly fetal cardiac anomalies, is essential. Optimal outcomes appear to be achieved with inpatient admission between 24 and 28 weeks of gestation, followed by betamethasone administration for fetal lung maturity, NICU consultation, and electronic fetal monitoring three times per day. The optimal timing of delivery is believed to be between 33 and 34 weeks of gestation, with delivery by elective cesarean.

TWIN-TWIN TRANSFUSION SYNDROME (TTTS)

Twin-twin transfusion syndrome (TTTS) is probably the most common complication in monochorionic twin pregnancies. It is caused by intraplacental arteriovenous shunts that are uncompensated and cause preferential blood flow. This results in one twin being an overall "arterial donor" while the co-twin is an overall "venous recipient." Unbalanced vascular communications are present in many monochorionic placentas, and as many as 15 to 30 percent of monochorionic twins have clinical evidence of some degree of TTTS.

The risk associated with TTTS is determined in large part by how early it is detected. If TTTS is diagnosed in the second trimester and is untreated, the loss rate for both twins approaches 100 percent.[16] TTTS accounts for 15 to 20 percent of all perinatal mortality in twin gestations, and for 50 percent of the perinatal mortality in monochorionic twins.

In the classic model, an artery from the donor twin flows to a portion of the shared placenta, which is drained by a vein to the recipient twin through a large placental arteriovenous anastomosis. The model is further complicated by the fact that numerous anastomoses are the rule rather than the exception in monochorionic placentas. Vascular anastomoses can be superficial or deep, and can be artery-to-artery, vein-to-vein, or arteriovenous. As opposed to what may be intuitive, the placentas of women with twin-twin transfusion syndrome actually have significantly fewer vascular anastomoses overall and a particular reduction in the number of artery-to-artery anastomoses. When anastomoses are present, they are more likely to be deeper and unidirectional compared with monochorionic placentas from unaffected pregnan-

---

16. Berghella V, Kaufmann M. Natural history of twin-twin transfusion syndrome without intervention. Journal of Perinatal Medicine 2001; 46:480–4.

cies. In normal monochorionic placentas, the greater number of anastomoses and much higher percentage of artery-to-artery anastomoses serve to restore the balance of bidirectional flow.

The arterial twin donor experiences anemia, hypovolemia, hypotension, and growth restriction. The anemia and hypovolemia reduce renal blood flow, causing a reduction in fetal urination. The low urinary output results in oligohydramnios, which can cause the amniotic membranes to lie in close apposition to the smaller fetus. The enveloping membrane restricts the donor fetus to the side of the uterine wall, causing what is referred to as a *stuck twin*. The stuck twin often appears to defy gravity and is sometimes misidentified as a monoamniotic twin. The organs of the donor twin are proportionately smaller, and the fetus may sustain ischemic injury involving the brain, kidneys, or intestines due to poor blood flow.

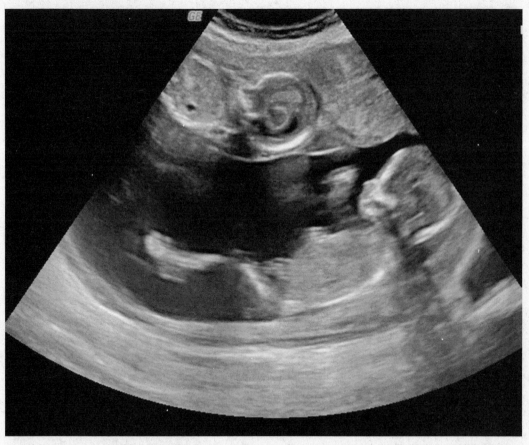

Diamniotic, monochorionic twin gestation with twin-twin transfusion syndrome. This ultrasound reveals a severe stuck twin *phenomenon where the visibly smaller Twin B is stuck against the anterior wall of the uterus by closely adherent amniotic membranes (visible surrounding Twin B). The amniotic fluid is significantly reduced around Twin B (oligohydramnios) and increased around Twin A (polyhydramnios).*

The venous twin recipient has hypervolemia, and this increased circulating blood volume leads to polyhydramnios because of increased renal blood flow and urination. The increased blood volume can also be hyperviscous, predisposing the recipient twin to thrombosis. The increased blood volume creates a strain on the heart of the recipient twin and can potentially result in cardiac hypertrophy, tricuspid insufficiency, and a high-output congestive heart failure, resulting in fetal hydrops (ascites, effusions, and skin edema). The polyhydramnios of the venous twin recipient can also cause other complications such as premature labor and premature rupture of the membranes.

Twin-twin transfusion syndrome is diagnosed according to the following ultrasonographic criteria:

1. A single placenta.
2. Polyhydramnios in one sac and oligohydramnios in the other (polyhydramnios is defined by a deepest vertical pocket of >8 cm, and oligohydramnios is defined by a deepest vertical pocket of <2 cm).
3. Twins of the same sex.
4. Possibly discordant for fetal size and placental echogenicity.
5. Recipient twin with persistently enlarged bladder.
6. Donor twin with a small or nonvisible bladder.

The prenatal diagnosis of TTTS is often presumptive. The most common competing diagnosis is intrauterine growth restriction that affects only one of the fetuses as a consequence of a placental factor or an abnormal umbilical cord insertion onto the placenta. This situation is often referred to as *selective IUGR* (sIUGR) and can usually be differentiated from TTTS by the absence of any differences in the amniotic fluid sacs and differences in umbilical artery Doppler studies.[17] Outcomes with sIUGR will be similar to those with singleton growth restriction and will vary with the severity of the growth restriction and abnormality of the Doppler flow studies.[18]

17. Gratacos E, Lewi L, Munoz B, et al. A classification system for selective intrauterine growth restriction in monochorionic pregnancies according to umbilical artery Doppler flow in the smaller twin. Ultrasound in Obstetrics & Gynecology 2007; 30:28–34.
18. Ishii K, Murakoshi T, Takahashi Y, et al. Perinatal outcomes of monochorionic twins with selective intrauterine growth restriction and different types of umbilical artery Doppler under expectant management. Fetal Diagnosis and Therapy 2009; 26:157–61.

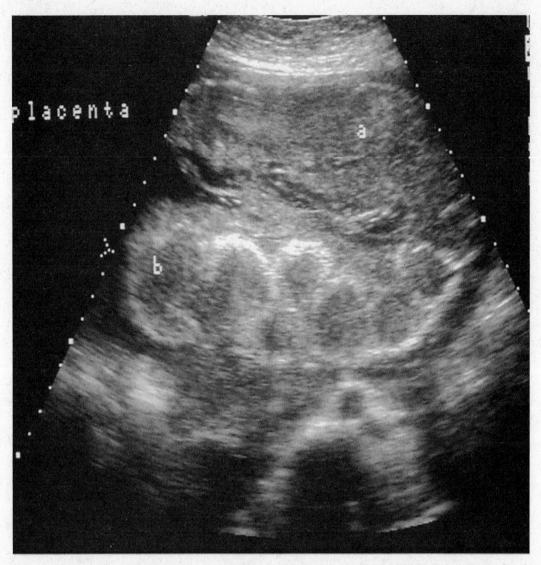

Diamniotic, dichorionic (di/di) twin gestation with selective intrauterine growth restriction (sIUGR) of Twin B. The ultrasound reveals the normal-appearing anterior placenta of Twin A and the heavily calcified placenta of a growth-restricted Twin B.

Even visualization of what appears to be a stuck twin is not definitive for a diagnosis of TTTS. A similar finding can be caused by a structural fetal abnormality such as renal agenesis, which results in an absence of amniotic fluid around the affected twin. Ruptured membranes and umbilical cord abnormalities such as velamentous insertion are other diagnostic possibilities to be considered.

One way to categorize TTTS is as mild, moderate, or severe on the basis of anticipated outcome. Severe TTTS is usually identified before 20 weeks' gestation and is frequently associated with severe polyhydramnios with one twin, along with a stuck co-twin. Without intervention, delivery usually occurs before 30 weeks' gestation due to either premature labor or premature rupture of the membranes. Fetal and/or neonatal mortality approaches 90 to 100 percent. In moderate TTTS, the diagnosis is usually made after 20 weeks, in the late second or early third trimester. Without intervention, the mortality rate for moderate TTTS ranges between 50 and 70 percent. Mild TTTS is the most benign. The diagnosis is usually made in the third trimester based on discrepant fetal weights and amniotic fluid volumes. The anticipated outcome of mild TTTS is reasonably good, similar to that of other twin pregnancies with selective growth restriction.

Because of the severity of early onset TTTS and the frequent rapid progression of the disorder, it is now recommended that monochorionic twins undergo ultrasound scanning every 2 weeks after 16 weeks of gestation. Growth assessments can continue to be performed every 4 weeks. However, every 2 weeks, the deepest vertical pocket of amniotic fluid in each sac should be measured, the presence or absence of fetal bladders in each twin assessed, umbilical artery Doppler studies performed to evaluate for placental dysfunction, and middle cerebral artery (MCA) peak systolic flow velocities performed to identify fetal anemia in the donor twin.[19]

If the diagnostic criteria for TTTS are identified, then staging should be performed using the Quintero criteria:[20]

- *Stage I:* Oligohydramnios (<2 cm) in one amniotic sac with polyhydramnios (>8 cm) in the other.
- *Stage II:* Discordant fluid volume as above and no bladder identified in the donor twin.
- *Stage III:* Abnormal Doppler studies. Absent or reversed blood flow in the umbilical artery or ductus venosus and pulsatile flow in the umbilical vein.
- *Stage IV:* Hydrops in one or both fetuses.
- *Stage V:* One or both fetuses have died.

The current Quintero classification system does not include an evaluation of fetal cardiac function. Other investigators have identified multiple abnormal cardiac findings particularly in the recipient twin, including ventricular hypertrophy, moderate to severe tricuspid regurgi-

---

19. American Congress of Obstetricians and Gynecologists (ACOG). Practice bulletin no. 144: Multifetal gestations: twin, triplet and higher order multifetal pregnancies. Obstetrics & Gynecology 2014; 123:1118–32.
20. Quintero RA, Morales WJ, Allen MH, et al. Staging of twin-twin transfusion syndrome. Journal of Perinatology 1999; 19:550–7.

tation, and ventricular systolic dysfunction.[21] Some investigators believe that an assessment of cardiac findings should be integrated into the Quintero criteria. While these are almost certainly important prognostic findings, there are insufficient data at the present time to recommend either revising or abandoning the Quintero staging criteria.

It is now well accepted that placental laser photocoagulation is considered the standard of care for those patients with Stage II–IV TTTS between 16 and 26 weeks of gestation.[22] At present, the use of intrauterine laser for TTTS is restricted to this gestational age window by the FDA. (Perinatal centers that specialize in fetoscopic laser therapy can be found on the website of the Twin-to-Twin Transfusion Syndrome Foundation at www.tttsfoundation.org.) With this technique, a fetoscopic laser is used to identify and ablate the vascular communication between the two fetuses. Studies are ongoing to determine whether laser photocoagulation offers a benefit to those cases with Stage I disease.

Laser photocoagulation should not be considered a panacea, however. Overall survival is about 65 percent; survival of both fetuses occurs in only about 50 to 60 percent of pregnancies, while survival of at least one fetus occurs in 80 to 90 percent of cases.[23] The survival rate is slightly better overall for the recipient twin compared to the donor. Later evidence of neurodevelopmental impairment is found in 10 to 20 percent of surviving twins, with a cerebral palsy rate of approximately 5 percent. Intact survival rates are higher for Stage I and II disease compared to Stage III and IV.

An alternative therapy for TTTS is large-volume reduction amniocentesis to remove fluid from the polyhydramniotic sac. However, it is clear that for Quintero Stage II–IV TTTS, laser photocoagulation results in superior outcomes compared to amnioreduction. The risk of dual death is reduced by about 67 percent, the risk of death of either twin is reduced by about 30 percent, the risk of neonatal death is reduced by about 71 percent, and the likelihood of being neurologically intact at six months of age is improved by 66 percent.[24, 25] At this point in time, amnioreduction is usually reserved for those cases beyond 26 weeks of gestation (when laser

21. Rychik J, Tian Z, Bebbington M, et al. The twin-twin transfusion syndrome: Spectrum of cardiovascular abnormality and development of a cardiovascular score to assess severity of disease. American Journal of Obstetrics & Gynecology 2007; 197:392 e1–e8.

22. Roberts D, Neilson JP, Kilby MD, Gates S. Interventions for the treatment of twin-twin transfusion syndrome. Cochrane Database of Systematic Reviews 2014; Jan 30; 1:CD002073.

23. Roberts D, Neilson JP, Kilby MD, Gates S. Interventions for the treatment of twin-twin transfusion syndrome. Cochrane Database of Systematic Reviews 2014; Jan 30; 1:CD002073.

24. Rossi AC, Vandrbilt D, Chamit RH. Neurodevelopmental outcomes after laser therapy for twin-twin transfusion syndrome. Obstetrics & Gynecology 2011; 118:1145–50.

25. Salomon LJ, Örtqvist L, Aegerter P, et al. Long-term developmental followup of infants who participated in a RCT of amniocentesis vs. laser photo coagulation for treatment of TTTS. American Journal of Obstetrics & Gynecology 2010; 203:444–51.

photocoagulation is not approved in the United States) with severe polyhydramnios, maternal respiratory difficulty, or preterm cervical shortening. It is also indicated for those cases with a stuck twin if the option for laser photocoagulation has passed. When performed, the average volume of amniotic fluid removed is between 1,500 and 2,000 ccs. The goal of amnioreduction is restitution of a normal amniotic fluid volume (deepest vertical pocket <8 cm) in the amniotic sac of the recipient twin.

Potential complications exist for both procedures. Laser photocoagulation involves the placement of a relatively large catheter through the uterine wall and into the amniotic sac to allow placement of the fetoscopic laser. This procedure is associated with perioperative rupture of the membranes in 15 to 30 percent of cases, leakage of amniotic fluid into the maternal abdomen in 7 percent of cases, placental abruption in 2 percent, intrauterine infection in 2 percent, and vaginal bleeding in 4 percent. Alternatively, amnioreductions have been associated with a complication rate of about 1.5 percent per procedure, with the complications being distributed between premature rupture of the membranes, abruption of the placenta, and intra-amniotic infection.

Another potential treatment option is that of septostomy, in which amniocentesis is performed to create holes in the membrane between the fetuses, allowing the amniotic fluid volumes to equalize. The donor fetus is then able to swallow the amniotic fluid, potentially correcting the hypovolemic state and increasing urine production. Unfortunately, this procedure does nothing to correct the underlying intraplacental shunts, and survival rates have not been substantially improved.[26] There also continues to be a relatively high rate of neurodevelopmental compromise in the surviving fetuses. Furthermore, there is a theoretical disadvantage to the procedure, which is the creation of monoamnionicity with resultant cord entanglement. Selective multifetal reduction has been described but is limited as an option because of the inevitable loss of the first twin. If selective reduction is performed, it must be by occlusion of that twin's umbilical cord in order to prevent subsequent acute injury to the surviving twin.

The long-term outcome among survivors needs more study. Concerns have been expressed over the possibility of ischemic brain injury to the donor twins and cardiomyopathy among surviving recipient twins. Neonatal hypertension has also been associated with TTTS especially in recipient twins. In addition, questions exist about the effect of this syndrome on hypertension late in childhood and adulthood.

---

26. Moise KJ, Dorman K, Lamvu G, et al. A randomized trial of amnioreduction versus septostomy in the treatment of twin-twin transfusion syndrome. American Journal of Obstetrics & Gynecology 2005; 193:701–7.

Twin Anemia-Polycythemia Sequence (TAPS)

Twin anemia-polycythemia sequence (TAPS) refers to the occurrence of a chronic and severe hemoglobin difference in a monozygotic/monochorionic twin pair in the absence of other criteria for TTTS. The diagnosis is made by an MCA peak systolic flow ≥1.5 multiple of the median (MoM) in one twin and a peak systolic flow MoM ≤1.0 in the co-twin. These changes are seen without the differences in amniotic fluid volumes that would meet the TTTS criteria. Postnatally, the criteria for anemia and polycythemia are an intertwin hemoglobin difference of at least 8.0 g/dl—that is, an anemic (donor) twin with a birth hemoglobin of 9 g/dl and a polycythemic (recipient) twin with a birth hemoglobin of 17 g/dl or greater. Isolated TAPS can occur spontaneously in monochorionic pregnancies. However, its reported frequency is much higher following laser photocoagulation for TTTS. The incidence of postlaser TAPS has been reported to be between 10 and 15 percent of cases.

TAPS is believed to be caused by the presence of only a few, very small arteriovenous anastomoses, allowing for a slow transfusion of blood from the donor to the recipient. The most common clinical scenario for TAPS occurs following laser photocoagulation where most, but not all, of the arteriovenous anastomoses have been ablated. As with TTTS, artery-to-artery anastomoses are believed to be important in equilibrating the blood flow between twins. Artery-to-artery anastomoses are seen in over 80 percent of uncomplicated monochorionic gestations. In contrast, these same artery-to-artery anastomoses are found in only about 25 percent of TTTS pregnancies and are even more rare (10 percent) in pregnancies complicated by TAPS. Because of the possibility of TAPS, an MCA peak systolic flow velocity should be included in the screening of all monochorionic gestations.

The ideal management of TAPS has not been defined. Both intrauterine transfusions and laser photocoagulation have been reported to be successful. Expectant management, however, may also be a reasonable option. Survival rates for twins complicated by TAPS, regardless of management, have been reported to range from 75 to 100 percent. The in utero interventions described previously have not been proven to be associated with either differences in survival or long-term outcomes.[27, 28]

27. Baschat AA, Oepkes B. Twin anemia-polycythemia sequence in monochorionic twins: Implications for diagnosis and management. American Journal of Perinatology 2014; 31:25–30.
28. Slaghekke F, Kist WJ, Oepkes D, et al. Twin anemia-polycythemia sequence: Diagnostic criteria, classification, perinatal management, and outcome. Fetal Diagnosis and Therapy 2010; 27: 181–90.

Intrauterine Fetal Death of One Twin: Acute Intertwin Transfusion

Acute intertwin transfusion occurs in monochorionic twin gestations after the intrauterine death of one of the twin pair. Excluding first-trimester losses, intrauterine demise of one fetus occurs in 2 to 5 percent of twin gestations and 14 to 17 percent of triplet gestations. The risk of second- and third-trimester fetal loss is several-fold higher for monochorionic twins than for dichorionic twins. In twin pregnancies complicated by the demise of one twin, intrauterine death of the co-twin occurs in 12 to 15 percent of monochorionic gestations but only 3 to 4 percent of dichorionic gestations.[29, 30] It is believed that the majority of these in utero deaths are the result of an acute transfusion of blood from the surviving twin into the circulation of the demised co-twin. This exsanguination into the circulation of the demised co-twin results in severe hypotension and possible ischemic injury to the survivor. In addition to the risk of fetal death, there is also a significant risk of prematurity, which probably reflects not only compromised fetal condition but also clinician concern for the surviving fetus.

Surviving co-twins of pregnancies complicated by a single IUFD are at risk for brain injury associated with the acute intertwin transfusion. In various prospective studies, 5 to 25 percent of surviving twins have evidence of ischemic brain injury. Most reported cases of fetal demise or neurologic injury have involved a third-trimester fetal death in utero. However, neurologic deficit in the surviving twin has been reported with demise of the co-twin as early as the beginning of the second trimester. An analysis of multiple studies reported on the rate of abnormal, postnatal (within four weeks of delivery) cranial imaging after a single fetal death. Abnormal cranial imaging was found in 34 percent of surviving monochorionic twins compared with only 16 percent for dichorionic twins. Later neurodevelopmental impairment following a single fetal death was found in 26 percent of the monochorionic twin survivors versus only 2 percent of the surviving dichorionic twins.[31]

Multicystic encephalomalacia is believed to be the precursor to infant and childhood cerebral impairment in most cases. This disorder results in cystic lesions within the cerebral white matter, distributed in areas supplied by the anterior and middle cerebral arteries, and is usually associated with profound neurologic handicap. It is difficult to predict which surviving

---

29. Ong S, Zamora J, Khan K, Kilby M. Prognosis for the co-twin following single-twin death: A systematic review. British Journal of Obstetrics and Gynaecology 2006; 113:992–8.
30. Hillman SC, Morris RK, Kilby MD. Co-twin prognosis after single fetal death: A systematic review and meta-analysis. Obstetrics & Gynecology 2011; 118:928–40.
31. Ibid.

monochorionic twin will develop brain injury. Ultrasound examination of the fetal brain may be suggestive of multicystic encephalomalacia, but it is not always definitive. Antenatal MRI of the fetal brain may be more useful in detecting encephalomalacia in utero.

We offer MRI to all women with monochorionic placentas approximately three weeks after the demise of one twin has been detected. Although it is unlikely that a normal MRI definitively rules out brain abnormalities, it is certainly a positive prognostic finding. On the other hand, detection of multicystic lesions would be predictive of a high rate of severe neurologic impairment. In addition to brain injury, a variety of other organ systems can be adversely affected in the surviving twin. These abnormalities may include ischemic bowel lesions, intestinal atresia, renal necrosis, and cystic renal dysplasia.

Two theories exist to explain the ischemic injury identified in the surviving monochorionic co-twin. The first theory is that the deceased fetus and its placenta produce thromboplastic substances that traverse the vascular communications between the twins, causing embolic infarcts in the survivor. This first theory is the older one and there is virtually no pathologic or physiologic evidence to support it. The second and more widely accepted hypothesis is that significant hypotension occurs at the time of the demise of the co-twin. After death of the first twin, the resulting low pressure in that twin's circulatory system results in blood from the survivor rapidly back-bleeding into the demised fetus. If the resulting hypotension is severe, the surviving twin is at risk for both demise and ischemic damage to vital organs. The brain is particularly at risk because of its high oxygen requirements. It should be stressed that since the injury is coexistent with the co-twin demise, rapid delivery of the surviving infant following a single IUFD will not improve outcome.

Pregnancy management after one fetus has died in utero depends on gestational age, chorionicity, maternal status, and the status of the surviving fetus. Knowledge of chorionicity is essential because the sequelae of acute intertwin transfusion depend on placental anastomoses that occur only in monochorionic twins. If expectant management is undertaken, close surveillance of the surviving fetus is required. Probably the greatest risk to the surviving twin is premature birth. In the presence of a single intrauterine fetal demise, referral to a tertiary care perinatal unit would be advisable. Serial ultrasonographic assessment of the surviving co-twin's growth is suggested, as is antenatal testing.

The 2011 joint publication of the National Institutes of Child Health and Human Development and the Society for Maternal-Fetal Medicine addressed the timing of indicated late preterm and early term birth following a single IUFD in a twin pregnancy.[32] If the IUFD

---

32. Spong CY, Mercer BM, D'Alton M, Kilpatrick S, Blackwell S, Saade G. Timing of indicated late preterm and early term birth. Obstetrics & Gynecology 2011; 118:323–33.

occurs at 34 weeks or beyond, delivery should be considered. A 2014 practice bulletin on multifetal gestations by the American Congress of Obstetricians and Gynecologists gave a similar recommendation stating that, in the absence of other indications, a single IUFD in a twin pregnancy less than 34 weeks should not prompt immediate delivery.[33] Vaginal delivery is not contraindicated, and cesarean delivery should be reserved for usual obstetric indications. The pregnancy history should be communicated to the pediatrician caring for the surviving co-twin because of the possibility of in utero vital organ injury.

In monochorionic pregnancies, an impending intrauterine fetal death is a much more complicated management issue. An impending IUFD of one fetus at a gestational age at which high survivability of the other twin can be presumed would justify immediate delivery. As a generalization, this would be about 34 weeks for a twin pregnancy. Delivery of twins between 30 and 34 weeks' gestation would be associated with a very high survival rate in most Level III centers, but would expose the newborns to the morbidity associated with iatrogenic prematurity. However, the morbidity expected as a consequence of delivery between 30 and 34 weeks' gestation appears to be less than that anticipated from a fetal demise and potential acute intertwin transfusion. For those multiples less than 30 weeks' gestation, the decision regarding delivery should be based on the anticipated neonatal outcome for the fetus in that particular hospital and whether or not it is superior to the anticipated sequelae of acute intertwin transfusion (approximately 25 percent fetal mortality and as high as a 25 percent risk of ischemic injury among survivors). If the risks of delivery are believed to be greater than the risk of acute intertwin transfusion, expectant management should be chosen.

Another alternative to consider when confronting a previable gestation with an impending demise of one twin is selective multifetal reduction. Intrauterine endoscopic occlusion of the umbilical cord of the compromised fetus has been successfully performed. Ligating the umbilical cord of the compromised fetus would prevent acute intertwin transfusion and the risk of demise or ischemic injury to the co-twin.

The final concern associated with intrauterine fetal demise of one twin is the possibility of a maternal consumptive coagulopathy. It has been previously estimated that there is an approximate 25 percent incidence of maternal disseminated intravascular coagulation abnormality when a single fetal demise occurs in a multiple gestation and that fetus is retained for at least four weeks. However, subsequent reviews have demonstrated that maternal coagulopathy has only rarely been reported. The 25 percent incidence seems to be a marked overestimation. Although uncommon, if expectant management is undertaken after intrauterine fetal demise, a

---

33. American Congress of Obstetricians and Gynecologists (ACOG). Practice bulletin no.144: Multifetal gestations: Twin, triplet and higher order multifetal pregnancies. Obstetrics & Gynecology 2014; 123:1118–32.

baseline maternal coagulation profile is recommended and follow-up testing performed only if maternal hemorrhagic symptoms develop. If a coagulopathy is detected, treatment with heparin has been reported to reverse the coagulation abnormality. Subsequent delivery after a remote intrauterine fetal demise of one twin should probably include a consideration of maternal coagulation status prior to delivery.

Assessing the Risk for Preterm Birth

Some multiples are delivered preterm because it is medically indicated—due to growth restriction, severe preeclampsia, twin-twin transfusion syndrome, and so on. However, approximately 70 percent of preterm births of multiples are spontaneous, resulting from either early rupture of the membranes or the early onset of labor. Most experts believe that uterine overdistension plays the greatest role in the etiology of preterm birth among multiples, although poor growth of one or more infants accounts for a substantial proportion as well.[34] The average gestational age at delivery decreases as the fetal number increases: 35.4 weeks of gestation for twins, 31.8 weeks of gestation for triplets, and 29.7 weeks of gestation for quadruplets. The increasing stretch on the uterine wall causes a number of biochemical and physiologic changes. These changes result in both an increased synchronization of uterine contractions as well as inflammatory changes in the cervix and fetal membranes, all contributing to a premature onset of the delivery process.

In vitro fertilization may be an independent risk factor for the early preterm delivery of multiples compared with those spontaneously conceived. Multifetal pregnancy reduction does not completely eliminate these risks, since it appears that there is a small increase in the rate of preterm delivery in higher-order multiples reduced to twins, compared with unreduced twins conceived using assisted reproductive technologies.

Far and away, the best screening test for the risk of preterm birth in a multiple gestation is a mid-trimester transvaginal cervical length measurement. A mid-trimester cervical length of <25 mm has been demonstrated to be the best predictor of preterm birth <32 weeks, <35 weeks, and <37 weeks—better than maternal history, digital cervical examination, the presence or absence of contractions, the fetal fibronectin test, or any other potential markers.[35] For instance, compared to a longer cervical measurement, a cervical length of <25 mm at 24 weeks' gestation in a multiple gestation is associated with an eightfold increased risk for delivery <35

---

34. Hediger ML, Luke B, Gonzalez-Quintero VH, Witter FR, Mauldin J, Newman RB. Fetal growth rates and very preterm birth of twins. American Journal of Obstetrics & Gynecology 2005; 193:1498–507.

35. Goldenberg RL, et al. The Preterm Prediction Study: The value of new versus standard risk factors in predicting early and all spontaneous preterm birth. American Journal of Public Health 1998; 88:233–8.

weeks. The risk of preterm birth increases markedly as the cervical length becomes shorter; risk also increases the earlier in gestation that the shortening of the cervix occurs. Among women carrying twins, those with a transvaginal cervical length of <10 mm at 23 weeks' gestation have a 60 to 70 percent risk of a spontaneous preterm birth <32 weeks' gestation.[36] Risk goes up to approximately 80 percent if cervical length is <10 mm by 16 to 20 weeks' gestation.

At MUSC, we routinely perform a transvaginal cervical length (TVCL) measurement on all patients carrying twins, triplets, or higher-order multiples during their routine ultrasound examinations between 18 and 24 weeks' gestation. A midtrimester TVCL >35 mm has been associated with only a 3 percent risk of spontaneous preterm birth <34 weeks' gestation.[37] Identifying a mid-trimester TVCL >35 mm provides significant reassurance to the patient—and allows for the avoidance of unnecessary limitations on activity, travel, work, or sexual relations.

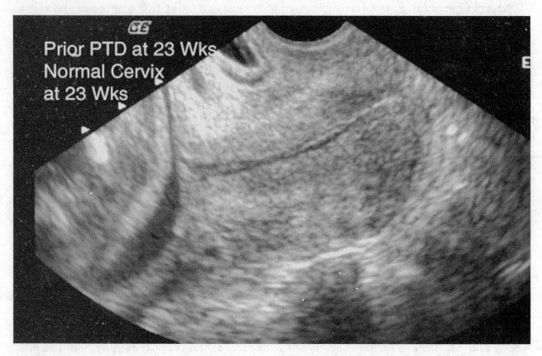

A normally long and closed cervix at 23 weeks' gestation by transvaginal ultrasound. This finding would be associated with a very low risk of spontaneous preterm birth.

36. Souka AP, Heath V, Flint S, et al. Cervical length at 23 weeks in twins in predicting spontaneous preterm delivery. Obstetrics & Gynecology 1999; 94:450–4.

37. Imseis HM, Albert TA, Iams JD. Identifying twin gestations at low risk for preterm birth with a transvaginal ultrasonographic cervical measurement at 24–26 weeks gestation. American Journal of Obstetrics & Gynecology 1997; 177:1149–55.

Alternatively, a shortened mid-trimester TVCL of <25 mm is known to correlate strongly with an increased risk of early preterm delivery in multiples.

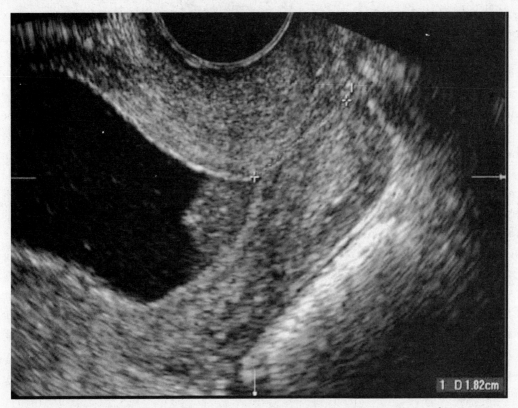

A remarkably short cervical length of less than 20 mm with pronounced funneling. There is also the presence of some sludge in the lower uterine segment, which further increases the risk of early preterm birth.

When a short cervix of <25 mm is identified in a multiple gestation, the management options are limited. Many obstetricians are of the opinion that there are no effective therapies to prevent preterm birth in twins or triplets. However, we disagree with that opinion. We believe there are several things that may help prolong the pregnancy. While the evidence supporting these interventions is not definitive, there are reasons to be optimistic about their chances for success. In the meantime, large multicentered trials are ongoing to better assess the effectiveness of most of these recommendations.

Reduced activity and increased rest are probably the most commonly prescribed interventions for multiple gestations. In the past, prescribing hospitalized bedrest at 26 weeks of gestation was a common treatment to help prevent preterm birth for twins and triplets. A meta-analysis of five randomized trials involving twins and two randomized trials involving triplets demonstrated that routine hospitalized bedrest did not reduce the risk of premature birth or perinatal mortality. Even when those twins whose mothers experienced dilation and effacement of the cervix were considered separately, there was still no improvement in any outcome.[38]

While hospitalized bedrest is now rarely recommended as a routine intervention for multiples, many providers still endorse restriction of strenuous activity and increased rest in multiples. Justification for this may come from other sources, especially for those multiples at higher risk based on maternal history, a shortened TVCL, or a plurality of triplets or greater. Some doctors say that there is scant evidence that reduced activity or increased rest is of any proven benefit. It should be noted that a recent secondary analysis of a prospective randomized trial of singleton (not multiple) gestations with a shortened cervix receiving progesterone therapy did not identify any benefit from a physician recommendation for home bedrest.[39] This study is limited by the fact that it was a postpartum questionnaire (recall bias) and there was no control for selection bias that would have favored a bedrest recommendation in the highest-risk cases. Indeed, it is disappointing to reflect on how little in medicine is *proven* to be beneficial. This problem is especially acute in obstetrics, where fewer randomized clinical trials are performed.

However, there is a difference between what can be proven in clinical trials and what we know from experience. After 30 years of practicing obstetrics and caring for more than a thousand women pregnant with multiples, I am certain that increased ambulatory activity, increased physical exertion, and increased stress all add to the risk of preterm delivery. Twenty-four-hour uterine monitoring studies have shown that maternal rest is associated with a reduction in uterine contraction frequency. Many studies looking at occupational fatigue have demonstrated a significantly increased risk of adverse pregnancy outcome, including preterm birth, associated with physically demanding work, prolonged standing, shift work, and night work.[40, 41, 42, 43]

38. Crowther CA, Han S. Hospitalization and bed rest for multiple pregnancy. Cochrane Database of Systematic Reviews 2010; 7:CD000110.
39. Grobman WJ, et al. Activity restriction among women with a short cervix. Obstetrics & Gynecology 2013; 121:1181–6.
40. Luke B, Mamelle N, Keith L, Munoz F, Minogue J, Papiernik E, et al. The association between occupational factors and preterm birth: A United States nurses' survey. American Journal of Obstetrics & Gynecology 1995; 173:849–62.
41. Mozurkewich EL, Luke B, Avni M, Wolfe FM. Working conditions and adverse pregnancy outcomes: A meta-analysis. Obstetrics & Gynecology 2000; 95:623–35.
42. Schneider KTM, Bollinger A, Huch A, Huch R. The oscillating "vena cava syndrome" during quiet standing—An unexpected observation in late pregnancy. British Journal of Obstetrics and Gynaecology 1984; 91:766–80.
43. Naeye RL, Peters EC. Working during pregnancy: Effects on the fetus. Pediatrics 1982; 69:724–7.

While these studies addressing occupational fatigue involved singleton gestations, it would be naïve to assume that a similar, if not magnified, effect did not occur in multiples.

After more than a decade of following changes in the cervical length by transvaginal ultrasound, I am convinced that unrestricted activity hastens cervical shortening, and that rest will slow that progression. Because of the frequency with which restriction of activity is advised, further research is needed to better define the effect of restricted activity and increased rest in high-risk mothers carrying multiples. However, in the meantime, we continue to believe that this is a wise and relatively safe intervention to help prolong pregnancy in those multiple gestations complicated by a significantly shortened mid-trimester cervical length.

When confronted with a mid-trimester TVCL <25 mm, another recommendation we make is to initiate treatment with daily vaginal progesterone. Again, the evidence is limited for the efficacy of vaginal progesterone in multiple gestations when a short cervical length is detected. However, a recent meta-analysis of all available prospective randomized trials, including twins, demonstrated a significant reduction of almost 50 percent in a composite of adverse neonatal outcomes and a nonsignificant but notable 30 percent reduction in preterm birth <33 weeks of gestation for those twins treated with vaginal progesterone.[44] A further study of 72 high-risk twin pregnancies with a cervical length at the 10th percentile or less (TVCL ≤30 mm) or with a history of prior preterm birth also showed a statistically nonsignificant but encouraging 37 percent decrease in the rate of preterm birth <34 weeks' gestation among women treated with vaginal progesterone.[45]

Most of these studies have been performed using a 200-mg progesterone vaginal suppository (Prometrium), although a 90-mg progesterone vaginal gel (Crinone) has also been used in some trials. None of the studies performed to date support the use of progesterone in unselected uncomplicated twins. Larger studies are currently ongoing to better assess the efficacy and benefits of vaginal progesterone among women with multiple gestations and shortened cervical length. A regimen of weekly injections of 17-alpha hydroxyprogesterone caproate (17P; 250 mg IM) between 16 and 36 weeks' gestation has been shown to reduce the risk of recurrent preterm birth among women with singleton gestations and a prior preterm delivery.[46] Conversely, based on multiple well-designed trials, there is no evidence that the prophylactic

44. Romero R, Nicolaides K, Aqudelo A, et al. Vaginal progesterone in women with an asymptomatic sonographic short cervix in the midtrimester decreases preterm delivery and neonatal morbidity: A systematic review and meta-analysis of individual patient data. American Journal of Obstetrics & Gynecology 2012; 206:124–39.

45. Klein K, Rode L, Nicolaides KH, et al. Vaginal micronized progesterone and risk of preterm delivery in high-risk twin pregnancies: Secondary analysis of a placebo-controlled randomized trial and meta-analysis. Ultrasound in Obstetrics and Gynecology 2011; 38:281–7.

46. Meis PJ, et al. Weekly 17-alpha hydroxyprogesterone for the prevention of recurrent preterm birth. New England Journal of Medicine 2003; 348:2379–85.

use of 17P is effective in preventing preterm birth in either twin or triplet gestations.[47, 48] The administration of 17P in a randomized fashion to unselected twin gestations, as well as to twin gestations with identified shortening of the cervical length, did not decrease the risk of spontaneous preterm delivery. In a recent study involving 165 twin pregnancies between 24 and 32 weeks of gestation whose mothers were identified as having a cervical length <25 mm, participants were randomized to 17P or placebo. The women also received a higher dose of 17P (500 mg twice weekly) due to concerns that women carrying twins might need a higher dose of medication. Unfortunately, no benefit to the therapy was seen. In fact, there was a significant increase in the rate of delivery <32 weeks of gestation in the 17P group compared to the group who received a placebo.[49]

Attempts have also been made to use oral beta mimetic tocolytics to prophylactically reduce the risk of preterm delivery. None of the published randomized trials involving these oral tocolytic agents demonstrated benefits when used in an unselected population of multiple gestations. Recently the U.S. Food and Drug Administration has warned against the use of terbutaline (the most popular beta mimetic tocolytic in the United States) during pregnancy in either the oral or the injectable form due to concerns over maternal cardiovascular complications and potential fetal effects. We no longer use oral or subcutaneous terbutaline for prophylaxis or long-term tocolytic therapy.

In the case of acute preterm labor, antenatal corticosteroids are administered to reduce the incidence of respiratory distress syndrome, intraventricular hemorrhage, and other complications of prematurity. The National Institutes of Health recommends administration of corticosteroids with preterm labor <34 weeks, and to women with preterm rupture of the membranes <30 to 32 weeks, regardless of plurality.[50]

An NIH-sponsored study identified a benefit associated with cerclage placement for women with a singleton gestation complicated by prior preterm birth and with a mid-trimester TVCL <25 mm.[51] This benefit was even greater if the TVCL was <15 mm. Cerclages

47. Rouse DJ, Caritis SN, Peaceman AM, et al. A trial of 17 alpha hydroxyprogesterone caproate to prevent prematurity in twins. New England Journal of Medicine 2007; 357:454–61.

48. Combs CA, et al. Failure of 17-hydroxyprogesterone to reduce neonatal morbidity or prolonged triplet pregnancy: A double blind randomized clinical trial. American Journal of Obstetrics & Gynecology 2010; 203:248 e1–e9.

49. Rouse DJ, Caritis SN, Peacemean AM, et al. A trial of 17 alpha-hydroxyprogesterone caproate to prevent prematurity in twins. New England Journal of Medicine 2007; 357:454–61.

50. Antenatal Corticosteroids Revisited: Repeat Courses. 2000. NIH Consensus Statement August 17–18; 17(2):1–18.

51. Owens J, et al. Multicentered randomized trial of cerclage for preterm birth prevention in high risk women with a shortened midtrimester cervical length. American Journal of Obstetrics & Gynecology 2009; 201:375.

have been shown to be beneficial in singleton pregnancies with a history of multiple prior mid-trimester losses consistent with a diagnosis of cervical insufficiency (CI). A woman with a twin or triplet gestation with the same history suggestive of CI would remain a candidate for a surgical cerclage.

Unfortunately, an ultrasound-indicated cerclage to prevent preterm birth in the face of a TVCL <25 mm has not been demonstrated to be of benefit in twin gestations. An analysis of all the available randomized trials of ultrasound-indicated cerclage placement in twin gestations demonstrated that the risks of preterm birth and perinatal mortality were actually increased in the cerclage group.[52] Similar findings have been found in smaller studies involving triplet gestations.[53] We restrict our use of cerclage to those twin gestations with either a classic history-based indication of cervical insufficiency or a physical exam–based indication, which is usually a significantly shortened and dilated cervix at a previable gestation that has failed both bedrest and vaginal progesterone.

There has been a recent resurgence of interest in the use of the vaginal pessary to reduce the risk of preterm birth in multiple gestations. The exact mechanism by which a cervical pessary may generate a beneficial effect is unknown. Some experts believe that pessaries may relieve direct pressure on the internal cervical os and redistribute the weight of the pregnancy onto the vaginal floor. Others believe that the pessary may compress the cervical canal, preventing loss of the cervical mucous plug, which plays a role in preventing ascending infection and the resultant inflammatory response.

A large study performed in 40 hospitals in the Netherlands recruited over 800 women pregnant with twins to a randomized trial of either the Arabin pessary (*n* = 401) or a standard care group (*n* = 407).[54] There was no difference in a composite of poor perinatal outcome between the two groups. However, among those multiple gestations with a cervical length at or below the 25th percentile (38 mm), the findings were more favorable. Both maternal and newborn outcomes were significantly improved in the subgroup of twin gestations in which mothers had a short cervix and also received a pessary. In addition, in the pessary group, the gestational age at delivery was significantly greater, and there was a lower risk of delivering <28 and <32 weeks of gestation. While the cervical pessary did not effectively prevent poor

52. Berghella V, et al. Cerclage for short cervix on ultrasonography: A meta-analysis of trials using individual patient level data. Obstetrics & Gynecology 2005; 106:181–9.
53. Rebarber A, et al. Prophylactic cerclage in the management of triplet pregnancies. American Journal of Obstetrics & Gynecology 2005; 193:1193–6.
54. Liem S, Schuit E, Hegeman M, et al. Cervical pessaries for the prevention of preterm birth in women with a multiple pregnancy (ProTwin): A multi-centre open label randomized controlled trial. Lancet 2013; 382:1341–9.

perinatal outcome or preterm birth among unselected twin gestations, it did seem to offer some benefit to those women with a shortened TVCL.

These promising findings with the use of a pessary in twins with a shortened mid-trimester cervical length need to be confirmed in future prospective trials. However, we are integrating the use of a pessary into our care of women pregnant with multiples. We are considering its use when the TVCL is significantly shortened and continues to shorten despite maternal rest and the use of vaginal progesterone.

Last, it should be mentioned that one of the simplest and, for the patient, most personally empowering options to prevent preterm birth is that of improved nutrition. Poor fetal growth in utero is clearly associated with an increase in both spontaneous and indicated preterm delivery. The early onset of restricted fetal growth is strongly associated with dangerous early preterm deliveries. Throughout this book, there is much discussion of the results from observational cohort studies revealing the benefits of a comprehensive nutritional program for multiples in prolonging pregnancy, reducing the risks of preterm birth, and improving infant outcomes. It has been repeatedly demonstrated that optimal maternal nutrition is associated with at least a 1- to 2-week longer duration of gestation in twin gestations, and with a potential for even greater improvement in triplet and higher-order multiple gestations.

Delivery of Multiples: Vaginal or Cesarean?

Several factors must be carefully weighed to best answer the question about the optimal mode of delivery for multiples, as well as the time interval between deliveries.

FETAL PRESENTATION

A primary factor in determining whether a patient pregnant with twins can deliver vaginally or will need a cesarean is fetal presentation. All combinations of intrapartum twin presentations can be classified into three groups: (1) Twin A vertex (also called cephalic)/Twin B vertex; (2) Twin A nonvertex/Twin B either vertex or nonvertex; (3) Twin A vertex/Twin B nonvertex. These presentations are found in approximately 40 percent, 20 percent, and 40 percent of cases, respectively. The current recommendations for each scenario are discussed in turn.

Vertex/vertex twins: A trial of labor and vaginal delivery is appropriate for all vertex-vertex twin gestations, regardless of gestational age or estimated fetal weight. No clear benefit to routine cesarean delivery of vertex-vertex twins has been identified, including for the birth of

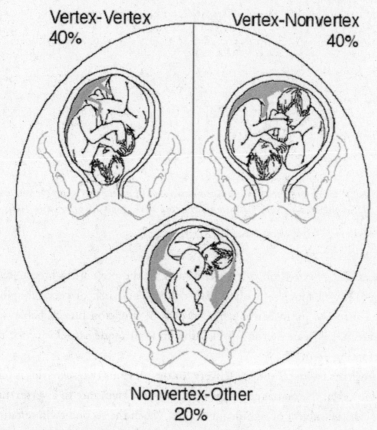

Vertex-Vertex
40%

Vertex-Nonvertex
40%

Nonvertex-Other
20%

Possible combinations of intrapartum twin presentations and the frequency with which they occur.

very-low-birthweight (<1,500 g) twins.[55] However, it's important to note that the presentation of the second twin may change in 5 to 10 percent of cases after delivery of the presenting twin. In most large series of twin births, the frequency of a vaginal delivery of Twin A followed by a cesarean delivery for Twin B is only 2 to 4 percent, which is a lower cesarean risk than for an uncomplicated singleton gestation in labor.

Non-vertex-presenting twin: Twin pregnancies with a non-vertex-presenting twin are nearly always managed by cesarean delivery. Historically, this was because of a fear of interlocking of the chins of a breech first twin and a vertex second twin at the time of delivery. Interlocking fetuses, however, are exceedingly rare.

55. Barrett JFR, Hannah ME, Hutton EK, et al. A randomized trial of planned cesarean or vaginal delivery for twin pregnancy. New England Journal of Medicine 2013; 369:1295–1305.

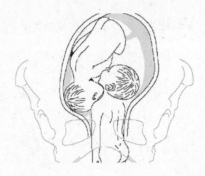

Delivery of a breech-presenting Twin A is interrupted by a cessation of progress when the chin of Twin A becomes interlocked with the chin of the cephalic-presenting Twin B.

More concerning is extension of the fetal head of the presenting breech twin. This extension predisposes to a more difficult breech delivery and risk of cervical spine injury for the first twin. Currently, in an era in which nearly all singleton breech babies are delivered by elective cesarean, cesarean delivery is also the optimal mode of delivery for twins with a non-vertex-presenting Twin A.

Vertex/nonvertex twins: Route of delivery for the previous two scenarios is relatively noncontroversial. However, the management of women whose twins are in a vertex/breech or vertex/transverse lie is the subject of significant debate. When the second twin remains nonvertex after delivery of the first twin, there are two options for vaginal delivery: breech extraction or external cephalic version.

External cephalic version is successful about 60–70 percent of the time and avoids having to deal with a breech delivery. Although external cephalic version is an acceptable strategy, it has been shown to be associated with more failures and delivery complications than primary breech extraction. One study analyzed 136 sets of vertex/nonvertex twins with a birthweight higher than 1,500 g in whom delivery of the second twin was managed by primary cesarean, external cephalic version, or primary breech extraction.[56] No differences were noted in the incidence of neonatal mortality or morbidity among the three delivery modes. However, external version was associated with a higher failure rate than breech extraction due to a higher rate of nonreassuring fetal heart rate patterns, cord prolapse, and compound presentation. The authors

56. Gocke SE, Nageotte MP, Garite T, Towers CV, Dorchester W. Management of the nonvertex second twin: Primary cesarean section, external version or primary breech extraction. American Journal of Obstetrics & Gynecology 1989; 161:111–14.

concluded that primary breech extraction of the second nonvertex twin weighing more than 1,500 g is a reasonable alternative to either cesarean delivery or external version. Therefore, provided that the obstetrician is sufficiently trained in breech extraction and the fetus is of appropriate size, breech extraction is the best option for achievement of a vaginal delivery with a nonvertex second twin.

Some obstetricians have concerns over the safety of breech extraction for the nonvertex second twin and have questioned whether outcomes are equivalent to cesarean delivery. There are many large retrospective series reporting on twin pregnancy outcomes, with some suggesting higher rates of newborn morbidity and mortality associated with breech extraction of the second twin, while others found no difference in outcomes between second twins delivered by breech extraction and by cesarean. Until recently, the only prospective randomized trial of cesarean delivery versus breech extraction for the nonvertex second twin supported the safety of vaginal breech delivery. Rabinovici and associates randomized 66 women with vertex/nonvertex twins of more than 35 weeks' gestation to vaginal delivery with breech extraction or elective cesarean delivery.[57] They found no differences in neonatal outcomes and no cases of either birth trauma or neonatal death. Not surprisingly, maternal fever and hospital length of stay were greater in the cesarean delivery group.

Two other studies on mode of delivery for twins lends further support to the safety of breech extraction for second twins under appropriate circumstances and with experienced obstetricians. Both studies were conducted in single institutions with strict protocols for labor management and immediate breech extraction of the nonvertex second twin. Schmitz and colleagues performed a retrospective study of 758 consecutive twin sets at more than 35 weeks' gestation with a cephalic-presenting Twin A.[58] These investigators found that neonatal morbidity for the second twin did not differ between planned cesarean and planned vaginal delivery. The second, more recent study by Fox and coworkers examined 287 twin pregnancies from an academic medical center.[59] Once again, following a strict labor management protocol, all nonvertex second twins underwent immediate breech extraction. The study found no difference in the rates of 5-minute Apgar scores lower than 7 or fetal acidosis between the planned vaginal delivery ($n = 130$) and the planned cesarean delivery groups ($n = 157$).

57. Rabinovici J, Barkai G, Reichman B, Serr DM, Mashiach S. Randomized management of the second non-vertex twin: Vaginal delivery or cesarean section. American Journal of Obstetrics & Gynecology 1987; 156:52–6.

58. Schmitz T, Carnavalet CdeC, Azria E, Lopez E, Cabrol D, Goffinet F. Neonatal outcomes of twin pregnancy according to the planned mode of delivery. Obstetrics & Gynecology 2008; 111:695–703.

59. Fox NS, Silverstein M, Bender S, Klauser CK, Saltzman DH, Rebarber A. Active second-stage management in twin pregnancies undergoing planned vaginal delivery in a US population. Obstetrics & Gynecology 2010; 115:229–33.

Useful information also comes from a recent multicenter study performed at eight hospitals in Ireland. Called the ESPRiT study, Breathnach and colleagues analyzed perinatal outcomes by mode of delivery in 971 diamniotic twin pregnancies.[60] Decisions on timing and mode of delivery were deferred to the lead clinician managing each case. Of those 971 pregnancies, 441 (45 percent) were deemed to be appropriate for trial of labor. Of those 441 women, 338 (77 percent) had a successful vaginal delivery of both twins. The most common indication for cesarean during a trial of labor was arrest of the first stage of labor. Breech extraction of the second twin was performed in 29 percent of those 338 successful vaginal deliveries. There were no differences in perinatal outcomes by planned mode of delivery. When they analyzed predictors of successful vaginal delivery for both babies, both multiparity and spontaneous conception were independently associated with successful vaginal birth. Four percent of women undergoing trial of labor had vaginal delivery of the first twin and cesarean delivery of the second twin.

The strongest data on this question come from a large prospective randomized trial of mode of delivery in twin pregnancies published in 2013.[61] This multicenter, multinational study randomized 2,804 women pregnant with diamniotic twins and a cephalic-presenting first twin after 32 weeks' gestation to either planned cesarean or planned vaginal delivery. The primary outcome was a composite of fetal or neonatal death or serious morbidity. In the planned cesarean group, 90 percent of women underwent cesarean delivery of both babies, and in the planned vaginal delivery group, 56 percent had successful vaginal delivery of both twins. In the planned vaginal group, 4.2 percent of women underwent vaginal delivery of the first twin and cesarean delivery of the second twin. The paper doesn't state specifically how many women had vaginal breech extraction of the second twin, but 36.4 percent of the planned vaginal delivery group had twins in a cephalic/noncephalic presentation at the time of delivery. The results showed no difference in the primary outcome between the planned cesarean and the planned vaginal groups, nor were there any differences in maternal morbidity between the groups. There were no differences in the primary outcome based on the presentation of the second twin (cephalic versus noncephalic).

The above retrospective and prospective data, including two randomized trials, on mode of delivery in diamniotic twin gestations with a cephalic-presenting first twin show that in selected women (near term and fetal weight >1,500 g), under appropriate conditions and with experienced obstetricians and supporting staff, there is no proven benefit to routine cesarean delivery. However, the importance of operator training and experience cannot be

60. Breathnach FM, McAuliffe FM, Geary M, et al. Prediction of safe and successful vaginal birth. American Journal of Obstetrics & Gynecology 2011; 205:237.e1–e7.
61. Barrett JFR, Hannah ME, Hutton EK, et al. A randomized trial of planned cesarean or vaginal delivery for twin pregnancy. New England Journal of Medicine 2013; 369:1295–1305.

underestimated as a factor affecting the safe vaginal delivery of twins, particularly when the second twin is in a nonvertex presentation. During the past decade, concerns about outcomes associated with singleton breech deliveries have led to virtual abandonment of vaginal delivery of breech-presenting singletons. As a consequence, fewer obstetricians are acquiring or maintaining the skills needed to safely perform vaginal breech extractions of nonvertex second twins.

Triplets: Although vaginal delivery is an option for triplets, there are no large prospective studies establishing its safety.[62] Adequate monitoring of three fetuses throughout labor and delivery is challenging. With triplets there is a much higher rate of malpresentation, as well as an increased likelihood of the triplets being very preterm or <1,500 g. As a result, elective cesarean delivery of patients with three or more live fetuses at a viable gestational age is the optimal management strategy in most cases. Vaginal delivery of triplets should probably be restricted to those cases with estimated fetal weights >2,000 g, at least the first two triplets presenting cephalic, and the obstetrician experienced in such deliveries.

Safe vaginal delivery of multiples requires careful preparation and multidisciplinary cooperation among obstetrics, anesthesia, nursing, and neonatology or pediatrics. On admission to labor and delivery, both fetal presentations should be confirmed by ultrasound. If a recent (within 1 to 2 weeks) ultrasound-estimated fetal weight for both babies is not available, this should also be obtained. As discussed earlier, knowledge of the presentation, gestational age, and estimated weight of each twin permits the establishment of a plan regarding the anticipated route of delivery.

HISTORY OF A PRIOR CESAREAN

Another important consideration in determining the method of delivery is the mother's obstetrical history. In singletons, the low transverse uterine incision is associated with a 0.5 to 1 percent risk of rupture in a future labor and up to 50 percent of those ruptures can be catastrophic. The risk of a low transverse uterine scar rupture in a twin gestation is not as well defined as it is for singletons, but most obstetricians believe that the risk is similar, at about 1 percent. After counseling, some women choose to have a trial of labor after their prior cesarean. However, given the baseline high risk of cesarean delivery for multiples and the potentially small increased risk of uterine rupture, most women with multiples and a prior cesarean opt to have a repeat cesarean.

---

62. Grobman WA, Peaceman AM, Haney EI, et al. Neonatal outcomes in triplet gestations after a trial of labor. American Journal of Obstetrics & Gynecology 1998; 179:942–5.

Time Interval Between Deliveries

Many investigators have historically considered the time interval between delivery of the first and second babies to be an important intrapartum variable affecting twin pregnancy outcome. After delivery of the first twin, uterine relaxation may develop, the umbilical cord of the second twin can prolapse, or placental abruption may occur, each posing a risk to the undelivered second twin. In addition, the cervix can constrict, making rapid delivery of the second twin impossible if nonreassuring fetal status develops. Many reports have suggested that the interval between deliveries should ideally be 15 minutes or less, and certainly not more than 30 minutes. Most of the data in support of this view, however, were obtained before the advent of continuous and dual intrapartum fetal monitoring capability.

Rayburn and associates reported the outcome of 115 second twins delivered vaginally at or beyond 34 weeks' gestation after vertex delivery of their co-twin.[63] Continuous monitoring of the fetal heart rate was performed in all cases. Pitocin was used if uterine contractions subsided within 10 minutes after delivery of the first twin. In this series, 70 second twins were delivered within 15 minutes of the first twin, 28 were delivered within 16 to 30 minutes, and 17 were delivered more than 30 minutes later. The longest interval between deliveries was 134 minutes. All these infants survived, and none had a traumatic delivery. All 17 of the neonates delivered more than 30 minutes after their co-twin had 5-minute Apgar scores of 8 to 10. In another series reported by Chervenak and colleagues, when the fetal heart rate of the second twin was monitored with ultrasound visualization throughout the period between twin deliveries, there was no relationship between the length of the interdelivery interval and low 5-minute Apgar scores.[64]

Although some second twins may require rapid delivery, most can be safely followed with fetal heart rate surveillance and remain undelivered for substantial periods of time. This less-hurried approach when the second twin is not demonstrating signs of nonreassuring fetal status may reduce the incidence of both maternal and fetal trauma associated with difficult deliveries performed to meet arbitrary deadlines.

63. Rayburn WF, Lavin JP Jr., Miodovnik M, Varner MW. Multiple gestation: Time interval between delivery of the first and second twin. Obstetrics & Gynecology 1984; 63:502–6.
64. Chervenak FA. The controversy of mode of delivery in twins: The intrapartum management of twin gestation (part II). Seminars in Perinatology 1986; 10:44–9.

For Additional Information

I am certain that not every obstetrician or maternal-fetal medicine specialist will necessarily agree with all of the management recommendations I've made here. I would be happy to personally confer with any health care provider regarding patients who are expecting multiples. I can be reached at DrRog@rogerbnewman.com.

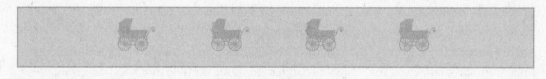

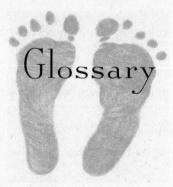

Glossary

abruptio placenta Condition in which the placenta separates from the uterus before birth.

acardiac twin *See* twin reversed arterial perfusion (TRAP) sequence.

acute intertwin transfusion A circulatory complication that can affect a surviving monochorionic twin after its co-twin dies in utero.

AGA *See* appropriate for gestational age.

alpha-fetoprotein A type of protein produced by an unborn baby or its yolk sac; a test of the mother's blood done at 15 to 18 weeks' gestation can suggest that more than one fetus is present, or that the fetus has an abnormality.

amino acids The structural components of protein.

amniocentesis A test done between 15 and 20 weeks' gestation to screen for certain genetic disorders; performed by inserting a needle through the mother's abdomen into the womb to withdraw a sample of amniotic fluid.

amnion The membrane closest to the unborn babies.

amniotic fluid The fluid within the uterus surrounding the unborn babies.

amniotic sac The fluid-filled, membranous sac within which the unborn baby grows, cushioned from shocks from the outside environment and kept at an even temperature; also called bag of waters.

analgesia Medication (usually a narcotic) that provides pain relief without total loss of sensation.

anemia *See* iron-deficiency anemia.

anesthesia Medication that provides pain relief by loss of sensation.

antenatal corticosteroid Medications given by injection to a pregnant woman at risk for preterm birth to hasten the maturation of the fetal lungs.

anthropometric measures The clinical assessments of body weight and measurements of upper-arm circumference, mid-thigh circumference, and skinfold thickness at various sites; used as indicators of nutritional status.

Apgar score A score given at one, five, and ten minutes after birth, summarizing a newborn's physical condition.

apnea The cessation of breathing for 15 to 20 seconds.

appropriate for gestational age (AGA) A newborn who weighs between the 10th and 90th percentiles for gestational age.

ART *See* assisted reproductive technologies.

assisted reproductive technologies (ART) The collective term for medications and therapies used to treat infertility.

bag of waters *See* amniotic sac.

betamethasone (Celestone) A steroid drug given to the mother by injection to speed maturation of the unborn babies' lungs.

bili-lights A bank of lights used for phototherapy in the treatment of hyperbilirubinemia.

biophysical profile A test combining information from the nonstress test with that of ultrasound; an assessment of the unborn babies' heart rates, breathing patterns, body movements, and muscle tone, and the amount of amniotic fluid surrounding each baby.

bloody show The blood-tinged mucous plug that is released when the cervix begins to dilate.

BPD *See* bronchopulmonary dysplasia.

Braxton-Hicks contractions Irregular contractions occurring throughout pregnancy that do not lead to effacement or dilation of the cervix.

breech extraction Vaginal, feet-first, physician-assisted delivery of a fetus in a breech position.

breech presentation The position of a fetus who is lying with his feet or buttocks closest to the cervix.

bronchopulmonary dysplasia (BPD) Damage to an infant's lungs caused by the use of a respirator.

cardiorespiratory monitor A piece of equipment that monitors a baby's heart and breathing rates.

catecholamines Hormones produced by the body during periods of stress.

Celestone *See* betamethasone.

cephalic presentation The position of a fetus who is lying head-down in the uterus.

cerclage A procedure to treat an incompetent cervix that involves stitching the cervix closed.

cervical insufficiency When the cervix opens spontaneously in early to mid-pregnancy, potentially resulting in a previable or early preterm birth.

cervix The opening at the bottom of the uterus that thins out (effaces) and opens (dilates) during labor and delivery.

chloasma An area of darkened pigmentation over the nose and cheeks that frequently appears during pregnancy.

chorioamnionitis Infection of the placental membranes.

chorion The membrane closest to the placenta.

chorionic villus sampling (CVS) A test of part of the chorion, performed at 10 to 12 weeks' gestation, to screen for a variety of potential congenital conditions.

chromosomes The genetic material contained in the mother's egg and the father's sperm that combines during fertilization.

chronic lung disease *See* bronchopulmonary dysplasia.

conception The fertilization of a woman's egg by a man's sperm.

conjoined twins A very rare condition of monoamniotic twin gestations in which the fetuses are partially fused and share certain organs or body parts.

contraction stress test A prenatal test in which a small amount of oxytocin is given to initiate uterine contractions, in order to evaluate how well the babies respond physically to the potential demands of labor.

corrected age The age a premature infant would have been if he had been born on his due date; for example, on his first birthday, a baby born two months premature has a corrected age of ten months.

crib death *See* sudden infant death syndrome.

CVS *See* chorionic villus sampling.

dexamethasone A corticosteroid sometimes used instead of betamethasone to enhance fetal lung maturity.

diamniotic Two amniotic placental membranes.

dichorionic Two chorionic placental membranes.

di/di *See* diamniotic *and* dichorionic.

dilation The progressive opening of the cervix during labor, measured in centimeters from 0 (not dilated) to 10 (fully dilated).

di/mo *See* diamniotic *and* monochorionic.

dizygotic Twins or higher-order multiples who develop from two separate zygotes; also called fraternal.

Doppler flow study Prenatal evaluation of the blood flow to the placenta.

ductus arteriosus A short vessel connecting the pulmonary artery to the aorta.

eclampsia The onset of seizures in a pregnant woman who developed preeclampsia.

ectopic pregnancy The implantation of an embryo in tissues other than the uterus, usually in the fallopian tube.

effacement The progressive thinning out of the cervix during labor.

electronic fetal monitoring Measurement of the fetal heart rates with external monitors before and during labor.

embryo The term for the developing baby prior to the third month of gestation.

endometrium The outer layer of the tissue lining the interior of the uterus.

epidural block A technique used to manage labor pain, in which analgesic medication is given via an epidural catheter inserted through a needle into the epidural space just outside the spinal cord.

episiotomy An incision made at delivery to widen the vaginal opening and prevent tearing as the baby emerges.

essential amino acids The components of proteins that cannot be produced by the body and must be supplied in the diet.

essential fatty acids The components of fats that cannot be produced by the body and must be supplied in the diet.

external cephalic version A procedure in which a health care provider manipulates the fetus by pressing on a pregnant woman's abdomen in an attempt to move a breech or transverse fetus into a head-first presentation.

extracorporeal membrane oxygenation (ECMO) A machine used in neonatal intensive care to provide cardiac and respiratory support.

fertilization When the mother's egg and the father's sperm unite; also known as conception.

fetal fibronectin A protein produced during pregnancy that functions like biological glue between the fetal membranes and the uterine lining. It is normally present in the cervical and vaginal secretions before 22 weeks' gestation and during the last 1 to 3 weeks before delivery. The presence of fetal fibronectin between 24 and 34 weeks' gestation, along with the symptoms of labor, is a positive sign of preterm labor.

fetus The term for the unborn child from the end of the embryonic period until delivery.

first trimester nuchal translucency (NT) screening A combination prenatal blood test and ultrasound exam that screens for Down syndrome and certain congenital heart defects.

fraternal Twins or higher-order multiples who develop from separate zygotes; also called dizygotic.

full term Delivery between 38 and 42 weeks' gestation, as calculated from the last menstrual period.

fundal height The distance from the fundus to the pelvic bone.

fundus The top of the uterus.

gavage feeding Infant feeding via a thin, flexible tube passed through either the nose or the mouth and into the stomach.

gestational age An unborn baby's age in weeks, as calculated from the mother's last menstrual period.

gestational age at birth The length of the pregnancy, as calculated from the mother's last menstrual period to the day of delivery.

gestational diabetes The development of diabetes during pregnancy.

HCG *See* human chorionic gonadotropin.

hematocrit The percentage of red blood cells in the blood.

hemoglobin The iron-containing component of red blood cells.

higher-order multiples A collective term for three or more babies resulting from one pregnancy; also called supertwins; includes triplets, quadruplets, quintuplets, sextuplets, septuplets, and so on.

human chorionic gonadotropin (HCG) A hormone produced by the chorion; it can be measured soon after conception to confirm a pregnancy.

human placental lactogen (HPL) A hormone that is produced by the placenta and affects metabolism.

hyperalimentation *See* parenteral nutrition.

hyperbilirubinemia Excessively high levels of bilirubin in the blood during the newborn period.

hypoglycemia Abnormally low blood sugar levels.

identical Twins or higher-order multiples who develop from a single zygote; also called monozygotic.

incompetent cervix *See* cervical insufficiency.

indomethacin *See* tocolytics.

intrahepatic cholestasis of pregnancy A liver disorder that causes intense itching and can increase the risk for preterm labor or stillbirth.

intrauterine growth restriction (IUGR) Birthweight of less than the 10th percentile for gestational age.

intraventricular hemorrhage Bleeding into the ventricles of the brain.

in utero Occurring in the uterus, before birth.

iron-deficiency anemia Abnormally low levels of red blood cells, which carry oxygen to the tissues.

IUGR *See* intrauterine growth restriction.

jaundice *See* physiologic jaundice.

kangaroo care The practice of having a parent hold a premature baby skin to skin against the chest, shown in studies to help the infant regulate his breathing and body temperature and to promote parent-infant bonding.

ketones A by-product of the breakdown of fat for energy.

ketosis A metabolic state in which there is an accumulation of excessive ketones in the body.

kilogram (kg) Unit of weight of the metric system, equivalent to 1,000 grams, or 2.2 pounds.

labor The process by which the cervix thins and opens to allow the babies to pass from the uterus through the vagina and be born.

large for gestational age (LGA) Birthweight above the 90th percentile for gestational age.

laser photocoagulation A fetal therapy in which a scope is placed into the uterine cavity to identify the arteriovenous connections on the placental surface that are causing twin-twin transfusion syndrome, and to ablate those connections using laser energy.

LBW *See* low birthweight.

let-down reflex The flow of milk into the ducts and collection areas behind the nipples, felt as a tingling sensation by the nursing mother.

LGA *See* large for gestational age.

lightening When the baby closest to the cervix settles deeper into the pelvis before delivery.

linea nigra A line of darkened pigment from the navel to the pubic bone that occurs in some women during pregnancy.

lipolysis The breakdown of fat into fatty acids.

low birthweight (LBW) A birthweight of less than 2,500 grams, or 5½ pounds.

magnesium sulfate Medication used in treating preeclampsia and preterm labor.

MBR *See* multiple birth ratio.

maternal-fetal medicine specialist An obstetrician who has completed a fellowship in the management of high-risk pregnancies.

metabolic programming The ways in which an individual's uterine environment and nutrition before birth can set the stage for the development of chronic diseases in adulthood.

mo/mo *See* monoamniotic *and* monochorionic.

monoamniotic A single inner placental membrane, indicating identical twins.

monochorionic A single outer placental membrane surrounding the fetuses, indicating identical twins.

monozygotic Twins or higher-order multiples who develop from a single zygote, which divided an extra time to result in two or more equal and matching embryos; also called identical.

multiple birth ratio (MBR) The number of multiple births per 1,000 total live births.

NEC *See* necrotizing enterocolitis.

necrotizing enterocolitis (NEC) A potential complication of prematurity that involves a gangrene-like condition of portions of the gastrointestinal tract.

neonatal intensive care unit (NICU) A specialized nursery staffed and equipped to care for seriously ill newborns.

neonatologist A pediatrician who specializes in the care of newborns.

neural tube defect A type of birth defect affecting the brain, spine, or spinal cord.

NICU *See* neonatal intensive care unit.

nifedipine *See* tocolytics.

nonstress test An evaluation of fetal movements and fetal heart rate using an electronic fetal monitor.

nosocomial infection An infection picked up from the hospital environment.

nuchal translucency *See* first trimester nuchal translucency (NT) screening.

nutritional supplements Specially formulated foods, usually in beverage form, that contain extra calories and/or protein.

OGTT *See* oral glucose tolerance test.

oral glucose tolerance test (OGTT) A test, often given prenatally, that involves ingesting a high-carbohydrate beverage and then having blood drawn at set intervals to determine blood glucose levels.

ovulation The release of a mature egg from the ovaries.

oxy-hood A plastic box or hood placed over the baby's head to deliver supplemental oxygen.

oxytocin A hormone that stimulates uterine contractions in pregnant and postpartum women, as well as the let-down reflex in breast-feeding women.

Pap smear A procedure that involves scraping a few cells from the cervix and examining them under a microscope to detect any abnormal changes.

parenteral nutrition A special formula for premature infants, given intravenously, that contains all essential nutrients; also called hyperalimentation.

patent ductus arteriosis (PDA) Condition in which the fetal connection between the aorta and the pulmonary artery fails to close after birth.

PDA *See* patent ductus arteriosis.

pelvic examination An internal examination performed manually to evaluate the cervix and uterus; may also involve using a vaginal probe for vaginal ultrasound.

perineum The area between the opening of the vagina and the rectum.

peripartum cardiomyopathy A rare form of congestive heart failure that develops during pregnancy or in the year after delivery.

phototherapy A treatment for hyperbilirubinemia that uses light waves to break down bilirubin so that it can be excreted in the urine.

physiologic jaundice A buildup of bilirubin in the blood during the newborn period, causing the skin to become yellow.

Pitocin *See* oxytocin.

placenta The outer layer of the fertilized egg; it develops into the vascular organ lining the uterus to supply the baby with nutrients and oxygen before birth.

placenta previa A condition in which the placenta lies partially or completely over the cervix, resulting in bleeding as the cervix dilates during labor and delivery.

placental abruption *See* abruptio placenta.

pneumonia Infection in the lungs.

polyhydramnios An excessive amount of amniotic fluid.

postpartum depression (PPD) A temporary feeling of depression after delivery, resulting from hormonal shifts and other factors.

postpartum psychosis The most serious form of postpartum mood disorder, characterized by a dangerous break with reality.

PPD *See* postpartum depression.

PPROM *See* preterm premature rupture of membranes.

preeclampsia A pregnancy complication in which there is protein in the urine, rapid weight gain, rise in blood pressure, and swelling from fluid retention; formerly called toxemia.

premature birth Birth prior to 37 full weeks of pregnancy.

presentation A fetus's position in the uterus, and one of the determining factors in whether a vaginal delivery is appropriate.

preterm birth Birth prior to 37 full weeks of pregnancy.

preterm labor Labor that begins prior to 37 full weeks of pregnancy.

preterm premature rupture of membranes (PPROM) Breaking of the membranes surrounding the fetus prior to 37 weeks' gestation.

pruritic urticarial plaques and papules of pregnancy (PUPPP) An itchy rash usually developing first on the abdomen or in the stretch marks in the third trimester.

Quad screening test A prenatal blood test that measures four separate substances to gauge the risk for Down syndrome and other genetic abnormalities.

radiant warmer A small open crib with an overhead heat source.

RDS *See* respiratory distress syndrome.

reduction *See* selective multifetal reduction.

respiratory distress syndrome (RDS) A common complication of prematurity in which lung tissue collapses on itself owing to lack of surfactant, the soaplike substance that helps to keep the lungs inflated.

retinopathy of prematurity (ROP) An eye complication of some premature babies in which blood vessels of the eye grow abnormally; also called retrolental fibroplasia.

retrolental fibroplasia *See* retinopathy of prematurity.

Rh factor A protein in red blood cells that can lead to complications if present in the blood of the unborn babies (Rh positive) but not in the mother (Rh negative).

RhoGAM A drug given to an Rh-negative woman to prevent her from making antibodies against an Rh-positive baby.

ritodrine *See* tocolytics.

ROP *See* retinopathy of prematurity.

rupture of membranes Breaking of the membranes surrounding the fetus, often at the onset of labor.

selective intrauterine growth restriction (sIUGR) Growth discordance in a multiple gestation, in which one fetus grows significantly more slowly than the other(s).

selective multifetal reduction A procedure by which one or more fetuses of a multiple gestation are selectively aborted in an attempt to improve the chances of survival and a better pregnancy outcome for the remaining fetuses.

sepsis Bacteria in the bloodstream.

SGA *See* small for gestational age.

SIDS *See* sudden infant death syndrome.

singleton A baby conceived and born alone.

small for gestational age (SGA) A newborn whose birthweight is below the 10th percentile for gestational age.

sonogram *See* ultrasound.

spina bifida A neural tube defect in which there is incomplete closing of the backbone and the membranes around the spinal column.

spinal block A pain-blocking technique used primarily during cesarean deliveries, in which anesthesia medication is injected into the spinal canal.

sudden infant death syndrome (SIDS) The death, during sleep and from unknown causes, of an infant who had appeared to be healthy; also called crib death.

supertwins A collective term for three or more babies resulting from one pregnancy; also called higher-order multiples; includes triplets, quadruplets, quintuplets, sextuplets, septuplets, and so on.

surfactant A fatty substance formed in the lungs that keeps the small air sacs, or alveoli, from collapsing.

tocolytics Drugs used to attempt to halt preterm labor.

TOLAC *See* trial of labor after cesarean.

toxemia *See* preeclampsia.

transition The end of the first stage of labor, when the cervix dilates from 8 to 10 centimeters.

transvaginal cervical length (TVCL) A measurement of cervical length that helps predict the risk of preterm labor.

transverse presentation The position of a fetus who is lying sideways in the uterus.

trial of labor An attempt to deliver vaginally in the presence of certain factors that could ultimately necessitate a cesarean delivery.

trial of labor after cesarean (TOLAC) An attempt to deliver vaginally after a previous cesarean birth.

trimester One of the three periods of pregnancy, each lasting about three months.

twin reversed arterial perfusion (TRAP) sequence A rare defect of monozygotic gestations in which one partially developed fetus lacks a heart and relies on its co-twin for its blood supply.

twin-twin transfusion syndrome (TTTS) A serious complication in some monochorionic pregnancies in which one twin receives too little blood, while the other receives too much.

twin type The identical or fraternal status of twins or higher-order multiples.

ultrasound Technology that bounces sound waves off the unborn babies and the surrounding fluid and membranes, then projects the resulting images onto a video screen; also called a sonogram.

umbilical arterial catheter A catheter threaded into a premature baby's umbilical artery in order to draw blood samples, give fluids and medications, and measure blood pressure.

urinary tract infection (UTI) Infection of the bladder or other structure of the urinary tract.

UTI *See* urinary tract infection.

vaginal birth after cesarean (VBAC) A vaginal delivery that follows a previous cesarean birth.

vasopressin A hormone similar to oxytocin that can trigger uterine contractions.

VBAC *See* vaginal birth after cesarean.

vertex presentation *See* cephalic presentation.

very low birthweight (VLBW) Birthweight of less than 1,500 grams, or 3 lb., 5 oz.

viability The gestational age at which a fetus may be expected to survive outside the uterine environment.

vital signs Pulse, temperature, and blood pressure.

VLBW *See* very low birthweight.

zygote The term for the fertilized egg prior to 12 weeks' gestation.

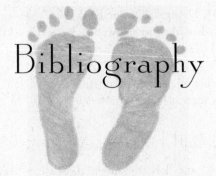

Bibliography

Alcohol and Smoking During Pregnancy

Ahluwalia IB, Merritt R, Beck LF, Rogers M. Multiple lifestyle and psychosocial risks and delivery of small for gestational age infants. Obstetrics & Gynecology 2001; 97:649–56.

Blake KV, Gurrin LC, Evans SF, Beilin LJ, Landau LI, Stanley FJ, et al. Maternal cigarette smoking during pregnancy, low birth weight and subsequent blood pressure in early childhood. Early Human Development 2000; 57:137–47.

Drews CD, Murphy CC, Yeargin-Allsopp M, Decoufle P. The relationship between idiopathic mental retardation and maternal smoking during pregnancy. Pediatrics 1996; 97:547–53.

Lampl M, Kuzawa CW, Jeanty P. Prenatal smoke exposure alters growth in limb proportions and head shape in the midgestation human fetus. American Journal of Human Biology 2003; 15:533–46.

Lorente C., Cordier S, Goujard J, Aymé S, Bianchi F, Calzolari E, et al. Tobacco and alcohol use during pregnancy and risk of oral clefts. American Journal of Public Health 2000; 90:415–19.

Mathews TJ. Smoking during pregnancy in the 1990s. National Vital Statistics Reports, vol. 49, no. 7. National Center for Health Statistics: Hyattsville, MD; 2001.

McDonald SD, Perkins SL, Jodouin CA, Walker MC. Folate levels in pregnant women who smoke: An important gene/environment interaction. American Journal of Obstetrics & Gynecology 2000; 187:620–5.

Pollack H, Lantz PM, Frohna JG. Maternal smoking and adverse birth outcomes among singletons and twins. American Journal of Public Health 2000; 90:395–400.

Shaw GM, Carmichael SL, Vollset SE, et al. Mid-pregnancy cotinine and risks of orofacial clefts and neural tube defects. Journal of Pediatrics 2009; 154:14–19.

Sørensen HT, Nørgård B, Pedersen L, Larsen H, Johnsen SP. Maternal smoking and risk of hypertrophic infantile pyloric stenosis: 10 year population based cohort study. British Medical Journal 2002; 325:1011–12.

Syme C, Abrahamowicz M, Mahboubi A, et al. Prenatal exposure to maternal cigarette smoking and accumulation of intra-abdominal fat during adolescence. Obesity 2010; 18:1021–5.

Tarter JG, Khoury A, Barton JR, Jacques DL, Sibai BM. Demographic and obstetric factors influencing pregnancy outcome in twin gestations. American Journal of Obstetrics & Gynecology 2002; 186:910–12.

Tong VT, Jones JR, Dietz PM, D'Angelo D, Bombard JM. Trends in smoking before, during, and after pregnancy—Pregnancy Risk Assessment Monitoring System (PRAMS), United States, 31 sites, 2000–2005. Morbidity and Mortality Weekly Report, Surveillance Summaries, vol. 58, no. SS-4, May 29, 2009.

Wisborg K, Henriksen TB, Secher NJ. Maternal smoking and gestational age in twin pregnancies. Acta Obstetricia et Gynecologica Scandinavica 2001; 80:926–30.

Bariatric Surgery and Pregnancy

American Society for Metabolic and Bariatric Surgery Guidelines. ASMBS allied health nutritional guidelines for the surgical weight loss patient. Surgery for Obesity and Related Diseases 2008; 4:S73–S108.

Beard JH, Bell RL, Duffy AJ. Reproductive considerations and pregnancy after bariatric surgery: Current evidence and recommendations. Obesity Surgery 2008; 18:1023–7.

Blankenship J. Pregnancy after surgical weight loss: Nutritional care and recommendations. Weight Management Newsletter, Summer 2005; vol. 3, no. 1. American Dietetic Association Dietetic Practice Group.

Ducarme G, Revaux A, Rodrigues A, Aissaoui F, Pharisien I, Uzan M. Obstetric outcome following laparoscopic adjustable gastric banding. International Journal of Gynaecology and Obstetrics 2007; 98:244–7.

Guelinckx I, Devlieger R, Vansant G. Reproductive outcome after bariatric surgery: A critical review. Human Reproduction Update 2009; 15:189–201.

Karkarla N, Dailey C, Marino T, Shikora SA, Chelmow D. Pregnancy after gastric bypass surgery and internal hernia formation. Obstetrics & Gynecology 2005; 105:1195–8.

Maggard MA, Yermilov I, Li Z, Maglione M, Newberry S, Suttorp M, et al. Pregnancy and fertility following bariatric surgery: A systematic review. Journal of the American Medical Association 2008; 300:2286–96.

Patel JA, Patel NA, Thomas RL, Nelms JK, Colella JJ. Pregnancy outcomes after laparoscopic Roux-en-Y gastric bypass. Surgery for Obesity and Related Diseases 2008; 4:39–45.

Roos N, Neovius M, Cnattingius S, et al. Perinatal outcomes after bariatric surgery: Nationwide population based matched cohort study. British Medical Journal 2013; 347:f6460.

Sheiner E, Levy A, Silverberg D, Menes TS, Levy I, Katz M, et al. Pregnancy after bariatric surgery is not associated with adverse perinatal outcome. American Journal of Obstetrics & Gynecology 2004; 190:1335–40.

Wax JR, Cartin A, Wolff R, Lepich S, Pinette MG, Blackstone J. Pregnancy following gastric bypass for morbid obesity: Effect of surgery-to-conception interval on maternal and neonatal outcomes. Obesity Surgery 2008; 18:1517–21.

Wax JR, Cartin A, Wolff R, Lepich S, Pinette MG, Blackstone J. Pregnancy following gastric bypass surgery for morbid obesity: Maternal and neonatal outcomes. Obesity Surgery 2008; 18:540–4.

Birth Defects, Infertility Treatments, and Multiples

Cox GF, Burger J, Lip V, Mau UA, Sperling K, Wu BL, et al. Intracytoplasmic sperm injection may increase the risk of imprinting defects. American Journal of Human Genetics 2002; 71:162–4.

Crane JP, LeFevre ML, Winborn RC, et al. A randomized trial of prenatal ultrasonographic screening: Impact on the detection, management, and outcome of anomalous fetuses. American Journal of Obstetrics & Gynecology 1994; 171:392–9.

De Kretser DM. The potential of intracytoplasmic sperm injection (ICSI) to transmit genetic defects causing male infertility. Reproduction, Fertility, and Development 1995; 7:137–42.

Gosden R, Trasler J, Lucifero D, Faddy M. Rare congenital disorders, imprinting genes, and assisted reproductive technology. Lancet 2003; 361:1975–7.

Hansen M, Bower C, Milne E, de Klerk N, Kurinczuk JJ. Assisted reproductive technologies and the risk of birth defects—a systemic review. Human Reproduction 2005; 20:328–38.

Hansen M, Kurinczuk JJ, Bower C, Webb S. The risk of major birth defects after intracytoplasmic sperm injection and in vitro fertilization. New England Journal of Medicine 2002; 346:725–30.

Luke B, Keith LG. Monozygotic twinning as a congenital defect and congenital defects in monozygotic twins. Fetal Diagnosis and Therapy 1990; 5:61–9.

Malone FD, Craigo SD, Chelmow D, D'Alton ME. Outcome of twin gestations complicated by a single anomalous fetus. Obstetrics & Gynecology 1996; 88:1–5.

Molloy AM, Kirke PN, Troendle JF, et al. Maternal vitamin B_{12} status and risk of neural tube defects in a population with high neural tube defect prevalence and no folic acid fortification. Pediatrics 2009; 123:917–23.

Reefhuis J, Honein MA, Schieve LA, Correa A, Hobbs CA, Rasmussen SA; National Birth Defects Prevention Study. Assisted reproductive technology and major structural birth defects in the United States. Human Reproduction 2009; 24:360–6.

Sutcliffe AG, D'Souza SW, Cadman J, Richards B, McKinlay IA, Lieberman B. Minor congenital anomalies, major congenital malformations and development in children conceived from cryopreserved embryos. Human Reproduction 1995; 10:3332–7.

Breast-Feeding

Academy of Nutrition and Dietetics. Position of the Academy of Nutrition and Dietetics: Promoting and supporting breastfeeding. Journal of the Academy of Nutrition and Dietetics 2015; 115:444–9.

American Academy of Pediatrics. Policy statement: Breastfeeding and the use of human milk. Pediatrics 2005; 115:496–506.

American Academy of Pediatrics. Policy statement. Breastfeeding and the use of human milk. Pediatrics 2012; 129:e827.

American College of Obstetricians and Gynecologists. Committee opinion. Breastfeeding: Maternal and infant aspects. Obstetrics & Gynecology 2007; 109:479–80.

American Dietetic Association. Position of the American Dietetic Association: Promoting and supporting breastfeeding. Journal of the American Dietetic Association 2005; 105:810–18.

Baker JL, Gamborg M, Heitmann BL, Lissner L, Sorensen TIA, Rasmussen KM. Breastfeeding reduces postpartum weight retention. American Journal of Clinical Nutrition 2008; 88:1543–51.

Collaborative Group on Hormonal Factors in Breast Cancer. Breast cancer and breastfeeding: Collaborative reanalysis of individual data from 47 epidemiological studies in 30 countries, including 50,302 women with breast cancer and 96,973 women without the disease. Lancet 2002; 360:187–95.

Gunderson EP. Breast-feeding and diabetes: Long-term impact on mothers and their infants. Current Diabetes Reports 2008; 8:279–86.

Karlson EW, Mandl LA, Hankinson SE, Grodstein F. Do breast-feeding and other reproductive factors influence future risk of rheumatoid arthritis? Results from the Nurses' Health Study. Arthritis & Rheumatology 2004; 50:3458–67.

Schwarz EB, Brown JS, Creasman JM, et al. Lactation and maternal risk of type 2 diabetes: A population-based study. American Journal of Medicine 2010; 123:863.e1–6.

Schwarz EB, Ray R, Stuebe AM, Allison MA, Ness RB, Freiberg MS, et al. Duration of lactation and risk factors for maternal cardiovascular disease. Obstetrics & Gynecology 2009; 113:974–82.

Stuebe AM, Rich-Edwards JW. The reset hypothesis: Lactation and maternal metabolism. American Journal of Perinatology 2009; 26:81–8.

US Department of Labor. Fact sheet #73: Break time for nursing mothers under the FLSA. Washington, DC; 2013. Available from: http://www.dol.gov/whd/regs/compliance/whdfs73.htm.

Calcium, Magnesium, Vitamin D, and Lead

American College of Obstetricians and Gynecologists. Committee opinion. Vitamin D: Screening and supplementation during pregnancy. Number 495, July 2011.

Atallah AN, Hofmeyr GJ, Duley L. Calcium supplementation during pregnancy for preventing hypertensive disorders and related problems. Cochrane Database of Systematic Reviews 2000; 3:CD001059.

Belizán JM, Villar J, Bergel E, del Pino A, Di Fulvio S, Galliano SV, et al. Long-term effect of calcium supplementation during pregnancy on the blood pressure of offspring: Follow up of a randomized controlled trial. British Medical Journal 1997; 315:281–5.

Bergel E, Barros AJ. Effect of maternal calcium intake during pregnancy on children's blood pressure: A systematic review of the literature. BioMed Central Pediatrics 2007; 7:15.

Bodnar LM, Catov JM, Roberts JM, Simhan HN. Prepregnancy obesity predicts poor vitamin D status in mothers and their neonates. Journal of Nutrition 2007; 137:2437–42.

Bodnar LM, Catov JM, Simhan HN, Holick MF, Powers RW, Roberts JM. Maternal vitamin D deficiency increases the risk of preeclampsia. Journal of Clinical Endocrinology & Metabolism 2007; 92:3517–22.

Bodnar LM, Krohn MA, Simhan HN. Maternal vitamin D deficiency is associated with bacterial vaginosis in the first trimester of pregnancy. Journal of Nutrition 2009; 139:1157–61.

Bodnar LM, Platt RW, Simhan HN. Early-pregnancy vitamin D deficiency and risk of preterm birth subgroups. Obstetrics & Gynecology 2015; 125:439–47.

Bodnar LM, Rouse DJ, Momirova V, et al. Maternal 25-hydroxyvitamin D and preterm birth in twin gestations. Obstetrics & Gynecology 2013; 122:91–8.

Bodnar LM, Simhan HN, Powers RW, Frank MP, Cooperstein E, Roberts JM. High prevalence of vitamin D insufficiency in Black and White pregnant women residing in the northern United States and their neonates. Journal of Nutrition 2007; 137:447–52.

Chappell LC, Seed PT, Briley AL, et al. Effect of antioxidants on the occurrence of pre-eclampsia in women at increased risk: A randomized trial. Lancet 1999; 354:810–16.

Chappell LC, Seed PT, Kelly FJ, et al. Vitamin C and E supplementation in women at risk of pre-eclampsia is associated with changes in indices of oxidative stress and placental function. American Journal of Obstetrics & Gynecology 2002; 187:777–84.

Conde-Agudelo A, Romero R. Antenatal magnesium sulfate for the prevention of cerebral palsy in preterm infants less than 34 weeks' gestation: A systematic review and meta-analysis. American Journal of Obstetrics & Gynecology 2009; 200:595–609.

Crowther CA, Middleton PF, Wilkinson D, et al. Magnesium sulphate at 30 to 34 weeks' gestational age: Neuroprotection trial (MAGENTA)-study protocol. BMC Pregnancy and Childbirth 2013; 13:91.

Doyle LW, Crowther CA, Middleton P, Marret S, Rouse D. Magnesium sulphate for women at risk of preterm birth for neuroprotection of the fetus. Cochrane Database of Systematic Reviews 2009; CD004661.

Ettinger AS, Hu H, Hernandez-Avila M. Dietary calcium supplementation to lower blood lead levels in pregnancy and lactation. Journal of Nutritional Biochemistry 2007; 18:172–8.

Ettinger AS, Lamadrid-Figueroa H, Téllez-Rojo MM, Mercado-Garcia A, Peterson KE, Schwartz J, et al. Effect of calcium supplementation on blood lead levels in pregnancy: A randomized placebo-controlled trial. Environmental Health Perspectives 2009; 117:26–31.

Ettinger AS, Téllez-Rojo MM, Amarasiriwardena C, Peterson KE, Schwartz J, Aro A, et al. Influence of maternal bone lead burden and calcium intake on levels of lead in breast milk over the course of lactation. American Journal of Epidemiology 2006; 163:4856.

Ginde AA, Sullivan AF, Mansbach JM, Camargo CA. Vitamin D insufficiency in pregnant and non-pregnant women of childbearing age in the United States. American Journal of Obstetrics & Gynecology 2010; 202:e1–e8.

Hernández-Avila M, Gonzalez-Cossio T, Hernández-Avila JE, Romieu I, Peterson KE, Aro A, et al. Dietary calcium supplements to lower blood lead levels in lactating women: A randomized placebo-controlled trial. Epidemiology 2003; 14206–12.

Hernandez-Avila M, Sanin LH, Romieu I, Palazuelos E, Tapia-Conyer R, Olaiz G, et al. Higher milk intake during pregnancy is associated with lower maternal and umbilical cord lead levels in postpartum women. Environmental Research 1997; 74:116–21.

Hofmeyr GJ, Atallah AN, Duley L. Calcium supplementation during pregnancy for preventing hypertensive disorders and related problems. Cochrane Database of Systematic Reviews 2006; 3:CD00159.

Hofmeyr GJ, Duley L, Atallah AN. Dietary Calcium Supplementation for Prevention of Pre-eclampsia and Related Problems: A Systematic Review and Commentary. British Journal of Obstetrics and Gynaecology 2007; 114:933–43.

Hollis BW. Circulating 25-hydroxyvitamin D levels indicative of vitamin D sufficiency: Implications for establishing a new effective dietary intake recommendation for vitamin D. Journal of Nutrition 2005; 135:317–22.

Hollis BW, Wagner CL. Assessment of dietary vitamin D requirements during pregnancy and lactation. American Journal of Clinical Nutrition 2004; 79:717–26.

Hollis BW, Wagner CL. Vitamin D requirements during lactation: High-dose maternal supplementation as therapy to prevent hypovitaminosis D for both the mother and the nursing infant. American Journal of Clinical Nutrition 2004; 80 (Suppl):1752S–8S.

Hu H, Téllez-Rojo MM, Bellinger D, Smith D, Ettinger AS, Lamadrid-Figueroa H, et al. Fetal lead exposure at each stage of pregnancy as a predictor of infant mental development. Environmental Health Perspectives 2006; 115:1730–5.

Hypponen E, Laara F, Reunanen A, Jarvelin MR, Virtanen SM. Intake of vitamin D and risk of type 1 diabetes: A birth-cohort study. Lancet 2001; 358:1500–3.

Javaid M, Crozier S, Harvey N, et al. Maternal vitamin D status during pregnancy and childhood bone mass at 9 years: A longitudinal study. Lancet 2006; 367:36–43.

Jelliffe-Pawlowski LL, Miles SQ, Courtney JG, Materna B, Charlton V. Effect of magnitude and timing of maternal pregnancy blood lead (Pb) levels on birth outcomes. Journal of Perinatology 2006; 26:154–62.

Johnson MA. High calcium intake blunts pregnancy-induced increases in maternal blood lead. Nutrition Reviews 2001; 59:152–6.

Koo WW, Walters JC, Esterlitz J, Levine RJ, Bush AJ, Sibai B. Maternal calcium supplementation and fetal bone mineralization. Obstetrics & Gynecology 1999; 94:577–82.

Liu PT, Stenger S, Li H, et al. Toll-like receptor triggering of a vitamin D–mediated human antimicrobial response. Science 2006; 311:1770–3.

Ogueh O, Khastgir G, Abbas A, et al. The feto-placental unit stimulates the pregnancy-associated increase in maternal bone metabolism. Human Reproduction 2000; 15:1834–7.

Okah FA, Tsang RC, Sierra R, Brady KK, Specker BL. Bone turnover and mineral metabolism in the last trimester of pregnancy: Effect of multiple gestation. Obstetrics & Gynecology 1996; 88:168–73.

McGrath J. Does "imprinting" with low prenatal vitamin D contribute to the risk of various adult disorders? Medical Hypotheses 2001; 56:367–71.

Mulligan ML, Felton SK, Riek AE, Bernal-Mizrachi C. Implications of vitamin D deficiency in pregnancy and lactation. American Journal of Obstetrics & Gynecology 2010; 202:429e1–9.

Polyzos NP, Anckaert E, Guzman L, et al. Vitamin D deficiency and pregnancy rates in women undergoing single embryo, blastocyst stage, transfer (SET) for IVF/ICSI. Human Reproduction 2014; 29:2032–40.

Rouse DJ, Hirtz DG, Thom E, et al.; for the Eunice Kennedy Shriver NICHD Maternal-Fetal Medicine Units Network. A randomized, controlled trial of magnesium sulfate for the prevention of cerebral palsy. New England Journal of Medicine 2008; 359:895–905.

Villar J, Abdel-Aleem H, Merialdi M, Mathai M, Ali MM, Zavaleta N, et al.; World Health Organization Calcium Supplementation for the Prevention of Preeclampsia Trial Group. American Journal of Obstetrics & Gynecology 2006; 194:639–49.

Wagner CL, McNeil R, Hamilton SA, et al. A randomized trial of vitamin D supplementation in 2 community health center networks in South Carolina. American Journal of Obstetrics & Gynecology 2013; 137:137–44.

Childhood Health After Infertility Treatment

Brandes JM, Scher A, Itkovits J, et al. Growth and development of children conceived by in vitro fertilization. Pediatrics 1992; 90:424–9.

Ludwig AK, Katalinic A, Thyen U, Sutcliffe AG, Diedrich K, Ludwig M. Neuromotor development and mental health at 5.5 years of age of singletons born at term after intracytoplasmic sperm injection: Results of a prospective controlled single-blinded study. Fertility and Sterility 2009; 91:125–32.

Ludwig AK, Katalinic A, Thyen U, Sutcliffe AG, Diedrich K, Ludwig M. Physical health at 5.5 years of age of term-born singletons after intracytoplasmic sperm injection: Results of a prospective, controlled, single-blinded study. Fertility and Sterility 2009; 91:115–24.

Ludwig AK, Sutcliffe AG, Diedrich K, Ludwig M. Post-neonatal health and development of children born after assisted reproduction: A systemic review of controlled studies. European Journal of Obstetrics & Gynecology and Reproductive Biology 2006; 127:3–25.

Middelburg KJ, Heineman MJ, Bos AF, Hadders-Algra M. Neuromotor, cognitive, language and behavioural outcome in children born following IVF or ICSI—A systemic review. Human Reproduction 2008; 14:219–31.

Place I, Englert Y. A prospective longitudinal study of the physical, psychomotor, and intellectual development of singleton children up to 5 years who were conceived by intracytoplasmic sperm injection compared with children conceived spontaneously and by in vitro fertilization. Fertility and Sterility 2003; 80:1388–97.

Ponjaert-Kristoffersen I, Bonduelle M, Barnes J, et al. International collaborative study of intracytoplasmic sperm injection–conceived, in vitro fertilization–conceived, and naturally conceived 5-year-old child outcomes: Cognitive and motor assessments. Pediatrics 2005; 115:e283–9.

Saunders K, Spensley J, Munro J, Halasz G. Growth and physical outcome of children conceived by in vitro fertilization. Pediatrics 1996; 97:688–92.

Schieve LA, Rasmussen SA, Buck GM, Schendel DE, Reynolds MA, Wright VC. Are children born after assisted reproductive technology at increased risk for adverse health outcomes? Obstetrics & Gynecology 2004; 103:1154–63.

Squires J, Kaplan P. Developmental outcomes of children born after assisted reproductive technologies. Infants & Young Children 2007; 20:2–10.

Childhood Health of Multiples

Akerman BA, Thomassen PA. The fate of "small twins": A four-year follow-up study of low-birthweight and prematurely born twins. Acta Geneticae Medicae et Gemellologiae 1992; 41:97–104.

Glinianaia SV, Jarvis S, Topp M, Guillem P, Platt MJ, Pearce MS, et al; on behalf of the SCPE collaboration of European Cerebral Palsy Registers. Intrauterine growth and cerebral palsy in twins: A European multicenter study. Twin Research and Human Genetics 2006; 9:460–6.

Glinianaia SV, Pharoah POD, Wright C, Rankin JM; on behalf of the Northern Region Perinatal Mortality Survey Steering Group. Fetal or infant death in twin pregnancy: Neurodevelopmental consequences for the survivor. Archives of Diseases of Children Fetal and Neonatal Edition 2002; 86:F9–15.

Grether JK, Nelson KB, Cummins SK. Twinning and cerebral palsy: Experience in four northern California counties, births 1983 through 1985. Pediatrics 1993; 92:854–8.

Koivurova S, Hartikainen A-L, Sovio U, Gissler M, Hemminki E, Järvelin M-R. Growth, psychomotor development and morbidity up to 3 years of age in children born after IVF. Human Reproduction 2003; 18:2328–36.

Leonard CH, Piecuch RE, Ballard RA, Cooper BAB. Outcome of very low birthweight infants: Multiple gestation versus singletons. Pediatrics 1994; 93:611–15.

Luke B, Brown MB, Hediger ML, Misiunas RB, Anderson E. Perinatal and early childhood outcomes of twins versus triplets. Twin Research and Human Genetics 2006; 9:81–8.

Luke B, Brown MB, Hediger ML, Nugent C, Misiunas RB, Anderson E. Fetal phenotypes and neonatal and early childhood outcomes in twins. American Journal of Obstetrics & Gynecology 2004; 191:1270–6.

Luke B, Leurgans S, Keith LG, Keith D. The childhood growth of twin children. Acta Geneticae Medicae et Gemellologiae 1995; 44:169–78.

Matsubara M, Sono J. Comparison of motor development between twins and singletons in Japan: A population-based study. Twin Research and Human Genetics 2007; 10:379–84.

Petterson B, Nelson KB, Watson L, Stanley F. Twins, triplets, and cerebral palsy in births in Western Australia in the 1980s. British Medical Journal 1993; 307:1239–43.

Raznahan A, Greenstein D, Lee NR, Clasen LS, Giedd JN. Prenatal growth in humans and postnatal brain maturation into late adolescence. Proceedings of the National Academy of Sciences; 2012; USA. 109:11366–71.

Taylor CL, de Groot J, Blair EM, Stanley FJ. The risk of cerebral palsy in survivors of multiple pregnancies with cofetal loss or death. American Journal of Obstetrics & Gynecology 2009; 201:e1–6.

Wilson RS. Risk and resilience in early mental development. Developmental Psychology 1985; 21:795–805.

Yokoyama Y, Shimizu T, Hayakawa K. Incidence of handicaps in multiple births and associated factors. Acta Geneticae Medicae et Gemellologiae 1995; 44:81–91.

Yokoyama Y, Shimizu T, Hayakawa K. Prevalence of cerebral palsy in twins, triplets, and quadruplets. International Journal of Epidemiology 1995; 24:943–8.

Complications in Multiple Pregnancy

Arias, F. Delayed delivery of multifetal pregnancies with premature rupture of membranes in the second trimester. American Journal of Obstetrics & Gynecology 1994; 170:1233–7.

Berry SM, Puder KS, Bottoms SF, Uckele JE, Romero R, Cotton DB. Comparison of intrauterine hematologic and biochemical values between twin pairs with and without stuck twin syndrome. American Journal of Obstetrics & Gynecology 1995; 172:1403–10.

Burgess JL, Unal ER, Nietert PJ, Newman RB. Risk of late preterm stillbirth and neonatal morbidity for monochorionic and dichorionic twins. American Journal of Obstetrics & Gynecology 2014; 210: 578–86.

Coonrod DV, Hickok DE, Zhu K, Easterling TR, Daling JR. Risk factors for preeclampsia in twin pregnancies: A population-based cohort study. Obstetrics & Gynecology 1995; 85:645–50.

Eberle AM, Levesque D, Vinzileos AM, et al. Placental pathology in discordant twins. American Journal of Obstetrics & Gynecology 1993; 169:931–5.

Gardner MO, Goldenberg RL, Cliver SP, Tucker JM, Nelson KG, Copper RL. The origin and outcome of preterm twin pregnancies. Obstetrics & Gynecology 1995; 85:553–7.

Gonzalez-Quintero VH, Luke B, O'Sullivan MJ, et al. Antenatal factors associated with significant birthweight discordancy in twins. American Journal of Obstetrics & Gynecology 2003; 189:813–17.

Li D, Liu L, Odouli R. Presence of depressive symptoms during early pregnancy and the risk of preterm delivery: A prospective cohort study. Human Reproduction 2009; 24:146–53.

Lipitz S, Achiron R, Zalel Y, Mendelson E, Tepperberg M, Gamzu R. Outcome of pregnancies with vertical transmission of primary cytomegalovirus infection. Obstetrics & Gynecology 2002; 100:428–33.

Luke B, Brown MB, Misiunas RB, Mauldin JG, Newman RB, Nugent C, et al. Elevated maternal glucose concentrations and placental infection in twin pregnancies. Journal of Reproductive Medicine 2005; 50:241–5.

Luke B, Nugent C, van de Ven C, et al. The association between maternal factors and perinatal outcomes in triplet pregnancies. American Journal of Obstetrics & Gynecology 2002; 187:752–7.

Meis PJ, Klebanoff H, Thom E, et al. Prevention of recurrent preterm delivery by 17 alpha-hydroxy-progesterone caproate. New England Journal of Medicine 2003; 348:2379–85.

Menard MK, Newman RB, Keenan A, Ebeling M. Prognostic significance of prior preterm twin delivery on subsequent singleton pregnancy. American Journal of Obstetrics & Gynecology 1996; 174:1429–32.

Michaels WH, Schreiber FR, Padgett RJ, Ager J, Pieper D. Ultrasound surveillance of the cervix in twin gestations: Management of cervical incompetency. Obstetrics & Gynecology 1991; 78:739–44.

Myles TD, Gooch J, Santolaya J. Obesity as an independent risk factor for infectious morbidity in patients who undergo cesarean delivery. Obstetrics & Gynecology 2002; 100:959–64.

Newman RB, Godsey RK, Ellings JM, Campbell BA, Eller DP, Miller C. Quantification of cervical change: Relationship to preterm delivery in the multifetal gestation. American Journal of Obstetrics & Gynecology 1991; 165:264–71.

Petrini JR, Dias T, McCormick MC, Massolo ML, Green NS, Escobar GJ. Increased risk of adverse neurological development for late preterm infants. Journal of Pediatrics 2009; 154:169–76.

Sattar N, Clark P, Holmes A, Lean MEJ, Walker I, Greer IA. Antenatal waist circumference and hypertension risk. Obstetrics & Gynecology 2001; 97:268–71.

Sattar N, Greer IA. Pregnancy complications and maternal cardiovascular risk: Opportunities for intervention and screening? British Medical Journal 2002; 325:157–60.

Sicuranza GB, Weinstein L, Saltzman DH, Farmakides G, Maulik D. Incidence of gestational diabetes in multifetal gestations. Journal of Maternal-Fetal Investigation 1997; 7:115–17.

Skentou C, Souka AP, To MS, Liao AW, Nicolaides KH. Prediction of preterm delivery in twins by cervical assessment at 23 weeks. Ultrasound in Obstetrics and Gynecology 2001;17:7–10.

Souka AP, Heath V, Flint S, et al. Cervical length at 23 weeks in twins in predicting spontaneous preterm delivery. Obstetrics & Gynecology 1999; 94:450–4.

Tarter JG, Khoury A, Barton JR, Jacques DL, Sibai BM. Demographic and obstetric factors influencing pregnancy outcome in twin gestations. American Journal of Obstetrics & Gynecology 2002; 186:910–12.

Wolf EJ, Mallozzi A, Rodis JF, Campbell WA, Vintzileos AM. The principal pregnancy complications resulting in preterm birth in singleton and twin gestations. Journal of Maternal-Fetal Medicine 1992; 1:206–12.

Xiong X, Fraser WD, Demianczuk NN. History of abortion, preterm, term birth, and risk of preeclampsia: A population-based study. American Journal of Obstetrics & Gynecology 2002; 187:1013–18.

Yukobowich E, Anteby EY, Cohen SM, Lavy Y, Granat M, Yagel S. Risk of fetal loss in twin pregnancies undergoing second trimester amniocentesis. Obstetrics & Gynecology 2001; 98:231–4.

Corticosteroids Administered Prenatally

American Congress of Obstetricians and Gynecologists (ACOG). Committee opinion no. 273. Antenatal corticosteroid therapy for fetal maturation. May 2003.

Bloom SL, Sheffield JS, McIntire DD, Leveno KJ. Antenatal dexamethasone and decreased birth weight. Obstetrics & Gynecology 2001; 97:485–90.

Elliott JP, Radin TG. The effect of corticosteroid administration on uterine activity and preterm labor in high-order multiple gestations. Obstetrics & Gynecology 1995; 85:250–4.

Hashimoto LN, Hornung RW, Lindsell CJ, Brewer DE, Donavan EF. Effects of antenatal glucocorticoids on outcomes of very low birth weight multifetal gestations. American Journal of Obstetrics & Gynecology 2002; 187:804–10.

National Institutes of Health Consensus Development Panel. Antenatal corticosteroids revisited: Repeat courses—National Institutes of Health consensus development conference statement; August 17–18, 2000. Obstetrics & Gynecology 2001; 8:144–50.

Schaap AH, Wolf H, Bruinse HW, Smolders-De Haas H, Van Ertbruggen I, Treffers PE. Effects of antenatal corticosteroid administration on mortality and long-term morbidity in early, preterm, growth-restricted infants. Obstetrics & Gynecology 2001; 97:954–60.

Thorp JA, Jones PG, Knox E, Clark RH. Does antenatal corticosteroid therapy affect birth weight and head circumference? Obstetrics & Gynecology 2002; 99:101–8.

Thorp JA, Jones PG, Peabody JL, Knox E, Clark RH. Effect of antenatal and postnatal corticosteroid therapy on weight gain and head circumference growth in the nursery. Obstetrics & Gynecology 2002; 99:109–15.

Walfisch A., Hallak M, Mazor M. Multiple courses of antenatal steroids: Risks and benefits. Obstetrics & Gynecology 2001; 98:491–7.

Costs of Infertility and Multiple Pregnancies

Callahan TL, Hall JE, Ettner SL, et al. The economic impact of multiple-gestation pregnancies and the contribution of assisted-reproduction techniques to their incidence. New England Journal of Medicine 1994; 331:244–9.

Chelmow D, Penzias AS, Kaufman G, Cetrulo C. Costs of triplet pregnancy. American Journal of Obstetrics & Gynecology 1995; 172:677–82.

Goldfarb JM, Austin C, Lisbona H, Peskin B, Clapp M. Cost-effectiveness of in vitro fertilization. Obstetrics & Gynecology 1996; 87:18–21.

Lemos EV, Zhang D, Van Voorhis BJ, Hu XH. Healthcare expenses associated with multiple vs singleton pregnancies in the United States. American Journal of Obstetrics & Gynecology 2013; 209:586. e1–11.

Luke B, Bigger HR, Leurgans S, Sietsema D. The cost of prematurity: A case-control study of twins versus singletons. American Journal of Public Health 1996; 86:809–14.

Luke B, Brown MB, Alexandre PK, Kinoshi T, O'Sullivan MJ, Martin D, et al. The cost of twin pregnancy: Maternal and neonatal factors. American Journal of Obstetrics & Gynecology 2005; 192:909–15.

Neuman PJ, Gharib SD, Weinstein MC. The cost of a successful delivery with in vitro fertilization. New England Journal of Medicine 1994; 331:239–43.

Diet and Nutrition During Pregnancy

Academy of Nutrition and Dietetics. Position paper. Nutrition and lifestyle for a healthy pregnancy outcome. Journal of the Academy of Nutrition and Dietetics 2014; 114:1099–1103.

Academy of Nutrition and Dietetics. Practice paper. Nutrition and lifestyle for a healthy pregnancy outcome. July 2014: 1–13.

Akre O, Boyd HA, Ahlgren M, Wilbrand K, Westergaard T, Hjalgrim H, et al. Maternal and gestational factors for hypospadias. Environmental Health Perspectives 2008; 116:1071–6.

American Diabetes Association. Nutrition recommendations and interventions for diabetes—2006. Diabetes Care 2006; 9:2140–57.

American Dietetic Association. Position of the American Dietetic Association: Health implications of dietary fiber. Journal of the American Dietetic Association 2008; 108:1716–31.

American Dietetic Association. Position of the American Dietetic Association: Nutrition and lifestyle for a healthy pregnancy outcome. Journal of the American Dietetic Association 2008; 108:553–61.

American Dietetic Association. Position of the American Dietetic Association: Obesity, reproduction, and pregnancy outcomes. Journal of the American Dietetic Association 2009; 109:918–27.

DiGirolamo AM, Ramirez-Zea M. Role of zinc in maternal and child mental health. American Journal of Clinical Nutrition 2009; 89(suppl):940S–5S.

Evert AB, Boucher JL. New diabetes nutrition therapy recommendations: What you need to know. Diabetes Spectrum 2014; 27:121–30.

Evert AB, Boucher JL, Cypress M, et al. Nutrition therapy recommendations for the management of adults with diabetes. Diabetes Care 2013; 36:3821–42.

Gidding SS, Lichtenstein AH, Faith MS, et al. Implementing American Heart Association pediatric and adult nutrition guidelines. Circulation 2009; 119:1161–75.

Goodnight W, Newman R; for the Society for Maternal-Fetal Medicine. Optimal nutrition for improved twin pregnancy outcome. Obstetrics & Gynecology 2009; 114:1121–34.

Institute of Medicine, Food and Nutrition Board. Dietary Reference Intakes: Energy, Carbohydrates, Fiber, Fat, Fatty Acids, Cholesterol, Protein and Amino Acids. Washington, DC: National Academies Press; 2002.

Lichtenstein AH, Appel LJ, Brands M, et al. Diet and lifestyle recommendations revision 2006. A scientific statement from the American Heart Association Nutrition Committee. Circulation 2006; 114:82–96.

Ludwig DS. The glycemic index: Physiological mechanisms relating to obesity, diabetes, and cardiovascular disease. Journal of the American Medical Association 2002; 287:2414–23.

Luke B. The evidence linking maternal nutrition and prematurity. Journal of Perinatal Medicine. 2005; 33:500–5.

Luke B. Nutrition for multiples. Multiple pregnancy symposium. Newman RB, editor. Clinical Obstetrics and Gynecology. September 2015; 58:585–610.

Luke B. Nutrition in multiple gestations. Clinics in Perinatology 2005; 32:403–29.

Morrison JA, Glueck CJ, Wang P. Dietary trans fatty acid intake is associated with increased fetal loss. Fertility and Sterility 2008; 90:385–90.

North K, Golding J; ALSPAC Team. A maternal vegetarian diet in pregnancy is associated with hypospadias. British Journal of Urology International 2000; 85:107–13.

Palan PR, Mikhail MS, Romney SL. Placental and serum levels of carotenoids in preeclampsia. Obstetrics & Gynecology 2001; 98:459–62.

Pereira MA, Jacobs DR, Van Horn L, Slattery ML, Kartashov AI, Ludwig DS. Dairy consumption, obesity, and the insulin resistance syndrome in young adults: The CARDIA study. Journal of the American Medical Association 2002; 287:2081–9.

Roberts JM, Balk JL, Bodnar LM, Belizán JM, Bergel E, Martinez A. Nutrient involvement in preeclampsia. Journal of Nutrition 2003; 133:1684S–92S.

Ronnenberg AG, Goldman MB, Chen D, Aitken IW, Willett WC, Selhub J, et al. Preconception folate and vitamin B_6 status and clinical spontaneous abortion in chinese women. Obstetrics & Gynecology 2002; 100:107–13.

Wheeler ML, Dunbar SA, Jaacks LM, et al. Macronutrients, food groups, and eating patterns in the management of diabetes. Diabetes Care 2012; 35:434–45.

Exercise, Work, and Physical Activity During Pregnancy

American College of Obstetrics and Gynecologists. Opinion no. 267. Exercise during pregnancy and the postpartum period. Obstetrics & Gynecology 2002; 99:171–3.

Bonzini M, Coggon D, Palmer KT. Risk of prematurity, low birthweight and pre-eclampsia in relation to working hours and physical activity: A systematic review. Occupational and Environmental Medicine 2007; 64:228–43.

Brett KM, Strogatz DS, Savitz DA. Employment, job strain, and preterm delivery among women in North Carolina. American Journal of Public Health 1997; 87:199–204.

Campbell MK, Mottola MF. Recreational exercise and occupational activity during pregnancy and birth weight: A case-control study. American Journal of Obstetrics & Gynecology 2001; 184:403–8.

Croteau A, Marcoux S, Brisson C. Work activity in pregnancy, preventive measures, and the risk of preterm delivery. American Journal of Epidemiology 2007; 166:951–65.

Fortier I, Marcoux S, Brisson J. Maternal work during pregnancy and the risks of delivering a small-for-gestational-age or preterm infant. Scandinavian Journal of Work Environment & Health 1995; 21:412–18.

Gabbe SG, Turner LP. Reproductive hazards of the American lifestyle: Work during pregnancy. American Journal of Obstetrics & Gynecology 1997; 176:826–32.

Haelterman E, Marcoux S, Croteau A, Dramaix M. Population-based study on occupational risk factors for preeclampsia and gestational hypertension. Scandinavian Journal of Work Environment & Health 2007; 33:304–7.

Hatch M, Ji BT, Shy XO, Susser M. Do standing, lifting, climbing, or long hours of work during pregnancy have an effect on fetal growth? Epidemiology 1997; 8:530–6.

Lawson CC, Whelan EA, Hibert EN, Grajewski B, Spiegelman D, Rich-Edwards JW. Occupational factors and risk of preterm birth in nurses. American Journal of Obstetrics & Gynecology 2009; 200: Article no. 51.e1.

Luke B, Avni M, Min L, Misiunas R. Work and pregnancy: The role of fatigue and the "second shift" on antenatal morbidity. American Journal of Obstetrics & Gynecology 1999; 181(5):1172–9.

Luke B, Mamelle N, Keith L, Munoz F, Minogue J, Papiernik E, et al. The association between occupational factors and preterm birth: A United States nurses' survey. American Journal of Obstetrics & Gynecology 1995; 173 (3 Pt. 1):849–62.

Magann EF, Evans SF, Weitz B, Newnham J. Antepartum, intrapartum, and neonatal significance of exercise on healthy low-risk pregnant working women. Obstetrics & Gynecology 2002; 99: 466–72.

Meyer JD, Nichols GH, Warren N, Reisine S. Maternal occupation and risk for low birth weight delivery: Assessment using state birth registry data. Journal of Occupational and Environmental Medicine 2008; 50:306–15.

Mottola MF. Exercise prescription for overweight and obese women: Pregnancy and postpartum. Obstetrics and Gynecology Clinics of North America 2009; 36:301–20.

Mozurkewich EL, Luke B, Avni M, Wolfe FM. Working conditions and adverse pregnancy outcomes: A meta-analysis. Obstetrics & Gynecology 2000; 95(4):623–35.

Naeye RL, Peters EC. Working during pregnancy: Effects on the fetus. Pediatrics 1982; 69:724–7.

Newman RB, Gill PJ, Katz M. Uterine activity during pregnancy in ambulatory patients: Comparison of singleton and twin gestations. American Journal of Obstetrics & Gynecology 1986; 154:530–1.

Newman RB, Gill PJ, Wittreich P, Katz M. Maternal perception of prelabor uterine activity. Obstetrics & Gynecology 1986; 68:765–9.

Newman RB, Goldenberg RL, Moawad AH, Iams JD, Meis PJ, Das A, et al. Occupational fatigue and preterm premature rupture of membranes. American Journal of Obstetrics & Gynecology 2001; 184:438–46.

Niedhammer I, O'Mahony D, Daly S, Morrison JJ, Kelleher CC. Occupational predictors of pregnancy outcomes in Irish working women in the Lifeways cohort. British Journal of Obstetrics and Gynecology 2009; 116:943–52.

Pompeii LA, Savitz DA, Evenson KR, Rogers B, McMahon M. Physical exertion at work and the risk of preterm delivery and small-for-gestational age birth. Obstetrics & Gynecology 2005; 106:1279–88.

Saurel-Cubizolles MJ, Zeitlin J, Lelong N, Papiernik E, Di Renzo GC, Breart G. Employment, working conditions, and preterm birth: Results from the Europop case-control survey. Journal of Epidemiology and Community Health 2004; 58:395–401.

Savitz DA, Olshan AF, Gallagher K. Maternal occupation and pregnancy outcome. Epidemiology 1996; 7:269–74.

Schneider KTM, Bollinger A, Huch A, Huch R. The oscillating "vena cava syndrome" during quiet standing—An unexpected observation in late pregnancy. British Journal of Obstetrics and Gynaecology 1984; 91:766–80.

Spinillo A, Capuzzo E, Baltaro F, Piazzi G, Nicola S, Iasci A. The effect of work activity in pregnancy on the risk of fetal growth retardation. Acta Obstetricia et Gynecologica Scandinavica 1996; 75:531–6.

Spinillo A, Capuzzo E, Colonna L, Piazzi G, Nicola S, Baltaro F. The effect of work activity in pregnancy on the risk of severe preeclampsia. Australian & New Zealand Journal of Obstetrics and Gynaecology 1995; 35:380–5.

Walker SP, Permezel M, Brennecke SP, Ugoni AM, Higgins JR. Blood pressure in late pregnancy and work outside the home. Obstetrics & Gynecology 2001; 97:361–5.

Fetal Growth and Birthweight of Multiples

Bukowski R, Smith GCS, Malone FD, Ball RH, Nyberg DA, Comstock CH, et al. Fetal growth in early pregnancy and risk of delivering low birthweight infant: Prospective cohort study. British Medical Journal 2007; 334:836–40.

Elster AD, Bleyl JL, Craven TE. Birthweight standards for triplets under modern obstetric care in the United States, 1984–1989. Obstetrics & Gynecology 1991; 77:387–93.

Hediger ML, Luke B, Gonzalez-Quintero VH, Witter FR, Mauldin J, Newman RB. Fetal growth rates and very preterm birth of twins. American Journal of Obstetrics & Gynecology 2005; 193:1498–507.

Hediger ML, Luke B, van de Ven C, Nugent C. Mid-upper arm circumference (MUAC) changes in late pregnancy predict fetal growth in twins. Twin Research and Human Genetics 2005; 8:267–70.

Jones JS, Newman RB, Miller MC. Cross-sectional analysis of triplet birthweight. American Journal of Obstetrics & Gynecology 1991; 164:135–40.

Min S-J, Luke B, Gillespie B, et al. Birthweight references for twins. American Journal of Obstetrics & Gynecology 2000; 182:1250–57.

Min S-J, Luke B, Min L, Misiunas R, Nugent C, van de Ven C, et al. Birthweight references for triplets. American Journal of Obstetrics & Gynecology 2004; 191:809–18.

Newman RB, Jones JS, Miller MC. Influence of clinical variables on triplet birthweight. Acta Geneticae Medicae et Gemellologiae 1991; 40:173–79.

Fetal Loss and Fetal Reduction

Alexander JM, Hammond KR, Steinkampf MP. Multifetal reduction of high-order multiple pregnancy: Comparison of obstetrical outcome with nonreduced twin gestations. Fertility and Sterility 1995; 64:1201–3.

Berkowitz RL, Lynch L. Selective reduction: An unfortunate misnomer. American Journal of Obstetrics & Gynecology 1990; 75:873–4.

Berkowitz RL, Lynch L, Chitkara U, Wilkins IA, Mehalek KE, Alvarez E. Selective reduction of multifetal pregnancies in the first trimester. New England Journal of Medicine 1988; 318:1043–7.

Berkowitz RL, Lynch L, Stone J, Alvarez M. The current status of multi-fetal pregnancy reduction. American Journal of Obstetrics & Gynecology 1996; 174:1265–72.

Bollen N, Camus M, Tournaye H, Wisanto A, Van Steirteghem AC, Devroey P. Embryo reduction in triplet pregnancies after assisted procreation: A comparative study. Fertility and Sterility 1993; 60:504–9.

Boulot P, Hedon B, Pelliccia G, Peray P, Laffargue F, Viala JL. Effects of selective reduction in triplet gestation: A comparative study of eighty cases managed with and without this procedure. Fertility and Sterility 1993; 60:497–503.

Brandes JM, Itskovitz J, Scher A, Gershoni-Baruch R. The physical and mental development of co-sibs surviving selective reduction of multifetal pregnancies. Human Reproduction 1990; 5:1014–17.

Cheang C-U, Huang L-S, Lee T-H, Liu C-H, Shih Y-T, Lee M-S. A comparison of the outcomes between twin and reduced twin pregnancies produced through assisted reproduction. Fertility and Sterility 2007; 88:47–52.

Depp R, Macones GA, Rosenn MF, Turzo E, Wapner RJ, Weinblatt VJ. Multifetal pregnancy reduction: Evaluation of fetal growth in the remaining twins. American Journal of Obstetrics & Gynecology 1996; 174:1233–40.

Dickey RP, Taylor SN, Lu PY, Sartor BM, Storment JM, Rye PH, et al. Spontaneous reduction of multiple pregnancy: Incidence and effect on outcome. American Journal of Obstetrics & Gynecology 2002; 186:77–83.

Dimitriou G, Pharoah POD, Nicolaides KH, Greenough A. Cerebral palsy in triplet pregnancies with and without iatrogenic reduction. European Journal of Pediatrics 2004; 163:449–51.

Evans MI, Berkowitz RL, Wapner RJ, et al. Improvement in outcomes of multifetal pregnancy reduction with increased experience. American Journal of Obstetrics & Gynecology 2001; 184:97–103.

Evans MI, Dommergues M, Wapner RJ, et al. Efficacy of transabdominal multifetal pregnancy reduction: Collaborative experience among the world's largest centers. American Journal of Obstetrics & Gynecology 1993; 82:61–6.

Evans MI, Fletcher JC, Zador IE, Newton BW, Quigg MH, Struyk CD. Selective first-trimester termination in octuplet and quadruplet pregnancies: Clinical and ethical issues. Obstetrics & Gynecology 1988; 71:289–96.

Groutz A, Yovel I, Amit A, Yaron Y, Azem F, Lessing JB. Pregnancy outcome after multifetal pregnancy reduction to twins compared to spontaneously conceived twins. Human Reproduction 1996; 11:1334–6.

Haning RV, Seifer DB, Wheeler CA, Frishman GN, Silver H, Pierce DJ. Effects of fetal number and multifetal reduction on length of in vitro fertilization pregnancies. Obstetrics and Gynecology 1996; 87:964–8.

Luke B. Reducing fetal deaths in multiple births: Optimal birthweights and gestational ages for infants of twin and triplet births. Acta Geneticae Medicae et Gemellologiae 1996; 45:333–48.

Luke B, Brown MB, Grainger DA, Stern JE, Klein N, Cedars MI. The effect of early fetal losses on singleton assisted-conception pregnancy outcomes. Fertility and Sterility 2009; 91:2578–85.

Luke B, Brown MB, Grainger DA, Stern JE, Klein N, Cedars MI. The effect of early fetal losses on twin assisted-conception pregnancy outcomes. Fertility and Sterility 2009; 91:2586–92.

Lynch L, Berkowitz RL, Stone J, Alvarez M, Lapinski R. Preterm delivery after selective termination in twin pregnancies. Obstetrics and Gynecology 1996; 87:366–9.

Macones GA, Schemmer G, Pritts E, Weinblatt B, Wapne R Jr. Multifetal reduction of triplets to twins improves perinatal outcome. American Journal of Obstetrics & Gynecology 1993; 169:982–6.

Melgar CA, Rosenfeld DL, Rawlinson K, Greenberg M. Perinatal outcome after multifetal reduction to twins compared with nonreduced multiple gestations. Obstetrics & Gynecology 1991; 78:763–7.

Morrison JA, Glueck CJ, Wang P. Dietary trans fatty acid intake is associated with increased fetal loss. Fertility and Sterility 2008; 90:385–90.

Porreco RP, Burke MS, Hendrix ML. Multifetal reduction of triplets and pregnancy outcome. Obstetrics & Gynecology 1991; 78:335–9.

Rebarber A, Carreno CA, Lipkind H, Funai EF, Maturi J, Kuczynski E, et al. Cervical length after multifetal pregnancy reduction in remaining twin gestations. American Journal of Obstetrics & Gynecology 2001; 185:1113–17.

Silver RK, Helfand MT, Russell TL, Ragin A, Sholl JS, MacGregor SN. Multifetal reduction increases the risk of preterm delivery and fetal growth restriction in twins: A case-control study. Fertility and Sterility 1997; 67:30–3.

Smith-Levitan M, Kowalik A, Birnholz J, Skupski DW, Hutson JM, Chervenak FA, et al. Selective reduction of multifetal pregnancies to twins improves outcome over nonreduced triplet gestations. American Journal of Obstetrics & Gynecology 1996; 175:878–82.

Stone J, Ferrara L, Kamrath J, et al. Contemporary outcomes with the latest 1000 cases of multifetal pregnancy reduction (MPR). American Journal of Obstetrics & Gynecology 2008; 199:406.e1–e4.

Folate, Vitamins, and Antioxidants

Catov JM, Nohr EA, Bodnar LM, Knudson VK, Olsen SF, Olsen J. Association of periconceptional multivitamin use with reduced risk of preeclampsia among normal-weight women in the Danish National Birth Cohort. American Journal of Epidemiology 2009; 169:1304–11.

Chappell LC, Seed PT, Briley A, Kelly FJ, Hunt BJ, Charnock-Jones SC, et al. A longitudinal study of biochemical variables in women at risk of preeclampsia. American Journal of Obstetrics & Gynecology 2002; 187:127–36.

Chappell LC, Seed PT, Kelly FJ, Briley A, Hunt BJ, Charnock-Jones SC, et al. Vitamin C and E supplementation in women at risk of preeclampsia is associated with changes in indices of oxidative stress and placental function. American Journal of Obstetrics & Gynecology 2002; 187:777–84.

Kim H, Hwang J-Y, Ha E-H, et al. Association of maternal folate nutrition and serum C-reactive protein concentrations with gestational age at delivery. European Journal of Clinical Nutrition 2011; 65:350–6.

Molloy AM, Kirke PN, Troendle JF, et al. Maternal vitamin B_{12} status and risk of neural tube defects in a population with high neural tube defect prevalence and no folic acid fortification. Pediatrics 2009; 123:917–23.

Osterhues A, Holzgreve W, Michels KB. Shall we put the world on folate? Lancet 2009; 374:959–61.

Thompson JR, Gerald PF, Willoughby MLN, Armstrong BK. Maternal folate supplementation in pregnancy and protection against acute lymphoblastic leukaemia in childhood: A case-control study. Lancet 2001; 358:1935–40.

Ray JG, Meier C, Vermeulen MJ, Boss S, Wyatt PR, Cole DEC. Association of neural tube defects and folic acid food fortification in Canada. Lancet 2002; 360:2047–8.

Scholl TO, Hediger ML, Bendich A, Schall JI, Smith WK, Krueger PM. Use of multivitamin/mineral prenatal supplements: Influence on the outcome of pregnancy. American Journal of Epidemiology 1997; 146:134–41.

Scholl TO, Hediger ML, Schall JI, Khoo C-S, Fischer RL. Dietary and serum folate: Their influence on the outcome of pregnancy. American Journal of Clinical Nutrition 1996; 63:520–5.

Spinnato JA, Freire S, Pinto E, et al. Antioxidant therapy to prevent preeclampsia: a randomized controlled trial. Obstetrics & Gynecology 2007; 110: 1311–18.

Wald N. Prevention of neural tube defects: Results of the Medical Research Council Vitamin Study. Lancet 1991; 338:131–7.

Xu H, Perez-Cuevas R, Xiong X, et al. An international trial of antioxidants in the prevention of preeclampsia (INTAPP). American Journal of Obstetrics & Gynecology 2010; 202:239.e1–10.

Glucose and the Glycemic Index

Foster-Powell K, Holt SHA, Brand-Miller JC. International table of glycemic index and glycemic load values: 2002. American Journal of Clinical Nutrition 2002; 76:5–56.

Jenkins DJA, Wolever TMS, Taylor RH, Barker H, Fielden H, Baldwin JM, et al. Glycemic index of foods: A physiological basis for carbohydrate exchange. American Journal of Clinical Nutrition 1981; 34:362–6.

Jovanovic L, Knopp RH, Kim H, Cefalu WT, Zhu X-D, Lee YJ, et al. Elevated pregnancy losses at high and low extremes of maternal glucose in early normal and diabetic pregnancy. Diabetes Care 2005; 28:1113–17.

Luke B, Brown MB, Misiunas RB, Mauldin JG, Newman RB, Nugent C, et al. Elevated maternal glucose concentrations and placental infection in twin pregnancies. Journal of Reproductive Medicine 2005; 50:241–5.

Parretti E, Carignani L, Cioni R, Bartoli E, Borri P, La Torre P, et al. Sonographic evaluation of fetal growth and body composition in women with different degrees of normal glucose metabolism. Diabetes Care 2003; 26:2741–8.

Scholl TO, Sowers MF, Chen X, Lenders C. Maternal glucose concentration influences fetal growth, gestation, and pregnancy complications. American Journal of Epidemiology 2001; 154:514–20.

Shaw GM, Carmichael SL, Laurent C, Siega-Riz AM; the National Birth Defects Prevention Study. Periconceptional glycaemic load and intake of sugars and their association with neural tube defects in offspring. Paediatric and Perinatal Epidemiology 2008; 22:514–19.

Shaw GM, Quach T, Nelson V, Carmichael SL, Schaffer DM, Selvin S, et al. Neural tube defects associated with maternal periconceptional dietary intake of simple sugars and glycemic index. American Journal of Clinical Research 2003; 78:972–8.

Yazdy MM, Liu S, Mitchell AA, Werler MM. Maternal dietary glycemic intake and the risk of neural tube defects. American Journal of Epidemiology 2009; 171:407–14.

Incidence of Multiple Pregnancy

Fuster V, Zuluaga P, Colantonio S, de Blas C. Factors associated with recent increase of multiple births in Spain. Twin Research and Human Genetics 2008; 11:70–6.

Imaizumi Y. Trends of twinning rates in ten countries, 1972–1996. Acta Geneticae Medicae et Gemellolgiae 1997; 46:209–18.

Jewell SE, Yip R. Increasing trends in plural births in the United States. Obstetrics & Gynecology 1995; 85:229–32.

Kiely JL, Kleinman JC, Kiely M. Triplets and higher-order multiple births. American Journal of Diseases of Children 1992; 146:862–8.

Luke B. The changing pattern of multiple births in the United States: Maternal and infant characteristics, 1973 and 1990. Obstetrics & Gynecology 1994; 84:101–6.

Luke B, Martin JA. The rise in multiple births in the United States: Who, what, when, where, and why. Clinics in Obstetrics and Gynecology 2004; 47:118–33.

Martin JA, Hamilton BE, Osterman MJK, Curtin SC, Mathews TJ. Births: Final data for 2013. National Vital Statistics Report, vol. 64, no. 1, January 15, 2015.

Martin JA, MacDorman MF, Mathews TJ. Triplet births: Trends and outcomes, 1971–94. National Center for Health Statistics. Vital and Health Statistics. Vol. 21, no. 55. Hyattsville, MD: National Center for Health Statistics; 1997.

Martin JA, Taffel SM. Current and future impact of rising multiple birth ratios on low birthweight. Statistical Bulletin 1995; April–June:10–18.

Mushinski M. Trends in multiple births. Statistical Bulletin 1994; July–September:28–35.

Pison G, D'Addato AV. Frequency of twin births in developed countries. Twin Research and Human Genetics 2006; 9:250–9.

Reynolds MA, Schieve LA, Martin JA, Jeng G, Macaluso M. Trends in multiple births conceived using assisted reproductive technology, United States, 1997–2000. Pediatrics 2003; 111:1159–62.

Russell RB, Petrini JR, Damus K, Mattison DR, Schwarz RH. The changing epidemiology of multiple births in the United States. Obstetrics & Gynecology 2003; 101:129–35.

Taffel SM. Health and demographic characteristics of twin births: United States, 1988. DHHS pub. no. (PHS) 92–1928. Vital and Health Statistics, 1992; series 21, no. 50.

Wilcox LS, Kiely JL, Melvin CL, Martin MC. Assisted reproductive technologies: Estimates of their contribution to multiple births and newborn hospital days in the United States. Fertility and Sterility 1996; 65:361–6.

Infant Morbidity and Mortality

Buekens P, Wilcox A. Why do small twins have a lower mortality rate than small singletons? American Journal of Obstetrics & Gynecology 1993; 168:937–41.

Delbaere I, Goetgeluk S, Derom C, De Bacquer D, De Sutter P, Temmerman M. Umbilical cord anomalies are more frequent in twins after assisted reproduction. Human Reproduction 2007; 22:2763–7.

Fellman J, Eriksson AW. Estimation of the stillbirth rate in twin pairs according to zygosity. Twin Research and Human Genetics 2007; 10:508–13.

Fowler MG, Kleinman JC, Kiely JL, Kessel SS. Double jeopardy: Twin infant mortality in the United States, 1983 and 1984. American Journal of Obstetrics & Gynecology 1991; 165:15–22.

Franche RL. Psychologic and obstetric predictors of couples' grief during pregnancy after miscarriage or perinatal death. Obstetrics & Gynecology 2001; 97:597–602.

Hutzal CE, Boyle EM, Kenyon SL, et al. Use of antibiotics for the treatment of preterm parturition and prevention of neonatal morbidity: A metaanalysis. American Journal of Obstetrics & Gynecology 2008; 199:620.e1–e8.

Joseph KS, Marcoux S, Ohlsson A, et al. Preterm birth, stillbirth and infant mortality among triplet births in Canada, 1985–96. Paediatric and Perinatal Epidemiology 2002; 16:141–8.

Kaufman GE, Malone FD, Harvey-Wilkes KB, Chelmow D, Penzias AS, D'Alton ME. Neonatal morbidity and mortality associated with triplet pregnancy. Obstetrics & Gynecology 1998; 91:342–8.

Kiely JL. The epidemiology of perinatal mortality in multiple births. Bulletin of the New York Academy of Medicine 1990; 66:618–37.

Kiely JL. Time trends in neonatal mortality among twins and singletons in New York City, 1968–1986. Acta Geneticae Medicae et Gemellologiae 1991; 40:303–9.

Kiely JL, Kleinman JC, Kiely M. Triplets and higher-order multiple births: Time trends and infant mortality. American Journal of Diseases of Children 1992; 146:862–8.

Kilpatrick SJ, Jackson R, Croughan-Minihane MS. Perinatal mortality in twins and singletons matched for gestational age at delivery at thirty weeks or more. Obstetrics & Gynecology 1996; 174:66–71.

Luke B, Brown MB. The changing risk of infant mortality by gestation, plurality, and race: 1989–91 versus 1999–01. Pediatrics 2006; December; 118:2488–97.

Luke B, Brown MB. The effect of plurality and gestation on the prevention or postponement of infant mortality: 1989–1991 versus 1999–2001. Twin Research and Human Genetics 2007; June, 10: 514–20.

Luke B, Brown MB. Maternal morbidity and infant mortality in twin versus triplet and quadruplet pregnancies. American Journal of Obstetrics & Gynecology 2008; 198:401.e1–e10.

Luke B, Brown MB. Maternal risk factors for potential maltreatment deaths among healthy singleton and twin infants. Twin Research and Human Genetics 2007; October; 10:778–85.

Luke B, Minogue J. Contribution of gestational age and birthweight to perinatal viability in singletons versus twins. Journal of Maternal-Fetal Medicine 1994; 3:263–74.

Pharoah POD, Platt MJ. Sudden infant death syndrome in twins and singletons. Twin Research and Human Genetics 2007; 10:644–8.

Powers WF, Kiely JL. The risks confronting twins: A national perspective. American Journal of Obstetrics & Gynecology 1994; 170:456–61.

Powers WF, Wampler NS. Further defining the risks confronting twins. American Journal of Obstetrics & Gynecology 1996; 175:1522–8.

Zhang J, Bowes WA, Grey TW, McMahon MJ. Twin delivery and neonatal and infant mortality: A population-based study. Obstetrics & Gynecology 1996; 88:593–8.

Infertility Treatments and Multiple Pregnancy

Bernasko J, Lynch L, Lapinski R, Berkowitz RL. Twin pregnancies conceived by assisted reproductive techniques: Maternal and neonatal outcomes. Obstetrics & Gynecology 1997; 89:368–72.

Bonduelle M, Liebaers I, Deketelaere V, Derde M-P, Camus M, Devroey P, et al. Neonatal data on a cohort of 2,889 infants born after ICSI (1991–1999) and of 2,995 infants born after IVF (1983–1999). Human Reproduction 2002; 17:671–94.

Centers for Disease Control and Prevention. Contribution of assisted reproductive technology and ovulation-inducing drugs to triplet and higher-order multiple births—United States, 1980–1997. Morbidity and Mortality Weekly Report 2000; 49(24):535–8.

Centers for Disease Control and Prevention. Use of assisted reproductive technology surveillance—United States, 2006. Morbidity and Mortality Weekly Report 2009; vol. 58, no. SS-5:1–25.

Centers for Disease Control and Prevention; American Society for Reproductive Medicine; Society for Assisted Reproductive Technology. 2006 Assisted reproductive technology success rates: National summary and fertility clinic reports. Washington, DC: US Dept. of Health and Human Services; 2008.

Chan OTM, Mannino FL, Benirsschke K. A retrospective analysis of placentas from twin pregnancies derived from assisted reproductive technology. Twin Research and Human Genetics 2007; 10: 385–93.

Chandra A, Copen CE, Stephen EH. Infertility service use in the United States: Data from the National Survey of Family Growth, 1982–2010. National Health Statistics Report, no. 73, January 22, 2014.

Fujimoto VY, Luke B, Brown MB, Jain T, Armstrong A, Grainger DA, et al. Racial and ethnic disparities in assisted reproductive technology (ART) outcomes in the United States. Fertility and Sterility (forthcoming).

Haggarty P, McCallum H, McBain H, Andrews K, Duthie S, McNeill G, et al. Effect of B vitamins and genetics on success of in-vitro fertilization: Prospective cohort study. Lancet 2006; 367: 1513–19.

Helmerhorst FM, Perquin DAM, Donker D, Keirse MJNC. Perinatal outcome of singletons and twins after assisted conception: A systematic review of controlled studies. British Medical Journal 2004; doi: 10.1136/bmj.37957.560278.EE.

Källen B, Olausson PO, Nygren KG. Neonatal outcome in pregnancies from ovarian stimulation. Obstetrics & Gynecology 2002; 100:414–19.

Lambalk CB, van Hooff M. Natural versus induced twinning and pregnancy outcome: A Dutch nationwide survey of primiparous dizygotic twin deliveries. Fertility and Sterility 2001; 75:731–6.

Luke B, Brown MB, Gonzalez-Quintero VH, Nugent C, Witter FR, Newman RB. Risk factors for adverse outcomes in spontaneous vs. assisted-conception twin pregnancies. Fertility and Sterility 2004; 81:315–19.

Luke B, Brown MB, Grainger DA, Stern JE, Klein N, Cedars M. The effect of early fetal losses on singleton assisted-conception pregnancy outcomes. Fertility and Sterility 2009; 91:2578–85.

Luke B, Brown MB, Grainger DA, Stern JE, Klein N, Cedars M. The effect of early fetal losses on twin assisted-conception pregnancy outcomes. Fertility and Sterility 2009; 91:2586–92.

Luke B, Brown MB, Wantman E, Baker VL, Grow DR, Stern JE. Second try: Who returns for additional assisted reproductive technology treatment and the effect of a prior assisted reproductive technology birth. Fertility and Sterility 2013; 100:1580–4.

Luke B, Nugent C, van de Ven C, Martin D, O'Sullivan MJ, Eardley S, et al. The association between maternal factors and perinatal outcomes in triplet pregnancies. American Journal of Obstetrics & Gynecology 2002; 187:752–7.

Romundstad LB, Romundstad PR, Sunde A, von Düring V, Skjærven R, Gunnell D, et al. Effects of technology or maternal factors on perinatal outcome after assisted fertilization: A population-based cohort study. Lancet 2008; 372:737–43.

Romundstad LB, Romundstad PR, Sunde A, von Düring V, Skjærven R, Vatten LJ. Increased risk of placenta previa in pregnancies following IVF/ICSI: A comparison of ART and non-ART pregnancies in the same mother. Human Reproduction 2006; 21:2353–8.

Seoud MAF, Toner JP, Kruithoff C, Muasher SJ. Outcome of twin, triplet, and quadruplet in vitro fertilization pregnancies: The Norfolk experience. Fertility and Sterility 1992; 57:825–34.

Skupski DW, Nelson S, Kowalik A, et al. Multiple gestations from in vitro fertilization: Successful implantation alone is not associated with subsequent preeclampsia. American Journal of Obstetrics & Gynecology 1996; 175:1029–32.

Sunderam S, Kissin DM, Crawford S, Folger SG, Jamieson DJ, Warner L, et al. Assisted reproductive technology surveillance—United States, 2012. Morbidity and Mortality Weekly Report, vol. 64, no. 6, August 14, 2015; 1–29.

Wang YA, Sullivan EA, Black D, Dean J, Bryant J, Chapman M. Preterm birth and low birthweight after assisted reproductive technology-related pregnancy in Australia between 1996 and 2000. Fertility and Sterility 2005; 83:1650–8.

Wilcox LS, Kiely JL, Melvin CL, Martin MC. Assisted reproductive technologies: Estimates of their contribution to multiple births and newborn hospital stays in the United States. Fertility and Sterility 1996; 65:361–6.

Iron and Zinc

Merialdi M, Caulfield LE, Zavaleta N, Figueroa A, DiPietro JA. Adding zinc to prenatal iron and folate tablets improves fetal neurobehavioral development. American Journal of Obstetrics & Gynecology 1998; 180:483–90.

Plum LM, Rink L, Haase H. The essential toxin: Impact of zinc on human health. International Journal of Environmental Research and Public Health 2010; 7:1342–65.

Scholl TO. Iron status during pregnancy: Setting the stage for mother and infant. American Journal of Clinical Nutrition 2005; 81 (Suppl):1218S–22S.

Scholl TO, Hediger ML, Fischer RL, Shearer JW. Anemia vs. iron deficiency: Increased risk of preterm delivery in a prospective study. American Journal of Clinical Nutrition 1992; 55:985–8.

Scholl TO, Hediger ML, Schall JI, Fischer RL, Khoo C-S. Low zinc intake during pregnancy: Its association with preterm and very preterm delivery. American Journal of Clinical Nutrition 1993; 137:1115–24.

Wellinghausen N, Kirchner H, Rink L. The immunobiology of zinc. Immunology Today 1997; 18: 519–21.

Zimmerman MB, Hurrell RF. Nutritional iron deficiency. Lancet 2007; 370:511–20.

Male Gender

Divon MY, Ferber A, Nisell H, Westgren M. Male Gender Predisposes to Prolongation of Pregnancy. American Journal of Obstetrics & Gynecology 2002; 187:1081–3.

Luke B, Brown MB, Grainger DA, Baker VL, Ginsburg E, Stern JE. The sex-ratio of singleton offspring in assisted-conception pregnancies. Fertility and Sterility 2009; 92:1579–85.

Luke B, Hediger ML, Min S-J, Brown MB, Misiunas RB, Gonzalez-Quintero VH, et al. Gender mix in twins and fetal growth, length of gestation, and adult cancer risk. Paediatric and Perinatal Epidemiology 2005; 19(Suppl 1):41–7.

Steier JA, Ulstein M, Myking OL. Human chorionic gonadotropin and testosterone in normal and preeclamptic pregnancies in relation to fetal sex. Obstetrics & Gynecology 2002; 100:552–6.

Maternal Age, Race, and Ethnicity

Fujimoto VY, Luke B, Brown MB, Jain T, Armstrong A, Grainger DA, et al. Racial and ethnic disparities in assisted reproductive technology (ART) outcomes in the United States. Fertility and Sterility (forthcoming).

Gonzalez-Quintero VH, Tolaymat L, Luke B, Gonzalez-Garcia A, Duthely L, O'Sullivan MJ, et al. Outcome of pregnancies among Hispanics: Revisiting the epidemiologic paradox. Journal of Reproductive Medicine 2006; 51:10–14.

Haebe J, Martin J, Tekepety F, Tummon I, Sheperd K. Success of intrauterine insemination in women aged 40–42 years. Fertility and Sterility 2002; 78:29–33.

Luke B, Brown MB. Contemporary risks of maternal morbidity and adverse outcomes with increasing maternal age and plurality. Fertility and Sterility 2007; 88:283–93.

Luke B, Brown MB. Elevated risks of pregnancy complications and adverse outcomes with increasing maternal age. Human Reproduction 2007; 22:1264–72.

Luke B, Brown MB, Misiunas RB, Gonzalez-Quintero VH, Nugent C, van de Ven C, et al. The Hispanic paradox in twin pregnancies. Twin Research and Human Genetics 2005; 8:532–7.

Paulson RJ, Boostanfar R, Saadat P, et al. Pregnancy in the sixth decade of life. Journal of the American Medical Association 2002; 288:2320–3.

Rolett A, Kiely JL. Maternal sociodemographic characteristics as risk factors for preterm birth in twins versus singletons. Paediatric and Perinatal Epidemiology 2000; 14:211–18.

Zhang J, Meikle S, Grainger DA, Trumble A. Multifetal pregnancy in older women and perinatal outcomes. Fertility and Sterility 2002; 78:562–8.

Maternal and Paternal Obesity

Baeten JM, Bukusi EA, Lambe M. Pregnancy complications and outcomes among overweight and obese nulliparous women. American Journal of Public Health 2001; 91:436–40.

Blomberg MI, Källen B. Maternal obesity and morbid obesity: The risk for birth defects in the offspring. Birth Defects Research (Part A) 2010; 88:35–40.

Catalano PM, Ehrenberg HM. The short- and long-term implications of maternal obesity on the mother and her offspring. British Journal of Obstetrics and Gynaecology 2006; 113:1126–33.

Chen A, Feresu SA, Fernandez C, Rogan WJ. Maternal obesity and the risk of infant death in the United States. Epidemiology 2009; 20:74–81.

Cnattingius S, Bergström R, Lipworth L, Kramer MS. Prepregnancy weight and the risk of adverse pregnancy outcomes. New England Journal of Medicine 1998; 338:147–52.

Flegal KM, Carroll MD, Ogden CL, Curtin LR. Prevalence and trends in obesity among US adults, 1999–2008. JAMA 2010; 303:235–41.

Landres IV, Milki AA, Lathi RB. Karyotype of miscarriages in relation to maternal weight. Human Reproduction 2010; 25:1123–6.

Nguyen R, Wilcox A, Skjærven R, Baird DD. Men's body mass index and infertility. Human Reproduction 2007; 22:2488–93.

Nohr EA, Vaeth M, Rasmussen S, Ramlau-Hansen CH, Olsen J. Waiting time to pregnancy according to maternal birthweight and prepregnancy BMI. Human Reproduction 2009; 226–32.

Polotsky AJ, Hailpern SM, Skurnick JH, Lo JC, Sternfeld B, Santoro N. Association of adolescent obesity and lifetime nulliparity—The Study of Women's Health Across the Nation. Fertility and Sterility 2010; 93:200411.

Ramlau-Hansen CH, Thulstrup AM, Nohr EA, Bonde JP, Sørensen TIA, Olsen J. Subfecundity in overweight and obese couples. Human Reproduction 2007; 22:1634–7.

Ramsay JE, Ferrell WR, Crawford L, Wallace AM, Greer IA, Sattar N. Maternal obesity is associated with dysregulation of metabolic, vascular, and inflammatory pathways. Journal of Clinical Endocrinology & Metabolism 2002; 87:4231–7.

Ramsay JE, Greer I, Sattar N. Obesity and reproduction. British Medical Journal 2006; 333:1159–62.

Sattar N, Clark P, Holmes A, Lean MEJ, Walker I, Greer IA. Antenatal waist circumference and hypertension risk. Obstetrics & Gynecology 2001; 97:268–71.

Stothard KJ, Tennant PWG, Bell R, Rankin J. Maternal overweight and obesity and the risk of congenital anomalies. Journal of the American Medical Association 2009; 301:636–50.

Watkins ML, Rasmussen SA, Honein MA, Botto LD, Moore CA. Maternal obesity and risk for birth defects. Pediatrics 2003; 111:1152–8.

Maternal Weight Gain in Singleton and Multiple Pregnancy

Brown JE, Murtaugh MA, Jacobs DR, Margellos HC. Variation in newborn size according to pregnancy weight change by trimester. American Journal of Clinical Nutrition 2002; 76:205–9.

Brown JE, Schloesser PT. Prepregnancy weight status, prenatal weight gain, and the outcome of term twin gestations. American Journal of Obstetrics & Gynecology 1990; 162:182–6.

Dubois S, Dougherty C, Duquette M-P, Hanley JA, Moutquin J-M. Twin pregnancy: The impact of the Higgins Nutrition Intervention Program on maternal and neonatal outcomes. American Journal of Clinical Nutrition 1991; 53:1397–1403.

Fenton TR, Thirsk JE. Twin pregnancy: The distribution of maternal weight gain of non-smoking normal-weight women. Canadian Journal of Public Health 1994; 85:37–40.

Fox NS, Rebarber A, Roman S, et al. Weight gain in twin pregnancies and adverse outcomes examining the 2009 Institute of Medicine guidelines. Obstetrics & Gynecology 2010; 116:100–6.

Fox NS, Stern E, Saltzman DH, et al. The association between maternal weight gain and spontaneous preterm birth in twin pregnancies. Journal of Maternal-Fetal & Neonatal Medicine 2014; 27:1652–5.

Gonzalez-Quintero VH, Kathiresan ASQ, Tudela FJ, et al. The association of gestational weight gain per Institute of Medicine guidelines and prepregnancy body mass index on outcomes of twin pregnancies. American Journal of Perinatology 2012; 29:435–40.

Hedderson MM, Gunderson EP, Ferrara A. Gestational weight gain and risk of gestational diabetes mellitus. Obstetrics & Gynecology 2010; 115:597–604.

Hediger ML, Luke B, Gonzalez-Quintero VH, et al. Fetal growth rates and the very preterm delivery of twins. American Journal of Obstetrics & Gynecology 2005; 193:1498–1507.

Institute of Medicine. Weight gain during pregnancy: Reexamining the guidelines. Food and Nutrition Board, National Academy of Sciences. Washington, DC; 2009.

Lantz ME, Chez RA, Rodriguez A, Porter KB. Maternal weight gain patterns and birth weight outcome in twin gestation. Obstetrics & Gynecology 1996; 87:551–6.

Luke, B. Twin births: Influence of maternal weight on intrauterine growth and prematurity. Federation Proceedings 1987; 46:1015.

Luke B, Brown MB, Hediger ML, Nugent C, Misiunas RB, Anderson E. Fetal phenotypes and neo-natal and early childhood outcomes in twins. American Journal of Obstetrics & Gynecology 2004; 191:1270–6.

Luke B, Bryan E, Sweetland C, Leurgans S, Keith L. Prenatal weight gain and the birthweight of trip-lets. Acta Geneticae Medicae et Gemellologiae 1995; 44:93–101.

Luke B, Gillespie B, Min S-J, Avni M, Witter FR, O'Sullivan MJ. Critical periods of maternal weight gain: Effect on twin birthweight. American Journal of Obstetrics & Gynecology 1997; 177:1055–62.

Luke B, Hediger ML, Nugent C, Newman RB, Mauldin JG, Witter FR, et al. Body mass index-specific weight gains associated with optimal birth weights in twin pregnancies. Journal of Reproductive Medicine 2003; 48:217–24.

Luke B, Hediger ML, Scholl TO. Point of diminishing returns: When does gestational weight gain cease benefiting birthweight and begin adding to maternal obesity? Journal of Maternal-Fetal Medi-cine 1996; 5:168–73.

Luke B, Keith L, Johnson TRB, Keith D. Pregravid weight, gestational weight gain, and current weight of women delivered of twins. Journal of Perinatal Medicine 1991; 19:333–40.

Luke B, Keith L, Lopez-Zeno JA, Witter FR, Saquil E. A case-control study of maternal gestational weight gain and newborn birthweight and birth length in twin pregnancies complicated by pre-eclampsia. Acta Geneticae Medicae et Gemellologiae 1993; 42:7–15.

Luke B, Leurgans S. Maternal weight gains in ideal twin outcomes. Journal of the American Dietetic Association 1996; 96:178–81.

Luke B, Min S-J, Gillespie B, et al. The importance of early weight gain on the intrauterine growth and birthweight of twins. American Journal of Obstetrics & Gynecology 1998; 179:1155–61.

Luke B, Minogue J, Abbey H, Keith L, Witter FR, Feng TI, et al. The association between maternal weight gain and the birthweight of twins. Journal of Maternal-Fetal Medicine 1992; 1:267–76.

Luke B, Minogue J, Witter FR, Keith LG, Johnson TRB. The ideal twin pregnancy: Patterns of weight gain, discordancy, and length of gestation. American Journal of Obstetrics & Gynecology 1993; 169(3):588–97.

Luke B, Nugent C, van de Ven C, Martin D, O'Sullivan MJ, Eardley S, et al. The association between maternal factors and perinatal outcomes in triplet pregnancies. American Journal of Obstetrics & Gynecology 2002; 187:752–7.

Luke B, O'Sullivan MJ, Martin D, Nugent C, Witter FW, Newman RB. Outcomes in quadruplet pregnancies: Role of maternal nutrition. American Journal of Obstetrics & Gynecology 2001; 185:S105.

Naeye RL, Blanc W, Paul C. Effects of maternal nutrition on the human fetus. Pediatrics 1973; 52:494–503.

Pettit KE, Lacoursiere DY, Schrimmer DB, et al. The association of inadequate mid-pregnancy weight gain and preterm birth in twin pregnancies. Journal of Perinatology 2015; 35:85–9.

Strauss RS, Dietz WH. Low maternal weight gain in the second or third trimester increases the risk for intrauterine growth retardation. Journal of Nutrition 1999; 129:988–93.

Pederson AL, Worthington-Roberts B, Hickok DE. Weight gain patterns during twin gestation. Jour-nal of the American Dietetic Association 1989; 89:642–6.

Omega-3 Fatty Acids and Seafood

Adair CD, Sanchez-Ramos L, Briones DL, Ogburn P. The effect of high dietary n-3 fatty acid supplementation on angiotensin II pressor response in human pregnancy. American Journal of Obstetrics & Gynecology 1996; 175:688–91.

American Dietetic Association; Dietitians of Canada. Position paper: Dietary Fatty Acids. Journal of the American Dietetic Association 2007; 107:1599–1611.

Cetina I, Koletzko B. Long-chain omega-3 fatty acid supply in pregnancy and lactation. Current Opinion in Clinical Nutrition and Metabolic Care 2008; 11:297–302.

Chappell LC, Seed PT, Briley AL, et al. Effect of antioxidants on the occurrence of pre-eclampsia in women at increased risk: A randomized trial. Lancet 1999; 354:810–16.

Chappell LC, Seed PT, Kelly FJ, et al. Vitamin C and E supplementation in women at risk of pre-eclampsia is associated with changes in indices of oxidative stress and placental function. American Journal of Obstetrics & Gynecology, 2002; 187:777–84.

Food and Drug Administration Center for Food Safety and Nutrition. Draft risk and benefit assessment of quantitative risk and benefit assessment of consumption of commercial fish, focusing on fetal neurodevelopmental effects (measured by verbal development in children) and on coronary heart disease and stroke in the general population; www.cfsan.fda.gov/~dms/mehgrb.html.

Foreman-van Drongelen MMHP, Zeijdner EE, Houwelingen AC, et al. Essential fatty acid status measured in umbilical vessel walls of infants born after a multiple pregnancy. Early Human Development 1996; 46:205–15.

Golding J, Steer C, Emmett P, Davis JM, Hibbeln JR. High levels of depressive symptoms in pregnancy with low omega-3 fatty acid intake from fish. Epidemiology 2009; 20:598–603.

Hibbeln JR, Davis JM, Steer C, Emmett P, Rogers I, Williams C, et al. Maternal seafood consumption in pregnancy and neurodevelopmental outcomes in childhood (ALSPAC study): An observational cohort study. Lancet 2007; 369:578–85.

Institute of Medicine. Seafood choices: Balancing benefits and risks. Washington, DC: National Academy Press; 2006.

Jacobson JL, Jacobson SW, Muckle G, Kaplan-Estrin M, Ayotte P, Dewailly E. Beneficial effects of a polyunsaturated fatty acid on infant development: Evidence from the Inuit of Artic Quebec. Journal of Pediatrics 2008; 152:356–64.

Koletzko B, Cetin I, Brenna JT; for the Perinatal Lipid Intake Working Group. Consensus statement: Dietary fat intakes for pregnant and lactating women. British Journal of Nutrition 2007; 98:873–7.

Koletzko B, Lien E, Agostoni C, Böhles H, Campoy C, Cetin I, et al. The roles of long-chain polyunsaturated fatty acids in pregnancy, lactation and infancy: Review of current knowledge and consensus recommendations. Journal of Perinatal Medicine 2008; 36:5–14.

Krauss-Etschmann S, Shadid R, Campoy C, Hoster E, Demmelmair H, Jiménez M, et al.; Nutrition and Health Lifestyle (NUHEAL) Study Group. Effects of fish-oil and folate supplementation of pregnant women on maternal and fetal plasma concentrations of docosahexaenoic acid and eicosapentaenoic acid: A European randomized multicenter trial. American Journal of Clinical Nutrition 2007; 85:1392–1400.

Makrides M, Gibson RA, McPhee AJ, et al. Neurodevelopmental outcomes of preterm infants fed high-dose docosahexaenoic acid. Journal of the American Medical Association 2009; 301(2):175–82.

McCann JC, Ames BN. Is docosahexaenoic acid, an n-3 long-chain polyunsaturated fatty acid, required for development of normal brain function? An overview of evidence from cognitive and behavioral tests in humans and animals. American Journal of Clinical Nutrition 2005; 82:281–95.

Morse, N.L. Benefits of docosahexaenoic acid, folic acid, vitamin D and iodine on foetal and infant brain development and function following maternal supplementation during pregnancy and lactation. Nutrients 2012; 4:799–840.

Mozaffarian D, Rimm EB. Fish intake, contaminants, and human health. Journal of the American Medical Association 2006; 296:1885–99.

Oken E, Østerdal L, Gillman MW, et al. Associations of maternal fish intake during pregnancy and breastfeeding duration with attainment of developmental milestones in early childhood: A study from the Danish National Birth Cohort. American Journal of Clinical Nutrition 2008; 88:789–96.

Olsen SF, Secher NJ. Low consumption of seafood in early pregnancy as a risk factor for preterm delivery: Prospective cohort study. British Medical Journal 2002; 324:447–50.

Raymond LJ, Ralston NVC. Mercury:selenium interaction and health implications. Seychelles Medical and Dental Journal, Special Issue, 2004; 7:72–7.

Reece MS, McGregor JA, Allen KGD, Harris MA. Maternal and perinatal long-chain fatty acids: Possible roles in preterm birth. American Journal of Obstetrics & Gynecology 1997; 176:907–14.

Roman AS, Schreher J, Mackenzie AP, Nathanielsz PW. Omega-3 fatty acids and decidual cell prostaglandin production in response to the inflammatory cytokine IL-1beta. American Journal of Obstetrics & Gynecology 2006; 195:1693–9.

Strain JJ, Davidson PW, Thurston SW, et al. Maternal PUFA status but not prenatal methylmercury exposure is associated with children's language functions at age five years in the Seychelles. Journal of Nutrition 2012; 142:1943–9.

Velzing-Aarts F, van der Klis FRM, van der Dijs FPL, Muskiet FAJ. Umbilical vessels of preeclamptic women have low contents of both n-3 and n-6 long-chain polyunsaturated fatty acids. American Journal of Clinical Nutrition 1999; 69:293–8.

Weisinger HS., Armitage JA, Sinclair AJ, Vingrys AJ, Burns PL, Weisinger RS. Perinatal omega-3 fatty acid deficiency affects blood pressure later in life. Nature Medicine 2001; 7:258–9.

Williams MA, Zingheim RW, King IB, Zebelman AM. Omega-3 fatty acids in maternal erythrocytes and risk of preeclampsia. Epidemiology 1995; 6:232–7.

Zeijdner EE, Houwelingen ACV, Kester ADM, et al. Essential fatty acid status in plasma phospholipids of mother and neonate after multiple pregnancy. Prostaglandins, Leukotrienes, and Essential Fatty Acids 1997; 56:395–401.

Postpartum Depression

Choi Y, Bishai D, Minkovitz CS. Multiple births are a risk factor for postpartum maternal depressive symptoms. Pediatrics 2009; 123:1147–54.

Freeman MP, Hibbeln JR, Wisner KL, Brumbach BH, Watchman M, Gelenberg AJ. Randomized dose-ranging pilot trial of omega-3 fatty acids for postpartum depression. Acta Obstetricia et Gynecologica Scandinavica 2006; 113:31–5.

Josefsson A, Angelsioo L, Berg G, Ekstrom CM, Gunnervik C, Nordin C, et al. Obstetric, somatic, and demographic risk factors for postpartum depressive symptoms. Obstetrics & Gynecology 2002; 99:223–8.

Kozhimannil KB, Pereira MA, Harlow BL. Association between diabetes and perinatal depression among low-income mothers. Journal of the American Medical Association 2009; 301(8):842–7.

Pearlstein T, Howard M, Salisbury A, Zlotnick C. Postpartum depression. American Journal of Obstetrics & Gynecology 2008; doi:10.1016/j.ajog.2008.11.033.

Vadlimarsdottir U, Hultman CM, Harlow B, Cnattingius S, Sparen P. Psychotic illness in first-time mothers with no previous psychiatric hospitalizations: A population-based study. PLOS Medicine 2009; 6:194–201.

Postpartum Weight

Baker JL, Gamborg M, Heitmann BL, Lissner L, Sorensen TIA, Rasmussen KM. Breastfeeding reduces postpartum weight retention. American Journal of Clinical Nutrition 2008; 88:1543–51.

Butte NF, Ellis KJ, Wong WW, Hopkinson JM, Smith EO. Composition of gestational weight gain impacts maternal fat retention and infant birth weight. American Journal of Obstetrics & Gynecology 2003; 189:1423–32.

Gunderson EP, Murtaugh MA, Lewis CE, Quesenberry CP, West DS, Sidney S. Excess gains in weight and waist circumference associated with childbearing: The Coronary Artery Risk Development in Young Adults Study (CARDIA). International Journal of Obesity 2004; 28:525–35.

Herring SJ, Rich-Edwards JW, Oken E, Rifas-Shiman SL, Kleinman KP, Gillman MW. Association of postpartum depression with weight retention 1 year after childbirth. Obesity 2008; 16:1296–1301.

Linne Y, Dye L, Barkeling B, Rossner S. Long-term weight development in women: A 15-year follow-up of the effects of pregnancy. Obesity Research 2004; 12:1166–78.

Linne Y, Dye L, Barkeling B, Rossner S. Weight development over time in parous women—the SPAWN study—15 years follow-up. International Journal of Obesity 2003; 27:1516–22.

Linne Y, Rossner S. Interrelationships between weight development and weight retention in subsequent pregnancies: The SPAWN study. Acta Obstetricia et Gynecologica Scandinavica 2003; 82:318–25.

Rooney BL, Schauberger CW. Excess pregnancy weight gain and long-term obesity: One decade later. Obstetrics & Gynecology 2002; 100:245–52.

Schmitt NM, Nicholson WK, Schmitt J. The association of pregnancy and the development of obesity: Results of a systematic review and meta-analysis on the natural history of postpartum weight retention. International Journal of Obesity 2007; 31:1642–51.

Smith DE, Lewis CE, Caveny JL, Perkins LL, Burke GL, Bild DE. Longitudinal changes in adiposity associated with pregnancy: The CARDIA study. Journal of the American Medical Association 1994; 271:1747–51.

Villamor E, Cnattingius S. Interpregnancy weight change and risk of adverse pregnancy outcomes: A population-based study. Lancet 2006; 368:1164–70.

Prenatal and Perinatal Care and Multiple Pregnancy Outcomes

Albrecht JL, Tomich PG. The maternal and neonatal outcome of triplet gestations. American Journal of Obstetrics & Gynecology 1996; 174:1551–6.

American Academy of Pediatrics; American College of Obstetricians and Gynecologists. Guidelines for perinatal care. 7th edition. Elk Grove, IL; 2012.

Bivins HA, Newman RB, Ellings JM, Hulsey TC, Keenan A. Risks of antepartum cervical examination in multifetal gestations. American Journal of Obstetrics & Gynecology 1993; 169:22–5.

Bosque EP, Brady JP, Affonso DD, Wahlberg V. Continuous physiological measurements of kangaroo versus incubator care in a tertiary level nursery. Pediatric Research 1988; 23:402A.

Burgess JL, Unal ER, Nietert PJ, Newman RB. Risk of late-preterm stillbirth and neonatal morbidity for monochorionic and dichorionic twins. American Journal of Obstetrics & Gynecology 2014; 210:578.e1.

Charpak N, Ruiz-Peláez JG, Figueroa de C Z, Charpak Y. Kangaroo mother versus traditional care for newborn infants ≤2000 grams: A randomized, controlled trial. Pediatrics 1997; 100:682–8.

Chervenak FA. The controversy of mode of delivery in twins: The intrapartum management of twin gestation (part II). Seminars in Perinatology 1986; 10: 44–9.

Chien L-Y, Whyte R, Aziz K, Thiessen P, Matthew D, Lee SK. Improved outcome of preterm infants when delivered in tertiary care centers. Obstetrics & Gynecology 2001; 98:247–52.

Collins MS, Bleyl JA. Seventy-one quadruplet pregnancies: Management and outcome. American Journal of Obstetrics & Gynecology 1990; 162:1384–92.

Committee on Fetus and Newborn. Levels of neonatal care. Pediatrics 2012; 130:587–97.

Crowther CA, Verkuyl DAA, Ashworth MF, Bannerman C, Ashurst HM. The effects of hospitalization for bedrest on duration of gestation, fetal growth, and neonatal morbidity in triplet pregnancy. Acta Geneticae Medicae et Gemellologiae 1991; 40:63–8.

Dias T, Akolekar R. Timing of birth in multiple pregnancy. Best Practice & Research, Clinical Obstetrics and Gynaecology 2014; 28:319–26.

Dubois S, Dougherty C, Duquette M-P, Hanley JA, Moutquin J-M. Twin pregnancy: The impact of the Higgins Nutrition Intervention Program on maternal and neonatal outcomes. American Journal of Clinical Nutrition 1991; 53:1397–1403.

Eller DP, Newman RB, Ellings JM, et al. Modifiable determinants of birthweight variability in twins. Journal of Maternal-Fetal Medicine 1993; 2:254–9.

Ellings JM, Newman RB, Hulsey TC, Bivins HA, Keenan A. Reduction in very low birthweight deliveries and perinatal mortality in a specialized, multidisciplinary twin clinic. Obstetrics & Gynecology 1993; 81:387–91.

Elliott JP, Radin TG. Quadruplet pregnancy: Contemporary management and outcome. Obstetrics & Gynecology 1992; 80:421–4.

Fishman A, Grubb DK, Kovacs BW. Vaginal delivery of the nonvertex second twin. American Journal of Obstetrics & Gynecology 1993; 168:861–4.

Friedman SA, Schiff E, Kao L, Kuint J, Sibai BM. Do twins mature earlier than singletons? American Journal of Obstetrics & Gynecology 1997; 176:1193–9.

Garcia FAR, Miller HB, Huggins GR, Gordon TA. Effect of academic affiliation and obstetric volume on clinical outcome and cost of childbirth. Obstetrics & Gynecology 2001; 97:567–76.

Gardner MO, Amaya MA, Sakakini J. Effects of prenatal care on twin gestations. Journal of Reproductive Medicine 1990; 35:519–21.

Gocke SE, Nageotte MP, Garite T, Towers CV, Dorchester W. Management of the nonvertex second twin: Primary cesarean section, external version or primary breech extraction. American Journal of Obstetrics & Gynecology 1989; 161:111–14.

Greig PC, Veille J-C, Morgan T, Henderson L. The effect of presentation and mode of delivery on neonatal outcome in the second twin. American Journal of Obstetrics & Gynecology 1992; 167:901–6.

Hartley RS, Emanuel I, Hitti J. Perinatal mortality and neonatal morbidity rates among twin pairs at different gestational ages: Optimal delivery timing at 37 to 38 weeks' gestation. American Journal of Obstetrics & Gynecology 2001; 184:451–8.

Jauniaux E, Kilby M. Minimizing perinatal mortality in twins: Planned birth at 38 weeks of gestation for dichorionic and 36 weeks of gestation for monochorionic twins. British Journal of Obstetrics and Gynaecology 2014; 121:1284–90.

Luke B, Brown MB, Alexandre PK, Kinoshi T, et al. The cost of twin pregnancy: Maternal and neonatal factors. American Journal of Obstetrics & Gynecology 2005; 192:909–15.

Luke B, Brown MB, Misiunas R, et al. Specialized prenatal care and maternal and infant outcomes in twin pregnancy. American Journal of Obstetrics & Gynecology 2003; 189:934–8.

Miller DA, Mullin P, Hou D, Paul RH. Vaginal birth after cesarean section in twin gestation. American Journal of Obstetrics & Gynecology 1996; 175:194–8.

Newman RB, Ellings JM. Antepartum management of the multiple gestation: The case for specialized care. Seminars in Perinatology 1995; 19:387–403.

Peaceman AM, Dooley SL, Tamura RK. Antepartum management of triplet gestations. American Journal of Obstetrics & Gynecology 1992; 167:1117–20.

Pons JC, Nekhlyudov L, Dephot N, Le Moal S, Papiernik E. Management and outcomes of sixty-five quadruplet pregnancies: Sixteen years' experience in France. Acta Geneticae Medicae et Gemellologiae 1996; 45:367–75.

Prins RP. The second-born twin: Can we improve outcomes? American Journal of Obstetrics & Gynecology 1994; 170:1649–57.

Rayburn WF, Lavin JP Jr., Miodovnik M, Varner MW. Multiple gestation: Time interval between delivery of the first and second twin. Obstetrics & Gynecology 1984; 63:502–6.

Tomashek KM, Wallman C; Committee on Fetus and Newborn. Cobedding twins and higher-order multiples in a hospital setting. Pediatrics 2007; 120:1359–66.

Vergani P, Ghidini A, Bozzo G, Sirtori M. Prenatal management of twin gestation: Experience with a new protocol. Journal of Reproductive Medicine 1991; 36:667–71.

Vutyavanich T, Kraisarin T, Ruangsri R-A. Ginger for nausea and vomiting in pregnancy: Randomized, double-masked, placebo-controlled trial. Obstetrics & Gynecology 2001; 97:577–82.

Reduced Sleep and Weight Gain

Gangwisch JE, Malaspina D, Boden-Albala B, et al. Inadequate sleep as a risk factor for obesity: Analyses of the NHANES I. Sleep 2005; 28:1289–96.

Hasler G, Buysse DJ, Klaghofer R, et al. The association between short sleep duration and obesity in young adults: A 13-year prospective study. Sleep 2004; 27:661–6.

Patel SR, Malhotra A, White DP, Gottlieb DJ, Hu FB. Association between reduced sleep and weight gain in women. American Journal of Epidemiology 2006; 164:947–54.

Spiegel K, Tasali E, Penev P, et al. Sleep curtailment in healthy young men is associated with decreased leptin levels, elevated ghrelin levels, and increased hunger and appetite. Annals of Internal Medicine 2004; 141:846–50.

Taheri S, Lin L, Austin D, et al. Short sleep duration is associated with reduced leptin, elevated ghrelin, and increased body mass index. PLoS Medicine 2004; 1:e62.

Tocolytics

Conde-Agudelo A, Romero R. Antenatal magnesium sulfate for the prevention of cerebral palsy in preterm infants less than 34 weeks' gestation: A systematic review and metaanalysis. American Journal of Obstetrics & Gynecology 2009; doi: 10.1016/j.ajog.2009.04.005.

Couser RJ, Hoekstra RE, Ferrara TB, Wright GB, Cabalka AK, Connett JE. Neurodevelopmental follow-up at 36 months' corrected age of preterm infants treated with prophylactic indomethacin. American Journal of Public Health 2000; 154:598–602.

Doyle LW, Crowther CA, Middleton P, Marret S, Rouse D. Magnesium sulphate for women at risk of preterm birth for neuroprotection of the fetus. Cochrane Database of Systematic Reviews 2009, Issue 1. Art. No.: CD004661. DOI: 10.1002/14651858.CD004661.pub3.

Suarez RD, Grobman WA, Parilla BV. Indomethacin tocolysis and intraventricular hemorrhage. Obstetrics & Gynecology 2001; 97:921–5.

Suarez VR, Thompson LL, Jain V, et al. The effect of in utero exposure to indomethacin on the need for surgical closure of a patent ductus arteriosus in the neonate. American Journal of Obstetrics & Gynecology 2002; 187:886–8.

Twin-Twin Transfusion Syndrome

Bajoria R, Wigglesworth J, Fisk NM. Angioarchitecture of monochorionic placentas in relation to the twin-twin transfusion syndrome. American Journal of Obstetrics & Gynecology 1995; 172:856–63.

Chmait RH, Korst LM, Bornick PW, Allen MH, Quintero RA. Fetal growth after laser therapy for twin-twin transfusion syndrome. American Journal of Obstetrics & Gynecology 2008; 199:47.e1–e6.

De Lia JE, Kuhlmann RS, Harstad TW, Cruikshank DP. Fetoscopic laser ablation of placental vessels in severe previable twin-twin transfusion syndrome. American Journal of Obstetrics & Gynecology 1995; 172:1202–11.

Gray PH, Cincotta R, Chan FY, Soong B. Perinatal outcomes with laser surgery for twin-twin transfusion syndrome. Twin Research and Human Genetics 2006; 9:438–43.

Ultrasound Determination of Chorionicity

D'Alton ME, Dudley DK. The ultrasonographic prediction of chorionicity in twin gestation. American Journal of Obstetrics & Gynecology 1989; 160:557–61.

Monteagudo A, Timor-Tritsch IE, Sharma S. Early and simple determination of chorionic and amniotic type in multifetal gestations in the first fourteen weeks by high-frequency transvaginal ultrasonography. American Journal of Obstetrics & Gynecology 1994; 170:824–9.

Scardo JA, Ellings JM, Newman RB. Prospective determination of chorionicity, amnionicity, and zygosity in twin gestations. American Journal of Obstetrics & Gynecology 1995; 173:1376–80.

Sepulveda W, Sebire NJ, Odibo A, Psarra A, Nicolaides KH. Prenatal determination of chorionicity in triplet pregnancy by ultrasonographic examination of the ipsilon zone. Obstetrics & Gynecology 1996; 88:855–8.

Vayssière CF, Heim N, Camus EP, Hillion YE, Nisand IF. Determination of chorionicity in twin gestations by high-frequency abdominal ultrasonography: Counting the layers of the dividing membrane. American Journal of Obstetrics & Gynecology 1996; 175:1529–33.

Vanishing Twins

Landy H, Keith LG, Keith D. The vanishing twin. Acta Geneticae Medicae et Gemellologiae 1982; 31:179–94.

Pinborg A, Lidegaard Ø, la Cour Freiesleben N, Andersen AN. Consequences of vanishing twins in IVF/ICSI pregnancies. Human Reproduction 2005; 20:2821–9.

Pinborg A, Lidegaard Ø, la Cour Freiesleben N, Andersen AN. Vanishing twins: A predictor of small-for-gestational age in IVF singletons. Human Reproduction 2007; 22:2707–14.

Shebl O, Ebner T, Sommergruber M, Sir A, Tews G. Birthweight is lower for survivors of the vanishing twin syndrome: A case-control study. Fertility and Sterility 2008; 90:310–4.

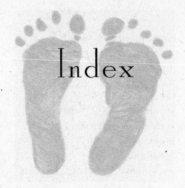

Index

anxiety
  deep breathing techniques for,
    180
  of fathers, 264
  about NICU, 309
  in reaction to multiples
    pregnancy, 257–60
Apgar score, 304–5, *305*, 558
aplasia cutis, 526
apnea, 166, 309, 318, 337
appetite
  depression and, 415
  multivitamins and, 131
  of newborns, 354
  postpartum, 348
  pregnancy and, 70, 100–1
  sleep disruption and, 384
  supplement drinks and, 144
aspirin, 163, 404
assisted reproductive technologies
    (ART)
  multiple births and, 11–12, 247,
    250
  parental bonding and, 411
  pregnancy weight gain and, 69
  preterm births and, 221
  ultrasounds and, 56
audiologists, 314

Baby-Friendly health care facilities,
    41–42, 342–43
baby gates, 405
baby monitors, 401
baby nurses, 386–87
baby-proofing, 404–6
babysitters, 387, 415
backaches
  during labor, 291
  during pregnancy, 172–75
  as preterm labor sign, 227
bacteria
  food-borne, 162
  in hospitals, 321
  infections from, 320–21
  in probiotics, 177
bag of waters, 20, 274
balance, center of gravity and,
    191

bargaining, in reaction to multiples
    pregnancy, 260–62
bariatric surgery, 160–62
Barker hypothesis, 64
bathing
  of babies, 306, 401, 406,
    409
  equipment for, 398
  during pregnancy, 173
  as sleep aid, 183
bedrest, 233–47
  benefits of, 233
  boredom and, 239–40
  childbirth classes and, 62
  after delivery, 301
  duration of, 247
  emotional issues with, 240–41,
    260–61
  exercise during, 241–46
  hospitalization for, 224, 236–37,
    238, 547–48
  levels of, 235–37
  muscle weakness and, 376
  practical management of,
    237–39
  resources for, 513
  vaginal bleeding and, 205
bedtime
  establishing rituals for, 391,
    394–95
  snacking at, 108, 367
behavioral problems, 164
belly bands, 174, 191
belly bulge, 383–84
bending during pregnancy,
    188
betamethasone, 232, 534
bilirubin, 316
biophysical profile, 60
birth
  handling of baby at, 304–6
  preparing plan for, 61, 273
  See also labor/delivery procedure
birth control pills
  breast-feeding and, 354
  multiple births and, 11
birth defects, 18
birthrates for multiples, 1, 10

birthweights
  bariatric surgery and, 160
  maternal alcohol use and, 165
  maternal smoking and, 166
  maternal weight gain and,
    71–72, 78–96
  for multiples vs. singletons, 24
  prenatal nutrition and, 63–66,
    71, 101
  prior pregnancies and, 44
  for triplets, *509–11*
  for twins, *507–8*
  zinc and, 137
bladder
  fetal defects of, 214
  infection of, 301
  pressure on, 178–79, 191, 274
bladder exstrophy, 525, 526
bleeding
  postpartum, 293, 300
  vaginal, 51, 56, 184, 192, 203–6
blood clots
  bedrest and, 236
  exercise and, 376
  vitamin K and, 305
blood glucose (blood sugar)
  fruit juice and, 128
  in gestational diabetes, 159
  glycemic index and, 113
  low, 100, 107
  morning sickness and, 147, 148
  of newborns, 316
  stabilizing, 78, 97–99, 105, 109,
    367, 368, 373, 374
  testing, 52
blood pressure
  of babies in NICU, 310
  after delivery, 301
  high (*see* hypertension)
  low (*see* hypotension)
  placental abruption and, 206
  prenatal checkup of, 51
  sleep position and, 181
blood pressure monitors, 310
blood supply
  fetal anomalies and, 214
  umbilical cord and, 60, 292
blood tests, 51

blood thinners, 163
blood type, 51, 308
bloody show, 274
body fat
  of babies, 316
  body mass index and, 73–74
  burning off, 373, 376
  ketones and, 109
  measuring, 379, *380–81, *382
  during pregnancy, 90, 365
body image
  changes in, 168–70
  emotional issues about, 270–72
  postpartum, 364, 384
  sexual activity and, 184
body mass index (BMI)
  postpartum, 382
  pregnancy diet and, 104
  pregnancy weight gain and, 67,
    73–74, *75–77*, 80–84, 89, 365
  vitamin D requirement and, 139
body temperature
  during exercise, 191
  illness and, 404
  postpartum, 301
  during pregnancy, 171, 180–81
  of premature babies, 309,
    316–17, 337
bonding with babies, 407–12
bottle-feeding, 311, 322, 360–63,
  389
bottle propping, 362
bottle warming, 362
bowel movements of newborns,
  353
Bradley Method, 61, 62
brain
  blood flow to, 214, 216
  development of, 21, 111, 112,
    118, 120, 325, 351
  injury to, 318, 542–43
  ultrasound checks of, 218, 312
bras for breast milk pumping, 359
Braxton-Hicks contractions, 227,
  275
Break Time for Nursing Mothers
  law, 360
breast abscesses, 358

breast cancer, 345
breast-feeding
  duration of, 343
  environmental contaminants
    and, 111
  frequency of, 355, 395
  instruction in, 41–42, 315, 341,
    343, 356–57
  legislation concerning, 359, 360
  maternal weight gain and, 68,
    73, 95, 271
  mechanics of, 354–60
  nutrition for, 345–54, 367, 369
  partner support for, 390
  resources for, 513–14
  supplementing, 360–61
  uterine cramps and, 301
  when to start, 311, 322
breast milk
  advantages of, 327–28, 342,
    343–45
  gavage delivery of, 322
  storing, 359–60
  supply of, 327, 346, 353–54, 358
breast pumps, 315, 340, 342, 354,
  357–59
breathing
  difficulty with (in mothers), 180,
    301
  difficulty with (in newborns),
    284, 309, 316–17
  relaxation exercises using, 180,
    259, 282
breech extractions, 287, 293,
  554–55, 557
breech presentations, 286–87, 295,
  554, *554*
Brethine (terbutaline), 231
bromocriptine (Parlodel), 342
bronchopulmonary dysplasia
  (BPD), 318
brown fat, 316
burping
  at bedtime, 395
  after feeding, 355, 363

caffeine, 128–29
calamine lotion, 404

calcium
  breast-feeding and, 322, 349,
    350–51
  caffeine and, 128–29
  for heartburn, 176
  nutritional function of, 107
  recommendation for pregnancy,
    104, 108, 122, 134–36
calorie requirements
  for breast-feeding mothers, 348,
    354
  for postpartum diets, 367, *368*,
    369
carbohydrates
  fluid retention and, 176
  function of, 105–6
  inadequate intake of, 100
  insulin sensitivity and, 374
  morning sickness and, 147
  recommendations for breast-
    feeding, *347*
  recommendations for
    postpartum diet, 367, *368*
  recommendations for pregnancy,
    99, *103*, 104
  in supplement drinks, 143,
    145–46
cardiac malformations, 214–15,
  525
cardiopulmonary resuscitation
  (CPR), 403
cardiorespiratory machines, 309
cardiovascular disease, 345
carpal tunnel syndrome, 175–76
carrying
  of babies, 398, 409
  of loads, during pregnancy, 188
car seats, 397
car travel, 195–96, 303
case managers, on health care
  team, 313
catecholamines, 186, 190, 233,
  258
Center for Loss in Multiple Birth
  (CLIMB), 335
Center for Postpartum Health, 418
center of gravity, pregnancy
  changes in, 172, 191

cephalic presentation, 285, 552–53
cerclage, 204–5, 226, 550–51
cerebral palsy, 136, 222, 232, 539
certified registered nurses (RNs), 313
cervical insufficiency (CI), 204–5, 226, 551
cervix
    constriction of, 558
    dilation of, 230, 274, *275*, 288, 295
    effacement of, 230, 274, *275*
    during labor, 290, 291
    length of, 50, 57, 223–26, 545–52, *546, 547*
cesarean delivery (C-section), 294–300
    for conjoined twins, 215
    emotional reaction to, 299–300
    frequency of, 62, 295
    hospital stay for, 307
    labor stages and, 289–90
    maternal bonding and, 407–8
    maternal history of, 288–89, 295, 557
    for monoamniotic twins, 532, 533, 534
    pain medication during, 283, 284
    placenta previa and, 205, 206
    postpartum care with, 302
    postpartum depression and, 416, 417
    presentation and, 285–88
    procedure for, 297–99
    risks with, 297
    scheduled vs. emergency, 296–97
    sexual activity and, 420
    vs. vaginal, 552–58
chairs
    high, 398
    for pregnancy comfort, 173, 187, 236
    rocking, 398
cheese, 105, 107, *114,* 122, 152, 153, 159, 162, 351

childbirth preparation
    classes for, 61–62
    resources for, 514
child care, 189, 387, 389, 399
chills, 291, 293, *294*
chiropractors, 175
chloasma (mask of pregnancy), 169
cholesterol, 110, 141–42
chorioamnionitis, 98, 320–21
chorion, 8, 9, 10, 16, 59, 213
chorionic villus sampling (CVS), 16, 56, 59
chromosomal abnormalities, 58
chromosomes, in fertilization, 8
chronic illness
    breast-feeding and, 345
    expectant mothers with, 263
chronic lung disease (CLD), 318
cigarettes. *See* smoking
circadian rhythms, 384, 394
circulatory system
    acardiac twins and, 526–27
    exercise and, 376
    stress on, 186
classes
    childbirth, 61–62
    prenatal exercise, 191
clefting (facial), 166, 214, 525, 526
clinical nurse specialists, 313
clothing
    bras for breast milk pumping, 359
    identical, for multiples, 409–10
    maternity, 149, 170–72, 177, 181
    for newborns, 333
    pajamas, for babies, 395
    sharing, among multiples, 399
clotrimazole, 163
cognitive behavioral therapy (CBT), 418
color of baby (Apgar score), 304, *305*
complications, 201–51
    bedrest for, 233–47
    delivery timing and, 281
    emergency C-sections and, 296

emotional response to, 257–60, 263, 416, 417
    fetal reductions and, 247–51, 526
    in monozygotic pregnancies, 213–20, 524–45
    neonatal, 315–22
    parental bonding and, 411–12
    with postmature fetus, 279
    postpartum, 300–2
    in preterm labor, 220–33
    symptoms/signs of, 203–13
    See also specific types
computed tomography (CT), 312
conception, process of, 8–10, 19
congestive heart failure, 215, 216
conjoined twins, 215–16, 526, 527–29, 530
constipation
    drinking water and, 127, 178
    exercise and, 241
    fiber and, 106, 109, 121
    multivitamins and, 132
    preventing, 179
continuous positive airway pressure (CPAP), 310
contraception. *See* birth control pills
contractions. *See* uterine contractions
corticosteroids, 232–33, 278, 416, 550
Coumadin, 163
cramps
    in legs, 173, 183, 195
    preterm labor and, 227
    uterine, 300–1
cribs, 395, 397, 406
crossed eyes (strabismus), 320
crowning, 291
crying
    nighttime, 396
    therapeutic touch and, 327
C-section. *See* cesarean delivery
cystic fibrosis, 58

daily log for households with multiples, 391, *392*

dairy foods
  bacteria and, 162
  menu suggestions with, 117
  morning sickness and, 147
  nutritional function of, 107–8,
    114, 122, 152, 153, 158
  recommendations for breast-
    feeding, *347,* 349, 351
  recommendations for
    postpartum diet, *368*
  recommendations for pregnancy,
    103, 105
Danish Twin Registry, 525
death of child
  breast-feeding and, 344
  coping with, 335–36, 516
  maternal weight gain and, 89
  preterm birth and, 220
  secondhand smoke exposure
    and, 166
  See also intrauterine fetal death;
    stillbirths
deep-breathing techniques, 180,
  259, 282
deep vein thrombosis (DVT),
  236
dehydration
  air travel and, 126
  breast-feeding and, 376
  constipation and, 178
  contractions and, 127, 275
  from diarrhea, 404
  from exercise, 191
  monitoring for, 128, 150
  preterm labor and, 227, 229,
    230
delivery. *See* cesarean delivery;
    labor/delivery procedure;
    vaginal delivery
denial, in reaction to multiples
    pregnancy, 254–57, 264
depression
  breast-feeding and, 354
  postpartum, 106, 123, 141,
    415–18
  in reaction to multiples
    pregnancy, 258
  sleep deprivation and, 384

developmental delays, 218, 220,
  319, 351, 411–12
developmental specialists, 314
dexamethasone, 232
diabetes
  adult-onset, 369
  breast-feeding and, 345
  placenta age and, 279
  postpartum depression and, 416
  prenatal nutrition and, 65
  See also gestational diabetes
diabetic diet, 97–98, 99–107, 367
diamniotic, dichorionic (di/di)
    twin pregnancies
  defined, 8, 10
  miscarriage risk for, 203
  prenatal checkups for, 56, 59
  selective intrauterine growth
    restriction in, *537*
  twin-peak sign in, *17*
diamniotic, monochorionic (di/
    mo) twin pregnancies
  complications in, 213
  defined, 9
  fetal reductions and, 248
  incidence of, 530
  prenatal checkups for, 56, 59
  twin-twin transfusion syndrome
    in, *535*
diaper bags, 398, 402
diapering
  at bedtime, 395
  instruction in, 306
  maternal bonding and, 309
  of premature babies, 326
diaper rash, 404
diarrhea
  with cramps, 227
  dehydration from, 404
  supplement drinks and, 144
diastasis recti, 383
Diclegis, 150
diet. *See* diabetic diet; nutrition
dietary reference intakes (DRIs),
  106–7, 346
dietary supplements
  bariatric surgery and, 162
  as beverages, 142–46

need for, 131–32
  resources for, 519
  vitamins, 132–42, 344
dietitians, 40–41, 314
dilation of cervix, 230, 274, *275,*
  288, 295
disease
  in family history, 44–45
  fetal determinants of, 64
dizygotic (DZ) twins, 10, 11. *See
  also* fraternal twins
dizziness
  bedrest and, 237
  circulatory stress and, 186
  during exercise, 192
  hypoglycemia and, 107
  postpartum anemia and, 300
docosahexaeonoic acid (DHA),
  111, 112, 141–42, 416
doctors
  patients' relationships with,
    43–49, 259–60, 328
  selection of, 31–37, 39
  See also specific types
donor eggs, 411
Doppler flow studies, 60–61, 217
Down syndrome (trisomy 21), 53,
  54, 58
driving, 195, 303
ductus arteriosus, 317
due date
  determining, 27–30, 55, 56, 63
  labor onset and, 278

e-cigarettes, 166–67
eclampsia, 136
edema, 175–76
Edwards syndrome (trisomy
  18), 58
effacement of cervix, 230, 274, *275*
eggs
  nutritional function of, 110, *114,*
    121, 123, 152, 153
  raw or undercooked, 162
  recommendations for breast-
    feeding, *347,* 351
  recommendations for pregnancy,
    103

fetal aneuploidy, 58
fetal anomalies
  ketosis and, 100
  structural defects, 213–18, 524–29
  testing for, 52, 53
fetal determinants of adult disease, 64
fetal distress, 281, 288, 295
fetal fibronectin, 57, 230, 278
fetal hypoxia, 219, 288, 295
fetal monitoring
  intrapartum, 292, 558
  during labor/delivery, 278, 289, 295
  outpatient, 281
fetal movement
  in biophysical profile, 60
  multiple births and, 14–15, 277
  start of, 22
fetal period, 21–27, 120
fetal reduction. *See* selective fetal reduction
fetal therapy resources, 515
fetal viability, 214, 221
fiber (dietary), 106–7, 108, 109, 121, 179, 373–74
financial concerns, 194, 196–97, 264–65, 315, 399, 416, 417
first aid, 403
first trimester
  fetal reduction during, 248
  menu suggestions for, 120
  nuchal translucency screening in, 54
  nutritional needs during, 118–19
fish, seafood
  menu suggestions with, 117
  nutritional function of, 110, 111–12, *114,* 121, 123, 153
  raw, 162
  recommendations for breast-feeding, *347,* 351
  recommendations for postpartum diet, *368,* 416
  recommendations for pregnancy, *103,* 105

fish oil, 141–42, 416
fluid retention, 176
folic acid, 108, 109, 118, 133–34, 166, 346, 525
fontanelle (soft spot), 319
food groups, *103,* 104, 107–112, *347, 368*
food poisoning, 162
foods
  allergies to, 344, 361
  heartburn-causing, 176–77
  nutritional high-performers, 113, *114–15,* 115–16, 424
  resources for, 515
  takeout, 125
footprints
  as mementos, 325, 336
  size comparison, *25–27*
  taken at birth, 305
foot swelling
  after delivery, 301
  during pregnancy, 171–72
foremilk, 355
formula
  as breast-milk supplement, 341, 346, 348, 357, 360–61
  calories in, 353
  nutritional value of, 361
fourth trimester. *See* postpartum period
fraternal twins
  assisted reproductive technologies and, 12
  birthrate for, 10, 11
  characteristics of, 10
  conception of, 8, 10
  DNA of, 17
  miscarriage risk for, 203
front packs for carrying babies, 398, 409
fruits
  fiber in, 374
  morning sickness and, 147
  nutritional function of, 108–9, *115,* 121
  recommendations for breast-feeding, *347*

recommendations for postpartum diet, *368*
recommendations for pregnancy, *103*
fundal height, 90, *91*
furniture
  for breast-feeding, 363
  cribs, 395, 397, 406
  high chairs, 398, 399
  nursery layout, 399–400
  for pregnancy comfort, 173, 187, 236
  rocking chairs, 398

gastroesophageal reflux disease (GERD), 176–77
gastrointestinal system
  anomalies in, 214, 525
  breast milk and, 344
  in premature babies, 321
gavage feeding, 38, 310–11, 322, 326, 357
gender
  birthweight and, 24
  determining via amniocentesis, 58
  determining via ultrasound, 56
genetics
  detecting abnormalities due to, 58
  postpartum depression and, 416
  pregnancies and, 44–45
germinal matrix, 318, 319
gestational age
  complications and, 315
  determining, 50
  fetal head size and, *234*
  hospital stays and, 222, *223*
  intrauterine growth and, *14, 20, 23,* 64, 129–30, 142
  optimal, *72,* 280–81
  prior pregnancies and, 44
  for quadruplets, 29, 221, 545
  for triplets, 29, 30, 221, 545
  for twins, 29, 30, 38, 221, 545
  weight gain and, 71, *81–83,* 84–85

gestational diabetes
    controlling, 159–60
    delivery method and, 295
    exercise and, 190
    postpartum depression and, 417
    postpartum diet and, 369
    screening for, 52, 98
ginger, for morning sickness, 148,
    149
glucose tolerance test, 52, 98
glycemic index, 113
grains
    fiber in, 373
    nutritional function of, 109, 115
    recommendations for breast-
        feeding, 347
    recommendations for
        postpartum diet, 368
    recommendations for pregnancy,
        103
    in vegetarian diet, 158
grandparents, 267–68, 324, 334,
    389
Grantly Dick-Read, 61
grief counseling, 335
    resources for, 516
Group B streptococcus (GBS), 320
growth. See intrauterine growth
guilt
    about babies in NICU, 333
    about hiring home help, 387
    about identity mix-ups, 410
    about nighttime feedings, 396
    toward older children, 413
    about reaction to multiples
        pregnancy, 258–59
Gyne-Lotrimin, 163

hair
    of fetus, 22
    of identical twins, 9
    during pregnancy, 169
hair dye, 169
handicapped parking, 195–96,
    235
head (baby's)
    circumference of, 234, 305
    position of, 274, 285–87

health care team
    assembling, 31–42
    for breast-feeding, 341
    for cesarean deliveries, 297
    as decision makers, 261–62
    for labor/delivery, 278–79, 289
    in NICU, 311–15, 328
health insurance
    for breast-feeding support, 359
    maternity leave and, 194,
        197–98
hearing
    neonatal complications with,
        320
    neonatal testing of, 314
heartbeats
    in embryonic period, 19
    during labor, 278
    multiple, 14
    nonstress test and, 60
heartburn, 136, 176–77
heart defects
    in newborns, 317
    preventing, 118
    screening for, 54
heart rate
    in Apgar score, 304–5, 305
    NICU monitoring of, 309
hemorrhages, intraventricular, 232,
    318–19, 320, 550
hepatitis B, 51
hernias, 383–84
herpes infections, 295
high chairs, 398, 399
hindmilk, 355
HIV, 51
holoprosencephaly, 526
home life with multiples, 385–406
    equipment for, 397–400
    health and safety issues of,
        402–6
    recruiting help with, 385–90
    schedules for, 390–92, 392
    sleep and, 393–97
hormones
    breast-feeding and, 354
    contractions and, 186, 190
    emotions and, 258

gastrointestinal effects of, 176
gestational diabetes and, 52
morning sickness and, 146, 150
multiple pregnancies and, 168
physical appearance and,
    169–70
postpartum depression and,
    416, 417
quad screening test and, 53
sleep disruption and, 384
urinary-tract infections and, 127
urination frequency and, 178
weight gain and, 70, 90
hospitals
    discharge from, 307, 325, 327,
        397
    infections acquired in, 321
    in labor/delivery plan, 273
    protocols for cesarean deliveries,
        297–99
    protocols for labor/delivery,
        278–79
    rooming-in at, 306–7, 342, 343
    selection of, 37–40, 289
    transfers from, 325
    See also neonatal intensive care
        units (NICUs)
human chorionic gonadotropin
    (HCG), 13, 19, 53, 54
human placental lactogen (HPL),
    52, 100
hunger. See appetite
hydration, 127–29, 178, 352–53,
    376
hydrocephaly, 319, 526
hydrocortisone cream, 404
hyperalimentation, 311
hyperbilirubinemia, 316, 318
hyperemesis gravidarum, 150
hypersomnia, 415
hypertension
    breast-feeding and, 345
    calcium and, 135
    placenta age and, 279
    placental abruption and, 206
    preterm births and, 51
Hypnobabies, 61, 62, 282
hypoglycemia, 100, 107

hypotension, 526
hypothyroidism, 305
hypoxia, 219, 288, 295

ibuprofen, 174, 301
identical twins
   assisted reproductive
      technologies and, 12
   birthrate for, 11
   birthweights of, 24
   characteristics of, 9
   complications with, 213–20,
      524–45
   conception of, 8
   DNA of, 17
   miscarriage risk for, 203
   optimal delivery time for,
      280–81
identity mix-ups, 410
illness
   calling doctor for, 404
   chronic, 245, 263
immune system
   exercise and, 376
   in premature babies, 320
incompetent cervix, 204–5, 226,
   551
incontinence, 179
incubators, 309, 310, 316, 333
indomethacin (Indocin), 231
Infant CPR Anytime Personal
   Learning Program, 403
infant seats, 398
infections
   of bladder, 301
   brain injury and, 318
   breast milk and, 327
   in breasts, 358
   cesarean delivery and, 302
   of eye, 305
   herpes, 295
   of kidney, 301
   neonatal, 320–21
   preventing, 324, 344
   of urinary tract, 50, 127, 178
   vaginal delivery and, 288
   yeast, 163, 207
   zinc and, 137

infertility treatments. *See* assisted
   reproductive technologies
Inhibin-A, 53
in-laws, 267–268, 334, 387
insomnia, 415
insulin sensitivity, 374
intelligence
   breast-feeding and, 344
   omega-3 fatty acids and, 351
interlocking, during delivery, 286,
   553, *554*
International Board Certified
   Lactation Consultants
   (IBCLCs), 41
International Childbirth
   Education Association, 62
International Lactation Consultant
   Association, 41, 356
intestinal obstruction, 526
intrahepatic cholestasis of
   pregnancy (ICP), 170
intrauterine crowding, 526
intrauterine fetal death (IUFD),
   217–18, 526, 542–45. *See also*
   stillbirths
intrauterine growth, 17–27
   discomfort from, 172–83
   fetal reductions and, 251
   gestational age and, 64, 129–30,
      142
   of head, *234*
   maternal weight gain and,
      79–80, 88, 90
   nutrition and, 552
intrauterine growth restriction
   (IUGR), 536
intravenous feeding, 311, 321
intraventricular hemorrhage
   (IVH), 232, 318–19, 320, 550
intubation, 310, 314
in vitro fertilization (IVF), 11,
   204, 221, 250, 258, 545
iodine, 352
ipecac, 404
iron (dietary), 99, 104, 110, 120–
   21, 128, 152, 158, 179, 367
iron-deficiency anemia, 51,
   120–21, 206, 300

irritability
   caffeine and, 128
   hypoglycemia and, 107
   during labor, 291
ischemic injuries, fetal anomalies
   and, 214
isolettes, 309, 310, 316, 333
itching, 170

jaundice, 316, 320
joint pain, 179, 417

kangaroo care, 327
Kegel exercises, 179
ketones, 50, 100, 109
ketosis, 100
kidney disease, 50, 65
kidneys, 178, 186, 233, 301

labor
   inducing, 279–83, 296
   triggers of, 274–78
   true vs. false, 275, *275*, 278
labor coaches, 291, 298
labor/delivery procedure, 273–303
   delivery method decision,
      284–85, 552–58
   hospital protocols for, 278–79
   interlocking during, 286, 553,
      554
   pain management during,
      282–84
   plan for, 273
   recovering from, 300–3
   timing of, 279–82
   See also cesarean delivery;
      vaginal delivery
lactation consultants, 42–43, 306,
   315, 341, 342, 359
Lactation Education Resources,
   357
lacto-engineering, 322
lacto-ovo-vegetarian diet, *151*
lacto-vegetarian diet, *151*
La Leche League International,
   356, 359
Lamaze International, 61, 62
lambda (twin peak) sign, 16

optimal delivery time for, 280–81

prenatal checkups for, 47, 56–57, 59–60

monosomy, 58

monozygotic (MZ) multiple pregnancies

   complications with, 213–20, 524–45

   defined, 8

   rate of, 11

mood disorders, postpartum, 414–18

morning sickness

   managing, 146–50

   maternal weight and, 72

   multiple births and, 13

mother's helpers, 387

Mothers of Multiples Club, 334, 387

mucous plug, 274

multiples

   distinguishing among, 410

   relationship among, 409

multiples births

   genetic tendency for, 10–11

   losses in, 335–36

   postpartum depression and, 417

   rates of, 10–12, 250

   resources for, 517

   risks with, 32

Multiples of America, 36, 189

multiples pregnancies

   blood glucose and, 100

   detecting complications with, 16

   detecting labor with, 277

   fetal development in, 24

   fetal postmaturity in, 279

   growth rate in, 24, 28

   intrauterine deaths in, 217–18

   sharing news of, 267–72

   signs of, 13

   weight gain and, 67

multivitamins

   problems with, 131–32

   recommendations for, 132–33

muscle tone (Apgar score), 304, *305*

naming children, 256, 410

nannies, 388

naps

   for babies, 394, 395

   for mothers, 400

nasogastric feeding. *See* gavage feeding

National Organization of Mothers of Twins Clubs, 36, 189

National Weight Control Registry, 366

nausea

   with analgesics, 282

   during labor, 291

   libido and, 184

   as multiples pregnancy symptom, 13, 146

   multivitamins and, 132

   supplement drinks and, 144

   with tocolytic medications, 231

   treatment for, 147–50

necrotizing enterocolitis (NEC), 321

neonatal dietitians, 314

neonatal intensive care units (NICUs)

   birthweights and, 89

   breast-feeding and, 342, 359–60

   complications treated in, 315–22

   discharge from, 336–38, 397

   equipment in, 309–11

   levels of, 39, 311

   parenting in, 322–36, 407

   preterm births and, 221

   protocols in, 307–9, 324, 333

   staff of, 311–15

   terminology used in, 329

neonatal nurse practitioners (NNPs), 313

neonatal nurses, 313

neonatologists, 39, 297, 304, 311, 313

neural tube defects, 58, 109, 118, 133, 134, 166, 525, 526

neurodevelopment

   assessment of, 312

   inequality of, among multiples, 411

nutrition and, 351

preterm birth and, 222, 232, 318–19

See also brain

new-baby blues. *See* postpartum depression

nicotine replacement products, 167

nifedipine (Procardia), 231

nipple feeding, 311, 322, 357

nipples (artificial), 343

nonstress test, 59–60, 278

North American Fetal Therapy Network, 215

nosocomial infection, 321

NSAIDs, 174

nuchal translucency (NT) screening, 54

nurse practitioners, 40, 304, 313

nurseries (home), 394, 395, 397, 399–400, 406

nursery levels of care (hospitals), 38–39, 307, 337

nurses

   during delivery, 289, 297, 304

   on health care team, 40

   for home help, 386–87

   in NICU, 313

   patients' relationships with, 328

nursing. *See* breast-feeding

nutrition, 97–130

   for breast-feeding mothers, 345–46, *347,* 348–54

   from breast milk, 327

   dietitians and, 40–41

   fetal complications and, 525

   food groups and, 107–12

   from high-performing foods, 113, *114–15,* 115–16

   maternal weight gain and, 63–66, 70, 95–96

   for newborns, 314

   postpartum depression and, 416

   for postpartum diet, 366, 367, *368,* 369–76

   preterm births and, 226, 396, 552

   recipes, 423–506

   recommended diet for, 99–107

nutrition *(cont'd)*
  resources for, 514–15, 517–19
  strategies for, 125–26, 368–70
  supplements (*see* dietary
    supplements; vitamins)
  trimester requirements for,
    118–24
  for vegetarians (*see* vegetarians)
  while on bedrest, 237–38
nuts
  nutritional function of, *114*
  recommendations for breast-
    feeding, *347*
  recommendations for
    postpartum diet, *368*
  recommendations for pregnancy,
    103

obesity
  bariatric surgery for, 160
  breast-feeding and, 344
  cesarean incisions and, 302
  postpartum weight and, 365
  pregnancy weight gain and, 74,
    76–77, 78, 89, 90
obstetricians
  childbirth preferences discussed
    with, 61
  delivery method and, 284, 287,
    295, 297, 557
  on health care teams, 40
  patients' relationships with, 43,
    259–60
  selecting, 32–34
occupational therapists (OTs),
  314
oils (dietary)
  recommendations for breast-
    feeding, *347*
  recommendations for
    postpartum diet, *368*
  recommendations for pregnancy,
    99, *103*, 109–10, 123, 124
omega-3 fatty acids
  postpartum depression and,
    106, 123, 416
  recommendations for breast-
    feeding, 351

recommendations for
  postpartum diet, 367
recommendations for pregnancy,
  99, 109, 110, 111, 123,
  141–42
oral glucose tolerance test
  (OGTT), 52
osteoporosis, 122
ovarian cancer, 345
overweight mothers
  birthweight and, 79
  body image and, 271
  body mass index for, 74, *76, 83*
  gestational diabetes and, 159
  pregnancy weight gain and,
    69, 72
ovo-vegetarian diet, *151*
ovulation, 8, 10, 19
ovulation induction, 11–12
oxyhoods, 310, 318
oxytocin, 127, 279, 301

pacifiers, 343
pain
  abdominal, 205, 210, 211–12
  after cesarean delivery, 302
  during labor, 282–84
  during pregnancy, 162, 172–75
  preterm labor and, 227, 228–29
  during sex, 183–84
Pap smear, 50
parenteral nutrition, 311
parent-infant bonding, 407–12
parenting
  in NICU, 322–36
  postpartum, 339, 421–22
Parlodel (bromocriptine), 342
Patau syndrome (trisomy 13), 58
patent ductus arteriosus (PDA), 317
paternity leave, 419
patient rights and responsibilities,
  43–44
Pedialyte, 404
pediatricians, 311, 402, 404
pediatric neurologists, 312
pediatric nurse practitioners
  (PNPs), 313
pediatric ophthalmologists, 312

pelvic examinations
  during labor, 278
  during pregnancy, 50
pelvic pressure, 50, 227
perineum, 291, 293
pessaries, 225–26, 551–52
pharmacists, 314
phenylketonuria, 305
phosphorus, 346
phototherapy, 316
physical activity. *See* exercise
physical therapists (PTs), 42, 175,
  314, 519
physicians. *See* doctors; *specific
  types*
physicians-in-training
  (residents), 66
Pilates, 191, 377
Pitocin, 279, 292, 293, 296, 298,
  558
placenta
  alcohol use and, 164
  delivery of, 293, 298
  determining age of, 279, *280*
  fetal reduction and, 249
  formation of, 8
  function of, 19, 28, 317
  glucose and, 100
  hormones produced by, 13,
    52, 53
  maternal diet and, 105, 119
  in monozygotic pregnancies, 213
  pain medications and, 282–83,
    284
  smoking and, 165
  structural survey of, 214
  twin type and, 9, 10, 16
  weight of, *73*
placental abruption, 205, 206,
  292, 558
placental laser photocoagulation,
  217
placenta previa, 205–6, 295
*Planning Your Pregnancy and
  Birth* (American College
  of Obstetricians and
  Gynecologists), 43
playpens, 398

pneumonia, 320, 344
poison control center, 402–3, 404
poisons, accessibility of, 405, 406
polyhydramnios, 215, 383
postmature fetus, 279
postpartum cardiomyopathy, 301
postpartum depression (PPD)
  causes of, 416–17
  omega-3 fatty acids and, 106,
    123, 141
  resources for, 520
  symptoms of, 415
  treatment for, 418
Postpartum Health Alliance, 418
postpartum period
  belly bulge in, 383–84
  bleeding in, 293
  dietary recommendations for,
    350–54, 364–76
  exercise during, 376–79
  recovery during, 300–3, 325
  rest during, 301, 384
  weight in, 71, 95, 98, 271, 345,
    348, 353, 379
postpartum psychosis, 417–18
Postpartum Support International,
  418
posture
  after cesarean delivery, 302
  to ease breathing, 180
  sitting, 173
  sleeping, 180–81
  standing, 172, 173–74, 187
  when lifting, 188, *188*
poultry
  menu suggestions with, 117
  nutritional function of, 110, 111,
    114, 121, 153
  raw, 162
  recommendations for breast-
    feeding, *347*
  recommendations for
    postpartum diet, *368*
  recommendations for pregnancy,
    103, 105, 112
preeclampsia
  blood pressure and, 51
  calcium and, 122

delivery method and, 295
indications of, 50
omega-3 fatty acids and, 106
postpartum treatment for, 301
protein in urine and, 50
stress and, 192
vitamins and, 135, 136, 137, 138
pregnancy
  discomfort during, 172–83
  embryonic period of, 18–21
  fetal period of, 21–27
  first vs. subsequent, 29
  memory loss and, 123
  patients' rights during, 43–44
  prior, 44, 205, 249, 288, 416,
    557
  start date of, 18
  termination of (*see* selective fetal
    reduction)
  See also multiples pregnancies
pregnancy-associated plasma
    protein-A (PAPP-A), 54
Pregnancy Discrimination Act,
  197–98
premature infants at home
  feeding schedule and, 396
  light exposure and, 397
  sleep schedule and, 396
Prenatal Care Fact Sheet, *48–49*
Prenatal Care Questionnaire, 44,
  45–46
prenatal checkups, 44–49
  components of, 47–48
  frequency of, *47*
  preparing for, 44–46, 48
Prenatal Cradle, 174, 191
prenatal exercise classes, 191
prenatal multiples resources,
  520–22
prenatal tests, 50–61
prepregnancy weight, 68–69,
  72, 74
presentation, 285–88, 289, 298,
  552–57
preterm births
  bariatric surgery and, 160
  cervical length and, 223–26
  complications with, 315–22

critical periods for, 221–22
death rate and, 220
dietary supplements and, 137,
  138, 139
fetal anomalies and, 215
frequency of, 220
intrauterine growth and, 64
NICU stays and, 308
parental bonding and, 411–12
postpartum depression and, 416
risk assessment for, 545–52
stress and, 192
tobacco and, 165, 167
See also premature infants at
  home
preterm labor, 220–33
  cervical length and, 57
  complications of, 550
  diagnosing, 230, 278
  hypoglycemia and, 100
  omega-3 fatty acids and, 123
  physical exertion and, 172, 186
  placental abruption and, 205
  stopping, 230, 231–33
  testing for risk of, 57, 58
  urinary-tract infections and, 127
  warning signs of, 50, 220,
    227–28
preterm premature rupture of
    membranes (PPROM),
    274–75
probiotics, 108, 177
Procardia (nifedipine), 231
progesterone, 19, 168, 176, 225,
  354, 549–50
Program Your Baby's Health (Luke
  and Eberlein), 66, 353
prostaglandins, 279
protein
  alcohol use and, 164
  food sources of, 108, 110–11,
    125
  function of, 105, *114*
  morning sickness and, 147
  recommendations for breast-
    feeding, *347*
  recommendations for
    postpartum diet, 367, *368*

protein *(cont'd)*
  recommendations for pregnancy,
    99, *103,* 104, 107
  in supplement drinks, 143,
    145–46
  for vegetarians, 151, 152–53,
    154–57, 158
pruritic urticarial papules and
  plaques of pregnancy
  (PUPPP), 170
pulmonary embolism, 236
pulse oximeter, 309
pyloric stenosis, 166
Pyridium, 301

quadruplets, quadruplet
  pregnancies
  birthrate for, 10
  birthweights of, 24
  breast-feeding of, 348, 354,
    360–61
  delivery method for, 284, 295,
    417
  gestational diabetes and, 52
  gestation time for, 29, 221, 275,
    281
  heartburn and, 176
  incidence of, 8
  infertility treatments and, 247
  intrauterine growth and, 70
  NICU stays for, 307–8
  postpartum dietary guidelines
    for, 369
  pregnancy dietary guidelines for,
    99, 101, *103,* 104
  preterm birth and, 220
  uterus size with, 13, *14,* 71, 168
  weight gain goals for, *68, 72, 82*
quad screening test, 53–54
quadshock, 385
Quintero criteria, 538–39
quintuplets, quintuplet pregnancies
  birthrate for, 10
  birthweights of, 24
  uterus size with, 13

race, multiple births and, 11
radiation, 18, 61, 312

radiologists, 312
recommended dietary allowances
    (RDAs)
  function of, 101
  for multivitamins, 132–33
reflex irritability (Apgar score),
    304, *305*
registered dietitians (RDs), 41
registered nurses (RNs), 313
relaxation techniques, 180, 259,
    282
renal dysplasia, 526
respirations (Apgar score), 304,
    305
respiratory distress syndrome
    (RDS), 318, 550
respiratory equipment, 310, 314
respiratory illness
  breast milk and, 344
  prematurity-related, 232, 318
  smoking and, 166
respiratory therapists, 314, 318
rest
  after delivery, 302, 384
  importance of, 186–87, 192
  for preterm birth risk, 224,
    547–49
  for working mothers, 193
  See also bedrest
restaurants, 125, 126
retinopathy of prematurity (ROP),
    312, 319–20
retrolental fibroplasia, 319
Reye's syndrome, 404
rheumatoid arthritis, 345
Rh factor, 51, 308
RhoGAM, 51
rights and responsibilities of
    patients, 43–44
risks to pregnancy
  from alcohol use, 163–65
  with multiples, 32
  preterm births and, 57–58,
    545–52
  from smoking, 165–67
rocking chairs, 398
rooming-in, 306–7, 342, 343
rubella, 51

ruptures
  of membranes, 58, 204, 215,
    216, 220, 274–75, 279,
    290–91, 293, 321, 536
  uterine, 288–89

safety issues. *See* baby-proofing
salads, *372–73*
schedules for households with
    multiples, 390–392, *392*
seafood. *See* fish, seafood
*Seafood Choices: Balancing Benefits
    and Risk* (Institute of
    Medicine), 112
secondhand smoke, 166
second trimester
  childbirth classes during, 62
  menu suggestions for, 121–22
  nutritional needs during, 120–21
seizures
  eclampsia and, 136, 210
  intraventricular hemorrhage
    and, 319
  magnesium sulfate and, 301
selective fetal reduction, 59, 214,
    247–51, 526, 540, 544, 545
selective intrauterine growth
    restriction (sIUGR), 536,
    537, 538
selective serotonin reuptake
    inhibitors (SSRIs), 418
sepsis, 320
serving sizes (food), 104
sexual activity, 183–85, 206, 420
shock (emotional), 253–54, 264,
    385
shoes, for pregnancy, 171–72
shortness of breath, 180, 301
showering, 173, 175, 183, 236,
    358, 393–94
siblings of multiples, 413–14
sickle-cell disease, 58
side aches, 175
Sidelines High Risk Pregnancy
    Support, 241
silver nitrate, 305
simultaneous nursing, *355,* 356,
    360, 409